Abnormal Cortical Development and Epilepsy

From basic to clinical science

Fondazione Pierfranco e Luisa Mariani – ONLUS
viale Bianca Maria 28
20129 Milan, Italy

Telephone: +39 (02) 795458
Fax: +39 (02) 76009582
Internet: www.fondazione–mariani.org
e-mail: info@fondazione–mariani.org

Abnormal Cortical Development and Epilepsy

From basic to clinical science

Editors
Roberto Spreafico, Giuliano Avanzini
and Frederick Andermann

Mariani Foundation Paediatric Neurology Series: 7
Series editor: Maria Majno

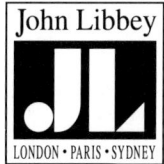

British Library Cataloguing in Publication Data

Abnormal cortical development and epilepsy
  Mariani Foundation paediatric neurology series; 7
  1. Epilepsy in children
  I. Spreafico, Roberto II. Avanzini, G. III. Andermann, Frederick IV. Mariani Foundation
  618.9'2853

ISSN: 0969-0301
ISBN: 0 86196 579 5

Cover illustration:
Retrogradely labelled cortical neurones.
Microphotograph by Roberto Spreafico

Published by
John Libbey & Company Ltd, 13 Smiths Yard, Summerley Street,
London SW18 4HR, England. Telephone:
Telephone +44(0) 181-947 2777 — Fax: +44(0) 181-947 2664
John Libbey & Company Pty Ltd, Level 10, 15/17 Young St., Sydney, NSW 2000, Australia.
John Libbey Eurotext Ltd, 127 avenue de la Répulique, 92120 Montrouge, France.

©1999 John Libbey & Company Ltd. All right reserved.
Unauthorised duplication contravenes applicable laws.

Printed in Great Britain by WBC Book Manufacturers Ltd, Bridgend, Mid Glamorgan CF31 3YN.

Contents

Synopsis	Epilepsies and cerebral dysplasia *Giuliano Avanzini*	ix

Part I Introduction

Chapter 1	The cortical dysplasias and epilepsy: where have we been, where are we and where are we going? *Frederick Andermann*	3

Part II Cortical development

Chapter 2	The pioneering studies on neuronal migration in the developing cerebral cortex *Marina Bentivoglio and Paolo Mazzarello*	23
Chapter 3	Acquired neonatal encephalopathies: cortical vasculature, postinjury reorganization, and neurological sequelae *Miguel Marín-Padilla*	35
Chapter 4	Some principles in the organisation and development of cortical connections *Giorgio M. Innocenti*	55
Chapter 5	Maturation of cortical physiological properties relevant to epileptogenesis *Giuliano Avanzini, Giulio Sancini, Laura Canafoglia and Silvana Franceschetti*	63
Chapter 6	Mechanisms of corticogenesis: cell proliferation and death in the developing human central nervous system *Alessandro Simonati, Cinzia Tosati, Elena Piazzola and Nicolò Rizzuto*	77
Chapter 7	Preferential impairment of motor and somatosensory cortices in two murine models of human diseases: the ethanol-exposed rat and the dystrophic mdx mouse *Diego Minciacchi, Maria Laura Santarelli, Donatella Carretta, Riccardo Carrai, Alberto Granato and Francesco Pinto*	91

Part III Animal models

Chapter 8	The methylazoxymethanol (MAM) treated rat as an animal model for human development brain dysgeneses: morphological features *Claudia Colacitti, Giulio Sancini, Silvana Franceschetti, Flaminio Cattabeni, Roberto Spreafico, Monica Di Luca and Giorgio Battaglia*	109

Chapter 9	The methylazoxymethanol (MAM) treated rat as an animal model for the neuronal migration disorders: electrophysiological findings in identified pyramidal neurones	121
	Silvana Franceschetti, Giulio Sancini, Claudia Colacitti, Monica Di Luca, Tatiana Lavazza, Ferruccio Panzica, Roberto Spreafico, Giorgio Battaglia and Giuliano Avanzini	
Chapter 10	Epileptogenesis in the freeze model of cortical microgyria	133
	David A. Prince and Kimberle M. Jacobs	
Chapter 11	Neuronal development in an epileptic rat with cortical heterotopia	145
	Kevin S. Lee, Frank Schottler, Matthew J. Anzivino, Jennifer L. Collins, Eric A. Frankel, Zong-Fu Chen, Edward Bertram and Laila Zai	

PART IV Electroclinical, imaging and neuropathological studies

Chapter 12	Neuroradiology of malformations of cortical development: band heterotopia, hemimegalencephaly, and polymicrogyria	161
	A. James Barkovich	
Chapter 13	Neuroradiology of malformations of cortical development: schizencephaly, periventricular heterotopia	171
	Ludovico D'Incerti, Laura Farina, Tiziana Granata and Mario Savoiardo	
Chapter 14	Neuronal migration disorders and epilepsy in infancy	177
	Federico Vigevano	
Chapter 15	Schizencephaly: clinical and genetic findings in a case series	181
	Tiziana Granata, Ludovico D'Incerti, Elena Freri, Silvana Franceschetti, Giuliano Avanzini, Antonio Faiella, Carlo Lenti and Giorgio Battaglia	
Chapter 16	Polymicrogyria and epilepsy	191
	Renzo Guerrini	
Chapter 17	Periventricular nodular heterotopia: further delineation of the clinical syndromes	203
	François Dubeau, Li Min Li, Alexandre Bastos, Eva Andermann and Frederick Andermann	
Chapter 18	The clinical and pathophysiological relevance of evoked potentials study in neuronal migration disorders	219
	Vidmer Scaioli, Tiziana Granata, Giorgio Battaglia, Ludovico D'Incerti, Roberto Spreafico, Ferruccio Panzica, Giuliano Avanzini and Lucia Angelini	
Chapter 19	Surgical pathology of cortical dysplasia, tuberous sclerosis and dysembryoplastic neuroepithelial tumours: experience with 55 cases in a recent series of 230 patients with chronic epilepsy	227
	Basile Pasquier, Michel Peoc'h, Raphaelle Barnoud, Dominique Pasquier, Philippe Kahane, Dominique Hoffmann, Alim Louis Benabid and Claudio Munari	

Chapter 20	Immunocytochemical studies in epileptogenic dysplastic tissue *Rita Garbelli, Basile Pasquier, Lorella Minotti, Laura Tassi, Silvia De Biasi,* *Alim L. Benabid, Giorgio Battaglia, Claudio Munari and Roberto Spreafico*	241

PART V   Genetic studies in neuronal migration disorders

Chapter 21	The role of homeobox genes in NMDs *Edoardo Boncinelli, Antonio Faiella, Michela Zortea, Francesca Albani*	253
Chapter 22	The genetic basis of malformations of neuronal migration: molecular mechanisms and clinical correlation *William B. Dobyns*	261

Part VI   Surgical approaches – how, why, when?

Chapter 23	Surgical treatment of cortical dysplasias and migration disorders *André Olivier, Warren Boling, Frederick Andermann and François Dubeau*	275
Chapter 24	Surgical management of severe partial epilepsy symptomatic of neuronal migration disorders: physiopathological considerations and perspectives of research *Claudio Munari, Lorella Minotti, Laura Tassi, Stefano Francione, Philippe Kahane, Carlo Alberto Galli, Nadia Colombo, Emilia Berta, Basile Pasquier, Giorgio Lo Russo, Dominique Hoffmann, Alim Louis Benabid, Roberto Spreafico*	303

Index   319

Epilepsies and cerebral dysplasia: a synopsis

Giuliano Avanzini

*Divisione di Neurofisiopatologia, Istituto Nazionale Neurologico C. Besta,
Via Celoria 11, 20133 Milan, Italy*

The impressive advances in neuroimaging techniques have substantially transformed our attitude towards partial cryptogenic epilepsies. A significant number of patients with partial epilepsies that would have previously been classified as cryptogenic, that is to say putatively determined by some types of undetectable brain pathology, are now identified as presenting well-defined early developmental defects responsible for their epilepsies.

On the one hand, this is having an important impact on our clinical approach especially as regard to surgical strategy; in adddition, it establishes a direct bridge with 'very basic' specialities, such as embryology and genetics, and provides new exciting insights into the neurobiology of epilepsies.

These considerations prompted Roberto Spreafico to design a meeting in which the topic of epileptogenic cortical developmental abnormalities could be addressed according to a multidisciplinary approach 'from basic to clinical science', an idea that was enthusiastically shared by Frederick Andermann and myself, whereas Giorgio Battaglia and Tiziana Granata contributed to the scientific organization. This volume is the result of this very meeting, held in Venice from October 2-4, 1997 within the framework of the Mariani Foundation Colloquia in Childhood Epilepsy, and under the aegis of the International School of Neurological Sciences in San Servolo. The highly professional work of the publisher John Libbey, the constant editorial assistance of the series editor Maria Majno and the generous support of the Mariani Foundation are gratefully acknowledged. The specific sections are preceded by the authoritative Introduction of Frederick Andermann, reviewing the historical development of our acquaintance with epileptogenic dysplasia since the 19th century, and highlighting the problems we are presently facing as well as future perspectives.

The following sections deal with cortical development, animal models of cerebral dysplasia, imaging, clinical neurophysiological and neuropathological studies, genetics and neurosurgery. The reader will enjoy learning from Marina Bentivoglio and Paolo Mazzarello's chapter that a pioneering account of radial arrangement of glial cells in mammalian foetuses had first been provided in 1888 by the Italian investigator Magini, whose drawings foreshadowed the then ubiquitously reproduced illustration by Rakic (1972). The way early subpial and white matter lesions could impair subsequent brain maturation, resulting in cortical and subcortical dysplasia, is analysed by Miguel Marín-Padilla on the basis of impressive autoptic material from the Paediatric Autopsy Service of

Dartmouth-Hitchcock Medical Center. The information drawn from impregnation methods capable of resolving the cytoarchitectural organization is correlated with the analysis of intracerebral vascular organization, and the latter's responsibility in determining cerebral maldevelopments is extensively discussed. For the outstanding experience of the Author in this field as well as the importance of the material on which it is based, this chapter serves as solid grounding for all other contributions. In the next chapter Giorgio Innocenti summarizes his longlasting engagement in investigating the development of cortical connectivity that led him in 1978 to put forward the fruitful concept of an early exuberant interhemisferic connectivity, to be reshaped during the following developmental stages. Novel observations on the morphogenetic role of vision are reported, based on high resolution techniques of single axon visualization and analysis.

How postnatal morphogenesis correlates with the maturation of physiological properties in the neocortex and how such maturational changes may affect the susceptibility to epileptogenic agents, the phenomenological expression of seizures and seizure-dependent brain damage is discussed in Chapter 5, prepared by Avanzini and co-workers. It reflects the effort of exploiting experimental results to improve our approach to the clinical problems related to childhood epilepsy.

The section is completed by the paper of Simonati et al. on the role of cell proliferation and death in corticogenesis, which supplements the previous chapters in creating a link between normal and pathological brain development. Cell proliferation and death are the morphogenetic events that determine the number of neurons in the cortical plate. Mutations of gene coding for protein involved in specific cell functions during development and pathological factors such as hypoxia-ischemia, radiation, drugs and toxic agents acting during gestation can interfere with the genetic development program, resulting in brain malformations. Significant advances in our understanding of epileptogenic mechanisms have arisen in the last fifty years from experimental studies carried out in animal models.This also explains the present interest in animal models of cerebral dysplasias that are the subject of the third part of the book. Results obtained in methylazoxymetanol (MAM)-induced dysgeneses, freeze model of cortical microgyria, tish mutant rat with cortical heterotopia, mdx mouse and ethanol-exposed rat are reported in this section. Minciacchi et al. (Chapter 7) found prenatal exposure to ethanol to affect terminal arborization of thalamo-cortical axons in rat somatosensory cortex, the same area where calcium-binding proteins were found underexpressed in mdx mice. Results of parallel morphological (Colacitti et al.) and neurophysiological (Franceschetti et al.) investigations on rats exposed in utero to MAM are reported in Chapter 8 and 9. This cytotoxic agent administered to pregnant rats on gestational day 15 selectively kills the cells committed to form the neocortex, giving rise to cortical layering abnormalities and subcortical nodules of gray matter similar to human brain dysgeneses that are known to be associated with intractable epilepsy. Changes in local GABAergic circuitry and/or impairment of K-dependent repolarizing mechanisms may explain the cellular hyperexcitability observed by the Authors. Particularly interesting is the evidence of a reciprocal connectivity between neuronal heterotopias and cortical areas, suggesting that heterotopic hyperexcitable neurons can participate into aberrant, potentially epileptogenic circuitry. Another interesting model of microgyria can be obtained in rats with transcranial freeze lesions made at birth or on postnatal day 1.

Evidence for structural reorganization of circuits in the microgyri and for an increased ratio between excitatory and inhibitory postsynaptic currents was obtained by David Prince and Kimberle M. Jacobs and is reported in the Chapter 10. Finally, a novel mutant animal (the tish rat) exhibiting bilateral subcortical band heterotopia and presenting with recurrent spontaneous seizures is described by Kevin Lee and associates, who demonstrate that misplaced cell proliferation, in addition to disturbed neuronal migration, contributes to the formation of cortical heterotopia.

The next section is devoted to neurophysiological (Granata et al. and Scaioli et al.), clinical (Vigevano, Granata et al., Guerrini, Dubeau et al.) imaging (Barkovich, D'Incerti et al.) and neuropathological (Pasquier et al., Garbelli et al.) studies, and provides a very interesting and updated account of the present possibilities of detecting and analysing cerebral dysplasia in patients referred to us for different neurological syndromes, often including epileptic seizures.

Thanks to the development of MRI, cerebral dysgeneses such as Taylor's focal cortical dysplasias, previously described on cerebral specimens extracted for epilepsy surgery, are now recognized as aetiological factors in an increasing number of patients with partial cryptogenic epilepsies on the basis of a proper MRI study suggested by clinical indications. Moreover, band heterotopia, also referred to as 'double cortex syndrome', was previously known only through neuropathological observations (Jakob Z. *Ges. Neurol. Psychiat.* 155, 1, 1936) until in 1989 Barkovich diagnosed it *in vivo* thanks to MRI. According to Vigevano (Chapter 14), brain dysgeneses that can now be detected by neuroradiological examination account for 3-4 percent of all epilepsies, and for 18-20 percent of severe epilepsies. Based on their important experience in this field, neuroradiologists and clinicians provide the reader with a detailed and comprehensive account of the epileptogenic dysgeneses most frequently encountered in a neurological setting. Although some clinical findings (namely severe partial (possibly multifocal) epilepsies with onset in childhood or adolescence associated with mental retardation and no other known etiological factor) might suggest an underlying brain dysgenesis, the spectrum of clinical manifestations is admittedly too broad to allow a definition of clinical syndromes consistently correlated with specific types of brain malformation. According to the clinical symptomatology, the epileptogenic zone seems in some cases to exceed the dysplastic areas shown by MRI, whereas in other cases it seems to be limited to part of the area with altered MRI signal. In general the topographic distribution of the epileptogenic zone cannot be assumed as simply coincidence with the morphologically altered cerebral areas displayed by MRI, and the severity of epilepsy is not necessarily proportioned to the extent of cerebral alterations. This is clearly the case of the schizencephaly-associated epilepsies which in Granata's series turned out to be more severe in patients with unilateral closure of small open cleft implying mild motor deficit, than in those with bilateral schizencephalies with severe neurological defects.

It is worth noting that the contribution of neurophysiological examinations is not limited to the current EEG findings (changes in background, focal slowing, intercritical or critical epileptiform activities) as reported in Granata's, Guerrini's and Dubeau's papers, but refers to some specific aspects such as the pronounced photic driving of background activity in periventricular nodular heterotopia previously reported by Battaglia et al. (*Epilepsia* 38, 1173, 1997). In addition, Scaioli reports in Chapter 18 the new exciting evidence of an extensive reorganization of cortical representation of certain sensory modalities in cortical dysgeneses, obtained by evoked potential study, a finding that neurosurgeons must take into account in designing surgical strategies.

Neuropathological aspects are addressed by Pasquier *et al.* on the basis of a series of 55 patients operated for pharmacoresistant epilepsies symptomatic of dysplastic lesions. This series confirms the high incidence of dysembryoplastic neuroepithelial tumors (DNETs) first described by Daumas-Duport *et al.* (*Neurosurgery* 23, 545, 1988) among the epileptogenic cortical lesions responsible for symptomatic epilepsies. The main features of DNETs are multinodular pattern with mucoid substance accumulation and proliferation of round oligodendrocyte-like cells. Surgical specimens from patients submitted to epilepsy surgery provide very valuable material for analysing circuit and cellular alterations relevant to epileptogenic mechanisms as it is clearly demonstrated by the presentation of Spreafico's team (Garbelli *et al.*). Although cortical lamination disruption is a common feature in focal cortical dysplasias, individual cases may differ significantly from each other in cell composition. According to this immunocytochemical study, the term of Taylor's focal dysplasia should be applied only to those cases where hypertrophic neurons filled with large amount of neurofilamented and balloon cells (incompletely differentiated elements with mixed glial and neuronal immunoreactive features) can be detected by immunocytochemistry. These histological characteristics correspond to a peculiar MRI picture, characterized by a blurring between gray and white matter that may allow to diagnose Taylor's displasia *in vivo*. Particularly interesting from the pathophysiological point of view is the finding of a reduction and abnormal distribution of immunoreactive neurons and neuropil observed with antibodies against calcium binding proteins, suggesting an abnormal organization of the intracortical GABAergic system. Cell proliferation in the periventricular germinal zone, migration to the cortical plate and cortical layering processes are under genetic control, and therefore the mutation of the relevant genes may result in different brain dysgeneses, depending on the developmental step that they are controlling. William Dobyns reviews the genes that have been found associated with human and mouse cortical malformations and reports in detail on the molecular genetics of classic lissencephaly and bilateral periventricular nodular heterotopia. His paper demonstrates the advantage for genetic studies of a classification of cerebral dysgeneses based on the affected embryological event.

The genetics of schizencephaly are addressed by Boncinelli *et al.*, who tell how, from a very general biological problem (the genetic control of the regionalization of CNS) a productive hypothesis had been generated, leading to the identification of an important group of homeobox genes. In particular Otx1, Otx2, Emx1 and Emx2 genes, expressed in vertebrate brain according to very precise regional and temporal patterns, have been demonstrated to establish the identity of various embryonic brain regions. Starting from the analysis of transgenic mice, lacking Emx2 gene, Boncinelli and associates hypothesized and subsequently demonstrated that mutations of Emx2 gene can result in schizencephaly in humans by affecting both proliferation and migration processes of cortical neurons.

These two papers take the reader to the most advanced frontiers of developmental neurobiology applied to human pathology. They demonstrate that the same cerebral dysgeneses may depend on gene mutations, a conclusion that does not rule out the possibility that acquired aetiological factors interfering at the same developmental stages may result in similar pictures. Distinctive clinical and neuroradiological criteria might be derived in future by a larger number of observations.

The book is concluded by two chapters on surgical management of severe epilepsies symptomatic of cortical dysplasias, by André Olivier and Claudio Munari and their teams. Olivier reviews the results of a series of 120 patients operated at the Montreal Neurological Institute, stressing the correlation between the extent of the lesion removal and the positive results. The main difficulty remains in accurately evaluating the localization and extent of the lesion: newer techniques such as three-dimensional MRI reconstruction look promising.

Claudio Munari's chapter is based upon personal experience on 30 patients out of 360 operated in the last seven years. The analysis of this material, part of which was used for. The study by Garbelli *et al.* confirms the conclusion that very often the dysplastic lesion, as it is depicted by MRI, is not coextensive with the epileptogenic zone. Therefore, a simple lesionectomy can be proposed only for those cases where the video-EEG ictal recording shows the topography of the ictal discharges to be strictly coincidental with the site of dysplasia, and when the clinical ictal semeiology does not conflict with this localization. In all other cases, the extent of the tissue to be removed should be decided on the ground of a clinico-neurophysiological evaluation, possibly including stereo-EEG ictal recording as is customary for cryptogenic epilepsies. A 'two-step' strategy, first limited to the MRI detectable lesion with the understanding that the removal of epileptogenic zone could be subsequently completed if seizures persist, can be proposed to informed patients and performed with their agreement. Munari's paper epitomizes the philosophy of the book by stressing the need of a strict interaction between clinical and basic science methodologies, in order to optimize the patient care on one side, and to deepen our knowledge on the neurobiology of cerebral dysplasia on the other. It appropriately concludes the book, which we are sure will be read with interest by both basic and clinical neuroscientists.

PART I

INTRODUCTION

Chapter 1

The cortical dysplasias and epilepsy: where have we been, where are we and where are we going?

Frederick Andermann

*Departments of Neurology and Paediatrics, McGill University,
Epilepsy Service, Montreal Neurological Institute and Hospital, 3801 University Street, Montreal, QC H3A ZB4, Canada*

The tradition of surgical treatment for intractable epilepsy at the Montreal Neurological Hospital goes back over 60 years. The resections were carried out by gyral emptying and the tissue obtained was not ideal for pathological analysis. In the United Kingdom, Murray Falconer, a New Zealander, developed surgical treatment at the Kings-Maudsley, a tradition which has been continued till now. He used a different technique. The epileptogenic tissue, electrically defined, was resected *en bloc* and was studied by the pathologists Clive Bruton and Nicholas Corsellis. They realized that some of the tissue obtained showed abnormal organization and these early patients were described by the neuropsychiatrist David Taylor in a paper entitled *Focal Dysplasia of the Cerebral Cortex in Epilepsy*. I quote from the original description: "An unusual microscopic abnormality has been defined in the lobectomy specimens removed surgically from the brains of epileptic patients. The abnormality could seldom be identified by palpation or by the naked eye. Histologically, it consisted of congregations of large neurons which were littered through all of the first cortical layer. In most, but not in all cases, grotesque cells, probably of glial origin, were also present in the depth of the affected cortex and in the subjacent white matter. This kind of abnormality appears to be a malformation. The picture is reminiscent of tuberous sclerosis but too many distinguishing features, both in the clinical and in the pathological aspects, make this diagnosis untenable. The cases are therefore looked on provisionally, since all but one are still alive, as comprising a distinct form of cortical dysplasia in which localized exotic populations of nerve cells underlie the electrical and clinical manifestations of certain focal forms of epilepsy." This definition has withstood the test of time and quite remarkably was made before modern imaging was available (Taylor *et al.*,1971). The description of the findings is hard to improve on and the most common form of cortical dysplasia is now described as the "Taylor type".

A number of years ago we were referred a young man with megalencephaly who had focal seizures involving the arm and leg on one side only. With most of these attacks he remained conscious but would occasionally fall, and he had mild hemiparesis. He had an extremely unusual ongoing or continuous focal epileptic abnormality over the contralateral central area. It consisted of moderate to high voltage sharp waves at 6–8 cycles per second. Dr. Rasmussen explored him and found that the epileptogenic abnormality arose in the greatly enlarged pre- and post- central gyri. Since the patient's hemiparesis was mild, he carried out only a resection anterior and posterior to this epileptogenic area and this had little effect on the seizures (Fig. 1A). Years later, a magnetic resonance scan was carried out which clearly showed the enlarged gyri. There was also lesser contralateral enlargement of the pre- and post-central gyry without, however, any epileptogenic abnormality arising in these (Fig. 1B). This patient showed the usual ongoing epileptic abnormalities associated with dysplasia which were much later identified and studied by Palmini and colleagues (1995). This was the first patient in whom we suspected that a dysplastic abnormality was the cause of the epilepsy.

The CT scan enabled recognition of some of the more gross structural developmental abnormalities, but it was the advent of magnetic resonance imaging which led to recognition of many more dysplastic lesions during life. An example of this distinction is provided by a young man who had focal seizures involving the foot and leg which caused frequent falls, making it impossible for him to attend school and leading to progressive weakness of the leg. Numerous high quality CT scans could not demonstrate an abnormality but the first MRI showed a focal lesion in the foot area (Fig. 2A). This turned out to be a benign glial tumour with dysplastic changes surrounding it, of a type later described by Prayson et al. (1993). The resection shown in Figure 2B led to considerable improvement and cessation of the attacks involving the lower extremities He now

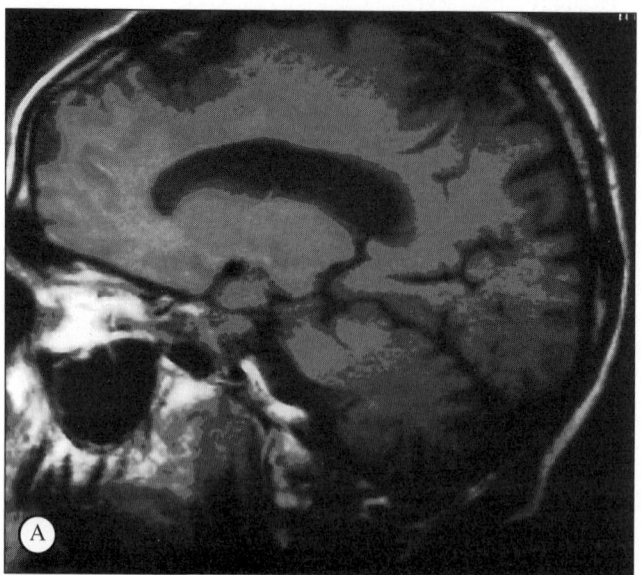
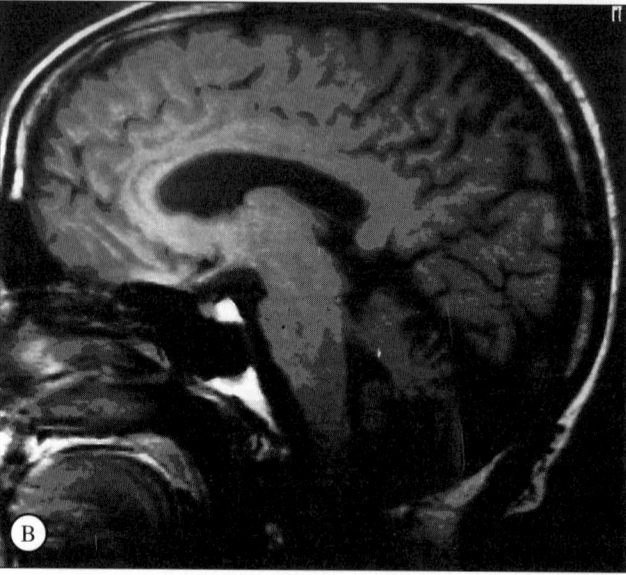

Fig. 1. (A) Sagittal MRI of a patient with megalencephaly. The pre- and post-central gyri are greatly increased in size. A resection was carried out in front and behind these gyri. The seizures were shown to originate in the enlarged gyri. (B) Contralateral sagittal section showing lesser enlargement of the pre- and post- central gyri. There was no epileptic abnormality arising on that side.

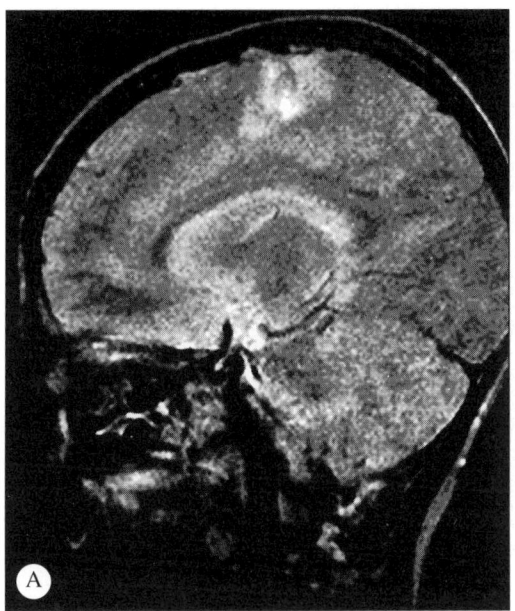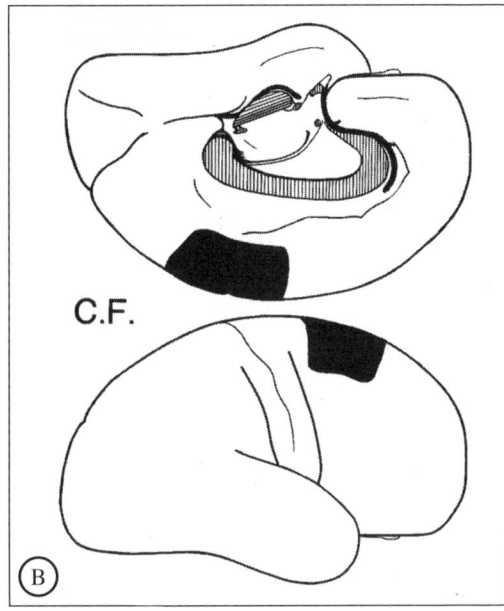

Fig. 2. (A) Sagittal MRI showing a benign glial tumour and surrounding cortical dysplasia in the foot area. This lesion was not visible on several high quality CT scans. (B) Resection of the lesion led to considerable improvement but no additional deficit in the foot.

requires a light plastic brace and has had no further increase in leg weakness. He continues to have seizures which now involve the upper extremities, but in these attacks he does not fall. This patient illustrates that residual dysplastic tissue may be present and still lead to recurrent seizures.

Cortical dysplasia may be associated with overlying skin changes such as the ectodermal dysplasia shown in the patient illustrated in Figure 3A. Underneath there was obvious thickening of grey matter and a calcification, a rather unusual finding in dysplasia (Fig. 3B). The resection (Fig. 3C) led to complete cessation of seizures and eventually gradual reduction and finally cessation of the medication by his neurologist. He had a recurrence, with a single seizure two years later. The medication was restarted in low doses and some days later he was found dead in bed, presumably due to a second and more severe seizure.

Other skin lesions associated with cortical dysplasia are multiple hemangiomata and in particular linear nevus sebaceous as illustrated in Figure 4A. This is not infrequently associated with hemimegalencephaly (Fig. 4B), as is achromic nevus of Ito. The skin lesions are usually over the head and neck but may involve other parts of the body and the underlying dysplastic abnormalities are usually ipsilateral but on occasion may be contralateral to the cutaneous abnormality. The changes of dysplasia are however not always visible on imaging and may produce epilepsia partialis continua even in the absence of recognizable MRI changes (Desbiens *et al.*, 1993). These changes may also be bilateral, although the severity of the epilepsy is not always the same on both sides. This issue requires further investigation. In one of our patients the contralateral dysplastic abnormality was only recognized at post mortem, although during life the seizures had been originating only on one side.

A major challenge has been the search for more and more subtle dysplastic abnormalities underlying intractable partial epilepsy. A recent important development was the introduction of surface coil MRI studies in which a 3D acquisition with appropriately placed surface coils is carried out. This

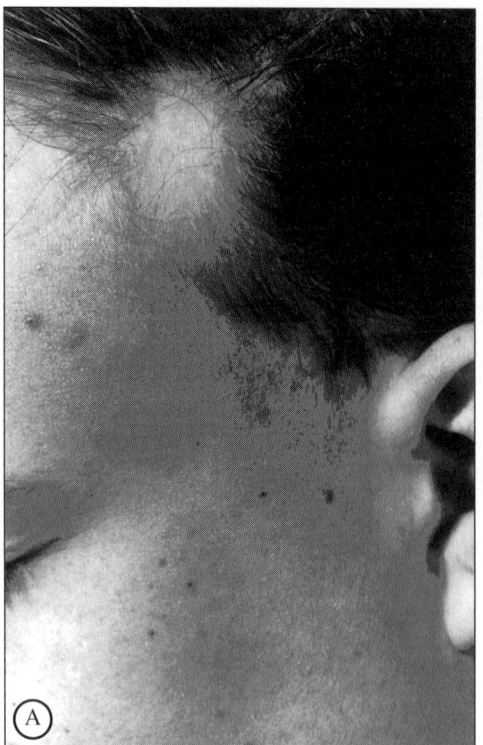
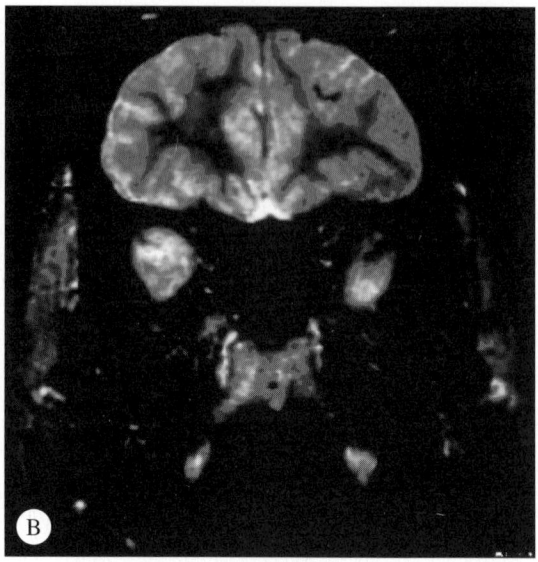
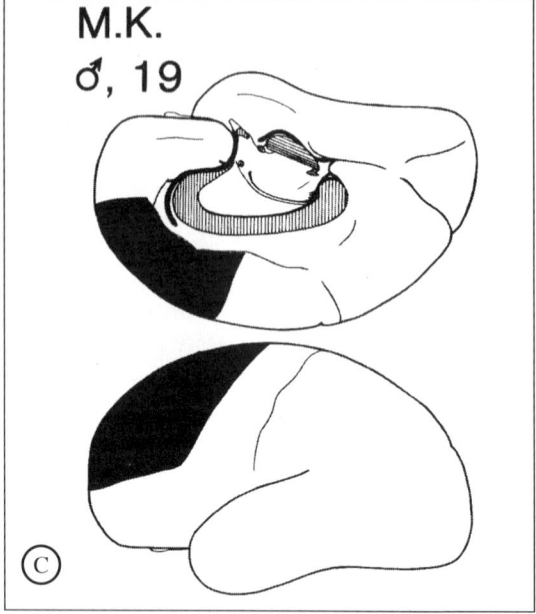

Fig. 3. (A) An area of frontal ectodermal dysplasia overlying a dysplastic lesion. (B) Thickening of the grey matter and calcification seen as a void signal in this coronal MR scan. Pathological diagnosis was cortical dysplasia of Taylor type. (C) Resection of the lesion led to cessation of attacks.

leads to an increased signal to noise ratio and to improved contrast between grey and white matter. It has enabled Dr. Barkovich and his group to recognize dysplastic lesions not otherwise seen with high quality MR imaging (Barkovich et al., 1995).

At the Montreal Neurological Institute, Alexandre Bastos has developed curvilinear reformatting based on a high quality 3D MR acquisition. Symmetrically curved slices are then obtained from a previously determined brain surface and can be rendered in 3D. The advantages of this technique

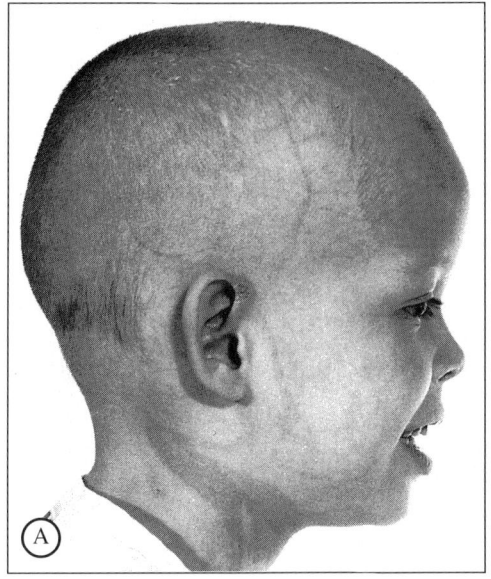
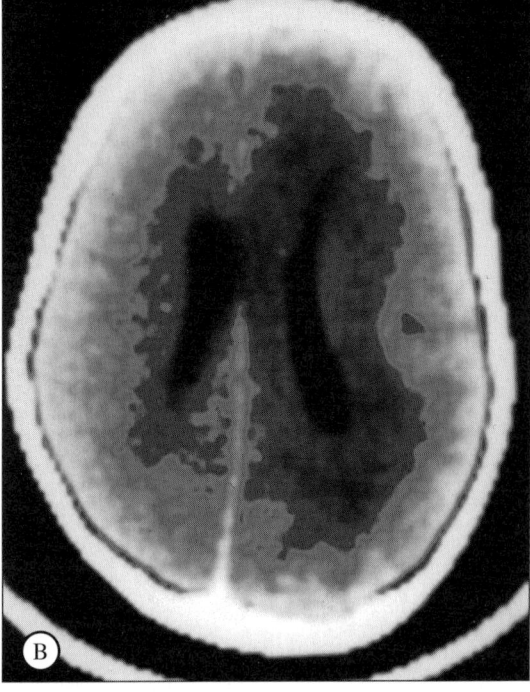

Fig. 4. (A) Linear nevus sebaceous of Jadassohn, on the neck of this young boy with intractable partial epilepsy. (B) Hemimegalencephaly on the side of the skin lesion.

are that it reduces partial volume effect, provides symmetric visualization of the cortical structures and preserves surface landmarks. The yield from this imaging technique is greater than can be obtained by studying orthogonal slices in which oblique cuts or slices along the long axis of a gyrus may create the false impression of gray matter thickening (Bastos et al., 1995). In a number of patients small dysplastic lesions could only be demonstrated by this technique.

The prospect for improved MR imaging in epilepsy includes also the utilization of morphometry as carried out by the group of Fish, Duncan and Shorvon at the National Hospital for Neurology and Neurosurgery (Sisodiya et al., 1995) and by Lee and Reutens at the Montreal Neurological Hospital (Lee et al., 1998). One can measure the gray and white matter volumes of a lobe and compare the gyral patterns of the two hemispheres. These approaches are time consuming and as yet do not have the practical significance of some of the other imaging methods.

Functional MRI as well as diffusion and perfusion studies may also be expected to provide as yet unsuspected information. Eventually one hopes to be able to visualize regional cerebral abnormalities which may be due to channel disorders.

Electrocorticography has shown an unusual pattern of virtually continuous but at times intermittent rhythmic epileptogenic discharge arising from dysplastic tissue (Fig. 5A). This was described by Palmini and colleagues and this abnormality was not found in patients who had seizures associated with tumours (Palmini et al., 1995). Whether other lesions can also produce this kind of abnormality remains as yet uncertain. The electroencephalogram also shows abnormalities of a very similar pattern (Fig. 5B) although these are less well defined compared with those seen at corticography (Gambardella et al., 1996). Thus it has become clear that this type of electrographic abnormality originates in dysplastic tissue itself, which distinguishes these abnormalities from classical glial tumours. The recognition of abnormalities of this type has considerable practical significance since it has been shown by Palmini et al. that not only maximal resection of the visible lesion, but

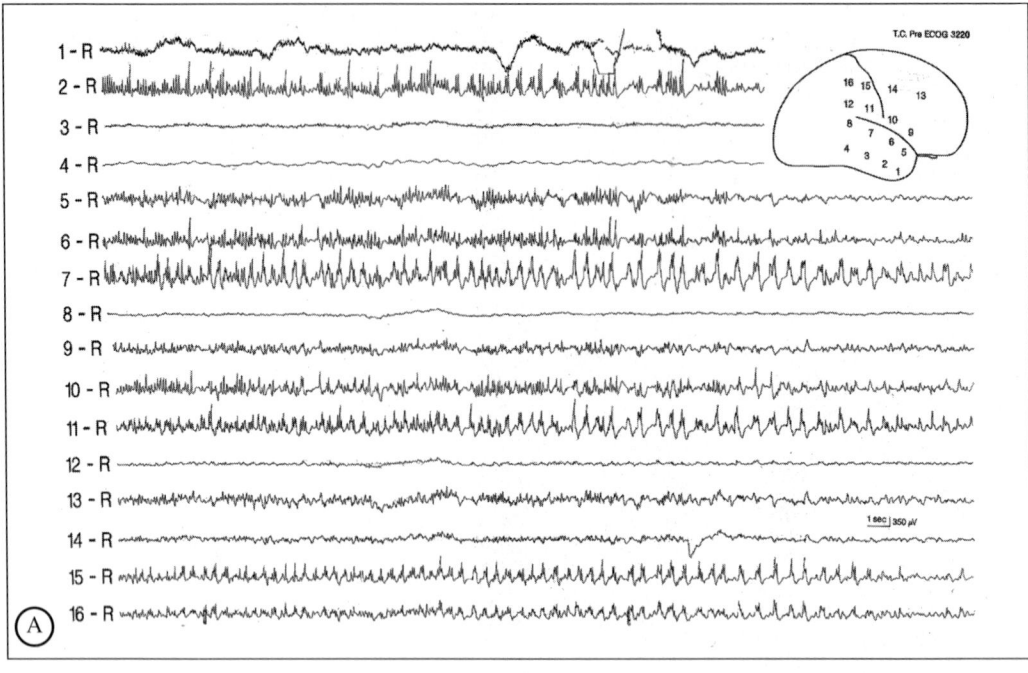

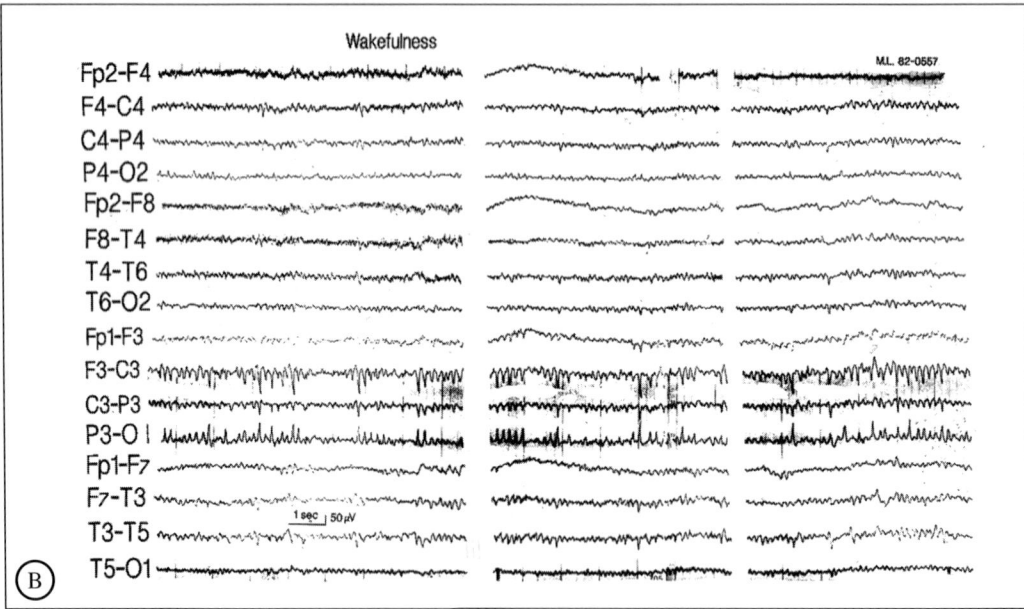

Fig. 5. (A) Virtually continuous epileptogenic interictal abnormality in the corticogram of a patient with cortical dysplasia of Taylor type. (B) An electroencephalogram from another patient with cortical dysplasia shows very similar, very abundant, almost rhythmic epileptogenic abnormality from areas overlying the dysplastic tissue.

additional resection of the area generating this type of continuous epileptiform discharge are required in order to obtain a good result (Palmini *et al.*, 1995).

These imaging and electrographic findings illustrate that there is a wide spectrum of dysplastic lesions ranging from small areas which can be completely resected with complete cessation of seizures, to more widespread abnormalities which cannot be seen by current imaging studies, ranging all the way to the diffuse hemispheral dysplastic abnormalities recognized by Chugani (1993) and also by our own group. These abnormalities, involving an entire hemisphere, are not necessarily associated with enlargement of the hemisphere.

Functional imaging has been helpful in some patients. It may show abnormalities which are not revealed by magnetic resonance imaging, as illustrated by a girl with intractable occipital seizures leading eventually to loss of the visual hemifield and whose MRIs were consistently normal. An interictal SPECT scan showed

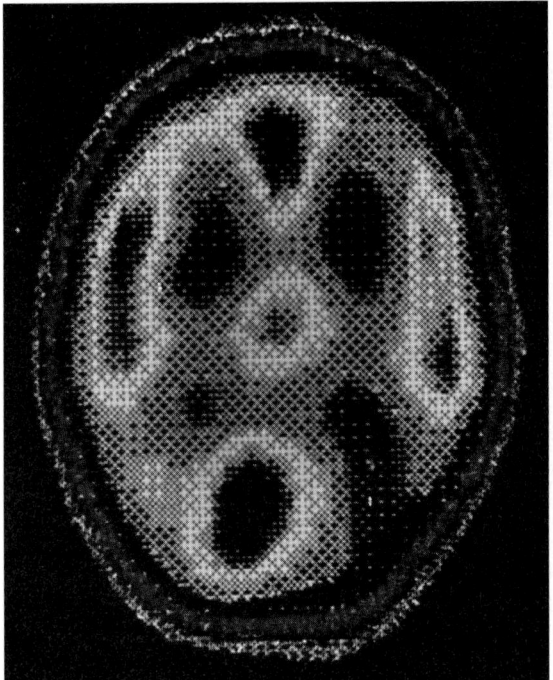

Fig. 6. An interictal SPECT scan of a patient with normal MRI and intractable parieto-occipital epilepsy leading to progressive loss of the visual field. The scan demonstrated focal hypoperfusion. The resected tissue showed cortical dysplasia.

evidence for hypoperfusion in the parieto-occipital region and the dysplastic nature of the abnormality was confirmed by pathological examination of the surgical specimen (Fig. 6). The interictal scans however are of limited value as a rule, even in patients with dysplasia whose ictal scans provide more useful information. Reduced flurodeoxyglucose (FDG) uptake may be shown in PET studies. This is illustrated in a young girl with a small cingulate, presumably dysplastic, lesion which led to more widespread frontal hypometabolism (Fig. 7).

In our centre, magnetic resonance spectroscopy carried out by Drs. Li, Arnold *et al.* (1998) has clearly demonstrated a maximal reduction of N-acetylaspartate in the lesional area with lesser reduction in the perilesional area of interest and minimal changes far from the lesion (Fig. 8).

Attempts have been made to grade the severity of dysplastic lesions. The least abnormality consists of vertical and horizontal dyslamination translating a disorder of migration. Abnormal neurons due to cortical malpositioning are most likely premature. In these lesions features of both migrational and maturational abnormality are present. Finally, differentiation abnormalities may be present in addition, leading to the occurrence of balloon cells. These are primitive elements not fully differentiated between glial and neuronal cell lines. The presence of balloon cells has been linked to the occurrence of the most severe epileptic abnormalities. As in other aspects of epilepsy no classification is likely to satisfy all workers in the field. However, the classification established by Barkovich and colleagues (1994) is workable and provides a useful framework on which to build.

In summary, dysplastic cortical abnormalities are characterized by thickening of the grey matter and poor grey white matter distinction. Small dysplastic abnormalities are frequently situated at this interface, in the bottom of sulci but occasionally in the crowns of gyri and may have variable extension.

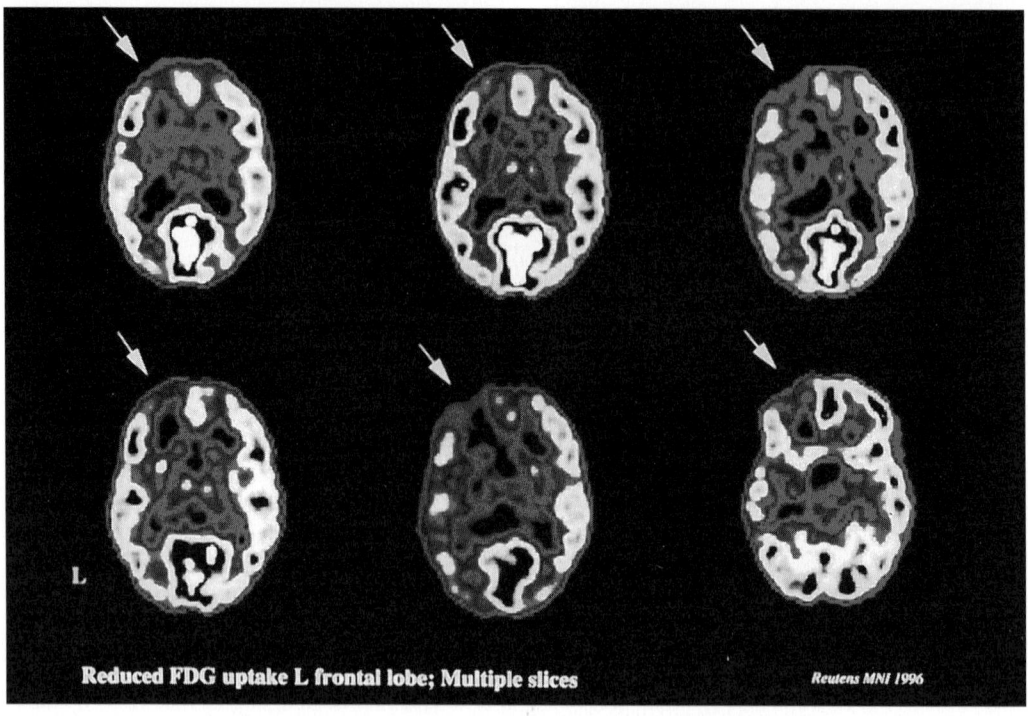

Fig. 7. FDG PET scan of a young girl with a small cingulate lesion showing widespread frontal hypometabolism.

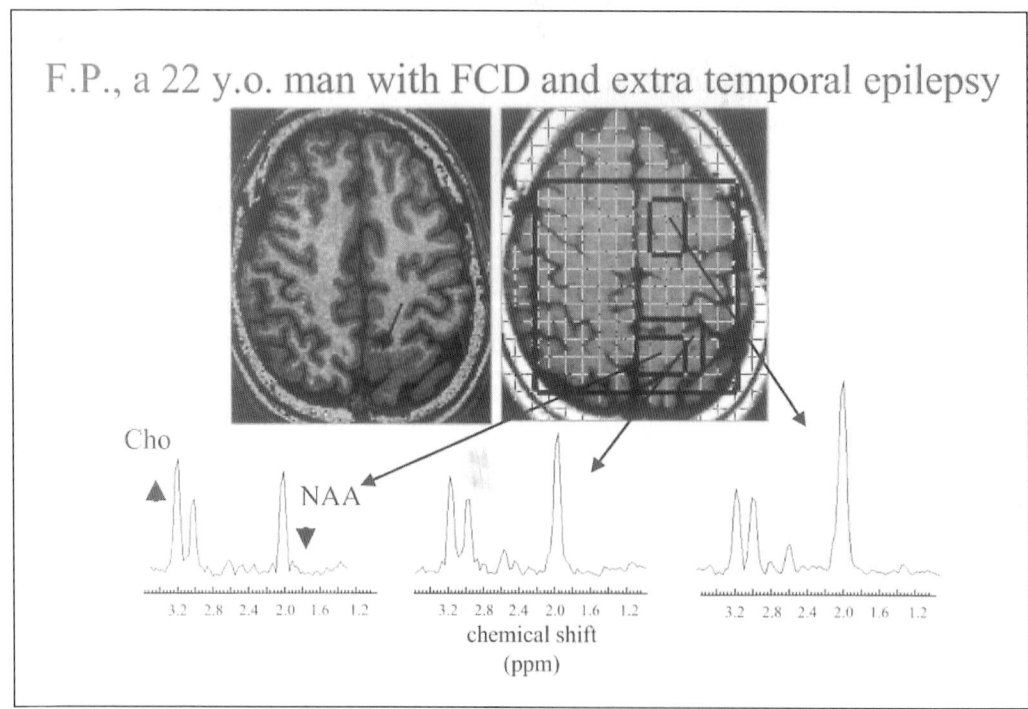

Fig. 8. Magnetic resonance spectroscopy shows the greatest decrease in N acetylaspartate in the dysplastic lesion, with lesser decrease in the surrounding tissue and only minimal changes far from the lesion.

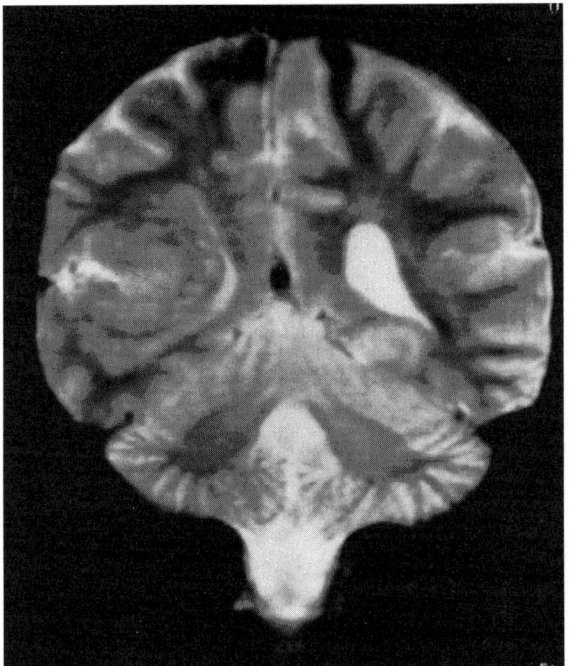

Fig. 9. *Large subcortical heterotopia and epilepsy. The lesion could not be excised since this would have led to unacceptable deficit. The seizures are imperfectly controlled by antiepileptic medication.*

Subcortical heterotopias are usually associated with some cortical abnormality as well. Their resection may be limited by the involvement of essential somatomotor, sensory, or language areas. This is illustrated by the MRI of a young woman whose heterotopia could not be resected because this would have led to unacceptable deficit (Fig. 9). Fortunately, her seizures were of less than maximal severity and she derived some benefit, although by no means full seizure control, from pharmacological treatment.

Periventricular nodular heterotopias are more common than suspected and may also be associated with intractable epilepsy. It is now clear that the epileptogenic abnormalities may occur at a distance from the periventricular nodules which tend to predominate over the posterior wall of the ventricular system (Fig. 10). Several centres have carried out temporal resections, sometimes without being aware of the presence of

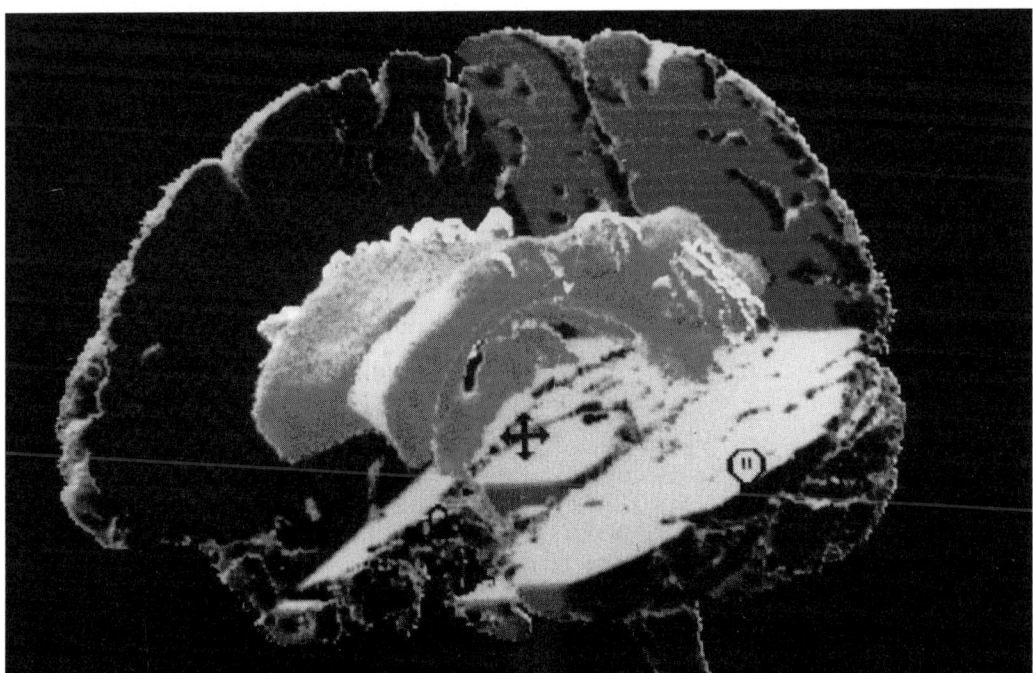

Fig. 10. *Reconstruction of the ventricles in a patient with periventricular nodular heterotopia. These predominate over the posterior aspect of the lateral ventricles and at times are found in the temporal horns as well.*

ABNORMAL CORTICAL DEVELOPMENT AND EPILEPSY

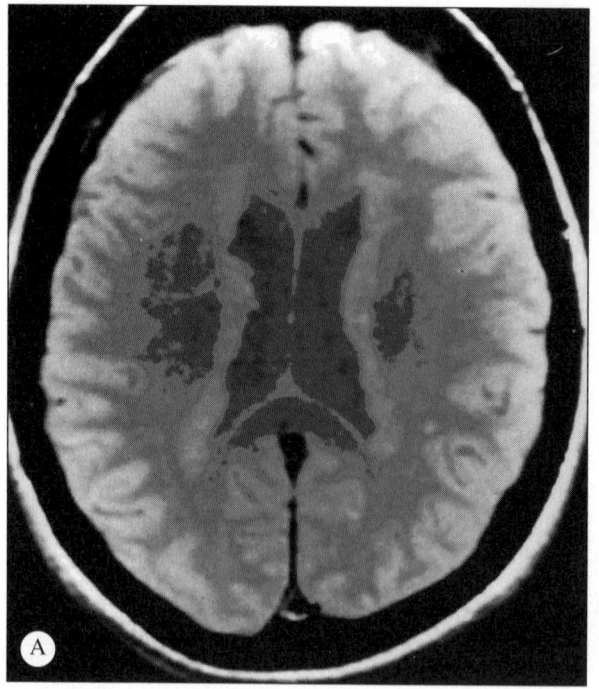

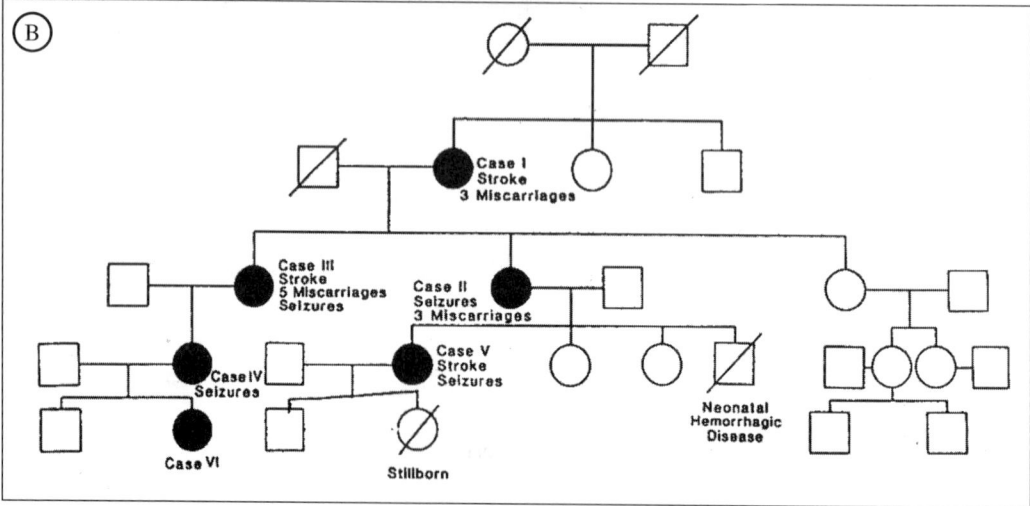

Fig. 11. (A) Contiguous periventricular nodular heterotopia. This abnormality may be inherited as sex-linked dominant. (B) Pedigree of a family described by Huttenlocher et al. Periventricular contiguous nodular heterotopia was found in members of four generations. There were no affected males in this pedigree, suggesting that the malformations may be lethal for male children. (Reproduced with permission.)

these nodules. The results have been unsatisfactory in the majority of cases and there is still considerable debate as to whether the lesions themselves are epileptogenic or whether it is the dysplastic overlying cortex which is responsible for the epileptic discharge. These patients now require invasive recording for clarification of the origin of the epileptic discharge (See Chapter 17 in this volume). Whether dual pathology, that is additional sclerosis of mesial temporal structures, is present in these patients is not entirely clear.

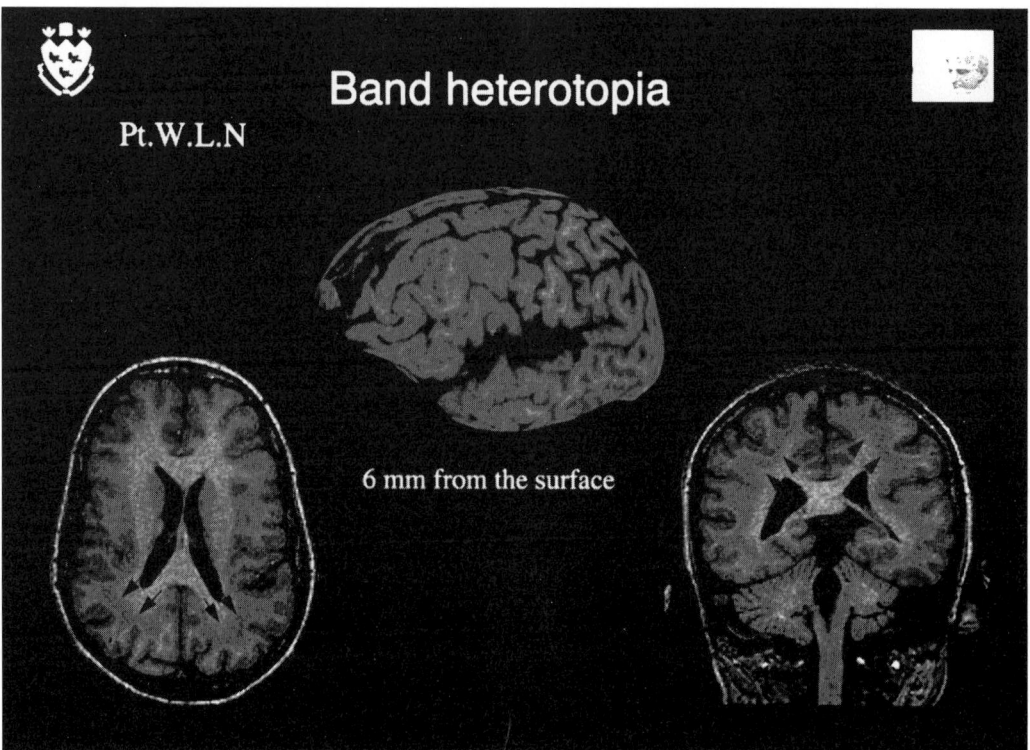

Fig. 12. Coronal and axial MRI and curvilinear reconstruction in a boy with band heterotopia. The band is separated from the cortex by a thin layer of white matter, best seen in the coronal plane. The curvilinear reconstruction is at 6 mm from the surface. The white matter is best seen behind the central sulcus. The findings suggest a degree of anterior pachygyria.

Contiguous periventricular nodules are often a manifestation of a sex-linked dominant disorder (Fig. 11 A). The first family, with the malformation in females spanning four generations, has been described by Huttenlocher *et al.* (1994). No living males were born to these women (Fig. 11 B) but they had an increased number of abortions. The abnormality seems to be lethal in male children although sporadic affected males with this abnormality have been described. The genetic basis of this abnormality has been clarified by the group of Walsh (1996).

Band heterotopia or the double cortex syndrome has been identified during life by Aicardi *et al.* (1990). Our own earliest description was inadequate since the quality of the imaging at that time did not permit recognition of the characteristic malformation consisting of a band of white matter underlying the cortex, with another band of grey matter below (Marchal *et al.*, 1989), shown in Figure 12. There is great variation in the degree of cortical abnormality associated with this subcortical migration defect. There is also considerable variation in the thickness and extent of the band (Barkovich *et al.*, 1994).

Most of the patients are female. Affected women may transmit the abnormality to daughters whereas the sons may have lissencephaly (Pinard *et al.*,1994). The underlying genetic abnormality has also been identified by Walsh *et al.* (1997) and the group of Pinard and Motte (1998).

Although the abnormalities are much rarer in males, it has now been described in 16 sporadic male epileptic patients with a considerable range in the severity of the epilepsy and of the associated cognitive abnormality. It has become clear that the band is not necessarily symmetrical and in one of our patients it was much thicker in one hemisphere compared with the other. Focal, or rather

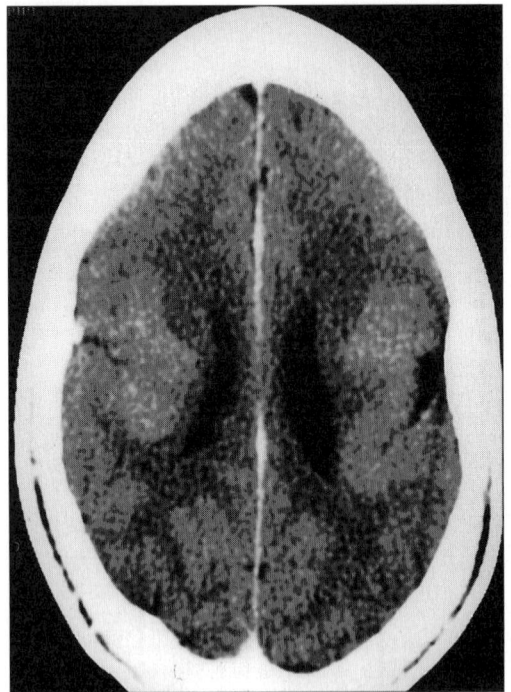

Fig. 13. A CT scan showing a thick band of grey matter surrounding a large sulcus. This was first interpreted as pachygyria and later shown to represent polymicrogyria.

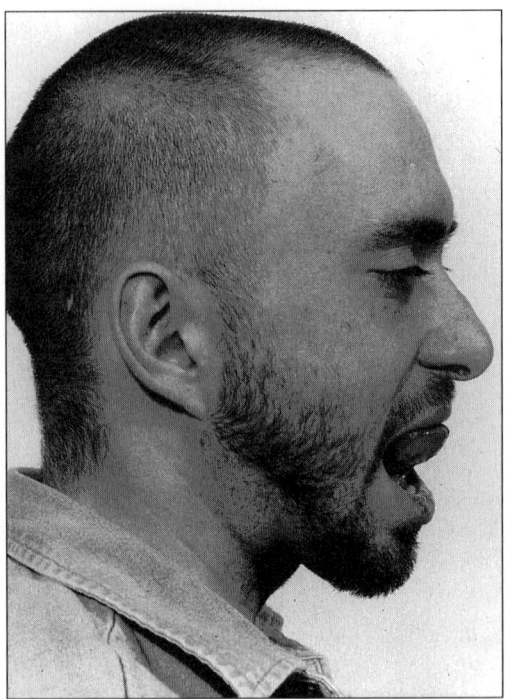

Fig. 14. A patient with bilateral perisylvian polymicrogyria during a maximal attempt of protruding his tongue.

pseudofocal, epileptic abnormalities may be encountered. Resection of more or less extended areas in three patients with such EEG findings may exceptionally be helpful. Extensive cortical transection in a patient with pseudofocal abnormalities carried out by Morrell and Whisler also did not result in a useful outcome.

Generalized pachygyria may present with severe and uncontrollable epileptic seizures. In one of our patients with this malformation and secondary generalized epilepsy a callosal section led to only very limited improvement in the attacks.

Micropolygyria is a disorder of cortical organization which occurs later in the pregnancy compared with the dysplastic lesions described above. Whether it can develop postnatally is still open to some discussion. These lesions have also been recognized during life with the help of modern imaging. In bilateral perisylvian micropolygyria the wide area of micropolygyria found on CT (Fig. 13) was first inter-

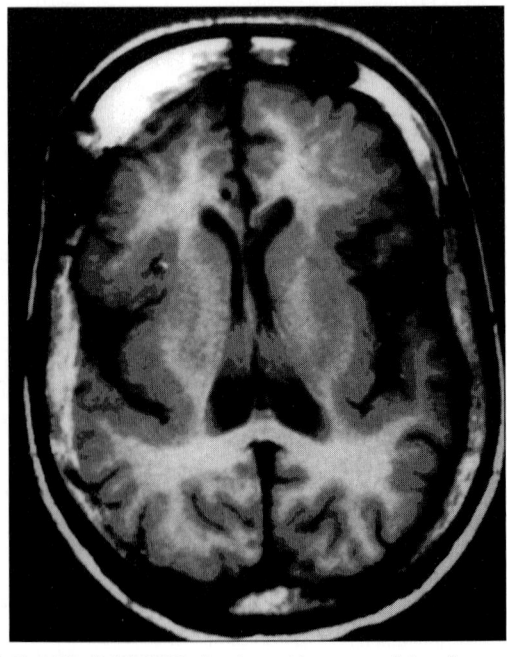

Fig. 15. Axial MRI showing wide open sylvian fissures and perisylvian polymicrogyria.

Chapter 1 The cortical dysplasias and epilepsy

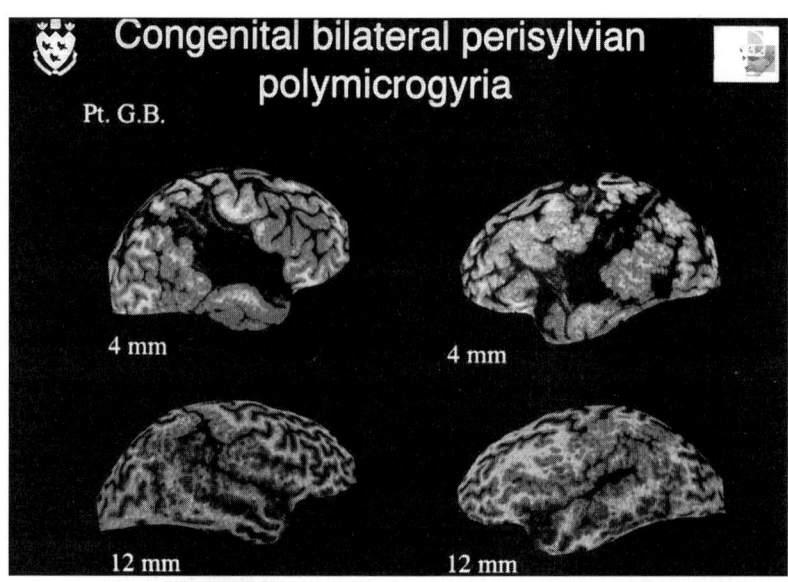

Fig. 16. *The polymicrogyria is best demonstrated by curvilinear reconstruction with cuts at different depths.*

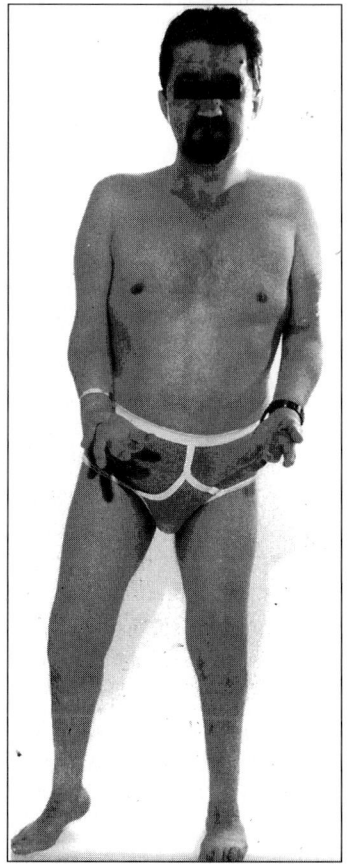

Fig. 17. *Patient with perisylvian polymicrogyria and arthrogryposis multiplex congenita.*

preted to represent pachygyria and only later was the nature of the abnormality correctly identified. The seizures are usually secondary generalized but in some patients consistently focal abnormalities may be found in addition, often originating in mesial temporal areas. The clinical abnormality consists of an at times very striking pseudobulbar palsy with complete anarthria but ability to pronounce vowels. The patients may not be able to protrude the tongue and usually can not move it sideways (Figs. 14-16). In other patients, presumably more in those whose abnormalities are not exactly homologous, the speech abnormality may be much milder or not at all noticeable. A mild hemiparesis with difficulty in rapid alternating movements of the fingers and in toe tapping may be present and this may be unilateral or bilateral. More recently, patients with neurological abnormalities of this type but without seizures have been described and emphasis has been placed on early recognition Miller *et al.* (1998). In about 10 per cent of patients there is associated arthrogryposis multiplex congenita (Fig. 17), and this may be due to an inflammatory process possibly involving both the peripheral and central nervous system. This however is still conjectural.

Here too magnetic resonance spectroscopy (Guerreiro, submitted) has shown reduction in NAA in the lesional area compared to perilesional or more remote regions of interest.

Poly-microgyria may also be inherited as a sex-linked dominant but perhaps other modes of inheritance may occur as well. It is likely that the early patients with pseudobulbar palsy described by Worster Drought may have had this malformation of cortical organization as well (Worster Drought, 1974).

Hypothalamic hamartoma has been a long-standing clinical puzzle. The early laughing attacks are often followed by considerable behavioural abnormalities and the development of a secondary generalized epileptic process. This occurs late in the first decade and there is deterioration in cognitive function with very striking and intractable aggression, hyperactivity and poor judgment. These abnormalities have been attributed to more widespread hemispheral changes but resection of focal areas showing at times interictal or ictal epileptogenic discharges has invariably led to failure (Cascino et al., 1993). That epileptogenic abnormalities can arise in the hamartoma itself has been shown by Munari and colleagues (1997). Surgical resection may lead to cessation of seizures or to considerable improvement. A series of six patients from four centres are currently being reported by Palmini et al. (in preparation). Radiosurgery has been employed as well by Kuzniecky and his group (1997) with good results.

Further confirmation that the hamartoma is in fact responsible for abnormality has been demonstrated by Tasch and colleagues (1998) who showed reduced N-acetylspartate in the hypothalamic lesions.

Not all patients with hypothalamic hamartoma, however, have severe epileptic or behavioural abnormalities. Berkovic and ourselves have recently studied two patients with very small hypothalamic lesions (± 5 mm in diameter) who merely had an urge to laugh, without more overt clinical manifestations.

Studies of neurotransmitter function in dysplastic tissue, based on histochemical analysis were performed in several patients by Spreafico and colleagues (See Chapter 20 in this volume). They have convincingly shown an increase in excitatory, glutaminergic function coupled with a decrease in GABAergic, inhibitory activity.

Concluding remarks

Since the 19th century various abnormalities of cortical development due to migration defects, disorders of maturation and disorders of cortical organization were described in brains at autopsy. Cortical dysplasia was then recognized in tissue resected during surgical treatment of patients with intractable epilepsy but this finding remained largely unappreciated until the development of modern imaging. CT allowed glimpses of the more obvious malformations but it was the advent of MRI which enabled recognition and classification of the different types of lesions.

In the Taylor type of cortical dysplasia it became clear that there was a wide range in the severity and above all in the extent of the abnormality. The lesions range from small areas, often difficult to identify, to extensive lesions surrounded by a halo or penumbra of presumably less severe, but still clinically significant, structural abnormality. Functional imaging with SPECT, PET and MRS have provided additional insights and led to improved strategies for surgical treatment. Even lesions involving the central strip may at times be successfully resected, but in such patients much depends on the preoperative neurological status.

The recognition of the fact that the dysplastic lesions are in themselves epileptogenic has been another milestone in our understanding of these abnormalities.

Subcortical heterotopias, and in particular periventricular nodular heterotopias, have been recognized as causing intractable epilepsy in some patients. Surgical approaches to these lesions are now being worked out. The hereditary nature of the lesions in some of these patients has explained the familial occurrence of epilepsy in a number of instances.

Generalized epileptic abnormalities and generalized disorders of migration and maturation have been described as band heterotopia or the double cortex syndrome. Here too, sex-linked dominant inheritance may occur and there has been progress in our understanding of the mechanisms of these genetically determined lesions. Focal resection in patients with band heterotopia however has been of questionable value to the small number of patients in whom it has been carried out.

Cortical malformations due to disorganization, occurring later in intrauterine life, are represented by micropolygyria. These lesions are often bilateral and perisylvian but at times they are unilateral and in some patients they may be occipital or frontal. Several syndromes have emerged, the most common being the one characterized by severe pseudobulbar palsy and mild pyramidal deficit (CBPS) (Kuzniecky et al., 1993). In some of these patients, particularly the ones with micropolygyria, the epilepsy may not be intractable and full control may be obtained by medical treatment (Ambrosetto et al. 1993).

Hypothalamic hamartomata and the associated epileptic syndrome have been better understood in recent years. Despite the risks of surgery, resection of the lesion offers hope of improvement in seizure control and in the often extremely severe behavioural abnormalities.

On the other hand, patients with small lesions leading only to a "need to laugh" without more overt epileptic or behavioural manifestations are now being recognized.

Finally, investigations have begun to uncover the transmitter abnormalities in patients with cortical dysplasia. An increase in excitatory glutaminergic activity and a decrease in inhibitory gabaergic activity have been identified in tissue from patients treated surgically for their intractable epilepsy (See Chapter 20 in this volume).

Recognition of the cortical dysplasias has turned over a new leaf in our understanding of intractable epilepsy in many individuals. This is best illustrated by a patient with focal seizures investigated by Dr. Rasmussen 25 years ago. No cause for his problem could be identified and Dr. Rasmussen suggested to the patient's parents that they might want to return in 25 years when advances in medicine could provide a clearer explanation of their son's epilepsy. The family literally accepted this advice and returned as suggested; 25 years later the MRI showed a typical example of transmantle dysplasia (Barkovich et al., 1997). In this man, rather exceptionally, the epileptic abnormality was not sufficient to justify surgical intervention and his seizures, though not of maximal severity, have continued.

Recognition of more subtle structural abnormalities, clarification of the significance of microdysgenesis and the search for rational therapy based on better understanding of the transmitter abnormalities are challenges for the present. Prevention of dysplastic abnormalities remains a challenge for the future and will depend on further progress in neuroscience.

References

Ambrosetto G. (1993): Treatable partial epilepsy and unilateral opercular neuronal migration disorder. *Epilepsia* **344(4)**, 604–608.

Barkovich A.J. Guerrini R., Battaglia G., Kalifa G., N'Guyen T., Parmeggiani A., Santucci M., Giovanardi-Rossi P., Granata T. & D'Incerti L. (1994): Band heterotopia: correlation of outcome with magnetic resonance imaging parameters. *Annals of Neurology* **36(4)**, 609–617.

Barkovich A.J., Rowley H.A. & Andermann F. (1995): MR in partial epilepsy: value of high-resolution volumetric techniques. *American Journal of Neuroradiology* **16(2)**, 339-343.

Barkovich A.J., Kuzniecky R.I., Dobyn W.B., Jackson G.D., Becker L.E. & Evrard P. (1996): A classification scheme for malformations of cortical development [Review]. *Neuropediatrics* **27(2)**, 59–63.

Barkovich A.J., Kuzniecky R.I. Bollen A.W., Grant P.E (1997): Focal transmantle dysplasia: specific malformation of cortical development. *Neurology* **49(4)**, 1148-1152.

Bastos A.C., Korah I.P., Cendes F., Melanson D., Tampiere D., Peters T., Dubeau F. & Andermann F. (1995): Curvilinear reconstruction of 3D magnetic resonance imaging in patients with partial epilepsy - A pilot study. *Magnetic Resonance Imaging* **13(8)**, 1107–1112.

Cascino G.D., Andermann F., Berkovic S.F., Kuzniecky R.I., Sharborough F.W. Keene D.L. Baldin P.F., Kelly P.J., Olivier A. & Feindel W. (1993): Gelastic seizures and hypothalamic hamartoma: evaluation of patients undergoing chronic intracranial EEG monitoring and outcome of surgical treatment. *Neurology* **43(4)**, 747–750.

Chugani H.T. (1993): PET in preoperative evaluation of intractable epilepsy. *Pediatric Neurology* **9(5)**, 411–413.

Desbiens R., Berkovic S.F., Dubeau F., Andermann F., Laxer K.D., Harvey S., Leproux F., Melanson D., Robitaille Y., Kalnins R. *et al.* (1993): Life-threatening focal status epilepticus due to occult cortical dysplasia. *Archives of Neurology* **50(7)**, 695-700.

Des Portes V., Pinad J.M., Billuart P., Vinet M.C., Koulakoff A., Carrie A., Gelot A., Dupuis E., Motte J., Berwald-Netter Y., Catala M., Kahn A., Beldjord C. & Chelly J. (1998): a novel CNA gene required for neuronal migration and involved in X-linked subcortical laminar heterotopia and lissencephaly syndrome. *Cell* **92(1)**, 51–61.

Eksioglu Y.Z., Scheffer I.E., Cardenas P., DiMario F., Ramsby G., Berg M., Kamuro K., Berkovic S.F., Duyk G.M., Parisi J., Huttenlocher P.R. & Walsh C.A. (1996): Periventricular heterotopia: an X-linked dominant epilepsy locus causing abberrant cerebral cortical development. *Neuron* **16(1)**, 77–87.

Gambardella A., Palmini A., Andermann F., Dubeau F., Da Costa J.C., Quesney L.F., Andermann E. & Olivier A. (1996): Usefulness of focal rhythmic discharges on scalp EEG of patients with focal cortical dysplasia and intractable epilepsy. *Electroencephalography and Clinical Neurophysiology* **98**, 243–249.

Guerreiro M.L., Andermann E., Guerrini R., Dobyns W.B. *et al.* (Submitted): Familial perisylvian polymicrogyria: a new familial syndrome of cortical maldevelopment.

Huttenlocher P.R., Taravath S. & Mojtahedi S. (1994): Periventricular heterotopia and epilepsy. *Neurology* **44(1)**, 51–55.

Kuzniecky R., Andermann F., Guerrini R. (1993): Congenital bilateral perisylvian syndome: study of 31 patients. The CBPS Multicenter Collaborative Study. *Lancet* **341(8845)**, 608–612.

Kuzniecky R., Guthrie B., Mountz J., Bebin M., Faught E., Gilliam F., Liu H.G. (1997): Intrinsic epileptogenesis of hypothalamic hamartomas in gelastic epilepsy *5-Ann Neuro* **42(1)**, 60–67.

Lee J.W., Andermann F., Dubeau F., Bernasconi A., Macdonald D., Evans A. & Reutens D.C. (1998): Morphic analysis of the temporal lobe in temporal lobe epilepsy. *Epilepsia* **39(7)**, 727–736.

Li L.M., Cendes F., Bastos A.C., Andermann F., Dubeau F. & Arnold D.L. (1998): Neuronal metabolic dysfunction in patients with cortical developmental malformations: a Proton magnetic resonance spectroscopic imaging study. *Neurology* **50(3)**, 755–759.

Livingston J.H., Aicardi J. (1990): Unusual MRI appearance of diffuse subcortical heterotopia or "double cortex" in two children. *Journal of Neurology, Neurosurgery & Psychiatry* **53(7)**, 617–620.

Marchal G., Andermann F., Donatella T., Robitaille Y., Melanson D., Sinclair B., Olivier A., Silver K. & Langevin P. (1989): Generalized cortical dysplasia manifested by diffusely thick cerebral cortex. *Archives of Neurology* **46(4)**, 430–434.

Miller S.P., Shevell M., Rosenblatt B., Silver K., O'Gorman A. & Andermann F. (1998): Congenital bilateral perisylvian polymicrogyria presenting as congenital hemiplegia. *Neurology* **50(6)**, 1866–1869.

Munari C., Tassi L., Berta E., Kahane P. & Quarato P.P. (1997): Case of a child with gelastic seizures and hypothalamic hamartoma [letter; comment]. *Epilepsia* **38(12)**, 1364–1365.

Palmini A., Gambardella A., Andermann F., Dueau F., Da Costa J.C., Olivier A., Tampoeri D., Gloor P., Quesney F., Andermann E., Paglioli E., Paglioli-Neto E., Coutinho L., Leblanc R. & Kim H-I. (1995): Intrinsic epileptogenicity of human dysplastic cortex as suggested by corticography and surgical results. *Annals of Neurology* **37**, 476-487.

Pinard J.M., Motte J., Chiron C., Brian R., Andermann E. & Dulac O. (1994): Subcortical laminar heterotopia and lissencephaly in two families: a single X linked dominant gene. *Journal of Neurology, Neurosurgery & Psychiatry* **57(8)**, 914–920.

Prayson R.A., Estes M.L. & Morris H.H.D. (1993): Coexistence of neoplasia and cortical dysplasia in patients presenting with seizures. *Epilepsia* **34(4)**, 609-615.

Ross M.E., Allen K.M., Srivastava A.K., Featherstone T., Gleeson J.G., Hirsch B., Harding B.N., Andermann E., Abdullah R., Berg M., Czapansky-Bielman D., Flanders D.J., Guerrini R., Motte J., Mira A.P., Scheffer I., Berkovic S., Scaravilli F., King R.A., Ledbetter D.H., Schlessinger D., Dobyns W.B. & Walsh C.A. (1997): Linkage and physical mapping of X-linked lissencephaly/SBH (XLIS): a gene causing neuronal migration defects in human brain. *Human Molecular Genetics* **6(4),** 555–562.

Sisodiya S.M., Free S.L., Stevens J.M., Fish D.R. & Shorvon S.D. (1995): Widespread cerebral structural changes in patients with cortical dysgenesis and epilepsy. *Brain* **118(Pt4),** 1039–1050.

Tasch E., Cendes F., Li L.M., Dubeau F., Montes J., Rosenblatt B., Andermann F., Arnold D. (1998): Hypothalamic hamartomas and gelastic epilepsy – A spectroscopic study. *Neurology* **51(4),** 1046–1050.

Taylor D.C., Falconer M.A., Bruton C.J. & Corsellis J.A.N. (1971): Focal dysplasia of the cerebal cortex in epilepsy. *J. Neurol. Neurosur. Psychiatry,* **34,** 369-387.

Worster-Drought C. (1974): Suprabulbar paresis, Congenital suprabulbar paresis and its differential diagnosis, with reference to acquired suprabulbar paresis. *Development Medicine & Child Neurology* **30 (Suppl)**,1–33.

PART II

CORTICAL DEVELOPMENT

Chapter 2

The pioneering studies on neuronal migration in the developing cerebral cortex

Marina Bentivoglio[1] and Paolo Mazzarello[2]

[1]Istituto di Anatomia e Istologia, Università di Verona, Strada Le Grazie 8, 37134 Borgo Roma, Verona, Italy
[2]Istituto di Genetica (IGBE), CNR, Pavia, Italy

Summary

Cortical morphogenesis started to be investigated in the last decades of the nineteenth century, and the basic events of cortical development, as well as the cell types colonizing the developing cerebral cortex, were long debated. Fundamental pioneering contributions, such as those provided by Kölliker, Vignal, His and Cajal, are outlined in this brief historical overview. In particular, following His' investigations Cajal worked out, with variants of the Golgi impregnation technique, details of neuronal and glial cell types of the developing cortex, and contributed greatly to the understanding of cortical shaping processes. The first Golgi impregnation of the cerebral cortex in foetuses was achieved by Giuseppe Magini, who clearly described a radial arrangement of glial cells. Magini also detected swellings with cell nuclei intercalated along the radial filaments, and hypothesized that these could represent developing nervous cells. The basic mechanisms of the outward displacement of young cortical neurones generated in the ventricular neuroepithelium, which was suggested by early studies, were elucidated on the basis of electron microscopy in the early 1970s by Pasko Rakic, who clarified that neuronal migration occurs along radial glia.

Introduction

'All neurones of the central nervous system are gypsies for some time of their career' wrote Gerald Edelman (1987) to emphasize that neuronal migration is the key mechanism of the developmental shaping of the nervous system, i.e. of the early steps of the career that nerve cells have to undertake to become functional neurones. During cortical development neurones are very active 'gypsies', and a spatially and temporally ordered sequence of migratory events is necessary to build up the cerebral cortex; the complexity of these mechanisms increases in the large cortex of primates. Disturbances of these processes can lead to a wide range of alterations, from severe brain malformations to local disruption of the cortical structure. Due to the rapid progress of brain imaging techniques, neuronal migration disorders are now diagnosed at a high resolution and, as will be dealt with extensively in this volume, they are at present at the focus of basic and clinical research on cortical excitability and epileptic phenomena.

We wish to point out in this introductory chapter that the understanding of the basic developmental events in the brain, including neuronal migration, has required a century of efforts, hypotheses and debates, which will be briefly outlined here. In order to proceed through the steps of the acquisition of knowledge on cortical development, we will ask the fundamental questions faced by neuroscientists towards the end of last century. What cell types can be identified during cortex formation? Do these cells move (i.e. do they migrate) in the developing cortex? And, if they migrate, how do they do this?

Methodological tools

Providing an answer to the above-mentioned questions requires not only a basic knowledge of the structure of the nervous system, but also the tools to process histologically very delicate material, such as embryonic and foetal brains, the staining of the sections and, finally, microscopic observation. In other words, in order to understand development of the nervous tissue, neuroscientists first needed to see it. A survey of the technological improvements that represented a breakthrough in histology in the nineteenth century goes beyond the purpose of this chapter. It should, however, be pointed out that a remarkable advance in the revelatory power of light microscopy was achieved only in the 1830s, when 'achromatic' instruments were introduced. Techniques for hardening tissue specimens (e.g. with alcohol or chromic acid) and stains of histological sections became available in the mid-nineteenth century, and were developed in the second half of the century. The use of formaldehyde, which is the most widely used fixative nowadays, was introduced only in 1893 (Blum, 1893), and fixation is considered to be a very critical procedure for handling a soft tissue such as that of the foetal brain.

The progress in the histological techniques brought about a revolution in the investigation of the nervous system. In particular, the use of stains based on carmine and hematoxylin greatly facilitated the study of histological preparations, and towards the end of the nineteenth century Franz Nissl introduced the stain of nerve tissue cells (Nissl, 1884, 1894) which still represents an effective and routinely used technique. The most revolutionary histological stain was, however, provided by the 'black reaction' (*reazione nera*) introduced by Camillo Golgi in 1873 (see Mazzarello, 1996, and Pannese, 1996 for historical accounts on the Golgi impregnation).

The Golgi stain is based on nervous tissue hardening in potassium dichromate and impregnation with silver nitrate, and visualizes at random individual elements, both neurones and glial cells. At the time of the introduction of the Golgi stain, the existence and features of different cell types in the nervous tissue were far from being defined, and the possibility of visualizing with Golgi impregnation individual nerve cell bodies to the full extent of their processes paved the way for modern neuroscience. The studies that led to the identification of the neuron as the anatomical, functional and ontogenetic unit of the nervous system are not the focus of the present overview, and the reader is referred to exhaustive accounts on the birth of the 'neuron doctrine' (Shepherd, 1991; Jacobson, 1993; Finger, 1994). On the other hand, it may be less known that in the last decades of the nineteenth century the Golgi technique, together with the above-mentioned advancements of histological methods, opened also the era of the studies on neural development, in which the investigations on the cerebral cortex played a central role. As will be emphasized further, the Golgi impregnation of glial elements greatly contributed to the understanding of cortical morphogenesis.

After the initial report of the chromoargentic impregnation, this technique was used for some years only in Camillo Golgi's laboratory at the University of Pavia (Mazzarello, 1996). The method then started to be applied in some Italian laboratories, but the Golgi stain became nationally and internationally renowned only in the mid-1880s; Camillo Golgi sent to the eminent histologist Albert Kölliker some of his stained preparations at the beginning of 1887 (Mazzarello, 1996). Santiago Ramón y Cajal observed Golgi-impregnated material for the first time in Madrid in 1887, and the view of these sections at the microscope was like a flash of lightning in his scientific life (see Cajal, 1996).

In the first half of the twentieth century the staining techniques of the nervous system were further refined and improved, but not much happened for about 60 years in the tools available for the study of the finest details of the developing nervous system. Finally, a revolutionary breakthrough was provided in the early 1950s by the introduction of the electron microscope, which opened entirely new perspectives in the cytology of neural development. At the end of the 1950s the use of tritiated thymidine allowed neuron birthdays and migration sites to be determined with autoradiography. Molecular biology also finally exploded in this field of research, and genes and molecules are now under scrutiny as protagonists of neural development. Fate mapping, tissue culture and transplantation are thus being examined with advanced molecular approaches.

Early studies on morphogenetic events and cell identity in the developing cerebral cortex

We now know that the cells destined to form the cortex are generated from proliferating cells in the pseudostratified neuroepithelium of the telencephalic ventricular zones. The young postmitotic neurones migrate outward from the ventricular zone along radial glial fibres across the cell-sparse intermediate zone (the future white matter) to the outer surface, where they form the primordial plexiform layer which represents the rudiment of the future layer I. Migratory neurones constitute the cortical plate, destined to form the layered adult cerebral cortex. The primordial plexiform layer is split by the cortical plate into two zones: the marginal zone, which will form layer I, and the subplate, a transient structure that will disappear.

The investigations that led to the understanding of these complex events started more than a century ago, and the findings relevant to neuronal migration are tightly linked to all the other data obtained in the early studies of cortical development. We wish to briefly outline first the pioneering contributions to the formation of the cortex, focusing then on migratory events.

The famous handbook of histology written by Kölliker had six editions between 1852 and 1896, and included a section on the development of the cerebral cortex, and Kölliker also focused on embryology (1879, 1882). In his studies, Kölliker (1879, 1882, 1896) described how in mammals, including man (he studied especially the developing cortex of the rabbit), the earliest formation in the future cortex was represented by a multilayered epithelium composed of cells that first exhibited an elongated shape and then became distinctly fusiform. The primitive epithelium was then divided into two main layers: a deep layer covering the ventricles maintained the primitive epithelial features, while an outer layer represented the first rudiment of the white matter. Through the subsequent transformation four layers were then subdivided: an external layer of white matter, a second layer and a third layer of gray and white matter, respectively, and the internal epithelial layer, which was the thickest portion of the developing cortex.

Probably influenced and stimulated by Kölliker's studies, Vignal, at the Laboratory of Histology of the Collège de France, published in 1888 a detailed account of the development of the mammalian cerebral cortex (Vignal, 1888a,b). As other neurohistologists who became interested in the developments, including Camillo Golgi (see below), Vignal (1884a,b) started investigating neural development in the spinal cord, and hypothesized that the rows of cells around the central canal could migrate towards the periphery to form the gray matter (a hypothesis which, however, Vignal doubted) or that the cells were multiplying at different sites in the gray matter. Vignal started then to investigate the cerebral cortex, publishing first a short note (1886), which was followed by extensive reports (1888a,b). In his study Vignal (1888a) compiled also a long section (10 pages) dedicated to 'history'. It was, however, a very recent history, since Vignal declared that the first work on the histogenesis of the elements of the brain had been published by Boll in 1874 (Boll's paper had actually appeared in 1873). Boll had investigated the brain of the chick embryo, and had stated the existence since the earliest developmental stages of two cell types, one destined to become nerve cells and the other 'connective' cells. In his review of previous studies, Vignal also quoted a paper dedicated to humans, and in particular to the study of the cerebral cortex in newborns (Besser, 1866), according to which the brain was formed at birth only by neuroglial cells.

Vignal (1888a) also extensively referred to the 'excellent' handbook of embryology written by Kölliker (1882), and he quoted the findings that Magini (see further) had just published.

In his studies Vignal (1888a,b) reported that the cells which form the cerebral vesicles rapidly lose their 'epithelial features' and become irregular cells with a well developed cytoplasm which constitute the embryonic gray matter, whereas the neuroglial cells are later differentiated from the embryonic cells. Vignal also outlined the presence in the developing cortex of a proliferating deep zone and morphogenetic events, including the relatively early appearance of a superficial first layer, the increase in width of the embryonic gray matter, and the development of the white matter.

In a series of fundamental contributions, His (1887; 1889a,b; 1904) proposed that the germinal epithelium, situated near the lateral ventricular surface of the developing cerebral wall, comprises two classes of precursor cells: the germinal cells near the ventricle produced neuronal cells (the neuroblasts), while the glial cells originated from different precursors (the spongioblasts), spanning the tickness of the developing nervous tissue. In contrast, Schaper (1897) suggested that the germinal zone consisted of a homogeneous precursor cell population, from which both neuronal and glial cells differentiated, and clearly stated that 'in all vertebrates at a certain period of their development the ventricular wall at all sections of the neural canal is the sole seat of the process of cell proliferation' (quoted by Paton, 1900). Paton (1900), who investigated the developing cerebral cortex of the pig and rabbit with several techniques, including the Golgi stain, was also fiercely opposed to His' views, stating that at the earliest stage the telencephalic wall was made up of three kinds of cells: the germinal cells, the spongioblasts and the indifferent cells (the former giving origin to the latter two). Paton could not distinguish any neuroblast among the germinal cells located close to the ventricle, whereas at later stages he found neuroblasts only at a considerable distance from the ventricle, so that he hypothesized the existence of an intermediate form between the germinal cell and the neuroblast. Overall the development of the cerebral cortex had to be ascribed, according to Paton (1900), to a regressive process of the glial cells and a growth of nerve cells. The cell movement in the developing cerebral cortex was also rather complicated in Paton's view, proposing a 'process of rotation' ('turn half-way round') of indifferent cells destined to become neuroblasts.

The debate on the precursors of cortical cell types has attracted a great deal of attention since these early studies, but a detailed account of these discussions would be too long and complicated, especially since, jumping one century ahead, such debate has not been entirely solved. The modern lineage studies have indicated that different cell types (neuronal subsets, astrocytes, oligodendrocytes) arise from distinct sets of progenitors in the cerebral cortex, but many questions about progenitor cell lineage and environmental determinants remain open (see McConnell, 1995, for review). Paton (1900), however, had concluded that 'A complete knowledge regarding the ultimate fate of the indifferent cells in the adult nervous system is not yet possible ... my belief is that a considerable number of them persist through life. The presence of these cells may have an important bearing in those pathological conditions which are characterized by an increase of the glia elements'. Thus, although Paton's ideas on the cell types and movements in the developing cortex were somewhat confused and confusing, at the beginning of the twentieth century he anticipated the interest in stem cells, which is now blooming at the end of the century with regard to repair in neural diseases or injuries (see McKay, 1997).

On the basis of the studies performed by His, the cerebral pallium was considered to consist exclusively of epithelial elements (i.e. elements deriving from the ectoderm), extending from the ventricular cavities to the brain surface. In addition, due to His' studies, it was made clear that the internal zone was made up by rapidly dividing germinal cells, capable of mitosis. When and where mitosis actually occurred was, however, a matter of debate, and Hatai (1902) described 'spherical cells or "germ cells" ' also in the most superficial layers of the cat developing cortex (Fig. 1).

It was noticed and emphasized by His (1887, 1889a,b, 1904) that in their displacement the cells formed a mass of 'bipolar' cells, which represented the first rudiment of the gray matter. The bipolar arrangement of young cells gave rise to a great debate: were the two extremities of the cells (which we now define as the trailing and leading processes) giving rise to dendrites, axons, or both? For example Hatai (1902) wondered whether an axon was developing out of the bipolar neurones or only dendrites could be seen in immature neurones (Fig. 1).

The studies performed by His exerted a profound influence on the earliest investigations pursued by Cajal with variants of the Golgi impregnation. Cajal (1904, 1911) clearly stated that the process of cell division occurred preferentially 'in the vicinity of the epithelium', and neuroblasts then migrated beneath the outer layer (the marginal veil, as the primordial plexiform layer was originally named).

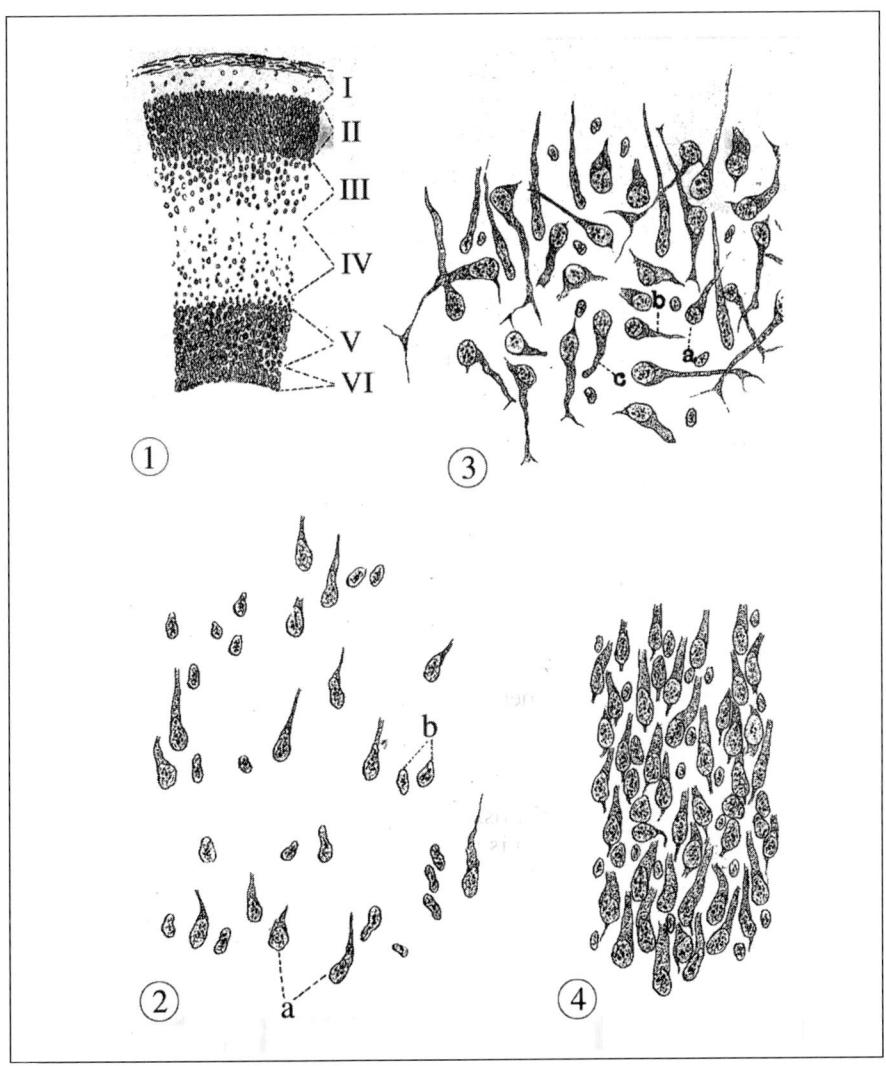

Fig. 1. Developing cortex of a cat foetus as drawn by Hatai (1902). (1) represents a transverse section, and (2), (3), and (4) illustrate, at higher magnification, details of layers III, IV and V, respectively. (Reproduced from Hatai, 1902.)

In his work on the cerebral cortex of human foetuses, Retzius (1893a) put emphasis on the large horizontal cells in the developing layer I, which Cajal had also described, and are now defined as the Cajal–Retzius cells. According to modern studies performed by Marín-Padilla with Golgi impregnation of the human developing cortex, layer I, and in particular the Cajal–Retzius cells, play a crucial role in cortical neuron differentiation (see Marín-Padilla, 1998).

Focusing on neuronal migration

Our brief historical outline points out that processes of cell division and the building up and constant variation of layers during cortical development were soon evident, and His emphasized that the germinal zone was continuing to produce neuroblasts which immediately acquired a bipolar form and were displaced towards the brain surface. His (1887; 1889a,b; 1904) also proposed that glial cells could help to guide the outward displacement of neuroblasts. However, the transition from the static microscopic observation to the full comprehension of the rapidly dynamic events occurring during development required a tremendous effort, to which the Golgi technique provided an important contribution.

'Convinced that the key for the solution of many questions is enclosed in the embryogenesis of nervous central organs' (Golgi, 1885), Camillo Golgi investigated with his method the developing nervous tissue. In 1885 (the volume was reprinted by a renowned publishing house in 1886), Golgi published the findings he had observed in the chick embryo, describing glial fibres 'radiating' from the central canal towards the periphery of the spinal cord: 'cylindric epithelial cells assume a clear black coffee-brown staining identical to that shown by the same staining in neuroglial cells. These cylindric cells traverse radially the plane of the section of the spinal cord, reaching its extreme peripheral border' (Golgi, 1885).

Radially elongated processes (defined as epithelial or ependymal elements) were soon detected in the embryonic spinal cord by means of the Golgi staining also by Lenhossék (1893) and Retzius (1893b).

Giuseppe Magini, who was working at the University of Rome, performed the first Golgi impregnation of the foetal cerebral cortex of several mammals, including humans. Magini's contributions, (1888a, 1888c) published in Italian, appeared also in French in the *Archives Italiennes de Biologie* (Magini, 1888b,d). He described how the 'cylindric epithelial cells' situated around the ventricular cavity proceeded 'like rays' towards the brain surface, and stated that the 'radiating neuroglial cells' exhibited a high number of 'varicosities' which he could not detect in the adult brain (Magini, 1888a). Very puzzled by the significance of these varicosities, Magini (1888a) hypothesized that they could represent developing nerve cells. In order to verify this assumption, Magini investigated whether the varicosities contained nuclei. To this purpose, he counterstained with hematoxylin the Golgi-impregnated tissue and clearly detected nuclei in the beads of the radial glia (Magini, 1888c). The figure which illustrated the contribution he presented at the Accademia dei Lincei (Magini, 1888c) was not published in the French translation of this paper (Magini, 1888d). However, this drawing (Fig. 2) demonstrates a remarkable insight into the structure of the developing cortex, and foreshadowed the data (and the famous illustration, see Fig. 3) provided by Rakic (1972) more than 80 years later.

Cajal was obviously aware of the work pursued by Golgi and Magini on embryonic tissue. Immediately after having seen Golgi-impregnated preparations of the nervous tissue, Cajal fully devoted himself to the study of the nervous system. Towards the end of 1888 Cajal initiated the study of embryonic material, and his first report, dedicated to the brain of the chick embryo, appeared at the beginning of 1889 (Cajal, 1889).

In his studies on the developing cerebral cortex, Cajal was impressed by the striking geometrical regularity of radial glia, and suggested that these cells may serve as a scaffolding for the embry-

Chapter 2 Pioneering studies on neuronal migration

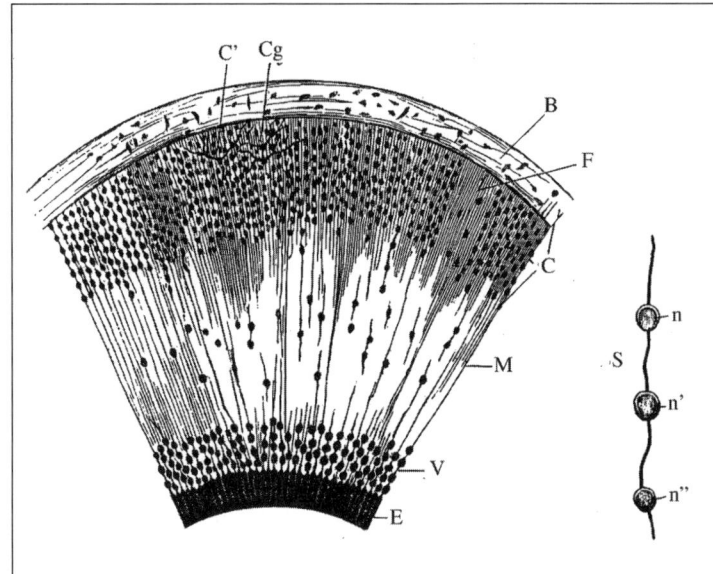

Fig. 2. Developing cortex of a calf foetus (4th month of gestation) impregnated with the Golgi stain and counterstained with hematoxylin, as drawn by Magini. In the original figure legend, the labels are indicated as follows: 'B, superficial zone of the white matter with very few filaments and rare spherical, fusiform, triangular cells; C, cortical matter rich in radial filaments and spherical cells; C' sketched nerve cell; Cg, twin nerve cells, whose division is not yet complete; M, medullary [myelinated] matter with radial filaments and scarce varicosities (spherical cells); V, varicosities (spherical cells) inserted in the filaments continuous with the epithelial cells'. On the right side: 'S: Three spherical cells of the cortical matter, with a big nucleus (n, n', n") surrounded by a rim of protoplasm, inserted on a filament'. (Reproduced from Magini, 1888c.)

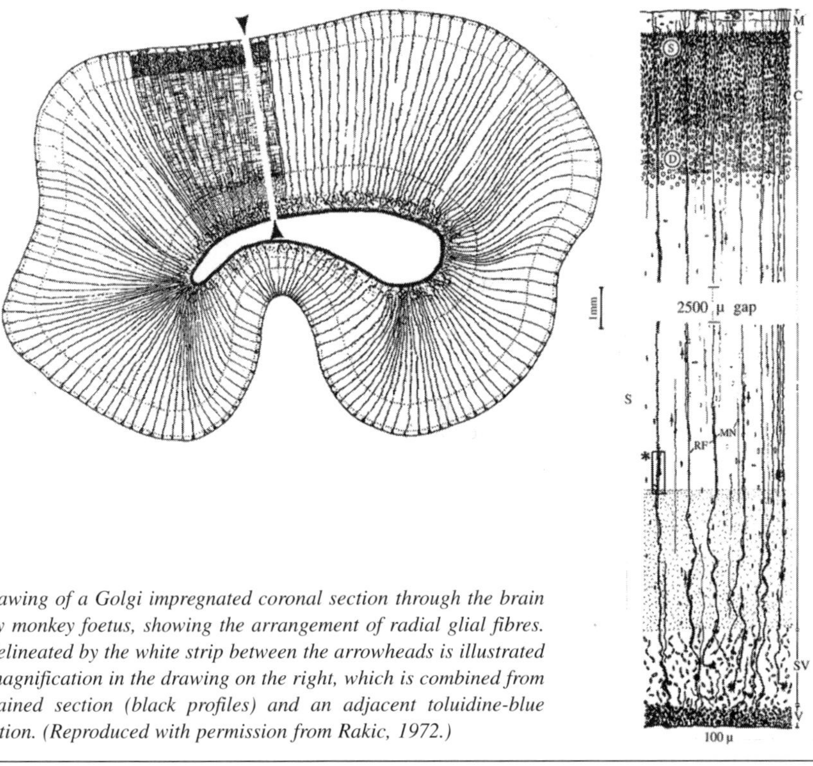

Fig. 3. Drawing of a Golgi impregnated coronal section through the brain of a 97-day monkey foetus, showing the arrangement of radial glial fibres. The area delineated by the white strip between the arrowheads is illustrated at higher magnification in the drawing on the right, which is combined from a Golgi-stained section (black profiles) and an adjacent toluidine-blue stained section. (Reproduced with permission from Rakic, 1972.)

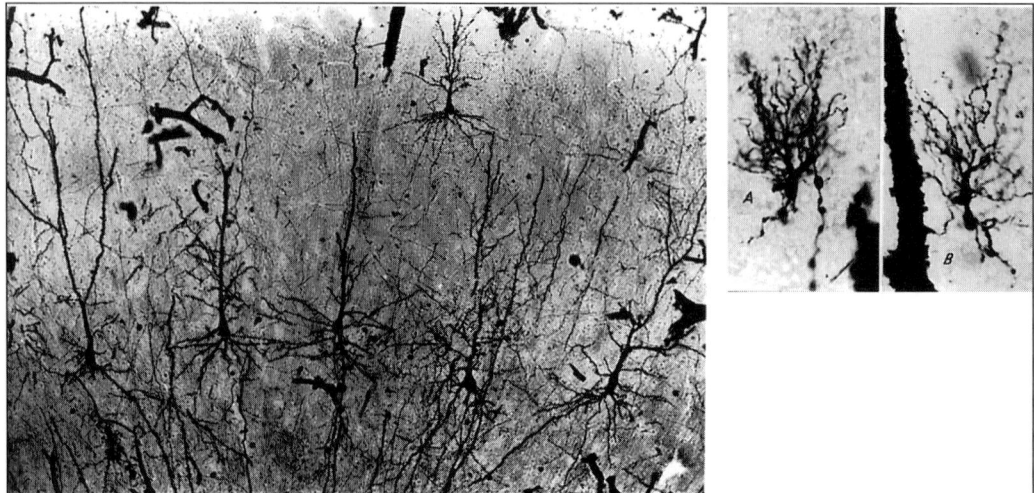

Fig. 4. Golgi impregnation of the developing cortex of the sheep. On the left: deep large pyramidal cells, and more superficially a middle-sized pyramidal neuron, already well differentiated in the motor cortex of a foetus of length 320 mm. On the right: neuroglial cells (foetus of length 100 mm.): A, cell with ascending processes; B, spider-like cell, some expansions reach the wall of a blood vessel. (Reproduced from Godina, 1951.)

onic tissue (Cajal, 1904, 1911). However, 'Ramón y Cajal had a hard time making up his mind as to the nature of "foetal radial cells" ' (Rakic, 1995). Cajal acknowledged Magini's findings on radial glial cells, but he severely criticized Magini's opinion that cells could be threaded in radial glia, and stated that the beads represented instead 'protoplasmic accumulations' (Cajal, 1904, 1911). However, Magini had indeed given a correct interpretation of his findings, as was ascertained much later (Rakic, 1971a, 1972).

The mechanisms of the outward displacement of neurones in the developing cortex remained unknown for decades, and apparently did not even receive much attention in the literature. One of the most extensive accounts on the development of the mammalian cerebral cortex based on the Golgi impregnation technique was provided by Godina (1951) in sheep, just before the era of electron microscopy. This detailed and careful study, which also contributed findings on neuronal migration, appeared only in Italian. Godina (1951) clearly described the early stages of the proliferative zone and the marginal veil, and the growing intermediate zone, invaded by afferent fibres and outward migrating neurones with a bipolar shape. Godina clearly described the maturation of neuroblasts which, after having reached the surface via their migration, then reached their final site with an outside-in gradient, assuming their pyramidal shape (Fig. 4). He also described how the 'ependymal fibres' were undergoing a regression and disappeared before birth, in agreement with modern studies indicating that the radial glia disappears at late developing stages (see Rakic, 1995). Godina (1951) hypothesized that glial cells were in part deriving from 'indifferent cells' migrating towards the surface, and in part by 'epithelial cells of the ependyma' which during ontogenesis moved away from the ventricular wall.

It finally became obvious in the 1960s in autoradiographic studies based on the incorporation of tritiated thymidine that cortical neurones were generated deeply into the cortex and were then taking up distant superficial positions constituting the cortical layers (see Rakic, 1972). However, still in the mid-1960s, it was believed that neurones did not undertake an active migration, but were instead translocating their nuclei within cylinders of cytoplasm extending from the ventricular zone to the cortical plate (Berry & Rogers, 1965; Morest, 1970).

The understanding of the displacement to the cortical plate of neurones generated in the ventricular and subventricular zones was finally guided by data on the migration of neurones along the

Bergmann glial fibres in the cerebellar cortex. In their detailed ultrastructural study of the development of the cerebellar cortex in the chick embryo, Mugnaini & Forstronen (1967) mentioned that vertically arranged bipolar migrating neurones were frequently apposed to the astrocytic Bergmann fibres, and hypothesized that movement of glial membranes could be implicated in neuronal migration.

In the cerebellar cortex Rakic (1971a) verified that granule cells were constantly apposed to the Bergmann glial fibres, and stated that 'the neuron–glia relationship apparently provides the necessary conditions for the migration of the young granule cell' (Rakic, 1971a). The intercellular relationships were finally clarified by Rakic (1971b, 1972) also in the developing cerebral cortex. By means of Golgi impregnation and electron microscopy, Rakic demonstrated in primates that 'late-arising cells find their way to the cortex by assuming a bipolar form and moving outward in direct and constant apposition to radial glial processes that span almost the entire width of the telencephalic wall' (Rakic, 1972). It has thus been finally established that 'The guided (radial glia) migration of neuronal precursors from the inner periventricular zone to the superficial neuropil and their subsequent collection into specific neuronal aggregates within it are universal processes in development of the central nervous system' (Marín-Padilla, 1998).

In his pioneering study on cortical development, Vignal (1888a) had humbly hoped that his anatomical work could represent 'one of the threads of the drill we throw unceasingly in this abyss that, until now, seems to us bottomless'. The bottom has certainly not been reached, but in the developing brain, as well as in neuroscience textbooks, young neurones can now happily and safely ride glial processes during their migration.

Acknowledgements

The authors are grateful to Prof. M. Lambiase for providing original reprints of some of the early studies, to Prof. E. Pannese for his advice, and to Prof. A. Barasa for providing the original photographs illustrating Godina's (1951) article.

References

Berry, M. & Rogers, A.W. (1965): The migration of neuroblasts in the developing cerebral cortex. *J. Anat.* **99**, 691–709.

Besser, L. (1866): Zur Histogenese der nervösen Elementartheile in den Centralorganen des neugeborenen Menschen. *Virchows Arch. Path. Anat.* **36**, 305–334.

Blum, F. (1893) Der Formaldehyd als Härtungsmittel. *Z. Wiss. Mikrosk.* **10**, 314–315.

Boll, F. (1873): Die Histologie und Histiogenese der nervösen Centralorgane. *Arch. Psychiat. Nervenkr.* **4**, 1–138.

Cajal, S. R. (1889): Coloracion por el método de Golgi de los centros nerviosos de los embriones de pollo. *Gaceta Médica Catalana* **12**, 6–8.

Cajal, S.R. (1904): *Textura del sistema nervioso de hombre y de los vertebrados*. Madrid: Moya.

Cajal, S.R. (1911): *Histologie du système nerveux de l'homme et des vertébrés*. Paris: Maloine.

Cajal, S.R. (1996): *Recollections of my life*. (Originally published as *Recuerdos di mi vida* in Madrid, 1901-1917) Translated by E. Horne Craigie; Cambridge, MA: MIT Press.

Edelman, G. (1987): *Neural Darwinism. The theory of neuronal group selection*. New York: Basic Books Inc.

Finger, S. (1994): *Origins of Neuroscience*. New York: Oxford University Press.

Godina, G. (1951): Istogenesi e differenziazione dei neuroni e degli elementi gliali della corteccia cerebrale. *Zeitsch. Zellforsch.* **36**, 401–435.

Golgi, C. (1873): Sulla struttura della sostanza grigia del cervello. *Gazzetta Medica Italiana, Lombardia* **33**, 244–246.

Golgi, C. (1885): *Sulla fina anatomia degli organi centrali del sistema nervoso.* Reggio Emilia: Tipografia Calderini (published again in 1886 Milan: Hoepli).

Hatai, S. (1902): Observations on the developing neurones of the cerebral cortex of foetal cats. *J. Comp. Neurol.* **12,** 199– 205.

His, W. (1887): Die Entwicklung der ersten Nervenbahnen beim menschlichen Embryo. Übersichtliche Darstellung. *Arch. Anat. Physiol. Leipzig Anat. Abth.* **92,** 368–378.

His, W. (1889a): Die Neuroblasten und deren Entstehung im embrionalen Mark. *Abh. Kgl. Sachs. Ges. Wissensch. Math. Phys. Kl.* **15,** 311–372.

His, W. (1889b): Die Formentwicklung des menschlichen Vorderhirns vom Ende des ersten bis zum Beginn des dritten Monats. *Abh. Kgl. Sachs. Ges. Wissensch. Math. Phys. Kl.* **15,** 673–736.

His, W. (1904): *Die Entwicklung des menschlichen Gehirns während der esten Monate.* Leipzig: Hirzel.

Jacobson, M. (1993): *Foundations of Neuroscience.* New York: Plenum Press

Kölliker, A. (1879): *Entwicklungsgeschichte des Menschen und der höheren Thiere.* Leipzig: Engelmann.

Kölliker, A. (1882): *Embryologie ou traité complet du développement de l'homme et des animaux supérieurs.* (Translated by A. Schneider from the 2nd German edition). Paris: Reinwald.

Kölliker, A (1896): *Handbuch der Gewebelehre des Menschen.* 6th edition, Vol. II. Leipzig: W. Engelmann.

Lenhossék, M. (1893): *Der feinere Bau des Nervensystems in Lichte neuester Forschung.* Fischer's Medizinische Buchhandlung. Berlin: H. Kornfeld.

Magini, G. (1888a): Nevroglia e cellule nervose cerebrali nei feti. In: *Atti del Dodicesimo Congresso della Associazione Medica Italiana,* Vol. I, pp. 28–291. Pavia: Tipografia Fratelli Fusi.

Magini, G. (1888b): Sur la névroglie et les cellules cérébrales chez le foetus. *Arch. Ital. Biol.* **9,** 59–60.

Magini, G. (1888c): Ulteriori ricerche istologiche sul cervello fetale. *Rendiconti della R. Accademia dei Lincei* **4,** 760–763.

Magini, G. (1888d): Nouvelles recherches histologiques sur le cerveau du foetus. *Arch. Iial. Biol.* **10,** 384–387.

Marín-Padilla, M. (1998): Cajal–Retzius cells and the development of the neocortex. *Trends Neurosci.* **21,** 64–71.

Mazzarello, P. (1999): *La struttura nascosta. La vita di Camillo Golgi.* Bologna: Cisalpino, Monduzzi. (*The Hidden Structure. The Life of Camillo Golgi.* Oxford University Press: in press.)

McConnell, S.K. (1995): Constructing the cerebral cortex: Neurogenesis and fate determination. *Neuron* **15,** 761–768.

McKay, R. (1997): Stem cells in the central nervous system. *Science* **276,** 66–71.

Morest, D.K. (1970): A study of neurogenesis in the forebrain of opossum pouch young. *Z. Anat. Entwickl.-Gesch.* **130,** 265–305.

Mugnaini, E. & Forstronen, P.F. (1967): Ultrastructural studies on the cerebellar histogenesis. I. Differentiation of granule cells and development of glomeruli in the chick embryo. *Z. Zellforsch. Mikrosk. Anat. Abt. Histochem.* **77,** 115–143.

Nissl, F. (1884): *Die patologischen Veränderungen der Nervenzellen der Grosshirnrinde.* Inaugural Dissertation. München: Med. Fakultät der Universität.

Nissl, F. (1894): Ueber die sogenannten Granula der Nervenzellen. *Neurol. Zbl.* **13,** 781–789.

Pannese, E (1996): The black reaction. *Brain Res. Bull.* **41,** 343–349.

Paton, S. (1900): The histogenesis of the cellular elements of the cerebral cortex. *Johns Hopkins Hospital Reports* **9,** 709–741.

Rakic, P. (1971a): Guidance of neurones migrating in the foetal monkey neocortex. *Brain Res.* **33,** 471–476.

Rakic, P. (1971b): Neuron-glia relationship during granule cell migration in developing cerebellar cortex. A Golgi and electronmicroscopic study in Macacus rhesus. *J. Comp. Neurol.* **141,** 283–312.

Rakic, P. (1972): Mode of cell migration to the superficial layers of foetal monkey neocortex. *J. Comp. Neurol.* **145,** 61–84.

Rakic, P. (1995): Radial glial cells: scaffolding for brain construction. In: *Neuroglial cells,* eds. H. Ketterman & B.R. Ransom, pp. 746–762. New York: Oxford University Press.

Retzius, G. (1893a): Die Cajal'schen Zellen der Grosshirnrinde beim Menschen und bei Säugethieren. In: *Biologische Untersuchungen,* Vol. V, pp. 1–8. Stockholm: Samson & Wallin.

Retzius, G. (1893b): Studien über Ependym und Neuroglia. In: *Biologische Untersuchungen.* Vol. V, pp. 9–26. Stockholm: Samson & Wallin.

Schaper, A. (1897): The earliest differentiation in the central nervous system of vertebrates. *Science* **5,** 430–431.

Shepherd, G.M. (1991): *Foundations of the Neuron Doctrine.* New York: Oxford University Press.

Vignal, W. (1884a): Formation et structure de la substance grise embryonnaire de la moelle épinière des vertébrés supérieurs. *Comp. Rend. Acad. Sci.* (Paris) **94,** 1526–1529.

Vignal, W. (1884b): Formation et développement des cellules nerveuses de la moelle épinière des mammifères. *Comp. Rend. Acad. Sci.* (Paris) **99,** 420–422.

Vignal, W. (1886): Sur le développement des éléments de la substance grise corticale des circonvolutions cérébrales. *Comp. Rend. Acad. Sci.* (Paris) **102,** 1332–1334.

Vignal, W. (1888a): Recherches sur le développement des éléments des couches corticales du cerveau et du cervelet chez l'homme et les mammifères. *Arch. Physiol. Norm. Pathol. (Paris)* **20,** 228–254.

Vignal, W. (1888b): Recherches sur le développement de la substance corticale du cerveau et du cervelet. *Arch. Physiol. Norm. Pathol. (Paris)* **20,** 311–338.

Chapter 3

Acquired neonatal encephalopathies: cortical vasculature, postinjury reorganization, and neurological sequelae

Miguel Marín-Padilla

Department of Pathology, Dartmouth Medical School, Hanover, New Hampshire 03755, USA

Summary

The neuropathology and developmental impact of acquired neonatal encephalopathies have been investigated in surviving infants in an attempt to determine their possible role in the pathogenesis of ensuing neurological sequelae, such as epilepsy, cerebral palsy, dyslexia and others disorders. Two basic types of acquired neocortical lesions has been explored: (A) subpial (layer I) haemorrhages with damage and reparation of the external glial limiting membrane and postinjury reorganization of the underlying gray matter; and (B) white matter damage with spearing and subsequent postinjury reorganization of the overlying gray matter. The outcome of either lesion is invariably an acquired cortical dysplasia which evolves from the postinjury reorganization of the surviving gray matter adjacent to the lesion. The subsequent maturation of the surviving gray matter either below a leptomeningeal heterotopia or above a white matter lesion is invariably altered. The postinjury cytoarchitectural alterations of this surviving gray matter are not static but evolving processes which continue to undergo transformations weeks, months, or even years, after the original injury. These acquired cortical dysplasias are characterized by: (a) neuronal displacement and disorientation; (b) alterations of the intrinsic circuitry; (c) alterations of the synaptic organization; (d) transformation of projective into local-circuit neurons; (e) isolated neuronal atrophy; (f) structural and functional hypertrophy of some intrinsic neurons; and (g) others less obvious dysplastic alterations difficult to ascertain. These postinjury dysplastic alterations are not static processes but evolving ones that continue to transform the structural and functional organization of the affected cortical region. It is proposed that it is not the original lesion but the progressive postinjury alterations of the affected cerebral cortex, the crucial underlying cause in the pathogenesis of the neurological sequelae, which affect some infants who survive neonatal brain damage.

Introduction

Neonatal encephalopathies constitute a heterogeneous group of congenital and/or acquired brain disorders characterized by variable distribution, severity, unsolved pathogenesis, and often a poor clinical outcome. Despite excellent clinical, pathological and radiological (imaging) reviews of these disorders, their impact on the subsequent maturation of the infant brain and their possible role in the pathogenesis of ensuing neurological sequelae remain poorly understood and inadequately studied. In this report, the evolving pathology and developmental impact of perinatally acquired cortical lesions are investigated in surviving infants. Acquired encephalopathies are associated with prematurity, respiratory difficulties (neonatal asphyxia), circulatory disturbances, monozygous twining (fetal transfusion syndrome), infections, trauma and/or labor complications (Schwartz, 1961; Banker & Larroche, 1962; Armstrong & Norman, 1974; Kissane, 1975; Larroche, 1977, 1991; Rorke, 1982; Volpe, 1987; Evrard et al., 1989; Friede, 1989; Reed & Claireaux, 1989; Takashima et al., 1989; Sarnat, 1992; Armstrong, 1995; Ravavi-Encha, 1995). Cortical damage can occur prenatally, during labor and/or postnatally, and its multifactorial pathogenesis is not yet clearly understood.

The clinical relevance of acquired encephalopathies is the fact that if the infant survives, the postinjury maturation of his/her brain may be altered and could result in cortical dysfunction. Moreover, infants who survive neonatal cortical lesions may subsequently develop a variety of neurological disorders, including epilepsy, cerebral palsy, dyslexia, mental retardation, poor school performance and minimal brain damage (Armstrong & Norman, 1974; Kissane, 1975; Clarren & Smith, 1978; Galaburda & Kemper, 1979; Wisniewski et al., 1983; Volpe, 1987; Friede, 1989; Reed & Claireaux, 1989; Robertson et al., 1989; Larroche, 1991; Sarnat, 1992; Marín-Padilla, 1993; Vinter et al., 1993; Armstrong, 1995; Mischel et al., 1995). Recent studies of infants who survived neonatal encephalopathies have shown postinjury cortical dysplasia which could play a role in the pathogenesis of neurological sequelae (Marín-Padilla, 1996, 1997). This report analyses, for surviving infants, the postinjury reorganization of the surviving cortex around acquired lesions and explores their clinical outcome.

Material and methods

From the Paediatric Autopsy Service of Dartmouth–Hitchcock Medical Center, 35 cases of infants who survived a variety of perinatally acquired cortical lesions have been selected (Table 1). Eventually, all infants died for a variety of reasons and complete postmortem studies were carried out. Their birth-ages range from 21 weeks of gestation to term. The infant survival, following the original lesion, ranges from a few hours to days, weeks, months, or years (Table 1). The evolving neuropathology of these cases has been studied with a variety of procedures: (1) routine stains (hematoxylin and eosin, Nissl, Bodian, and luxol-fast-blue); (2) immunohistochemical stains (glial fibrillary acidic proteins, anti-human non-phophorilated neurofilament proteins, palvalbumin, and synaptophysin); and (3) the rapid Golgi method (Table 1). The study of this material has permitted the evaluation of the evolving pathology of some lesions through their acute, subacute (healing) and chronic (reparation) stages, and the exploration of their corresponding impact on the maturation of adjoining and primarily undamaged regions of the infant developing neocortex.

Results

To understand the evolving pathology and developmental impact of any acquired cortical lesion it is necessary to evaluate: (a) its direct impact upon the affected region; (b) its subsequent pathologic evolution through its acute, subacute and chronic stages; (c) its indirect (postinjury) impact on the development of adjoining unaffected cortical regions; and (d) the residual dysplasia and its functional implications. Two basic types of acquired cortical lesions are explored herein: **(A)** subpial haemorrhages with external glial limiting membrane (EGLM) damage; and **(B)** white matter (WM) damage with preservation of overlying gray matter (GM).

(A) Layer I: subpial haemorrhage with EGLM damage

About 15 per cent of perinatally acquired hemorrhagic lesions of the neocortex are subpial haemorrhages (Friede, 1989). These hemorrhagic lesions are invariably associated with damage to the EGLM which must be promptly repaired to re-establish the neocortex's anatomical integrity.

The EGLM is an essential anatomical and functional component of the CNS which demarcates the nervous from the surrounding meningeal tissues. It is composed of closely apposed glial endfeet united by tight junctions and covered by the basal lamina (BL) material manufactured by them. Early in development, the EGLM is essentially composed and maintained by the endfeet of radial glial and those of a few layer I astrocytes (Marín-Padilla, 1990, 1993). After the completion of neuronal migration, the reabsorbing endfeet of degenerating radial glial are progressively replaced by those of additional layer I astrocytes (Marín-Padilla, 1990, 1995). During postnatal life, the small astrocytes of layer I become the EGLM essential components; although some fibrous astrocytes co-participate in its maintenance. The number of both layer I and fibrous astrocytes increases (reactive gliosis of layer I) in some pathologic conditions, including epilepsy (Rorke, 1982; Friede, 1989; Sarnat, 1992).

During the vascularization of the neocortex, the EGLM is progressively perforated by meningeal vessels. In this vascular perforation, the BLs of both the EGLM and the perforating vessel fuse at the site of entry, restoring the CNS anatomic integrity and permitting the perforating vessel to enter into the nervous tissue (Andres, 1976; Casley-Smith *et al.*, 1976; Krisch *et al.*, 1982, 1983; Pile-Spellman *et al.*, 1984; Marín-Padilla, 1988; Marín-Padilla & Amieva, 1989) The fusion of the BLs forms a pial funnel which accompanies the perforating vessel into the nervous tissue, thus establishing a perivascular compartment (Virchow–Robin space) around it (Marín-Padilla, 1987). This perivascular space remains open to the leptomeningeal space allowing meningeal (mesodermal) elements to enter through it and to contribute muscle cells to the growing vessel (Casley-Smith *et al.*, 1976; Pile-Spellman *et al.*, 1984; Marín-Padilla, 1988). Inflammatory cells also enter and exit the CNS through this perivascular space. Throughout the CNS terminal capillary plexus, this perivascular space disappears by fusion of both laminae into a single one which is, thereafter, manufactured and maintained by the endfeet of fibrous and protoplasmic astrocytes (Marín-Padilla, 1995). A similar type of fusion of BLs occurs between those of the CNS and the Schwann cells at the entrance and exit sites of nerves (Krisch *et al.*, 1982, 1983; Marín-Padilla & Amieva, 1989).

Subpial haemorrhages are invariably associated with damage and disruption of the EGLM. Small disruptions are repaired promptly by regenerating endfeet of local astrocytes and leave no residual lesion. The repair of large disruptions involves extensive cellular changes, causes secondary alterations in layer I and the underlying gray matter, and may result in permanent dysplastic lesions (Brun 1965a,b: Marín-Padilla, 1993).

Acute lesions
The earliest features of EGLM damage are glial endfeet edema with a mild separation of the pia from the underlying nervous tissue and elongation of the perforating vessels (Fig. 1A). Persistent edema causes glial endfeet disintegration, EGLM damage, rupture of perforating vessels and subpial haemorrhages (Fig. 1B). Cellular debris, reactive astrocytes, macrophages, and growing terminals from damaged axonic and glial fibres are recognized at the injured site.

Subacute (healing) lesions
The hemorrhagic site is filled with inflammatory cells with the removal of necrotic debris by microglia and macrophages. The perivascular space of undamaged vessels are filled with hemosiderin-laden macrophages travelling toward the pial surface and the perivascular lymphatics of meningeal vessels. Hemosiderin-laden macrophages may persist at the injured site, the Virchow-Robin space of uninjured vessels, and the overlying leptomeninges.

The free terminals of glial and afferent fibres damaged by the haemorrhage are recognized throughout the healing site. These regenerating terminals are covered by short and long sprouts with numerous filopodia (Fig. 2A). Some of these regenerating fibres regrow new endfeet which are incorporated into the damaged EGLM. Local layer I and fibrous astrocytes proliferate and also contribute endfeet to the EGLM reparation. The terminal dendritic bouquets of pyramidal cells

Table 1. Perinatal neocortical damage: clinical, neuropathological, staining and autopsy data from the 35 selected cases

Case	Born	Lived	Clinical findings	Stains	Autopsy findings (neocortex)
I. Acute stages					
1 9368	21 wg PCD	1h	Cardiac Ebstein Malformation	HE	PVH, PH, Focal WHM & GMH
2 8941	26 wg PCD	2h	RDS	HE & Golgi, Bodian	PVH, Focal WMH
3 8442	22 wg PCD	Aspiration meconium		HE & Golgi	Early multifocal PVH, PH
4 9379	24 wg PCD	3h	RDS	HE, Bodian	Early multifocal PVH, Focal WHM, PH
5 8460	27 wg PCD	4h	RDS	HE & Golgi	PVH, IVH
6 9548	24 wg PCD	17h	Fetal transfusion syndrome	HE	Anemic twin, Early multifocal PVH, Pletoric twin, severe PVH & IVH
7 8937	30 wg PCD	1 day	RDS	HE & Golgi Bodian	Early PVH, IVH, PH, Focal WMD & GMD
8 804439	26 wg PCD	1 day	RDS	HE & Golgi	PVH, Focal PVL, GMD
9 9353	25 wg PCD	3 days	RDS, Early BPD	HE, Bodian	Early PVH, PH, IVH, Focal WHM & GMH
II. Subacute (healing) stages					
10 91135	33 wg PCD	5 days	RDS, Aspiration meconium	HE	Multicystic encephalopathy, PVL, WMD, mild hydrocephalus
11 8845	28 wg PCD	5 days	RDS, prenatal WM damage	HE & Golgi Myelin, Bodian	LMH, Focal PH, Necrosis WM, Multicystic encephalopathy, Acute hydrocephalus
12 89129	26 wg PCD	10 days	RDS, BPD	HE, Bodian	PVH, Cerebral edema, WMD, Necrosis WM axons
13 804720	28 wg PCD	20 days	Enterocolitis Peritonitis	HE & Golgi	PVH, Early PVL
14 9045	38 wg PCD	12 days	RDS, BPD Prenatal WM damage	HE & Golgi	Multicystic encephalopathy, WMD, Early PVL, Focal LMH, Surviving GM
15 90108	28 wg PCD	15 days	BDP	HE & Golgi	WMD, Cerebral edema, PH GMH, IVH
16 9045	26 wg PCD	16 days	RDS, Pneumonia, Hypertermia	HE & Golgi	WMD, Subpial edema, PH, Early PVL, Hydrocephalus
17 8971	29 wg PCD	17 days	RDS, Early BPD	HE & Golgi	Recent MH, Early PVL
18 794170	34 wg PCD	18 days	RDS, Microcephaly, Retarded Growth Prenatal WM damage	HE & Golgi	Multicystic encephalopathy, Extensive LMH, Microgyria
19 722143	35 wg PCD	26 days	GI atresia surgically treated, BPD	HE, Golgi	Focal WMD & GMD
20 722143	31 wg PCD	26 days	RDS Pneumonia, Hypertermia	HE, Golgi	Focal WMD and edema GMD

Table 1. Continued

Case	Born	Lived	Clinical findings	Stains	Autopsy findings (neocortex)
III. Chronic (repaired) stages					
21 9478	32 wg PCD	4 days	Pletoric twin, Fetal transfusion, Prenatal WM damage	HE, GFAP, Neurofilament	Multicystic encephalopathy, Healed WMD, Surviving GM, Neocortical dysplasia
22 8941	30 wg PCD	32 days	Prenatal WM damage	HE & Golgi, Neurofilament	Multicystic encephalopathy, Healed WMD, Surviving GM
23 9210	39 wg PCD	5 weeks	Prenatal WM damage, Pneumonia, BPD	HE, GFAP	Focal microgyria, PVL, WMD, Multicystic encephalopathy,
24 907	28 wg PCD	3 months	Perinatal brain damage, Developmental delay, BPD	HE & Golgi Myelin, Neurofilament	WMD, PVL, Surviving GM, Hydrocephalus *ex-vacuo*, Neocortical dysplasia
25 96137	26 wg PCD	7 months	Perinatal brain damage, Developmental delay, BPD, *Seizures*	HE & GFAP, Neurofilament	Multicystic encephalopathy, Ulegyria, WMD, GMD, Neocortical dysplasia
26 8615	26 wg PCD	8 months	Perinatal brain damage, Developmental delay, BPD	HE & Golgi Bodian	Multicystic encephalopathy Focal microgyria, PVL Hydrocephalus *ex-vacuo*, Neocortical dysplasia, HN
27 8937	24 wg PCD	8 months	Perinatal brain damage, Developmental delay, BPD, *Seizures*	HE & Golgi GFAP Myelin, Neurofilament	GMD & WMD, PVL, LMH, Multicystic encephalopathy, Microgyria, Hydrocephalus, Neocortical dysplasia, HN
28 93209	26 wg PCD	2.5 days	Developmental delay, *Status epilepticus*	HE & Golgi, GFAP, Neurofilament	WMD, Focal ulegyria, *Ex-vacuo* hydranencephaly, Neocortical dysplasia, HN
29 8511067	32 wg PCD	5 years Alive	BPD, Cerebral palsy, *Epilepsy*, Mental retardation	HE & Golgi, Myelin, GFAP	Frontal Lobe Bx. (2.5 years), GMD, LMH, Neocortical dysplasia, HN
30 98147	Term Shaken 11 days PCD	7 years	Postnatal brain damage, Cerebral palsy, Blindness, *Epilepsy*, Mental retardation	HE, Myelin, GFAP, Bodian, Synaptophysin, Neurofilament	Fronto-temporal porencephaly, Hydrocephalus *ex-vacuo*, Ulegyria, PVL, Focal LMHs, Neocortical dysplasia, NH
31 88175	35 wg PCD	8 years	Prenatal WM damage, *Epilepsy*, Mental retardation, Drowning	Myelin, HE, Neurofilament, Bodian, HE, GFAP	Parieto-occipital porencephaly, Surviving GM. PVL, Extensive LMHs, Focal ulegyria, Neocortical dysplasia, HN
32 9517048	Term PCD	10 years Alive	Postnatal brain damage, *Epilepsy*, Left frontal trauma	HE, Golgi, Neurofilament	Frontal gliotic GM, WMD, Surviving GM, Multicystic encephalopathy, Neocortical dysplasia HN
33 9381	37 wg	11 years	Postnatal brain damage, Cerebral palsy, *Epilepsy*, Mental retardation	HE, GFAP, Myelin Neurofilament	Parieto-occipital porencephaly, PVL, LMHs, Surviving GM, Neocortical dysplasia, HN
34 97173	Term PCD	11 years	Peritonitis, Gastric perforation, Cerebral palsy, Mental retardation	HE, GFAP, Neurofilament	Left parieto-temporo-occipital porencephaly, Surviving GM, Atrophy corpus callosum
35 90108	Term	16 years Alive	Postnatal brain damage	HE, Golgi, GFAP	Right occipital porencephaly, Neocortical dysplasia, HN

Abbreviations: PCD = perinatal (prenatal, neonatal and/or postnatal) neocortical damage; RDS = respiratory distress syndrome; PRM = premature rupture of membranes; BPD = bronchopulmonary dysplasia; PH = pial haemorrhages; PVH = periventricular (matrix) haemorrhages; WMH = white matter haemorrhages; GMH = grey matter haemorrhages; IVH = intraventricular haemorrhages; GM = grey matter, WHD = white matter damage; GMD = grey matter damage; PVI = periventricular infarct; HN = hypertrophic neurons; HE = hematoxylin and eosin; Golgi = rapid Golgi method; GFAP = glial fibrillary acidic proteins.

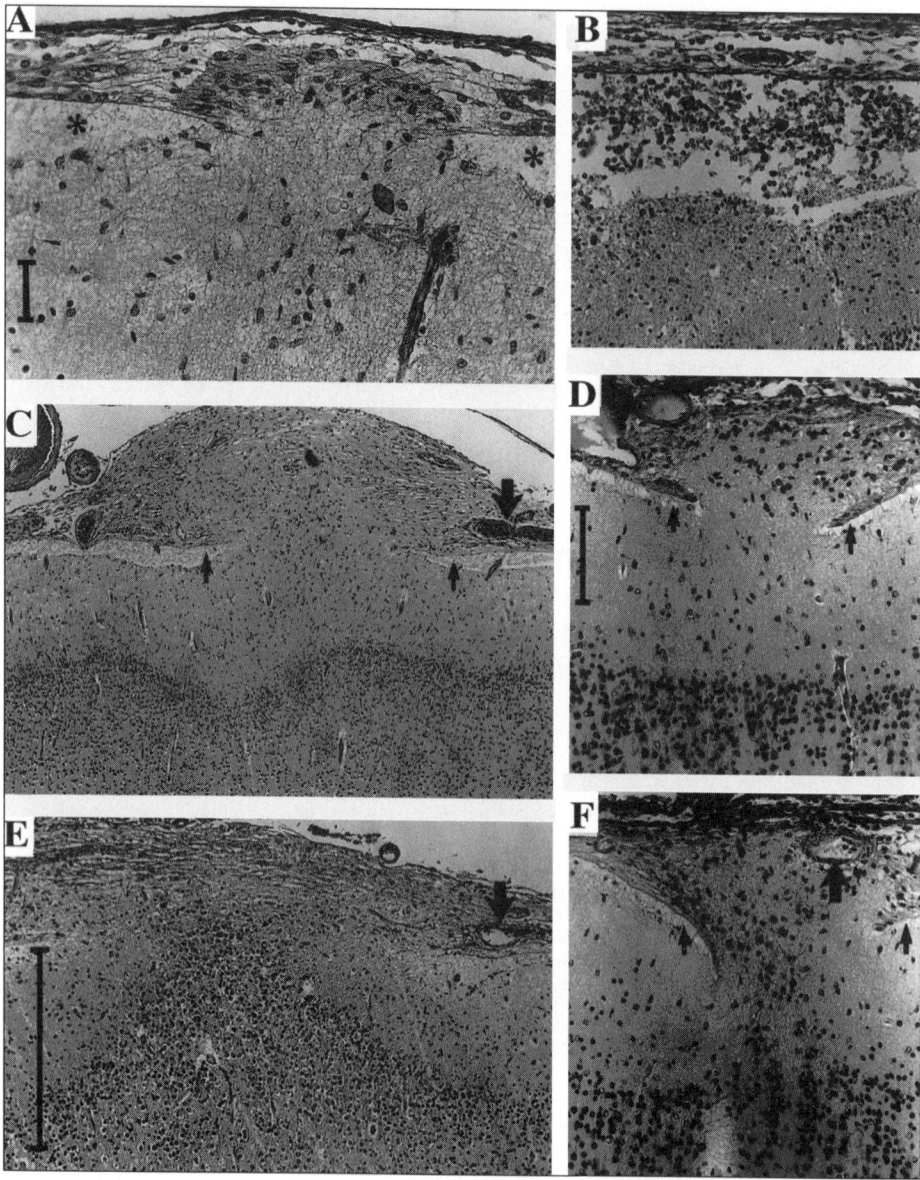

Fig. 1. Composite figure showing various pathologic stages of subpial (layer I) haemorrhages with EGLM disruption and repair, formation of superficial heterotopias, and postinjury reorganization of the underlying cortex. (A) Repair of small EGLM disruption with a microscopic leptomeningeal heterotopia (LMH) composed of glial elements probably without clinical significance and marked edema (asterisks) of adjacent glial endfeet (case 14). (B) Recent subpial haemorrhage with rupture of perforating vessels, EGLM disruption and layer I damage (case 1). (C) Verrucous LMH with adjacent glial endfeet edema (small arrows), extensive postinjury cytoarchitectural alterations of both layer I and the underlying gray matter, pial vessels buried (large arrow) by heterotopia, and partial obliteration (acquired marginal heterotopia) of layer I (case 14). (D) Small LMH with disruption of the EGLM persistent glial endfeet edema (small arrows) and absence of obvious postinjury alterations in the underlying cortex (case 18). (E) Extensive LMH showing the EGLM disruption, displacement of cellular elements into the leptomeningeal space, and extensive postinjury alterations in both layer I (obliteration) and underlying gray matter (case 26). (F) Large LMH showing the EGLM disruption site with adjacent glial endfeet edema (small arrow), columnar displacement of the cellular elements of the underlying gray matter, and a pial vessel buried by the lesion (case 24). Scales = 100 μm. (from Marín-Padilla, 1996.)

may also be severed (pruned) by the haemorrhage. Some pyramidal cells survive this dendritic pruning and assume new stellate morphologies (Fig. 2B). These alterations cause postinjury modifications in the organization of both layer I and the underlying GM which are better recognized in chronic lesions.

Chronic (repaired) lesions
The repair of large EGLM disruptions implies significant postinjury cellular modification, including proliferation of local astrocytes, survival and transformation of partially damaged neurons, cytoarchitectural alterations in both layer I and underlying GM, eventual reparation of the EGLM which often occur within the leptomeningeal space, and the formation of residual superficial dysplastic lesion (Fig. 1A, C–F).

These superficial dysplastic lesions have been described in the literature by a variety of terms such as: 'brain warts', 'marginal heterotopias', 'sulci fusion', and some types of focal microgyria, agyria, and pachygyria (Brun, 1965a,b; Friede, 1989; Morgan & Marín-Padilla, 1992; Marín-Padilla, 1993, 1995). I prefer the term 'leptomeningeal heterotopia' (LMH), because they result from the reparation of a damaged EGLM within the leptomeningeal space (Marín-Padilla, 1993). Their size varies from microscopic lesions without dysplastic changes to extensive superficial dysplasia with significant alterations of the underlying cortex (compare Figs. 1C–F). LMHs are recognized by their protrusion above the surrounding cortex, their avascular verrucous surface, and by the abrupt disappearance of pial capillaries (covered by the lesion) at the edge of the lesion (Figs. 1C–F). LMHs are characterized by a disorganized admixture of blood vessels, glial cells, displaced neurons, diffused gliosis, and the tortuous terminals of axonic and glial fibres (Fig. 3). In addition to reactive gliosis, LMHs are also characterized by reactive fibrosis with collagen manufactured by local meningeal fibroblasts.

Beneath a large LMH, the cytoarchitecture of layer I and the GM may be permanently altered (Morgan & Marín-Padilla, 1992; Marín-Padilla, 1993). The horizontal axons of Cajal–Retzius cells are bent toward the disruption but do not penetrate into the LMH (Figs. 1C, E, F and 3). The horizontal pathway of these axons is well established within layer I prior to the EGLM injury and, therefore, they remain unaffected by the lesion (Fig. 3). Postinjury alterations of the GM include: neuronal disorganization and displacement; fibrillar, glial and vascular disorganization; alterations of the intrinsic circuitry; and the presence of both atrophic and hypertrophic neurons and of bundles of myelinated fibres. Displaced neurons change their intrinsic circuitry and their morphology may be secondarily altered. Following dendritic pruning, some affected pyramidal cell (layers II and III) are transformed into stellate neurons and their connectivity is modified. While some GM neurons become atrophic with short dendrites and a few spines, others become hypertrophic with long and complex dendrites covered by countless spines and an axon that often arises from one of its dendrites and is locally distributed (Fig. 3 asterisk). Hypertrophic cells are believed to be postinjury transformed local-circuit neurons. Some hypertrophic neurons are strongly positive in neurofilament preparations. Some of these GM alterations may be indistinguishable from those described in neuronal migration anomalies (Mischel *et al.*, 1995).

In principle, any of these postinjury alterations should be sufficient to cause cortical dysfunction and could eventually play a role in the pathogenesis of neurological sequelae. LMHs have been described in a variety of neurologic disorders, including dyslexia, cerebral palsy, epilepsy and fetal alcohol syndrome (Brun, 1965a,b; Taylor *et al.*, 1971; Clarren & Smith, 1978; Galaburda & Kemper, 1979; Wisniewski *et al.*, 1983; Galaburda *et al.*, 1985; Evrard *et al.*, 1989; Morgan & Marín-Padilla, 1992; Marín-Padilla, 1993; Mischel *et al.*, 1995).

(B) Acquired white matter damage with sparing of gray matter

The developing WM is particularly vulnerable to perinatal asphyxia, hypoxia, ischemia, circulatory disturbances and/or trauma. Its vulnerability may be due to its rapid growth, active metabolic rate,

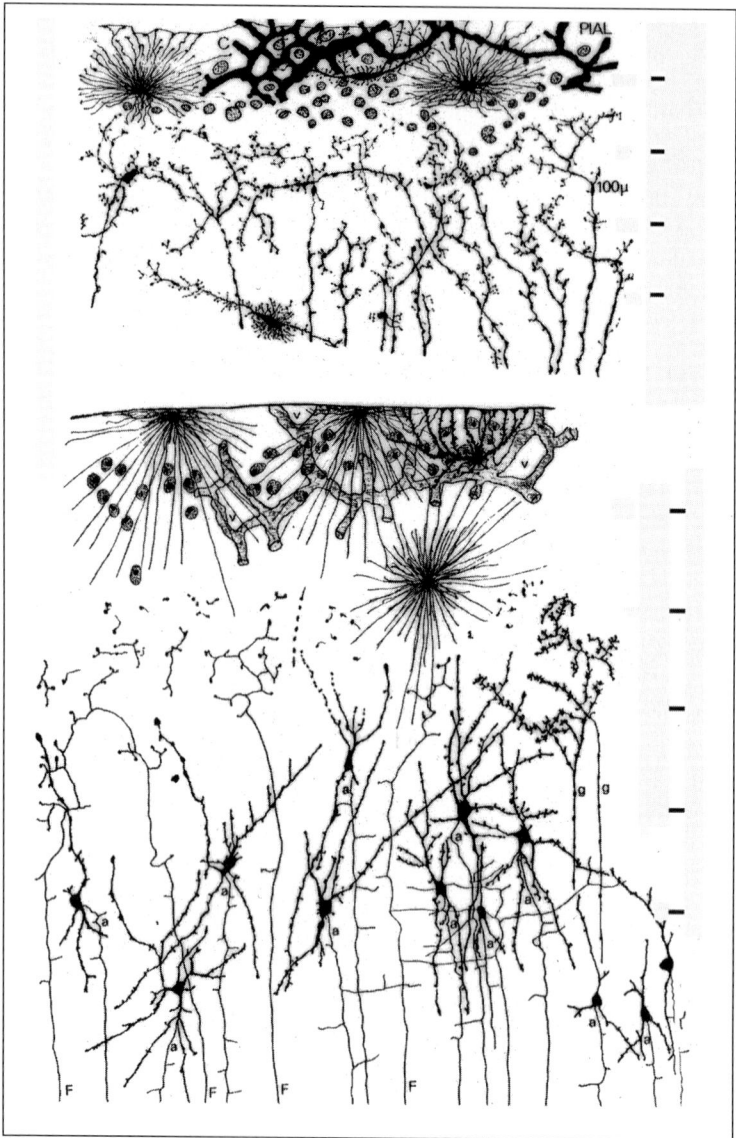

Fig. 2. Composite figure of camera lucida drawings from rapid Golgi preparations showing the essential glial and neuronal alterations observed during the subacute or healing stages of subpial (layer I) haemorrhages. (A) Detail of a healing subpial hemorrhagic injury showing the terminal regeneration of radial glial fibres damaged (severed) by the haemorrhage, hemosiderin-laden macrophages, postinjury revascularization, and local proliferation of fibrous and layer I astrocytes co-participant in the EGLM reparation. (B) Detail of the healing stage of layer I (subpial) hemorrhagic injury showing the terminal dendritic pruning of pyramidal neurons damaged (severed) by the haemorrhage and their subsequent postinjury transformation into stellate neurons. Also illustrated are the terminal regeneration of radial glial (g) and afferent (F) fibres damaged (severed) by the haemorrhage, the scattered fragments of degenerating neuronal and glial elements, local proliferation of layer I and fibrous astrocytes, hemosiderin-laden macrophages, and post-injury revascularization (v) of the region. Some developing neurons partially damaged by terminal dendritic pruning survive and are morphologically transformed into stellate cells. Other damaged neurons undergo atrophic and/or hypertrophic changes, and still others may regenerate new dendritic and axonic (a) terminals. Some of these postinjury transformed neurons may persist within the affected cortex (acquired cortical dysplasia) resulting in alterations of the cytoarchitecture and intrinsic circuitry of the affected cortex which could cause cortical dysfunction and play a role in the pathogenesis of ensuing neurological sequelae. Scale: inter-bar interval = 100 μm. (From Marín-Padilla, 1996.)

and its increasing distance from additional perforating vessels by the intervening expansion of the overlying GM (Banker & Larroche, 1962; Rorke, 1982; Marín-Padilla, 1997).

The developing WM is vascularized by an expanding short-linked anastomotic capillary plexus formed between adjacent perforating vessels (Wolff et al., 1975; Duvernoy et al., 1981; Marín-Padilla, 1985, 1987, 1988, 1995, 1997; Akina et al., 1986; Nakamura, et al. 1994). The first anastomotic plexus is formed throughout the periventricular zone and, subsequently, new plexuses are progressively established from lower to upper regions of the WM paralleling its ascending maturation. The capillaries of these plexuses undergo continuous remodelling by both capillary angiogenesis and reabsorption adjusting to the structural and functional needs of the growing cortex. The distance between perforating vessels ranges from 150 to 300 µm and is maintained relatively constant during neocortical development. Consequently, the number of vessels entering and exiting the neocortex increases gradually paralleling both its pre and postnatal expansions (Marín-Padilla, 1987). The number of interconnecting arterio-venous capillary loops formed between new and pre-existing perforating vessels also increases progressively maintaining, at all times, the developing neocortex well vascularized.

The vascularization of the GM is a late developmental process which starts after the completion of neuronal migration and progresses from lower to upper regions paralleling its ascending maturation. It is also carried out by arterio-venous capillary loops established between pre-existing and new perforating vessels (Duvernoy et al., 1981; Marín-Padilla, 1985, 1987, 1988). The GM, which represents the neocortex's neuronal anlage, is more directly (new perforators), better (new arterio-venous capillary loops) and more profusely (additional perforators) vascularized than the underlying WM. Therefore, the GM may be better equipped than the underlying WM to endure temporary hypoxia, ischemia and/or circulatory disturbances. Perhaps these vascular features could explain why the GM is often spared in WM lesions and able, in surviving infants, to continue its (albeit altered) structural and functional maturation. The vascular destruction which characterizes WM lesions does not necessarily affect the GM arterio-venous capillary loops which remain essentially intact thus permitting the circulation of blood.

Acute lesions
A softer and poorly outlined area with subtle colour changes may be the first indication of a WM lesion. As the lesion ages, its softness, borders and colour changes become better defined and focal haemorrhages may appear. Early lesions are characterized by edema, loss of architecture and microvacuolization. Thereafter, tissue disintegration becomes apparent, empty spaces start to appear throughout the damaged tissue, and the number of inflammatory, microglia, macroglia and reactive glial cells increases.

The essential feature of any WM lesion is the local destruction of axis-cylinders from corticipetal, corticofugal and association fibres. Damaged WM fibres are clearly recognized with special procedures, such as the rapid Golgi, neurofilament and silver methods. Damaged axons disintegrate rapidly and are reduced to small fragments which are heavily stained with these methods. These fragments are rapidly phagocytized by intrinsic microglia, extrinsic macrophages and phagocytic astrocytes which also become heavily stained. There are no recognizable GM alterations overlying acute WM lesions.

Subacute (healing) lesions
The healing stage of WM lesions evolves through a series of rapidly succeeding events, including edema, necrosis, liquefaction, reabsorption and removal of debris by macrophages, and eventual cavitation. Irregular spaces start to appear within the damaged WM which, at first, lack distinct borders and may be empty and/or fluid filled and may have inflammatory cells. These spaces are surrounded by minimal or no reactive gliosis and are separated by glio-vascular trabeculi which may carry surviving axonic fibres. In surviving infants, the size of spaces increases, some coalesce into larger ones and, eventually, they are transformed into cystic cavities lined by minimal reactive

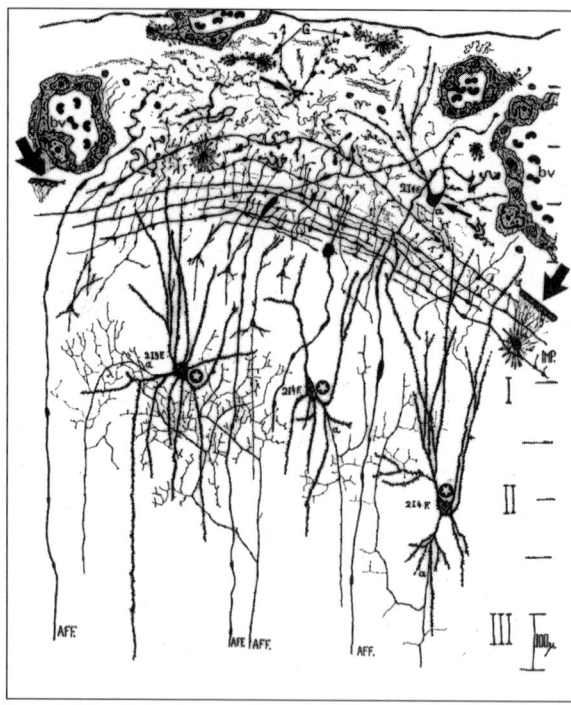

Fig. 3. Mosaic of camera lucida drawings from rapid Golgi preparations (case 18) showing some of the postinjury cytoarchitectural alterations of the developing neocortex underlying a LMH caused by a subpial hemorrhagic lesion with EGLM disruption. The EGLM disruption site is located between the remnants of the original pial surface marked by thick arrows. The residual dysplastic lesion is formed within the leptomeningeal space and contains an admixture of displaced neuronal, fibrillar, glial and vascular elements, including: displaced neurons (small arrows), tortuous terminals of both axonic (F) and glial fibres, buried pial vessels with red cells, bending of the horizontal (tangential) axons of Cajal–Retzius neurons, and large hypertrophic neurons (*) with long dendrites (some reaching into the LMH) covered with numerous spines and axons arising from one of the dendrites in the underlying gray matter. There are also atrophic and displaced neurons. Some of these postinjury dysplastic alterations may persist within the damaged region, altering its structural organization and functional activity permanently and could play a role in the pathogenesis of subsequent neurologic sequelae. Scale: inter-bar interval = 100 μm. (From Marín-Padilla, 1993.)

gliosis. If the ependymal epithelium was also damaged, these cystic cavities become connected with the ventricular system (e.g. porencephalies). Connected and unconnected cavities may develop concomitantly.

Rapid Golgi and neurofilament preparations demonstrate the extent of fibre destruction within the lesion as well as a significant reduction of fibres throughout adjacent and distant, primary undamaged, WM regions. The fibre reduction away from the original lesion is caused by the ensuing antero- and retrograde degeneration of corticipetal, corticofugal and association fibres destroyed. Consequently, a generalized reduction of axonic fibres, hydrocephalus *ex-vacuo*, is a direct consequence of any acquired WM lesion. The degree of hydrocephalus *ex-vacuo* depends on the number of fibres originally destroyed.

An important feature of some WM lesions is the sparing of the overlying GM (Fig. 4). This spared GM retains its vasculature and is capable, in surviving infants, of continuing its structural and functional development (Fig. 4A). The surviving vasculature of the spared GM supplies the growing needs of the infant neocortex (Fig. 4). Eventually, long horizontal anastomoses are formed above the border of the necrotic zone which represent the lower limit of the spared GM vascular system (Fig. 4A, curved arrow).

Despite the retention of its vascular system, the postinjury maturation of the GM overlying WM lesions is often altered for several reasons. The spared GM will be deprived of afferent terminals from corticipetal and association fibres destroyed by the underlying WM lesion; and some of its projective neurons will fail to reach their functional targets because their efferent axons (corticofugal fibres) have also been destroyed. Damaged (severed) corticofugal fibres undergo retrograde (as well as anterograde) degeneration up to the origin of their collaterals which survive as well as the parent neuron. Some axotomyzed neurons survive and their axonic collaterals continue to grow within the GM, their number may increase, and their intracortical distribution assumes new patterns. Consequently, surviving axotomyzed pyramidal cells are, postinjury,

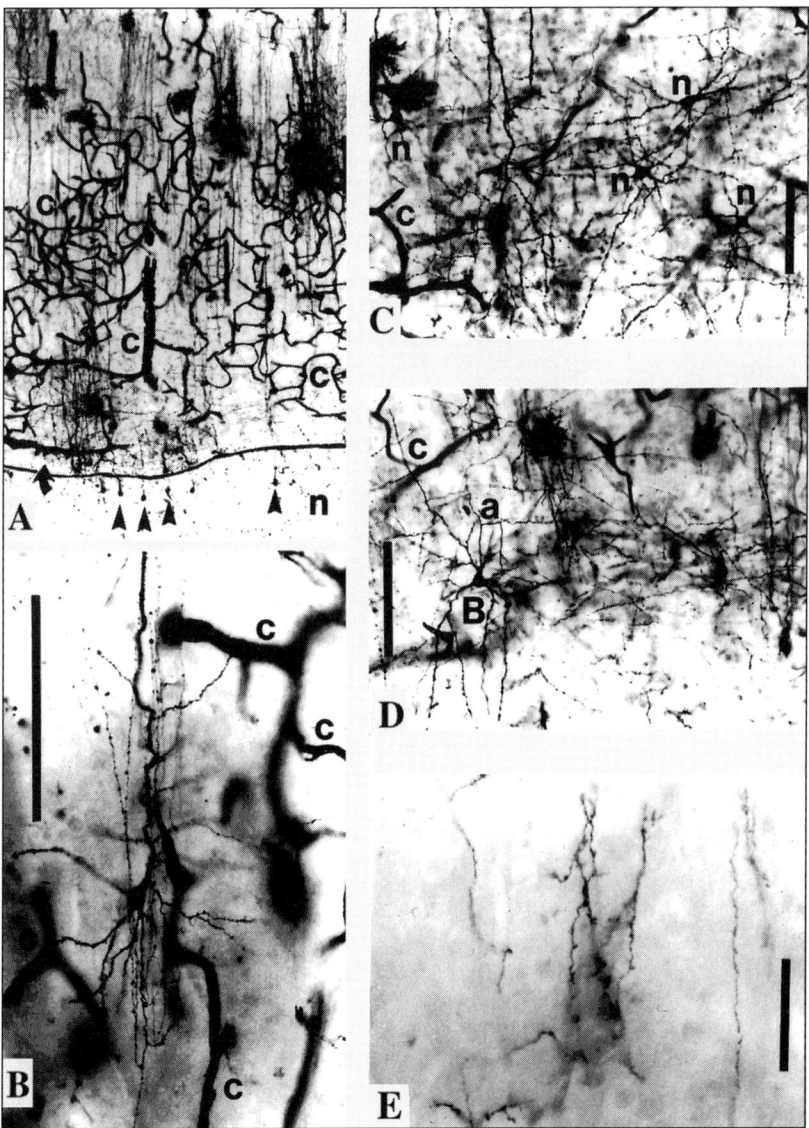

Fig. 4. Composite figure from rapid Golgi preparations (case 14) showing various postinjury alterations affecting the spared and still developing gray matter (GM) overlying an extensive white matter lesion (see Figs. 5A and 6). (A) Lower power microscopic view (¥50) of the GM overlying a subcortical WM necrosis (n) showing its intact intracortical vasculature and anastomotic capillary plexus (c), the long horizontal anastomotic vessel bordering the necrotic area (arrow) representing the lower limit of the GM vasculature, several deep-sited neurons (arrowheads) damaged by the lesion, and the limit of the necrosis outlined by an india-ink line (see Fig. 6). (B) Detail of an axotomyzed pyramidal cell transformed into a local-circuit neuron with several ascending collaterals arising from its proximal axonic stump (scale bar = 100 μm). (C) Microscopic view of layer V showing the morphology of several surviving stellate neurons (n) and its intact capillary (c) plexus (scale bar = 100 μm). (D) Microscopic view of a large unaffected basket cell (B) of layer V with an ascending axon (a), several long horizontal collaterals, and various terminal pericellular (baskets) nests (scale bar= 100 μm). (E) Detail of a pericellular basket (from cell depicted in D) formed around the unstained body of a pyramidal neuron (invisible in this Golgi-preparation) showing various axo-somatic terminal contacts 'en-passant' (scale bar = 50 μm). Despite the extensive necrosis of the underlying WM and because of the retention of its independent blood supply, most cellular elements of the spared GM survive and undergo postinjury transformations which result in a residual (permanent) cortical dysplastic lesion (see also Figs. 5 and 6). (From Marín-Padilla, 1997.)

transformed from projective into local-circuit neurons, altering both their morphology and intrinsic connectivity (Figs. 4B and 6).

Some deep-sited axotomyzed pyramidal neurons develop long horizontal axonic collaterals which expand paralleling the border of the necrotic zone (Fig. 6a). Some of these long horizontal collaterals may become incorporated into the residual WM retransforming the original cell into a projective neuron. The surviving axonic collaterals of other axotomyzed pyramidal neurons arch upwardly, ascend vertically for a long distance, and bifurcate several times (Figs. 5B–D and 6b). These ascending collaterals are extremely thin and finely beaded, suggesting active growth (Fig. 5B). The axonic collaterals of other axotomyzed cells are short, irregular and coarsely beaded, suggesting postinjury regressive changes. Another feature of this partially isolated GM is the hypertrophy of some of its intrinsic neurons, including basket cells characterized by long horizontal axonic collaterals and numerous baskets (Figs. 4D, E and 6c).

Despite the absence of afferent terminals and possibly because of it, the intrinsic circuitry of this partially isolated GM increases. The deprivation of afferent terminals throughout the spared GM seems to stimulate the postinjury expansion of its intrinsic circuitry. Synaptic sites vacated by the destruction of afferent fibres may be progressively re-established by terminals from intrinsic fibres. Also, the postinjury rewiring of neurons throughout the spared GM may contribute to their survival.

Chronic (repaired) lesions

The repaired stages of perinatally acquired WM lesions are represented by three distinct entities: multicystic encephalopathy (Figs. 5A, C), porencephaly (Fig. 5B), and hydranencephaly (Figs. 5D, E), and/or combinations of these disorders (Friede, 1989; Armstrong, 1995; Ravira-Encha, 1995; Marín-Padilla, 1997). Despite obvious pathologic differences, the pathogenesis of these entities is similar and they share the following features: (a) focal and/or extensive destruction of the WM with formation of residual cystic cavities connected and/or unconnected to the ventricular system; (b) universal reduction of WM fibres throughout the cerebral hemispheres (hydrocephalus *ex-vacuo*); (c) persistence of a thin band of WM tissue with long projective fibres; (d) periventricular gliosis with remnants of ependymal epithelium and glial nodules; (e) persistence of gliovascular trabeculi with surviving axonic fibres; and (f) the survival of overlying GM (Fig. 5 white and black arrows). The cortical dysplasia which evolve progressively in the spared GM is also essentially similar in the three entities. Moreover, epilepsy, cerebral palsy, mental retardation and other neurological sequelae can subsequently occur in any of these pathologic entities (Table 1).

In multicystic encephalopathies, porencephalies, and hydranencephalies, the overlying spared GM survives despite its partial isolation from sensory inputs (corticipetal fibres destruction) and inability to reach distant functional targets (corticofugal fibres destruction). Although capable of continuing its maturation, the overall cytoarchitectural organization of the spared GM may be progressively altered. Weeks, months, or even years after the original WM insult, this partially isolated GM continues to reorganize its neuronal, fibrillar, vascular and glial elements. Although the GM laminations and distribution of its elements may appear to be within normal limits, the usage of specific neurohistological methods discloses a variety of postinjury alterations. Frequently described cytoarchitectural alterations include: the presence of large stellate interneurons (Fig. 7); the presence of large neurons at the GM/WM border surrounded by the nuclei of several satellite glial cells; aggregation of neurons into small groups separated by cell-free zones; disorientation of some neurons; focal obliteration of some laminations; and increase of the intrinsic neuropil.

Rapid Golgi preparations of the spared GM have shown morphologic alterations in many neurons, structural disorganization and increase in the intrinsic neuropil. The presence of scattered large interneurons with long dendrites and intracortical distribution of their axon is another prominent feature (Fig. 3). Often, the axon of some of these large neurons arises from one of the dendrites at a significant distance from the soma. These large neurons are considered to be hypertrophic interneurons and more prominent throughout the supragranular layers (Figs. 3 and 7). Large polymorphous neurons with long dendrites are also found at the GM/WM border as well as within the residual WM (unpublished observations). Local disorientation of neurons, neuronal atrophy and degenerative dendritic changes in some neurons have been also described. These alterations are associated with modifications in the intrinsic circuitry of the affected region.

Neurofilament preparations confirm the presence of intrinsic circuitry anomalies as well as the presence of large and strongly positive stellate interneurons (Fig. 7). Large hypertrophic stellate neurons are particularly prominent in layers II and III (Figs. 3 and 7). The strong neurofilament staining of these neurons is probably due to an actual increase in the number of intrinsic filaments in both their enlarged soma and long dendrites. Hypertrophic neurons may participate in the postinjury synaptic reorganization of the spared GM, reconnecting synapses vacated by the degenerating afferent fibres destroyed by the underlying WM lesion. The presence of myelinated and strongly positive bundles of fibres contribute to the abnormal circuitry of the spared GM. These bundles of fibres cross the cortex in different direction, some accumulate near and/or within layer I, and many of them reach the residual band of WM.

All of these alterations constitute a postinjury cortical dysplasia with variable severity ranging from minimal to severe. This type of acquired cortical dysplasia results from the postinjury reorganization of the spared and partially isolated GM overlying WM lesions and is associated with some degree of cortical dysfunction. These dysplastic changes continue to evolve modifying progressively the organization of the affected region, and they will undoubtedly play a significant role in the pathogenesis of ensuing neurological sequelae.

Conclusions

In acquired neonatal encephalopathies, spared regions of the GM retain their blood supply, continue their development and, despite partial functional isolation, they are able to reorganize their intrinsic circuitry. The number of possible cytoarchitectural alterations which can evolve in this spared GM during its postinjury maturation could be extraordinary. Those described herein are but a few of the most prominent ones. These postinjury alterations are not static processes but ongoing ones which started after the injury and continue to evolve throughout weeks, months or years following the original brain injury. During the postinjury maturation of the spared GM, additional structural and functional alterations might evolve from pre-existing ones, making it difficult to distinguish original from superimposed alterations. Moreover, the cortical organization of an infant who eventually develops epilepsy (or other neurological sequelae) might undergo further additional (secondary) alterations caused by the seizures themselves. It must be emphasized that, in both normal and/or abnormal conditions, the intrinsic organization of the developing human neocortex undergoes progressive transformations throughout the life of the individual.

In subpial haemorrhages, many pyramidal cells survive the pruning of terminal dendrites, are transformed into stellate neurons, and undergo modification of their intrinsic synaptic organization. Following a WM injury, axotomyzed neurons of the overlying GM are transformed from long-projective into local-circuit neurons. Their damaged (severed) efferent axons undergo retrograde degeneration up to the origin of their collaterals. The number of surviving collaterals arising from their proximal axonic stump may increase in some neurons while decrease in others. Although partially deprived of sensory inputs and unable to reach distant targets, these axotomyzed neurons survive and continue to modify both their structure and intrinsic functional neuropil. Cajal (1968) described similar neuronal transformations in the developing neocortex and cerebellum of young kittens following an experimental injury. Pyramidal and Purkinje cells recently axotomyzed by a surgical cut of the WM are progressively transformed from long-projective into local-circuit neurons and assume new patterns of axonic distribution.

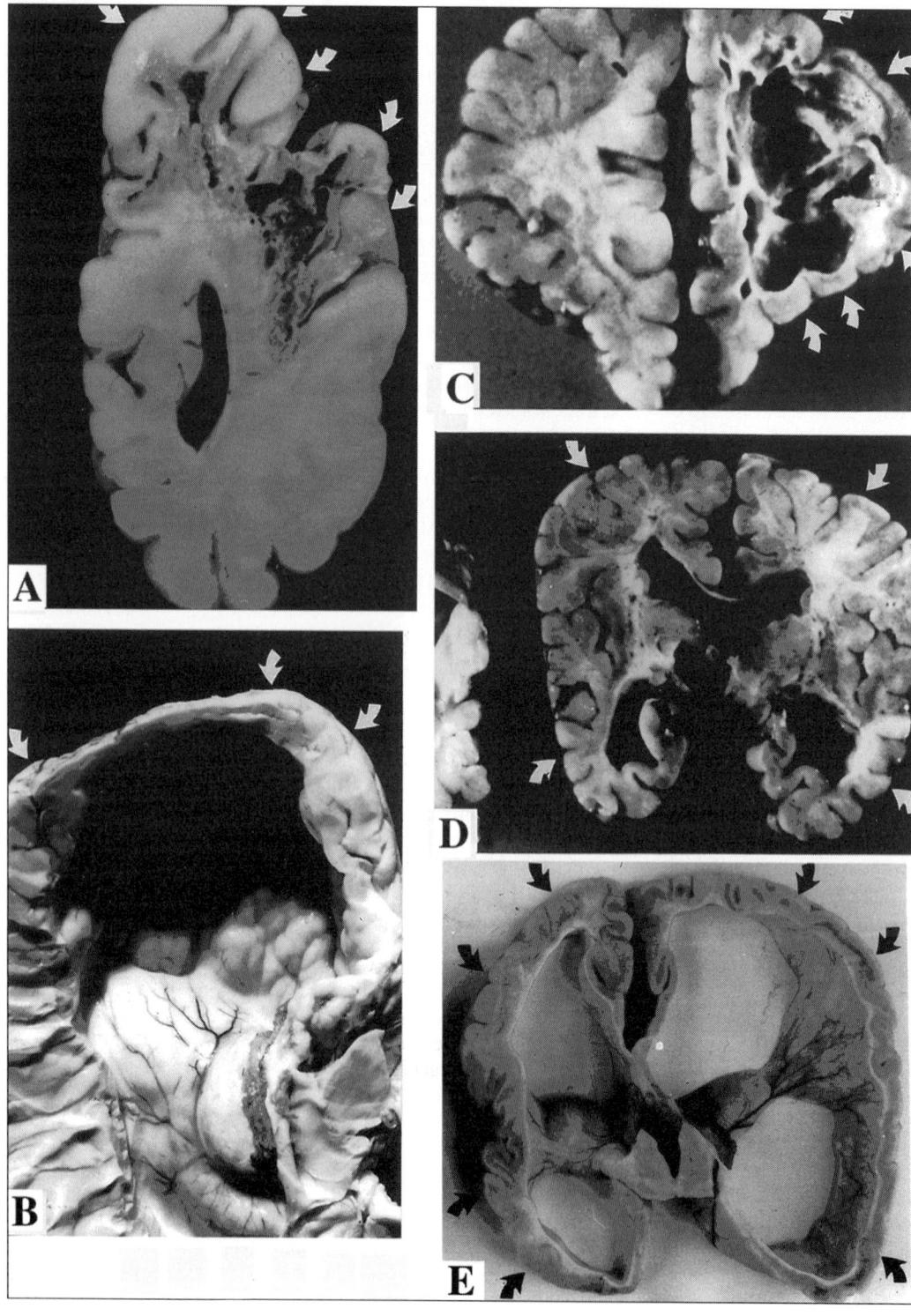

Fig. 5. (Opposite) Composite figure illustrating the essential pathologic features of subacute and chronic white matter lesions with the sparing of the overlying gray matter (GM). (A) Detail of the healing stage of a subacute multicystic encephalopathy (case 14) showing extensive WM necrosis, tissue disintegration, and early cavitation. While most of the overlying GM has remained unaffected (white arrows), in some areas the GM has been also damaged (infarcted) by the primary insult (see Fig. 4A). (B) View of an unilateral occipital lobe porencephaly (case 30) resulting from an extensive WM lesion showing the cystic enlargement of the connected ventricle, the marked reduction of WM tissue, and the survival of the overlying GM (white arrows). (C) Detail of an unilateral multicystic encephalopathy (case 25) showing multiple WM cavities unconnected to the ventricular system and separated by glio-vascular trabeculi, the survival of the overlying GM (white arrows), and the unaffected left frontal lobe. (D) Detail of an hydrocephalus ex-vacuo (case 24) caused by a diffused WM lesion showing universal attenuation of WM tissue, marked atrophy of the corpus callosum, generalized dilatation of the ventricular system, and the survival of the overlying GM (white arrows). (E) Detail of an hydranencephaly (case 27) caused by extensive WM lesion showing severe universal hydrocephalus ex-vacuo, generalized attenuation of WM tissue, severe atrophy of the corpus callosum, and near universal survival of the overlying GM (black arrows). All cases are also characterized by a residual thin band of WM tissue, a thick periventricular gliotic scar, and subpial (layer I) reactive gliosis. In all cases, the gyral patterns of the spared GM have evolve within normal limits (white and black arrows). In some cases (B and E), the spared GM is attenuated in some regions. Despite the extent and severity of the original WM lesions, the overlying GM has retained essentially intact both its independent leptomeningeal blood supply and intracortical anastomotic vasculature. Although, the spared GM above WM lesions is capable of continuing its development its subsequent structural and functional maturation will certainly be altered. Severe attenuation of WM tissue and the formation of a thick periventricular glial scar with focal calcifications (periventricular leukomalacia) is commonly associated with both poor prognosis and devastating neurologic sequelae. Postinjury epilepsy occurred in cases 24, 27 and 30. (From Marín-Padilla, 1997.)

Many local-circuit neurons survive cortical damage, develop long dendrites heavily stained in neurofilament preparations, and participate in the reorganization of the GM intrinsic neuropil. Some of these local-circuit neurons develop large bodies with an enlarged nucleus, long dendrites covered with numerous dendritic spines, and an expanded axonic territory (Marín-Padilla, 1993, 1996, 1997). Their heavy neurofilament staining remains unexplained (Adams *et al.*, 1992; Vinter *et al.*, 1993) . In my opinion, and that of others, the number of their intrinsic neurofilaments increases, reflecting postinjury structural and functional hypertrophy (Bignami *et al.*, 1968; Taylor *et al.*, 1971; Manz *et al.*, 1979; De Rosa *et al.*, 1992; Doung *et al.*, 1994; De Felipe *et al.*, 1996). In WM lesions, the degeneration of extrinsic terminals will leave numerous synaptic sites vacant throughout the surviving GM which may be capable of re-establishing functional contacts with intrinsic fibres. Local-circuit neurons with appropriate receptors may develop additional presynaptic terminals reconnecting vacant synaptic sites and subsequently undergoing both structural and functional hypertrophy (Bignami *et al.*, 1968; Manz *et al.*, 1979; Ferrer *et al.*, 1992; Armstrong, 1993; Marín-Padilla, 1993, 1997; Doung *et al.*, 1994). Nuclear polyploidy has been suspected in some of these large neurons which further supports their postinjury functional hypertrophy (Manz *et al.*, 1979).

Seven of the infants studied (cases 27–33) developed epilepsy, two cerebral palsy (cases 28, 32) and three were mentally retarded (cases 28–30). The epilepsy in these cases is considered to be a consequence of the postinjury structural and functional reorganization of the surviving GM rather than a direct consequence of the original injury. Each case represents a distinct and unique clinical entity which reflects the particular postinjury reorganization of its surviving GM. The literature concerning the association between epilepsy and cortical dysplasia is vast, complex, unclear, and in need of delineation and standardization (Vinter *et al.*, 1993). Epilepsy has been reported in many different conditions, including congenital encephalopathies, metabolic disorders, anomalies of neuronal migration, sequelae of perinatal brain damage, tumours, infections, pachygyria-agyria syndromes, megalencephalic syndromes and trauma. It might be impossible to establish a common denominator for epilepsy from such a heterogeneous group of disorders. However, most of these disorders could cause, directly and/or indirectly, alterations on the developing neocortex which could, in the course of its subsequent maturation, result in acquired cortical dysplasia and eventual dysfunction. The different types of epilepsies, rather than being the direct consequence of each particular condition, could be the outcome of the evolving, postinjury reorganization of their affected neocortex and could, in this sense, share a common pathogenesis.

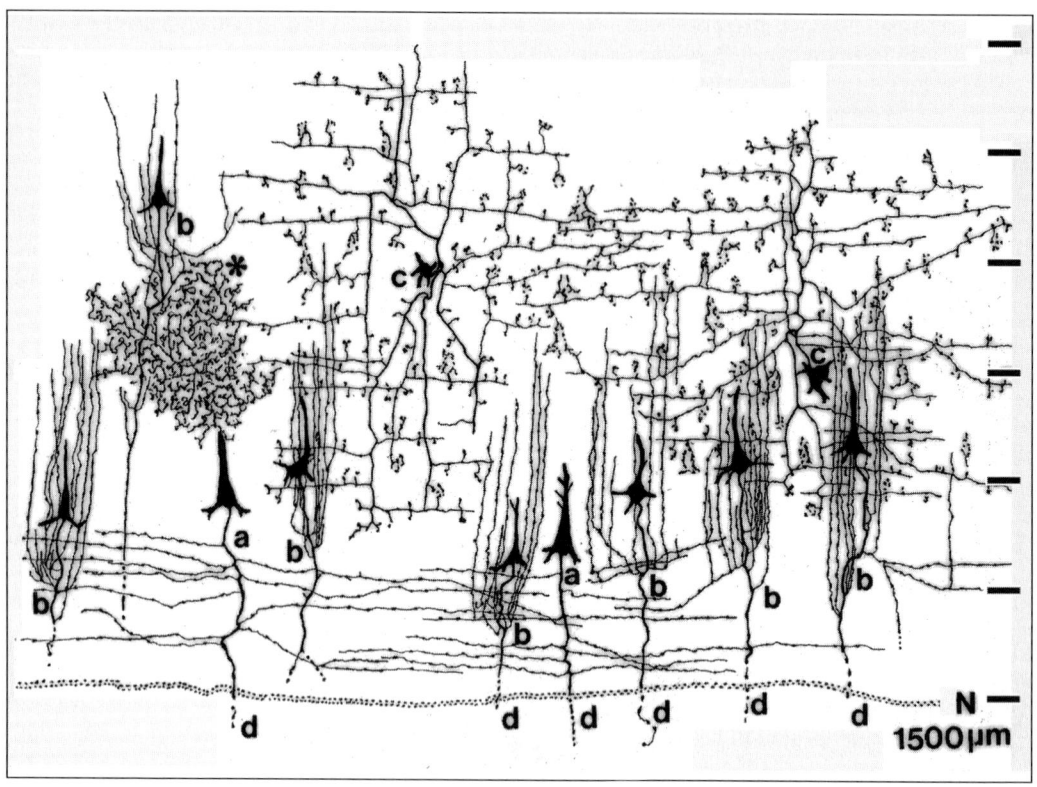

Fig. 6. Mosaic of camera lucida drawings from rapid Golgi preparations (case 14) showing some of the postinjury cytoarchitectural alterations observed in the spared gray matter (GM) overlying a subacute white matter (WM) lesion (see Figs. 4A and 5A). The following gray matter (GM) elements are illustrated: the axonic profiles of two axotomyzed pyramidal neurons (a) characterized by long horizontal collaterals bordering the necrotic zone (n); the axonic profiles of seven axotomyzed pyramidal neurons (b) with long ascending (arcuate) collaterals; the axonic profiles of two large (hypertrophic) basket cells (c) with long horizontal collaterals and numerous terminal pericellular baskets; and the complex intracortical axonic profiles (*) of unidentified local-circuit neurons. Within the necrotic zone (N), the retrograde degeneration (fragmentation) of some efferent fibre (d) progresses up to the origin of axonic collaterals transforming surviving projective pyramidal cells into intrinsic local-circuit neurons. The upper border of the necrotic zone (N) has been marked with a double ink-line. The location (depth) of the necrotic zone of the subcortical WM lesion is about 1500 μm from the pial surface and roughly at the border between layers V and VI. Scale bar = 100 μm. (From Marín-Padilla, 1997.)

The infant's brain represents an evolving entity characterized by progressive and unique organization of its neurons, blood vessels, glial elements, defensive elements and eventual functional connectivity. Any lesion (congenital or acquired) affecting the developing infant neocortex will have repercussions on its subsequent structural and functional maturation and will result in modifications throughout its evolving neuropil. While some of these postinjury modifications may be clinically silent, others may be compensated, and still others may be manifested via cortical dysfunction, such as mental retardation, dyslexia, cerebral palsy, epilepsy, speech impairment, poor school performance, blindness, various developmental delays, as well as many other neurological disturbances. The altered functional activity of a postinjury transformed neocortex may be blocked, failing to reach lower centres (e.g. cerebral palsy), may be discharged via abnormal motor activity (e.g. epilepsy), may result in visual errors (e.g dyslexia), and/or may result in various other types of clinical disorders. What must be emphasized concerning perinatal brain damage is the following:

(a) the intrinsic neuropil of spared GM regions is progressively transformed; (b) this postinjury reorganization will result in variable degrees of cortical dysplasia with their corresponding dysfunction; and, (c) these evolving postinjury alterations play a significant role in the pathogenesis of ensuing neurological sequelae.

The need to study the human brain with procedures capable of demonstrating its normal and/or abnormal cytoarchitectural organization cannot be overemphasized. A neuron is an independent entity characterized by unique features: (1) unique spatial location and orientation; (2) unique three-dimensional distribution of its dendritic and axonic arborizations; (3) unique distribution and organization of its synapses; and (4) unique array of axonic connections with many other neurons. Throughout the life of the individual, these four features evolve and modify progressively from the interplay of each neuron's genetic make-up, unique environment and unique interneuronal connectivity (Cajal, 1911; Higgins et al., 1997). Any genetic and/or acquired alteration affecting the brain will result in changes which will certainly modify the features of each affected neuron. If any affected neuron survives, it will assume new, unique and evolving features which will have repercussions through the overall organization of the brain. Consequently, it is crucial to use, in addition to routine methods, procedures capable of demonstrating: (a) the complete neuron, its location, its dendritic and axonic arbors, its three-dimensional spatial distribution and its interrelationships (rapid Golgi method); as well as (b) the organization of its evolving intrinsic circuitry (neurofilament stains). Only the use of these additional methods will provide a clear understanding of the evolving, normal and/or abnormal, structural and functional organization of the developing human brain.

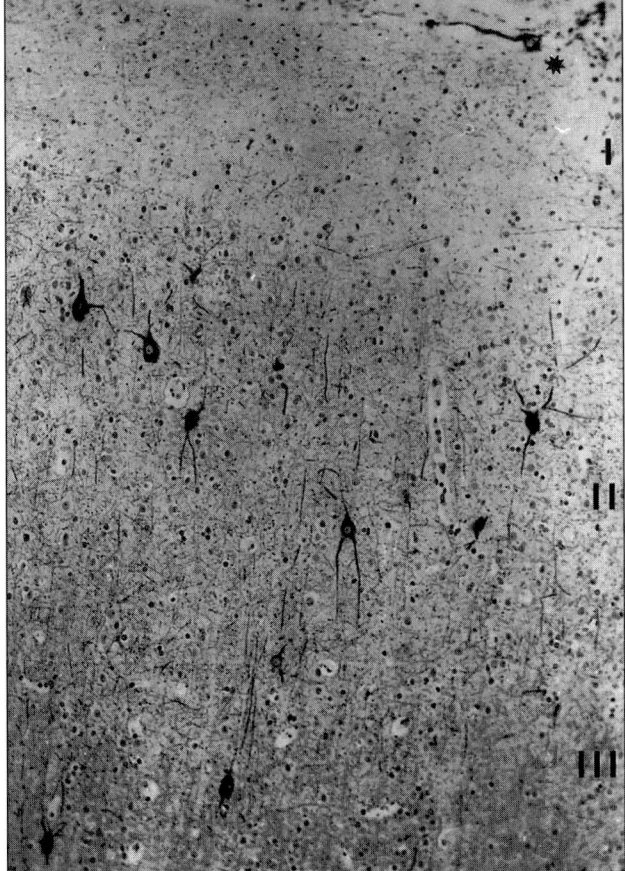

Fig. 7. Microscopic view, from neurofilament preparations, of the upper region of the spared GM overlying a parieto-occipital porencephalic cyst (case 33) showing several strongly positive intrinsic hypertrophic stellate neurons throughout layers II and III and a Cajal–Retzius cell in layer I (asterisk). These hypertrophic neurons are considered to represent postinjury transformed local-circuit neurons which participate in the rewiring of the intrinsic neuropil of the spared gray matter (GM) which is partially deprived of afferent fibres and unable to rich distant functional targets by the destruction of corticipetal and corticofugal by the underlying white matter (WM) lesion. The progressive postinjury dysplastic changes of the spared GM, including its hypertrophic neurons, are believed to play a significant role in the pathogenesis of neurological sequelae. Case 33 represents an eleven year-old epileptic girl.

Acknowledgements

This work was supported by a Jacob Javits Neuroscientist Investigator Award, from the NINCDS grant NS-22897, NIH, USA.

References

Adams, C., Hwang, P.A., Gilday, D.L., Armstrong, D.D., Becker, L.E. & Hofman, H.J. (1992): Comparison of SPECT, EEG, CT, MRI, and pathology in partial epilepsy. *Pediatr. Neurol.* **8,** 97–103

Akina, M., Nonaka, H., Kagesawa, M. & Tanaka, K. (1986): A study on the microvasculature of the cerebral cortex. Fundamental architecture and its senile changes in the frontal cortex. *Lab. Invest.* **55,** 482–89

Andres, K.H. (1967): Über die Feinstruktur der Arachnoidea und Dura Mater von Mammalian. *Z. Zellforsch.* **79,** 272–295.

Armstrong, D. (1995): Neonatal encephalopathies. In: *Pediatric Neuropathology,* ed. S. Ducket, pp. 334–351. Baltimore: Williams & Wilkins Publications.

Armstrong, D. & Norman, M.G. (1974): Periventricular leukomalacia in neonates. Complications and sequelae. *Arch. Dis. Child* **49,** 367–375.

Armstrong, D. D. (1993): The neuropathology of temporal lobe epilepsy. *J. Neuropath. Exp. Neurol.* **52,** 433–443.

Banker, B.Q. & Larroche, J.-C. (1962): Periventricular leukomalacia of infants. A form of neonatal anoxic encephalopathy. *Arch. Neurol.* **7,** 386–410.

Bignami, A., Palladini, G. & Zappella, M. (1968): Unilateral megalencephaly with nerve hypertrophy. An anatomical and quatitative study. *Brain Res.* **9.** 103–114.

Brun, A. (1965a): Marginal glioneuronal heterotopias of the central nervous system. *Acta Pathol. Microbiol. Scand.* **65,** 221–233.

Brun, A. (1965b): The subpial granular layer of the foetal cerebral cortex. *Acta Pathol. Microbiol. Scand.* 79 **(Suppl. 179)**, 1–89.

Cajal, S. R. (1911): *Histologie du système nerveux de l'homme et des vertébrés* (reprinted in 1972), pp. 520–532, 836–846. Madrid: Consejo Superior Investigaciones Cientificas.

Cajal, S. R. (1968): *Degeneration & regeneration of the nervous system* (translated from the 1928 Spanish edition by R. M. May). pp. 617–677. London: Hafner Publishing Company.

Casley-Smith, E., Földi-Börcsök, E. & Földi, M. (1976): The prelymphatic pathway of the brain as revealed by cervical lymphatic obstruction and the passage of particles. *Br. J. Exp. Path.* **57,** 179–188.

Clarren, S.K. & Smith, D.W. (1978): The fetal alcohol syndrome. *New England J. Med.* **298,** 1063–1068.

De Felipe, J., Sola, R.G. & Marco, P. (1996): Changes in excitatory and inhibitory synaptic circuits in the human epileptic cortex. In: *Excitatory amino acids and the cerebral cortex,* eds. F. Conti & T.P. Hicks, pp. 299–312. Cambridge MA: MIT Press.

De Rosa, M.J., Ferrel, M.A., Burke, M.M., Secor, D.L. & Vinters, H.V. (1992): An assessment of the proliferative potential of 'balloon cells' in focal cortical resection performed for childhood epilepsy. *Neuropath. Appl. Neurobiol.* **18,** 566–574.

Doung, T., De Rosa, M.J., Poukens, V., Vinters, H.V. & Fisher, R.S. (1994): Neuronal cytoskeletal abnormalities in human cerebral cortical dysplasia. *Acta Neuropath.* **87,** 493–503.

Duvernoy, H.M., Delon, S. & Vannson, J.L. (1981): Cortical blood vessels of the human brain. *Brain Res. Bull.* **7,** 519–579.

Evrard, P., Saint-Geoges, D., Kadhim, H.J. & Gadisseux, J-F. (1989): Pathology of prenatal encephalopathies. In: *Child neurology and developmental disabilities. Proceedings of the fourth international child neurology congress*, ed. J.H. French, pp. 153–176. Baltimore: P.H. Brooks.

Ferrer, I., Pineda, M., Tallada, M., Oliver, B., Russi, A., Oller, L., Noboa, R., Zujar, M.J. & Alcantara, S. (1992): Abnormal local-circuit neurons in epilepsia partialis continua associated with cortical dysplasia. *Acta Neuropath.* **83,** 647–652.

Friede, R.L. (1989): *Developmental neuropathology,* pp. 27–97. Berlin: Springer-Verlag.

Galaburda, A.M. & Kemper, T.L. (1979): Cytoarchitectonic abnormalities in developmental dyslexia: a case study. *Ann. Neurol.* **6**, 94–100.

Galaburda, A.M., Sherman, G.F., Rosen, G.D., Aboitiz, F. & Geschwind. N. (1985): Developmental dyslexia: four consecutive patients with cortical anomalies. *Ann. Neurol.* **18**, 222–233.

Higgins, D., Burack, M., Lein, P. & Banker, G. (1997): Mechanisms of neuronal polarity. *Current opinions in neurobiology* **7**, 599–604.

Kissane, J.M. (1975): *Pathology of infancy and childhood,* pp.117–148. St Louis: C.V. Mosby Company.

Krisch, B., Leonhardt, H. & Oksche, A. (1982): The meningeal compartment of the median eminence of the cortex. A comparative analysis in the rat. *Cell Tissue Res.* **228**, 597–640.

Krisch, B., Leonhardt, H. & Oksche, A. (1983): Compartments and vascular arrangement of the meninges covering the cerebral cortex of the rat. *Cells Tissue Res.* **238**, 459–474.

Larroche, J-C. (1977): *Developmental pathology of the neonate,* pp. 399–446. Amsterdam: Excerpta Medica.

Larroche, J-C. (1991): Fetal and perinatal brain damage. In: *Textbook of fetal and perinatal pathology.* eds. J.S. Wigglesworth, & D.B. Singer, pp. 807–838. Boston: Blackwell Scientific Publications.

Manz, H.J., Phillips, T.M., Towden, G. & McCullough, D.C. (1979): Unilateral megalencephaly, cerebral cortex dysplasia, neuronal hypertrophy and heterotopia. Cytomorphometric, fluorimetric cytochemical, and biochemical analyses. *Acta Neuropath.* **45**, 97–103.

Marín-Padilla, M. (1985): Early vascularization of the embryonic cerebral cortex: a Golgi and electron microscopic study. *J. Comp. Neurol.* **241**, 237–249.

Marín-Padilla, M. (1987): Embryogenesis of the early vascularization of the central nervous system. In: *Microneurosurgery, Vol. III: Clinical considerations and microsurgery of racemous angiomas,* ed. M. G. Yasargil, pp. 23–47. Stuttgart: Thieme-Verlag.

Marín-Padilla, M. (1988): Embryonic vascularization of the mammalian cerebral cortex. In: *Cerebral Cortex, Vol. 7, Development and maturation of cerebral cortex.* eds. A. Peters, & E.G. Jones, pp. 479–509. New York, Plenum Press.

Marín-Padilla, M. (1990): Three-dimensional structural organization of layer I of the human cerebral cortex. A Golgi study. *J. Comp. Neurol.* **229**, 89–105.

Marín-Padilla, M. (1993): Pathogenesis of late-acquired leptomeningeal heterotopias and secondary cortical alterations. A Golgi study. In: *Dyslexia and development: neurobiological aspects of extra-ordinary brains,* eds. A.M. Galaburda, & T.L. Kemper, pp. 64–88. Cambridge MA: Harvard University Press.

Marín-Padilla, M. (1995): Prenatal development of fibrous (white matter), protoplasmic (gray matter), and layer I astrocytes in the human cerebral cortex: a Golgi study. *J. Comp. Neurol.* **357**, 554–572.

Marín-Padilla, M. (1996): Developmental neuropathology and impact of perinatal brain damage. I. Hemorrhagic lesions of neocortex. *J. Neuropath. Exp. Neurol.* **55**, 758–773.

Marín-Padilla, M. (1997): Developmental neuropathology and impact of perinatal brain damage. II. White matter lesions of the neocortex. *J. Neuropath. Exp. Neurol.* **56**, 219–235.

Marín-Padilla, M. & Amieva, M.R. (1989): Early neurogenesis of the mouse olfactory nerve: Golgi and electron microscopic studies. *J. Comp. Neurol.* **288**, 339–352.

Mischel, P.S., Nguyen, L.P. & Vinters, H.V. (1995): Cerebral cortical dysplasia associated with pediatric epilepsy. Review of neuropathologic features and proposal for a grading system. *J. Neuropath. Exp. Neurol.* **54**, 137–153.

Morgan, J.T. & Marín-Padilla, M. (1992): Cortical repair and reorganization following traumatic microinjury in the developing rat neocortex (Abstract). *Soc. Neurosc.* **18**, 601A.

Nakamura, Y., Okudera, T. & Hashimoto T. (1994): Vascular architecture in white matter of neonates: its relationship to periventricular leukomalacia. *J. Neuropath. Exp. Neurol.* **53**, 582–589.

Pile-Spellman, J.M., McKusic, K.A., Strauss, H.W., Coony, J. & Taveras, J.M. (1984): Experimental *in vivo* imaging of the cranial perineural lymphatic pathway. *Am. J. Neuroradiol.* **5**, 539–545.

Ravavi-Encha, F. (1995): Fetal neuropathology. In: *Pediatric neuropathology,* ed. S. Ducket, pp. 108–122. Baltimore: Williams & Wilkins Publications.

Reed, G.B.& Claireaux, A.E. (1989): *Diseases of the fetus and newborn. Pathology, imaging, genetics and management,* pp. 432–437. London, Chapman & Hall Medical.

Robertson, C.M.T., Finer, N.N. & Grace, M.G.A. (1989): School performance of survival of neonatal encephalopathy associated with asphyxia at term. *J. Pediatr.* **114,** 753–760.

Rorke, J.B. (1992): *Pathology of perinatal brain injury,* pp. 45–130. New York: Raven Press.

Sarnat, H.B. (1992): *Cerebral dysgenesis. Embryology and clinical expression,* pp. 89–134. Oxford: Oxford University Press.

Schwartz, P. (1961): *Birth injuries of the newborn. Morphology, pathogenesis, clinical pathology and prevention.* pp. 73–90. New York: Hafner Publishing Company.

Takashima, S., Mito, T. & Ando, Y. (1989): Pathogenesis of periventricular white matter haemorrhages in preterm infant. *Brain Dev.* **8,** 25–30.

Taylor, D. C., Falconer, M.A., Bruton, C.J. & Corsellis, J.A.N. (1971): Focal dysplasia of the cerebral cortex in epilepsy. *J. Neurol. Neurosurg. Psychiatry,* **34,** 369–387.

Vinter, H.V., De Rosa, M.J. & Farrel, M.A. (1993): Neuropathologic study of resected cerebral tissue from patients with infantile spasms. *Epilepsia,* **34,** 772–779.

Volpe, J.J. (1987): *Neurology of the newborn,* pp. 160–181. Philadelphia: WB Saunders Company.

Wisniewski, K., Dambska, M., Sher, J.H. & Qazi, Q. (1983): A clinical neuropathological study of fetal alcohol syndrome. *Neuropediat.* **4,** 197–201.

Wolff, J.R., Bär, Th. & Güldner, F.H. (1975): Common morphogenetic aspects of various organotypic microvascular patterns. *Microvascular Res.* **10,** 373–395.

Chapter 4

Some principles in the organisation and development of cortical connections

Giorgio M. Innocenti

Institute for Cell Biology and Morphology, University of Lausanne, Switzerland, and Division of Neuroanatomy and Brain Development, Department of Neuroscience, Karolinska Institut, S-17177 Stockholm, Sweden

Summary

Cortical neurones are heavily interconnected and this constitutes a fundamental trait of cortical organisation. Beyond their own importance in cortical function, connections between neurones of the two hemispheres provide a model for the study of normal organisation, development and function of cortico-cortical connections. Inter-hemispheric connections are degenerate, in the sense that two areas are potentially interconnected by a number of different axonal systems. Axon types involved in these connections can be identified on the grounds of their specific distributions. They have highly complex arbors and appear to be suited to perform transformations of a computational kind. A functional assay of visual callosal connections can be obtained from the changes of inter-hemispheric EEG coherence during visual stimulation. Indeed, stimuli which activate callosal connections increase EEG coherence between visual areas of the two hemispheres in animals and man. Callosal connections develop due to a combination of cell-intrinsic and cell-extrinsic factors, the latter including visual experience. Axons specifically aimed at different cortical areas are found early in development and this suggests that each cortical area might contain multiple sets of neurones, each specified for targeting different contralateral sites. The terminal arbors of callosal axons differentiate through a series of growth stages which overproduce axons, axonal branches and synapses, and require subsequent refinement by selective deletions. The existence of cell-intrinsic determinants of callosal connections is also inferred from the quantitative study of the phenotype of callosal axons, in comparison with that of other axon types. Visual experience appears to validate the differentiation of the callosal axons as soon as they have established their first synaptic contacts. This early validation is sufficient to ensure a subsequent nearly normal differentiation of the axons.

Introduction

Connections among cortical neurones constitute an enormously complex network characterised by specificity and degeneracy. *Specificity* is reflected in the fact that the connections of each cortical neurone are the expression of its phenotype (e.g. pyramidal or non-pyramidal cell), and of its belonging to a certain area, column or layer. *Degeneracy* (Edelman, 1978) is suggested by the fact that, in general, two points in cortex can, at least in principle, be interconnected by multiple direct, or more or less indirect pathways. The activation of one or the other of these pathways, however, does not correspond to the same brain state, a condition which would be better characterised as redundancy. Instead, different brain states including internal representations parallel the activation of one or the other pathway, although the result may be isofunctional under sufficiently slack environmental conditions (see also Mayr, 1994 and the ensuing debate).

The subtle dynamic balance between excitatory and inhibitory connections presumably ensures the shifts in the activation of different configurations of cortical neurones, the neuronal assemblies, which since Hebb (1949) and Milner (1974) have been identified as a probable basis for cortical function (Edelman, 1978; Von der Malsburg & Schneider, 1986; Singer & Gray, 1995). The balance is destroyed in epilepsy and presumably, in different ways, in other frequent human pathologies such as dementia and schizophrenia. It is therefore important to understand how and when cortical networks develop and how modifiable they may be in development.

Over the last 20 years callosal connections have provided a model for the analysis of cortical connections in development. The analysis is far from being complete but it can already provide general concepts, most of which appear to apply to other cortical connections (discussed in Innocenti, 1995; Innocenti & Tettoni, 1997).

The organisation of callosal connections

In all species, the majority of callosal axons originate from pyramidal neurones in layer III. The infragranular layers V and VI contribute axons to some callosal projections, particularly to feedback projections from higher to lower areas (reviewed in Innocenti, 1986; Kennedy et al., 1991). The available electrophysiological and neurochemical evidence unequivocally demonstrates that the vast majority of these axons establish excitatory synapses. However, some axons probably terminate on inhibitory neurones and therefore have inhibitory action on the target sites (reviewed in Innocenti, 1986; Conti & Manzoni, 1994; Payne, 1994). The existence of a few directly inhibitory callosal axons seems probable (Hughes & Peters, 1992).

The analysis of the distribution of populations of callosally projecting neurones or axons and the visualisation, three-dimensional reconstruction and computer analysis of individual axons indicate that callosal connections are organised according to a number of specific rules.

First, each cortical area is connected with the corresponding area (homotopic callosal connections) and with its own characteristic set of other areas in the contralateral hemisphere (heterotopic callosal connections). The analysis of individual callosal axons originating from visual areas 17 and 18 in the cat (Houzel et al., 1994; Bressoud & Innocenti, 1998 and unpublished) has shown that these areas have separate connections to the contralateral 17/18 (type O, axons), and to a number of extrastriate areas, i.e. the 19/21a or 7 border region (type IE axons), and the PMLS/PLLS border region (IIE axons). In addition, they send diverging axons to combinations of the same extrastriate areas (the PMLS/PLLS *and* PMLS/21a borders, as well as the PMLS/PLLS *and* 19/21a or 7 borders; types EIII and EIV axons, respectively). This organisation suggests that areas of the two hemispheres can become functionally interconnected in couples, or in larger assemblies. This exemplifies one aspect of the degeneracy of cortico-cortical connections. It should be added that, in general, areas which are callosally connected are also connected intra-hemispherically. Therefore, neurones in the opposite hemispheres might become functionally interconnected by a number of alternative intra- and inter-hemispheric routes.

Second, callosal connections are unevenly distributed across the cortical areas (reviewed in Innocenti, 1986; Kennedy et al., 1991). In the visual system, callosal connections are restricted near the border between areas 17 and 18. This region represents the vertical meridian of the visual field and, in the cat, up to 20 degrees of visual field along it (Payne, 1994). A similar restricted distribution of callosal connections is found in the primary somatosensory areas, along the representation of the body midlines. In agreement with what has been mentioned above, different densities of callosally projecting neurones were found in regions of the primary visual and somatosensory areas representing different sectors of the sensory peripheries (Innocenti & Fiore, 1976; Caminiti et al., 1979; Innocenti, 1980; Kennedy et al., 1986). This suggested that the maps generated by thalamic afferents in the somatosensory areas are rescaled in the corpus callosum by virtue of the distribution of its neurones of origin (Innocenti, 1978).

Third, callosal connections conform to the columnar organisation of the cortex. Callosally projecting neurones and terminating callosal axons are often segregated in discrete columns or patches, and this applies both to primary sensory or motor areas as well as to non-primary areas (reviewed in Innocenti, 1986; Houzel et al., 1994). In the visual system callosal axons appear to interconnect columns specifically responsive to the same orientation of the visual stimulus (discussed in Houzel et al., 1994; Bressoud & Innocenti, unpublished).

The studies mentioned above suggested that callosal connections perform specific transformations of the cortical maps and therefore, in a broad sense, operations of a computational kind. It was also suggested that individual callosal axons perform at least three types of operations. In summary, by the geometry of their arbors, they create complex projection maps which relate to the retinotopy as well as to other properties of the projecting cortex and of its target areas. By virtue of the differential distribution of synaptic boutons within their terminal territory, axons can differentially amplify, for different targets, the messages generated at their cell body. Finally, length and calibre of branches can influence the timing of activation of the different targets. Therefore axons can operate transformations, in the spatial (mapping), intensity (weighting) and temporal (synchronisation or desynchronisation) domains (Innocenti, 1995) whose importance for cortical function remains to be explored.

A functional assay of callosal connections

New impetus to the study of callosal function came from the work of Singer and collaborators (Engel et al., 1991) showing that the interruption of callosal connections eliminates the synchronous oscillatory and stimulus-dependent activation of neurones in the primary visual areas of the two hemispheres. Similar findings were reported by others (Munk et al., 1995; Nowak et al., 1995). The importance of the finding is related to the "binding problem", i.e., in its simplest expression, the problem of interconnecting perceptual elements coded by separate neurones in the same or in different cortical areas. Consensus is beginning to emerge among several laboratories that the "binding problem" might be solved with the creation of highly dynamic assemblies of coactive cortical neurones, via cortico-cortical connections. Callosal connections provide an ideal system to test such a hypothesis since they are beginning to be known in detail and are easily interrupted or manipulated.

A further advantage of the callosal connections is that they link broadly spatially separate neurones in the two hemispheres. This allows the use of non-invasive EEG techniques that, in principle, could assay the state of callosal connections in normal and pathological conditions. To this end, we have recently undertaken an analysis of inter-hemispheric EEG coherence in ferrets and in man under stimulus conditions which, based on the morphological knowledge mentioned above, either activate callosal connections or do not (Kiper et al., 1998). The results of this study show that, as expected, inter-hemispheric coherence increases between symmetrical electrodes placed on the visual areas of the two hemispheres, for identically oriented stimuli projected near the vertical meridian of the visual field. In humans, but not in ferrets, the increase is obtained only with stimuli which are perceived as continuous across the vertical meridian of the visual field even though the continuity may be cognitive, rather than sensory in nature (Kiper et al., 1998).

Stages of axonal differentiation in the development of callosal connections

In the development of visual callosal axons five growth-stages can be identified (Aggoun-Zouaoui & Innocenti, 1994; Innocenti, 1995; Aggoun-Zouaoui et al., 1996).

The first stage consists of the elongation of axons between the hemispheres and up to the target areas. The second stage is characterised by axonal collateralisation in the white matter, underneath the target cortex. The third and fourth stages involve cortical ingrowth and branching in the grey matter. The fifth stage is characterised by synaptogenesis. Most of these growth stages cause overproduction of axonal components, i.e. of axons of their branches in the white and the grey matter, and of synapses. They are followed by selection of the components to be maintained and by elimination of the others. On average, the elimination is in the order of at least 60-70 per cent of the peak reached in development and it applies both to axons aimed at extrastriate areas and to those aimed at striate areas (Berbel & Innocenti, 1988; Aggoun-Zouaoui & Innocenti, 1994; Aggoun-Zouaoui et al. 1996; Bressoud & Innocenti, 1998). The stages of exuberant growth and the subsequent

partial deletions progressively focus the topography of callosal connection. At synaptogenesis the connections are already restricted to their adult territories. Therefore, the subsequent synaptic reduction appears not to sharpen significantly their topography. Instead, it is possible that, at this stage, the strength of the connections becomes finely tuned, a view compatible with the available electrophysiological evidence on the development of callosal connections (Milleret et al., 1994). If this view is correct, and if similar concepts can be generalised to other cortico-cortical connections, one might infer that this stage of development could also be critical for the development of epileptic symptoms. It is certain, in man, that regressive events comparable to those described in animals take place, and in particular that an important elimination of synaptic contacts occurs (Huttenlocher, 1979; Huttenlocher et al., 1982), and a massive elimination of callosal axons is probable (Clarke et al., 1989).

Cell-intrinsic vs. extrinsic determinants of callosal connections

The concept that connections are largely the consequence of the differentiation of a highly specialised part of the neurone, the axon, spurs questions on the cell-intrinsic vs. cell-extrinsic determinants of cortical connectivity. In order to answer such questions we have analysed a number of morphological parameters in two sets of axons subserving different connections in different species and systems: the thalamo-cortical connections to the barrel-field of the mouse and the visual callosal connections of the cat (Tettoni et al., 1998). We found that these two axonal systems are identical in a number of parameters, including the topological organisation of the arbors, the distribution of boutons, and the angles of branching. We suggest that these parameters may be determined by cell intrinsic constraints, possibly common to all axons. Instead, thalamo-cortical axons bear a larger number of boutons than callosal axons, and this is mainly due to the fact that their bouton-bearing branches are longer. This trait too, might be largely determined by intrinsic factors although some influence of extrinsic factors cannot be excluded (discussed in Tettoni et al., 1998).

Another hint suggesting the existence of cell-intrinsic determinants of callosal connections came from the finding that the different types of callosal axons (described above) and interconnecting the primary visual areas to homotopic or higher-order visual areas, or to combinations of them, appear early in development. Indeed, the different axonal types can be identified as early as when the axons have reached the contralateral targets and have begun to branch subcortically (Bressoud & Innocenti, 1998). Interestingly, the different types of axons originate not only from sites destined to remain callosally connected but also from sites which lose callosal connections in development. These findings suggest that different sets of cell types exist in areas 17 and 18, each specified early to send an axon to a different contralateral target or set of targets.

It has been known for a number of years that callosal connections require normal visual experience in order to attain normal development (Innocenti & Frost, 1979, 1980; Innocenti et al., 1985; Olavarria, 1995). In the absence of visual experience, in particular in kittens raised with binocular deprivation of vision by eyelid suture, a condition mimicking congenital cataract, a larger number of callosal connections are eliminated than in normal kittens. The concept that the development of callosal connections is controlled by experience was later generalised to other cortico-cortical connections (Luhman et al., 1986, 1990; Callaway & Katz, 1991; Mc Casland et al., 1992; Löwel

& Singer, 1992; Price et al., 1994; Schmidt et al., 1997; Zufferay & Innocenti, unpublished). An exaggerated loss of callosal connections was obtained with other forms of input deprivation, in particular, binocular enucleation (Innocenti & Frost, 1980) and early interruption of the optic chiasm (Boire et al., 1995). The task of maintaining the transient callosal connection has met with a limited amount of success in studies in the cat. Indeed, only a moderate enlargement of the callosal efferent zone (the region containing the cell bodies of callosally projecting neurones) and of the callosal terminal territory (the region containing the termination of callosal axons) could be obtained by early strabismus or enucleation (Innnocenti & Frost, 1979; Lund & Mitchell, 1979; Berman, 1991) although one study failed to replicate the finding (Olavarria & Van Sluyters, 1995). A more conspicuous enlargement of the region of callosal connections was obtained by enucleation in rodents (e.g. Cusick & Lund, 1982; Rhoades et al, 1984, 1987; Fish et al., 1991).

The studies mentioned raised the question of the role of visual experience in the development of cortical connections, i.e. whether vision has a morphogenetic role, in the sense that it can finely shape the development of callosal connections either by stimulating the growth of axons or by selectively validating axons and axonal components formed in excess at the stages of exuberant growth. Alternatively, the role of vision could be that of validating developmental processes based on rules and mechanisms intrinsic to the neurones and/or to the cortex. This question was recently addressed by studying the role of vision in the differentiation of visual axons which interconnect the primary visual areas (type O axons, see above). We investigated these axons in kittens deprived of pattern vision during the period of arbor formation and synaptogenesis (Jin et al., unpublished). We found stunted terminal arbors in kittens continuously deprived of vision. This was already noticeable at the end of the first postnatal month, i.e. at a time when the axons have just begun to form their arbors and the first synapses. Apparently, in the absence of pattern vision, most axons undergo only limited growth and do not form their characteristic terminal columns. Many of these axons are subsequently eliminated. This finding seems to support a morphogenetic role of vision. However, unexpectedly, eight days of vision beginning at natural eye opening, at a time when axons have only begun to form their first synapses, caused a nearly normal development of the arbors in spite of a subsequent long visual deprivation extending over the period of arbor formation.

These findings confirm previous indications that vision validates callosal connections at early stages of their development (Innocenti et al., 1985). In addition, it now appears that the vision-dependent validation is necessary and sufficient for the further growth and differentiation of the arbors. These can then continue autonomously, in the absence of vision.

Conclusions and perspectives

The work summarised above demonstrates that cortical connections can now be studied at unprecedented levels of morphological resolution, taking advantage of the techniques of single axon visualisation and analysis. These techniques have generated not only new data but, more importantly new morphological, functional and developmental concepts relating to the axon. Axons can now be viewed as performing a number of transformations of a computational kind, in the spatial, temporal and amplitude domains (see Innocenti, 1995). These transformations depend largely on the axon's morphological phenotype. Therefore, the development of connections should be studied from the point of view of the axonal phenotype. Several stages can be identified in the processes that lead to axonal differentiation. These are presumably the expression of cell-intrinsic constraints, as are several aspects of the mature axonal phenotype. Experience has the ultimate power of validating axonal phenotype. How tight and detailed this validation is cannot yet be stated with certainty. It appears that the consequences of vision outlast vision itself and appear to trigger events which can lead to a nearly normal autonomous differentiation of the axons. The critical question now is how precise the axonal phenotype needs to be in order for the cortical network in which it is embedded to function. It is very unlikely that this question could be tackled by animal experimentation only. Instead, a tighter integration between the animal and the human work appears to be necessary. As far as cortico-cortical connections are concerned, one of the techniques which could bridge the gap between the animal and the human work is probably EEG coherence analysis. The fact that this technique appears to provide information related not only to the morphology of cortico-cortical connectivity, but also to the activation of the connections during cognitive processes, should be taken as an additional challenge.

Acknowledgements

Supported by Swiss National Research Foundation grants 31-39707. 93, 31-050566. 97 and 4038-43990.

References

Aggoun-Zouaoui, D. & Innocenti, G. M. (1994): Juvenile visual callosal axons in kittens display origin- and fate-related morphology and distribution of arbors. *Eur. J. Neurosci.* **6**, 1846–1863.

Aggoun-Zouaoui, D., Kiper, D. C. & Innocenti, G. M. (1996): Growth of callosal terminal arbors in primary visual areas of the cat. *Eur. J. Neurosci.* **8**, 1132–1148.

Berbel, P. & Innocenti, G. M. (1988): The development of the corpus callosum in cats: a light- and electron-microscopic study. *J. Comp. Neurol.* **276**, 132–156.

Berman, N. E. J. (1991): Alterations of visual cortical connections in cats following early removal of retinal input. *Dev. Brain Res.* **63**, 163–180.

Boire, D., Morris, R., Ptito, M., Lepore, F. & Frost, D. O. (1995): Effects of neonatal splitting of the optic chiasm on the development of feline visual callosal connections. *Exp. Brain Res.* **104**, 275–286.

Bressoud, R. & Innocenti, G. M. (1998): Organization and target-aimed growth of visual callosal axons. *Soc. Neurosci. Abstr.* **24**, 124–19, 308.

Callaway, E. M. & Katz, L. C. (1991): Effects of binocular deprivation on the development of clustered horizontal connections in cat striate cortex. *Proc. Natl. Acad. Sci. USA* **88**, 745–749.

Caminiti, R., Innocenti, G. M. & Manzoni, T. (1979): The anatomical substrate of callosal messages from SI and SII in the cat. *Exp. Brain Res.* **35**, 295–314.

Clarke, S., Kraftsik, R., Van der Loos, H. & Innocenti, G. M. (1989): Forms and measures of adult and developing human corpus callosum: is there sexual dimorphism? *J. Comp. Neurol.* **280**, 213–230.

Conti, F. & Manzoni, T. (1994): The neurotransmitters and postsynaptic actions of callosally projecting neurones. *Behav. Brain Res.* **64**, 37–53.

Cusick, C. G. & Lund, R. D. (1982): Modification of visual callosal projections in rats. *J. Comp. Neurol.* **212**, 385–398.

Edelman, G. M. (1978): Group selection and phasic reentrant signaling a theory of higher brain function. In: *The mindful brain*, eds. G. M. Edelman & V. B. Mountcastle, pp. 51–100. Cambridge (USA) and London: The MIT Press.

Engel, A. K., König, P., Kreiter, A. K. & Singer, W. (1991): Interhemispheric synchronization of oscillatory neuronal responses in cat visual cortex. *Science* **252**, 1177–1179.

Fish, S. E., Rhoades, R. W., Bennett-Clarke, C. A., Figley, B. & Mooney, R. D. (1991): Organization, development and enucleation-induced alterations in the visual callosal projection of the hamster: single axon tracing with *Phaseolus vulgaris* leucoagglutinin and Di-I. *Eur. J. Neurosci.* **3**, 1255–1270.

Hebb, D. O. (1949): *Organization of behavior*, pp. 1–335. New-York: John Wiley & Sons.

Houzel, J. -C., Milleret, C. & Innocenti, G. (1994): Morphology of callosal axons interconnecting areas 17 and 18 of the cat. *Eur. J. Neurosci.* **6**, 898–917.

Hughes, C. M. & Peters, A. (1992): Symmetric synapses formed by callosal afferents in rat visual cortex. *Brain Res.* **583**, 271–278.

Huttenlocher, P. R. (1979): Synaptic density in human frontal cortex - Developmental changes and effects of aging. *Brain Res.* **163**, 195–205.

Huttenlocher, P. R., De Courten, C., Garey, L. J. & Van der Loos, H. (1982): Synaptogenesis in human visual cortex - Evidence for synapse elimination during normal development. *Neurosci. Lett.* **33**, 247–252.

Innocenti, G. M. (1978): Postnatal development of interhemispheric connections of the cat visual cortex. *Arch. Ital. Biol.* **116**, 463–470.

Innocenti, G. M. (1980): The primary visual pathway through the corpus callosum: morphological and functional aspects in the cat. *Arch. Ital. Biol.* **118**, 124–188.

Innocenti, G. M. (1986): General organization of callosal connections in the cerebral cortex. In: *Cerebral Cortex, Vol. 5*, eds. E. G. Jones & A. Peters, pp. 291–353. New York: Plenum Publishing Corporation.

Innocenti, G. M. (1995): Exuberant development of connections, and its possible permissive role in cortical evolution. *TINS* **18**, 397–402.

Innocenti, G. M. & Fiore, L. (1976): Morphological correlates of visual field transformation in the corpus callosum. *Neurosci. Lett.* **2**, 245–252.

Innocenti, G. M. & Frost, D. O. (1979): Effects of visual experience on the maturation of the efferent system to the corpus callosum. *Nature* **280**, 231–234.

Innocenti, G. M. & Frost, D. O. (1980): The postnatal development of visual callosal connections in the absence of visual experience or of the eyes. *Exp. Brain Res.* **39**, 365–375.

Innocenti, G. M. & Tettoni, L. (1997): Exuberant growth, specificity and selection in the differentiation of cortical axons. In: *Normal and abnormal development of cortex*, eds. A. M. Galaburda & Y. Christen, pp. 99–120. Berlin, Heidelberg, New York: Springer-Verlag.

Innocenti, G. M., Frost, D. O. & Illes, J. (1985): Maturation of visual callosal connections in visually deprived kittens: a challenging critical period. *J. Neurosci.* **5**, 255–267.

Kennedy, H., Dehay, C. & Bullier, J. (1986): Organization of the callosal connections of visual areas V1 and V2 in the macaque monkey. *J. Comp. Neurol.* **247**, 398–415.

Kennedy, H., Meissirel, C. & Dehay, C. (1991): Callosal pathways and their compliancy to general rules governing the organization of corticocortical connectivity. In: *Vision and visual dysfunction, Vol. 3: Neuroanatomy of the visual pathways and their development*, eds. B. Dreher & S. Robinson, pp. 324–359. London: Macmillan.

Kiper, D. C., Knyazeva, M., Tettoni, L., Maeder, M., Despland, P. A. & Innocenti, G. M. (1998): Interhemispheric EEG coherence during visual stimulation. *Invest. Ophtalmol. Vis. Sci.* **39**, S324.

Löwel, S. & Singer, W. (1992): Selection of intrinsic horizontal connections in the visual cortex by correlated neuronal activity. *Science* **255**, 209–212.

Luhmann, H. J., Millán, L. M. & Singer, W. (1986): Development of horizontal intrinsic connections in cat striate cortex. *Exp. Brain Res.* **63**, 443–448.

Luhmann, H. J., Singer, W. & Martínez-Millán, L. (1990): Horizontal interactions in cat striate cortex: I. Anatomical substrate and postnatal development. *Eur. J. Neurosci.* **2**, 344–357.

Lund, R. D. & Mitchell, D. E. (1979): Asymmetry in the visual callosal connections of strabismic cats. *Brain Res.* **167**, 176–179.

Mayr, E. (1994): Population thinking and neuronal selection: metaphors or concepts? In: *Selectionism and the brain*, eds. O. Sporns & G. Tononi, pp. 27-34. San Diego, New York, Boston, London, Sydney, Tokyo, Toronto: Academic Press.

McCasland, J. S., Bernardo, K. L., Probst, K. L. & Woolsey, T. A. (1992): Cortical local circuit axons do not mature after early deafferentation. *Proc. Natl. Acad. Sci. USA* **89**, 1832–1836.

Milleret, C., Houzel, J. C. & Buser, P. (1994): Pattern of development of the callosal transfer of visual information to cortical areas 17 and 18 in the cat. *Eur. J. Neurosci.* **6**, 193–202.

Milner, P. M. (1974): A model for visual shape recognition. *Psychological Review* **81**, 521–535.

Munk, M. H. J., Nowak, L. G., Nelson, J. I. & Bullier, J. (1995): Structural basis of cortical synchronization. II. Effects of cortical lesions. *J. Neurophysiol.* **74**, 2401–2414.

Nowak, L. G., Munk, M. H. J., Nelson, J. I., James, A. C. & Bullier, J. (1995): Structural basis of cortical synchronization. I. Three types of interhemispheric coupling. *J. Neurophysiol.* **74**, 2379–2400.

Olavarria, J. (1995): The effect of visual deprivation on the number of callosal cells in the cat is less pronounced in extrastriate cortex than in the 17/18 border region. *Neurosci. Lett.* **195,** 147–150.

Olavarria, J. F. & Van Sluyters, R. C. (1995): Overall pattern of callosal connections in visual cortex of normal and enucleated cats. *J. Comp. Neurol.* **363,** 161–176.

Payne, B. R. (1994): Neuronal interactions in cat visual cortex mediated by the corpus callosum. *Behav. Brain Res.* **64,** 55–64.

Price, D. J., Ferrer, J. M. R., Blakemore, C. & Kato, N. (1994): Postnatal development and plasticity of corticocortical projections from area 17 to area 18 in the cat's visual cortex. *J. Neurosci.* **14,** 2747–2762.

Rhoades, R. W., Mooney, R. D. & Fish, S. E. (1984): Comparison of visual callosal organization in normal, bilaterally enucleated and congenitally anophtalmic mice. *Exp. Brain Res.* **56,** 92–105.

Rhoades, R. W., Fish, S. E., Mooney, R. D. & Chiaia, N. L. (1987): Distribution of visual callosal projection neurones in hamsters subjected to transection of the optic radiations on the day of birth. *Dev. Brain Res.* **32,** 217–232.

Schmidt, K. E., Kim, D. S., Singer, W., Bonhoeffer, T. & Löwel, S. (1997): Functional specificity of long-range intrinsic and interhemispheric connections in the visual cortex of strabismic cats. *J. Neurosci.* **17,** 5480–5492.

Singer, W. & Gray, C. M. (1995): Visual feature integration and the temporal correlation hypothesis. *Ann. Rev. Neurosci.* **18,** 555–586.

Tettoni, L., Gheorghita-Baechler, F., Bressoud, R., Welker, E. & Innocenti, G. M. (1998): Constant and variable aspects of axonal phenotype in cerebral cortex. *Cerebral Cortex,* **8,** 543–522.

Von der Malsburg, C. & Schneider, W. (1986): A neural cocktail-party processor. *Biol. Cybern.* **54,** 29–40.

Chapter 5

Maturation of cortical physiological properties relevant to epileptogenesis

Giuliano Avanzini, Giulio Sancini, Laura Canafoglia and Silvana Franceschetti

Divisione di Neurofisiopatologia, Istituto Nazionale Neurologico C. Besta, Via Celoria 11, 20133 Milan, Italy

Summary

The infantile brain differs from the adult one both in its susceptibility to epileptogenic agents and the phenomenological expression of the seizures. The high incidence of epilepsy in early infancy is partially accounted for by the frequency of epileptogenic pathologies affecting the perinatal and early postnatal periods. In addition, some physiological characteristics of the immature brain can contribute to making it prone to epilepsy.

The immaturity of intrinsic cellular excitable properties and the facilitation of the excitatory amino-acid mediated neurotransmission insufficiently counteracted by the immature GABA system in the early postnatal stages predispose the infantile brain to hyperexcitable events. On the other hand, the fatiguability of the excitatory synaptic transmission, the limitation in the ability to sustain long-lasting discharges and the immaturity of bursting mechanisms account for a reduced probability of highly synchronized sustained discharges. An important turning point is related to the maturation of a subpopulation of neocortical pyramidal neurons endowed with bursting properties. It is estimated to occur around the third/fourth month of human postnatal life and is correlated with the ability to produce the high voltage cortical activity underlying hypsarrhythmia.

Another important developmental step is related to the maturation of the thalamo-cortical system enabling the infantile brain to produce bilateral synchronous spike-wave discharges.

The potentially harmful effect of epileptic discharges on the developing brain is still controversial. Some experimental results suggest that the immature brain is more protected against seizure-induced brain damage. However, even subtle biological changes either due to the epilepsy *per se* or to the antiepileptic drug side effects may have an appreciably negative impact on the intellectual and behavioral functions in a critical period such as the developmental one.

Maturational changes in cortical excitable properties may affect the susceptibility to epileptogenic agents, the phenomenological expression of seizures and consequently seizure-dependent brain damage (Mares, 1991). It is therefore not surprising that infantile epilepsies differ from the adult ones in terms of frequency, semiology and prognosis inasmuch as some etiological factors are particularly frequent in infancy.

Hereafter, some age-related changes relevant to epileptogenesis will be discussed. Since most of this information is drawn from experimental studies in animals, it is particularly important to establish some correlation between human and animal (namely the rat's) postnatal developmental stages. Based on anatomical studies of callosal reshaping, changes in neocortical synaptic density and myelination (Innocenti, 1986), the following correspondences can be drawn.

At birth, the rat neocortex is more immature that the human one and reaches a comparable stage around postnatal day 5, corresponding to about one month of human postnatal life. From this point onwards, developmental rates in rat and in man diverge significantly so that the 3rd human postnatal month corresponds to days 13-15 in the rat, while the first year of human postnatal life does not outlast the 25th day of the rat.

Postnatal developmental changes in the neocortex

Morphology

During the first month of postnatal life, the rat neocortex undergoes important architectural changes. At birth, only two definitive immature layers (I and II) are recognizable in the somatosensory cortex. By postnatal day two (P2) layer V is completely separate from a still undifferentiated cortical plate and by P3 the trilaminar structure of the cortical plate becomes evident (Rice *et al.*, 1985) and differentiates further during the next few days under the influence of the ingrowth of thalamo-cortical and callosal fibers (Wise & Jones, 1976, 1978).

Most of the morphogenetic processes affecting pyramidal cell bodies, dendrites and axons also occur after birth during postnatal weeks 1-4 (Miller & Peters, 1981; Miller, 1988) and result in a tremendous increase in the volume of the neuropil, due in large part to the growth of dendrites (Eayers & Goodhead, 1959; Peters & Feldman 1973; Feldman & Peters, 1978; Miller, 1981). During the first postnatal week, both pyramidal and local circuit neurons show evidence of somatic spines (Parnavelas *et al.*, 1978) which are transient features of immature pyramidal neurons, since they are rare or absent on mature elements, while some persist on mature local circuit neurons. Concomitant changes in the physiological properties of rat neocortical neurons have been analysed by Kriegstein *et al.*, (1987) McCormick & Prince (1987), Avanzini *et al.*, (1992) and Franceschetti *et al.*, (1993, 1995) and will be summarized in the next paragraphs.

Passive properties

During the first postnatal week the resting membrane potential in rat pyramidal neurons is slightly but significantly lower than in adults, while membrane resistance and time-constant are more than twice as high as the corresponding values in mature neurons (Fig. 1). The values approach mature levels during the first three postnatal weeks, with the most pronounced changes occurring in the initial 8-10 postnatal days. Electrotonic length increases also significantly in the same period of time, implying less attenuation of the incoming signals in the early postnatal stages.

Increase in cell body size and the elaboration of dendritic arborization can largely account for these changes; in particular the increase in electrotonic length is mainly influenced by the geometry of dendritic arborization. It has to be borne in mind, however, that the density and distribution of ionic channels (McCormick & Prince, 1987) and electrogenic pump activity (Fukuda *et al.*, 1992) change markedly during the first 3-4 postnatal weeks: these events may also contribute to the progressive evolution of resting membrane potential and input resistance.

Voltage dependent channels

Pyramidal neurons recorded during the first week of post-natal life were able to respond consistently to supra-threshold depolarizing pulses with overshooting action potentials. Immature action potentials are rather long, due to a slow rise time and slow repolarization (Kriegstein *et al.*,

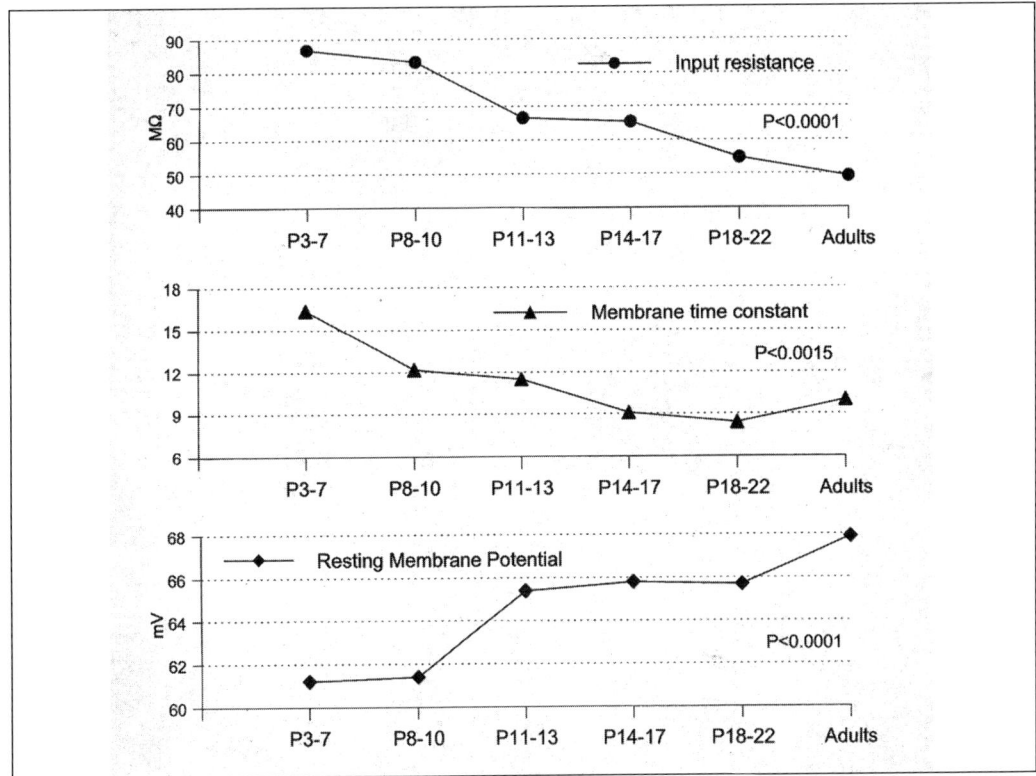

Fig. 1. Time course of resting potential input resistance and electronic length during the three first postnatal weeks in rats.

1987, McCormick & Prince, 1987). The steepness of the depolarizing phase increases markedly until the first days of the third week, then slowly takes up the adult form; while action potential repolarization shows a more regular trend to its mature form (Fig. 2). The progressive increase in Na$^+$ channel density, without significant changes in fast Na$^+$ current (Inap) kinetics, that has been reported in neocortical neurons during post-natal development (Huguenard et al., 1988; Alzheimer et al., 1993) accounts for the progressive increase in the steepness of Na$^+$ action potentials. The peculiar role of the persistent fraction of Na$^+$ current (Inaf) in the maturation of pyramidal cell properties will be discussed. Various types of immature K$^+$ current patterns have also been reported in different neuronal types, including hippocampal and neocortical neurons (Zona et al, 1988; Klee et al., 1995). In particular the mean closing time of Ca^{2+} activated K$^+$ channels after birth is lower than in adults and tends to shorten during the first post-natal month (Kang et al., 1996). The resulting changes in K$^+$ currents together with the progressive increase in channel density could contribute significantly to the maturational shaping of action potential repolarization.

In immature pyramidal neurons, Ca^{2+} spikes can be consistently evoked when the Na$^+$ current has been blocked by tetrodotoxin and K$^+$ hyperpolarizing currents have been partially removed using tetraethylammonium as a non-specific extracellular blocker. These Ca^{2+} spikes have a slower rise time than in adult animals, indicating a lower density of Ca^{2+} channels (McCormick & Prince, 1987). A regular increase in the somatic Ca^{2+} current amplitude (and hence estimated Ca^{2+} channel density) has recently been demonstrated in postnatal rat neurons by Lorenzon & Foehring (1995); these authors did not find significant changes in the proportions of different types of Ca^{2+} currents. The maturation of T-type Ca^{2+} current (I$_T$) was analyzed in isolated neurons from rat thalamic reticular nucleus (R$^+$) (Tsakiridou et al., 1995) which is involved in rhythmic synchronous

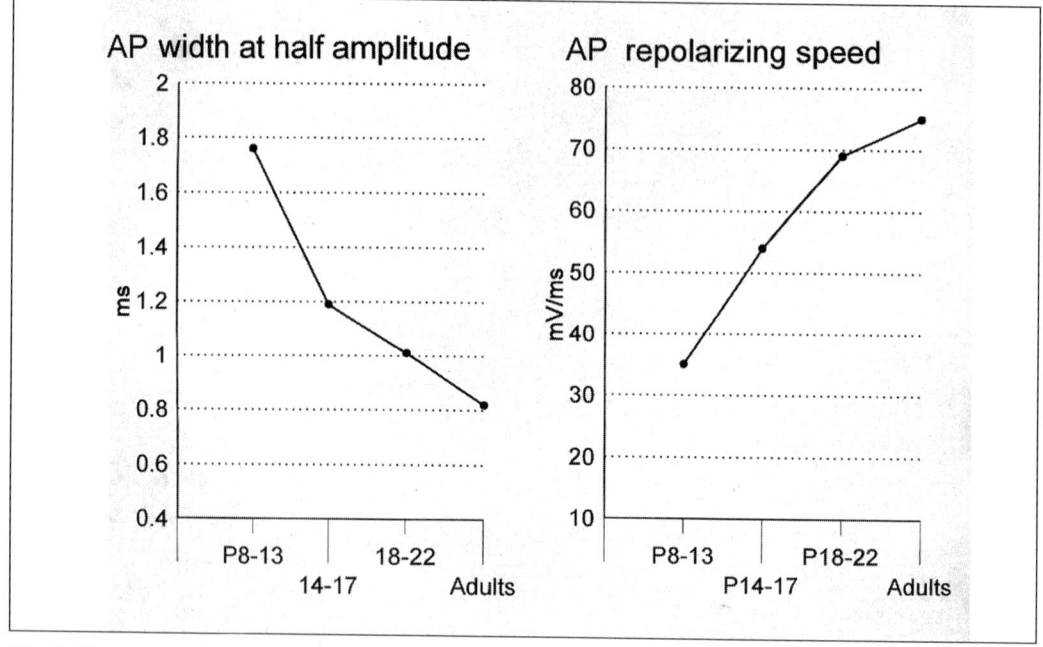

Fig. 2. Time course of action potential (AP) width and repolarizing speed during the three first postnatal weeks in rats. (Modified from Franceschetti et al., 1997.)

thalamocortical activities (Mulle et al., 1986, Avanzini et. al., 1989). A significant increase in I_T amplitude was found to occur between P11 and P18 when it attains the adult values.

Firing characteristics

During the first week of post-natal life, pyramidal neurons require rather large depolarizing pulses to elicit a train of action potentials; however the train rarely exceeds 250 ms in duration from the onset of depolarization. During the train of discharges, the steepness of the rising phase declines slightly and there is a slight initial decrease in firing frequency following the first inter-spike interval. This behaviour was described by McCormick & Prince (1987), and attributed by Lorenzon & Foehring (1993) to the strong expression of a long-lasting post-train after-hyperpolarization due to a K^+Ca^{2+} dependent current present in very immature animals (see above). However, it is also possible that partially defective spike generation due to the physiologically low density of Na^+ channels (Kriegstein et al., 1987; Huguenard et al., 1988) may prevent the generation of long-lasting trains of action potential at this stage in development.

The initial discharge rate in response to depolarizing current pulses quickly increases during the second week, and at the end of the third week pyramidal neurons acquire the ability to discharge with a frequency close to that of cells in adult animals. Concurrently with the increase in firing frequency, spike frequency adaptation develops and provides increasingly efficient capacity to modulate the discharge in response to incoming depolarizations (Fig. 3). The progressive development of this phenomenon can be appreciated starting from the second week, when most pyramidal neurons acquire the ability to discharge with a long-lasting train in response to a long-lasting steady state depolarization.

In mature rats, the firing response to 400-1000 ms depolarizing current pulses provided a means of classifying pyramidal neurons into different subtypes. On this basis Connors & Gutnick (1990) identified regular spiking (RS) and intrinsically bursting (IB) pyramidal neurons. In RS neurons,

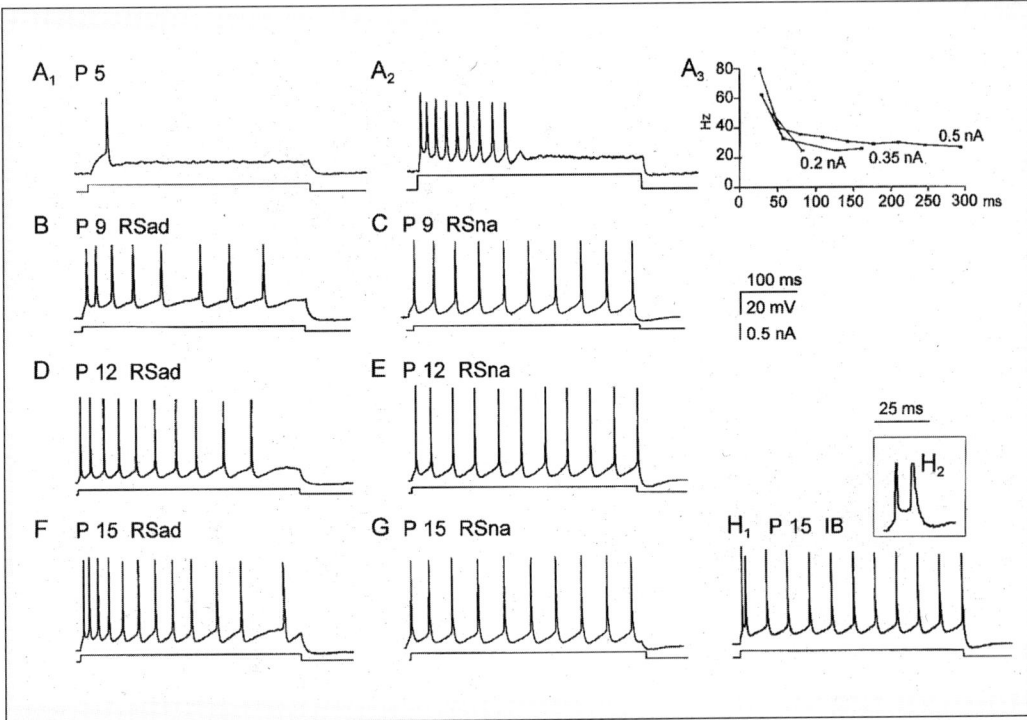

Fig. 3. Firing characteristics in response to the intracellular injection of long-lasting depolarizing pulses in rat neocortical neurons of the postnatal ages P5, P9, P12, P15. Regular spiking (RS) neurons have been further subclassified as adapting (RSad) or non-adapting (RSna) according to the degree of spike frequency adaptation (spa). Note in A3 that spa is already present during the first postnatal week and that intrinsically bursting (IB) neurons are evident only at the end of the second postnatal week (H1, H2). (From Franceschetti et al., 1998.)

threshold depolarization evokes a single action potential, while supra-threshold depolarizing current pulses evoke long trains of action potentials, each individual action potentials being followed by a hyperpolarizing after-potential.

The firing mode that distinguishes IB neurons becomes evident only at the end of the second postnatal week, when 23 per cent of the neurons in layer V start to discharge with two closely spaced action potentials in response to supra-threshold depolarization. This immature burst discharge attains a more mature appearance during the third week, but the full characteristics of a mature burst (including the ability to discharge with more than three action potentials) appears only at the end of the first month. A typical example of an immature IB burst recorded at P15 is shown in Fig. 3. In more mature neurons, concomitantly with the appearance of the more mature burst, the depolarizing after-potentials increase, both in amplitude and duration. The resting membrane potentials in neurons with IB or RS firing type do not differ; membrane input resistance in IB neurons is slightly but not significantly lower than in RS neurons (Franceschetti *et al.*, 1993, 1995).

In mature neurons, bursting activity in IB neurons is insensitive to various Ca^{2+} channel blockers, but is abolished using the Na^+ channel blocker tetrodotoxin (Franceschetti *et al.*, 1995). This finding supports the explanation that both the fast spike and slow depolarizing potential giving rise to the burst are sustained by Na^+ currents, as recently suggested for bursting neurons in other cortical structures, such as CA1 pyramidal neurons in subiculum and hippocampus (Mattia *et al.*, 1993, Azouz *et al.*, 1996). The persistent fraction of the Na^+ current, which has been demonstrated to contribute significantly to the firing properties of neocortical pyramidal neurons (Stafstrom *et al.*, 1985), appears

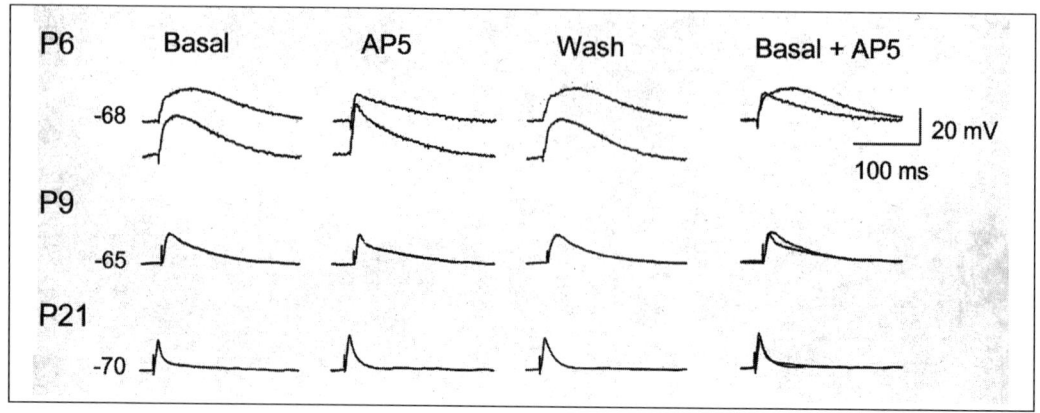

Fig. 4. *Postnatal maturation of excitatory postsynaptic potentials (EPSPs) in rats. Note that long-lasting EPSPs during the first postnatal week contain an APV-sensitive NMDA mediated component (see superimposition) which persists even when the membrane is artificially hyperpolarized.*

to be the best candidate for the generation of the neocortical burst. Interestingly, the maturational profile of the persistent Na^+ current (Huguenard *et al.*, 1988; Alzheimer *et al.*, 1993) fits well with the relatively late appearance of the bursting behavior in neocortical neurons (Franceschetti *et al.*, 1998).

Receptor-mediated activities

In spite of the presence of GABA immunoreactive neurons, hyperpolarizing inhibitory postsynaptic potentials (IPSPs) are not detectable during the first postnatal week. On the contrary, an immature excitatory aminoacid (EAA)-mediated neurotransmission is already effective during the first days of life. Immature excitatory postsynaptic potentials (EPSPs) are highly fatiguable, long lasting and contain a N-methyl-D-aspartate (NMDA) component (Fig. 4) which is less sensitive to the voltage-dependent Mg^{2+} block than in adults (Avanzini *et al.*, 1992).

During the second week GABA-mediated IPSPs become more and more pronounced. EAA-mediated monosynaptic EPSPs become shorter, although a late NMDA-mediated component is still evident at VM until P10-15 (Fig. 4). In addition, the multisynaptic multiphasic EPSPs can be orthodromically elicited from P8 to P15 (Fig. 5), due to the relative immaturity of GABA-mediated inhibition, which fails to counteract them effectively (Luhman & Prince, 1991). Fast-firing (FS) putative GABAergic interneurons IB cells can occasionally be recorded.

During the third week NMDA-mediated neurotransmission evolves rapidly toward its mature characteristic (i.e. voltage-dependent Mg^{2+} sensitivity).

Cortical rhythms

In discussing the physiological properties of the neocortex, it should be borne in mind that cortical activities are by no means independent of subcortical, namely thalamic, influences that are particularly relevant to the generation of thalamo-cortical rhythms (e.g. sleep spindles). It has been shown that thalamic rhythmogenesis depends on the reciprocal interaction between thalamic reticular nucleus (Rt) and the other thalamic nuclei projecting to the neocortex (thalamo-cortical nuclei: TC; Mulle *et al.*, 1986; Avanzini *et al.*, 1989). Thanks to a set of Ca^{2+}/K^+ membrane currents Rt neurons are in fact able to generate sequences of bursts-hyperpolarization complexes resulting in membrane rhythmic oscillations that are then transmitted to TC nuclei.

The interaction between Rt and TC depends on their reciprocal interconnections including the GABAergic (inhibitory) Rt-TC projection and the glutamatergic (excitatory) TC-Rt projection established by the axon collaterals of TC neurons. As already said above, the I_T current which is

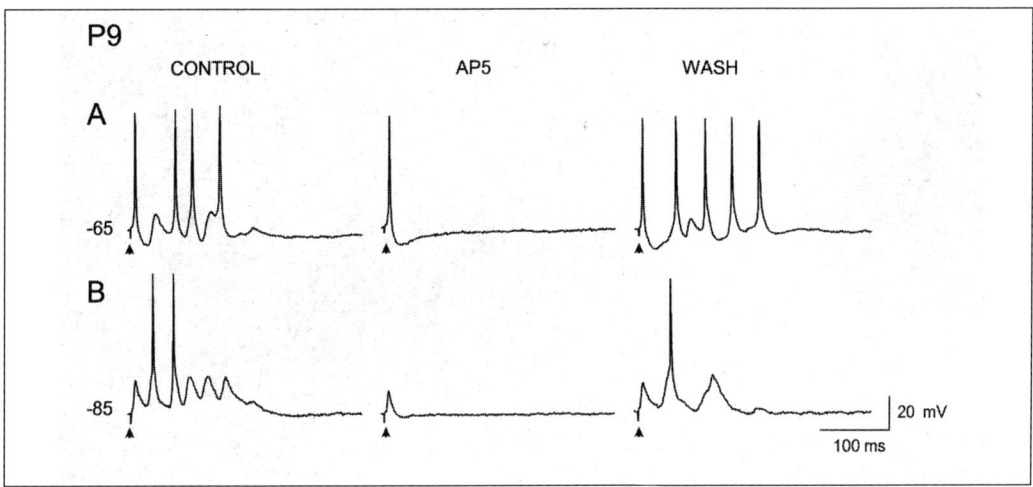

Fig. 5. Multiphasic EPSPs in a P9 rat. Note that the late EPSPs are blocked by APV, demonstrating their NMDA dependency.

responsible for Rt rhythmogenic properties matures during the third postnatal week (Tsakiridou et al., 1995); during the same period the synaptic organization of both TC collaterals to Rt and Rt projection fibres to TC nuclei develops considerably, reaching the adult morphological features by P21 (De Biasi et al., 1996).

Intracortical mechanisms operated by IB and local circuit neurons may also contribute to some extent to generate regional EEG synchronous activities. IB neurons have been shown to generate a strong synchronized output which can recruit a large neuronal population through their arising from GABAergic neurons which are known to contribute to sculpting synchronous discharges. The ineffectiveness of these two synchronizing mechanisms in the immature cortex accounts for the asynchronous erratic character of EEG activities in early infancy.

Age-related etiological factors

Although in symptomatic epilepsy the seizure onset can be considerably delayed with respect to the time of the brain insult, congenital and perinatal brain defects are associated with infantile epilepsies with much higher frequency than with the adult forms (Hauser et al., 1993).

The following pathological conditions are particularly relevant for infantile epilepsies (Volpe, 1995):

(1) Hypoxic-ischemic encephalopathy

(2) Intracranial haemorrhages

(3) Metabolic disturbances

(4) Intracranial infections

(5) Developmental brain abnormalities: cerebral malformations and dysplasias, neurocutaneous syndromes

(6) Genetic disorders.

Hypoxic-ischemic encephalopathy may result from antepartum events (toxemia; maternal hypotension), intrapartum events (traumatic delivery or prolonged labour; acute placental or cord disturbances) or both situations. Postnatal hypoxic insults (severe apnoeic spells or cardiac failure) can be mainly found in premature infants.

Two types of intracranial haemorrhages are mostly involved in the genesis of seizures: germinal matrix-intraventricular and subdural haemorrhages. The germinal matrix-intraventricular haemorrhage is principally a lesion of the premature infant and can occur with or without periventricular (parenchimal) hemorrhagic infarction. The subdural haemorrhage is commonly due to a traumatic event and is usually associated with a cerebral contusion.

Metabolic disturbances most frequently include aberrations in levels of glucose (hypoglycemia), especially in low-birth-weight infants or children of diabetic mothers, and alterations of divalent cations (hypocalcemia and hypomagnesemia). Other causes involve pyridoxine dependency, hyponatremia, disturbances of amino acid and organic acid metabolism, and disorders of glucose transport from blood to brain (Volpe, 1995).

Intracranial infections such as meningitis, encephalitis and abscess may be caused by several bacterial, viral, fungal and protozoan agents. The infant is prone to develop infections during the intrauterine development (CNS infections by viruses, Toxoplasma and Treponema), in association with the birth process (Herpes virus) and in the first postnatal period. Later in childhood, acute encephalitis may occur after exanthematous diseases and immunizations. Rarely subacute encephalitis (e.g. subacute sclerosing panencephalitis) can occur in childhood.

Many developmental brain defects can result in seizures, especially cerebral cortical dysgenesis, related to a disturbance of neuronal migration. These may present a hereditary pattern or be secondary to teratogenic insults from various pathogens during the developmental period (e.g. congenital Cytomegalovirus infection).

Genetic disorders can be associated with distinct syndromes which have epilepsy as a prevalent or secondary component (epileptogenic encephalopathies). Single-gene disorders and multigenic inheritance are also involved in determining 'idiopathic' epilepsies with specific age-related expression during infancy, childhood and adolescence.

Age-dependent susceptibility to epileptogenesis

Passive properties, voltage-dependent current characteristics (on which neuronal firing depends) and receptor-mediated activities in immature neurons concur in making the cerebral cortex particularly susceptible to epileptogenic agents.

The relatively depolarized resting potential present in immature animals holds the neuron close to the threshold for action potential generation; furthermore, the higher membrane resistance to input may act in conjunction with the rather short electrotonic length to amplify incoming depolarizing signals. This tendency is further enhanced by the immaturity of firing properties, i.e. the less effective repolarization following action potential and the delayed maturation of firing frequency adaptation.

In addition, the NMDA-mediated neurotransmission is relatively facilitated due to its incomplete sensitivity to voltage-dependent Mg^{2+} block (Avanzini et al., 1992). Concurrently GABA transmission is poorly effective in earliest stages and tends to induce depolarizing rather than hyperpolarizing IPSPs (Luhman & Prince, 1991).

Age-dependent expression of infantile epilepsies

Two main forms are known to develop in newborns or infants aged less than three months: the *early myoclonus encephalopathy* (EME; Aicardi & Gouthieres, 1978) and the *early infantile encephalopathy with suppression bursts* (EIEE; Ohtahara et al., 1976; Ohtahara, 1978). These two syndromes occur in infants with a severe neurological impairment. Both are associated with the suppression-burst (SB) EEG pattern but present with different types of seizures: mainly spasms in EIEE; partial motor seizures, tonic spasms (uncommon before four to five months of age) and myoclonus in EME, which is therefore particularly relevant to our topic. SB are commonly attributed to a disconnection of the cortex from subcortical (namely thalamic) afferents. This could release an 'idiocortical' rhythmic activity responsible for SB. Alternatively, SB have been suggested to be triggered by brainstem rhythmogenic structures that can influence the cortical activities through direct projections ending in the superficial cortical layers. The brainstem hypothesis for SB pathogenesis is therefore compatible with a cortical disconnection from thalamic structures. In any case, the discontinuous character of SB resulting from high amplitude or rhythmic bursts of cortical activities interspersed by flat EEG correlates very well with the above reported physiological properties of immature cortical neurons. The facilitation of EAA-mediated neurotransmission (due to the incomplete sensitivity to the voltage-dependent Mg^{2+} block of NMDA receptors) and the poor inhibitory effectiveness of GABA transmission (due to GABA depolarizing responses), together with the immaturity of intracortical IB dependent synchronizing mechanisms, would account for the characteristics of the bursts. The remarkable fatiguability of excitatory mechanisms would explain the suppression of the EEG activities following the bursts, which has been shown to reflect on inhibitory status of cortical neurons (Steriade *et al.*, 1994). The thalamo-cortical disconnection may result from different pathological mechanisms including the persistence of primitive spiny neurons in the white matter preventing the thalamic afferents from reaching their cortical target (Spreafico *et al.*, 1993).

West syndrome is often considered as synonymous for infantile spasms (IS), a unique form of seizure disorder occurring in infants during the first year of life. Its usual age of onset is between three and seven months. Spasms consist of sudden bilateral symmetrical or asymmetrical contractions of neck, trunk and arm muscles. They can predominantly involve either flexor or extensor muscle and can be unilateral in 6-8 per cent of the cases. IS are typically associated with the interictal pattern of hypsarrhythmia consisting of a very high-voltage slow EEG activity, irregularly interspersed with spikes and sharp waves occurring randomly in all cortical areas. Atypical patterns include preservation in the awake-EEG. The most common ictal pattern is a high-voltage, frontal dominant generalized slow-wave transient, followed by profound voltage attenuation.

The age range of expression of hypsarrhythmia correlated well with the differentiation of the intracortical synchronizing mechanism provided by IB neurons. The ability of such a subpopulation of layer V pyramidal neurons to recruit large populations of cortical neurons in synchronous activities may account for the generation of high-voltage slow and sharp waves or spikes. The erratic character of hypsarrhythmia is due to the persisting immaturity of projection TC systems capable of a more widespread synchronizing effect of different cortical regions.

As already said, TC projection systems mature after P21 in rats (De Biasi *et al.*, 1996) corresponding to the last part of the second semester of postnatal life in human, but only during the second year of postnatal life does it attain progressively a sufficient degree of maturation to support sustained rhythmic discharges of spikes and waves. This time corresponds to the earlier expression of the *Lennox-Gastaut syndrome* and *myoclonic astatic epilepsy* (Beaumanoir, 1985; Doose, 1985), both characterized by atypical absences, axial tonic, atonic and myoclonic seizures that may occur either in previously normal children or as an evolution of a pre-existing encephalopathy. Both are characterized by diffuse interictal spike-wave complexes which should be less than 2.5 Hz in frequency in the Lennox-Gastaut syndrome (Gastaut *et al.*, 1966) but can be faster in myoclonic astatic epilepsy (Doose, 1985). Doose *et al.*, (1970) also emphasize the interictal pattern of monomorphic parietal theta rhythm as the hallmark of a genetic susceptibility to this form. The ability to generate bilateral synchronous spike-wave activities can be correlated with the progressive maturation of the TC synchronizing system.

Age-related changes in seizure-induced brain damage

A progressive course of an epilepsy leading to intractability of the seizures and to neurological and cognitive deterioration is rather frequently observed. Although the possibility of an evolutionary course of the underlying encephalopathy should always be taken into account, there are evidences that seizures may *per se* induce secondary damages in the brain, thus promoting a progressive course of the neurological disorder. The problem has been intensively studied in the animal model: the most interesting pathogenetic information that can be drawn from chronic models concerns how acute epileptic conditions can induce lesion and seizure-dependent rearrangements of brain circuits that lead to permanent epileptogenic changes. The time course of the experimental epilepsies induced by pilocarpine, tetanus toxin, kainic acid and electrical stimulation has a characteristic profile consisting of an early acute stage, followed by a chronic phase after a more or less prolonged delay. The acute phase terminates with a winding down of the direct effect of the epileptogenic factor or intervening compensatory mechanisms. The degenerative and regenerative events that start during the acute phase and further progress during a latent period eventually lead to the permanent changes in the brain excitability on which the chronic phase depends. The biologic bases of these long-term changes have been particularly studied in the hippocampus and consist of a more or less selective degeneration of hilar cells and the sprouting of dentate granule cell axons. Their epileptogenic role has been suggested on the basis of two different interpretations.

Dormant basket cell hypothesis

The sustained release of excitatory amino acid from granule cell terminals in the hilar region induces an excitatory degeneration of the highly vulnerable population of hilar mossy cells, which normally excite GABA-containing basket interneurons, and mediate granule cell feed-forward and feedback inhibition. Deprived of their major excitatory stimulus, the basket cells become tonically less active and are no longer capable of decreasing granule cell excitability (Sloviter, 1991). This hypothesis is consistent with the above-mentioned observations made in kainic acid and electrical stimulation models, and could account for the permanent hippocampal epileptogenic changes induced by the acute experimental procedures (Sloviter, 1994).

Mossy fibre sprouting and excitatory synaptic reorganization

After the first demonstration of mossy fibre sprouting and recurrent granule cell reinnervation in rats treated with kainic acid (Tauck & Nadler, 1985), similar patterns have been reported in pilocarpine-treated (Cavalheiro *et al.*, 1991) and kindled (Ben-Ari & Represa, 1990) animals. Mossy fiber sprouting has been found to be associated with the monosynaptic re-excitation of granule cells (Tauck & Nadler, 1985; Isokawa & Levesque, 1991) thought to underlie chronic hippocampal seizures (Mathern *et al.*, 1993). Ben-Ari and Represa (1990) have outlined the cascade of events set in motion by a seizure-dependent Ca^{2+} influx into hippocampal neurons involving the activation of immediate-early genes and leading to a dramatic increase in the mRNA of nerve growth factor, which may contribute to seizure-induced mossy fibre sprouting. Newly formed axon collaterals tend to reinnervate the inner molecular layer of the fascia dentata that has been deprived of the projections of the degenerated hilar cells.

Either mechanism (or both) may participate in making dentate granule cells permanently active. It is important to stress the striking similarities between the degenerative/regenerative changes reported in models and those found in hippocampal tissue taken from epileptic patients, thus suggesting that the chronic model is particularly suited to improving our understanding of human temporal lobe epilepsies.

Conclusions

More than two-thirds of human epilepsies begin during childhood and adolescence while the anatomo-functional organization of the brain is still in evolution (Commission on Classification and Terminology of the ILAE, 1989). The high incidence of epilepsy during infancy is partially accounted for by the high frequency of congenital and perinatal risk factors. The peculiar susceptibility of infantile brain to epileptogenic agents should also be taken into account. The immaturity of intrinsic cellular excitable properties and the facilitation of the EAA-mediated neurotransmission, insufficiently counteracted by the immature GABA system in the early postnatal stages, predispose the infantile brain to hyperexcitable events. On the other hand, the fatiguability of the excitatory synaptic transmission, the limitation in discharge duration during sustained stimulation and the immaturity of bursting mechanisms are expected to reduce the probability of highly synchronized sustained discharges. This may explain the fragmentary erratic character of epileptic discharges in the epilepsies of the first year of life.

The issue of a potential harmful effect of epileptic discharges on the developing brain is a controversial one. The experimental results have shown the immature brain to be more protected against seizure-induced brain damage. It needs to be considered however that even subtle brain damages may have a crucial negative impact on the intellectual and behavioural functions in a critical period such as the developmental one. Moreover the additional negative effect of antiepileptic drugs should also be taken into account (Holmes, 1997).

Further studies may contribute to the clarification of this point as well as other poorly understood aspects of infantile epilepsies, namely the delayed onset of idiopathic epilepsies suggesting that the underlying genetically determined defect requires some additional developmentally regulated factors for its clinical expression.

Acknowledgements
The editorial assistance of Metella Paterlini is gratefully acknowledged.

References

Aicardi, J. & Gouthieres, F. (1978): Encéphalopatie myoclonique néonatale. *Rev. EEG Neurophysiol* **8**, 99–101.

Alzheimer, C., Schwindt, P.C. & Crill, W.E. (1993): Postnatal development of a persistent sodium current in pyramidal neurons from rat sensorimotor cortex. *J. Neurophysiol.* **69**, 290–292.

Avanzini, G., Franceschetti, S., Panzica, F. & Buzio, S. (1992): Age-dependent changes in excitability of rat neocortical neurons studied in vitro. In: Molecular neurobiology of epilepsy, eds. J. Engel, C. Wasterlain, A. Cavalheiro, U. Heinemann & G. Avanzini. *Epilepsy Res.* **(Suppl.) 9**, 95–105.

Avanzini, G., De Curtis, M., Panzica, F. & Spreafico, R. (1989): Intrinsic properties of nucleus reticularis thalami neurons of the rat studied in vitro. *Journal of Physiology* **416**, 111–133.

Azouz, R., Jensen, M.S. & Yaari Y. (1996): Ionic basis of spike after-depolarization and burst generation in adult rat hippocampal CA1 pyramidal cells. *Journal of Physiology* **492**, 211–223.

Beaumanoir, A. (1985): The Lennox-Gastaut syndrome. In: *Epileptic syndromes in infancy, childhood and adolescence*, eds. J. Rogers, C. Dravet, M. Bureau, F.E. Dreifuss & P. Wolf, pp. 89–99. London: John Libbey.

Ben-Ari, Y., & Represa, A. (1990): Brief seizures episodes induce long-term potentiation and mossy fibre sprouting in the hippocampus. *Trends Neurosci.* **13**, 312–318.

Cavalheiro, E.A., Leite, J.P., Bortolotto, Z.A., Turski, W.A., Ikonomidou, C. & Turski L. (1991): Long-term effects of pilocarpine in rats: structural damage of the brain triggers kindling and spontaneous recurrent seizures. *Epilepsia* **32**, 778–782.

Commission on *Classification and Terminology of the International League Against Epilepsy* (1989): Proposal for revised classification of epilepsy and epileptic syndromes. *Epilepsia* **30**, 389–99.

Connors, B.W. & Gutnick, M.J. (1990): Intrinsic firing patterns of diverse neocortical neurons. *Trends Neurosci* **13**, 99–104.

De Biasi, S., Amadeo, A., Arcelli, P., Frassoni, C., Meroni, A. & Spreafico, R. (1996): Ultrastructural characterization of the postnatal development of the thalamic ventrobasal and reticular nuclei in the rat. *Anat. Embryol.* **193**, 341–353.

Doose, H. (1985): Myoclonic astatic epilepsy of early childhood. In: *Epileptic syndromes in infancy, childhood and adolescence*, eds. J. Rogers, C. Dravet, M. Bureau, F.E. Dreifuss & P. Wolf, pp. 78–88. London: John Libbey.

Doose, H., Gerken, H., Leohardt, R., Volzke, E. & Volz, C. (1970): Centrencephalic myoclonic-astatic petit mal. *Neuropediatrie* **4**, 162–171.

Eayers, J.T. & Goodhead, B. (1959): Postnatal development of the cerebral cortex of the rat. *J. Anat.* **93**, 385–402.

Feldman, M. & Peters, A. (1978): The forms of non-pyramidal neurons in the visual cortex of the rat. *J. Comp. Neurol.* **179**, 761–794.

Franceschetti, S., Buzio, S., Sancini, G., Panzica, F. & Avanzini, G. (1993): Expression of intrinsic bursting properties in neurons of maturing sensorimotor cortex. *Neurosci. Lett.* **162**, 25–28.

Franceschetti S., Guatteo E., Panzica F, Sancini G., Wanke E., & Avanzini G. (1995): Ionic mechanisms underlying burst firing in pyramidal neurons: intracellular study in rat sensorimotor cortex. *Brain Res.* **696**, 127–139.

Franceschetti, S., Panzica, F., Sancini, G. & Avanzini, G. (1997): Postnatal neocortical development: maturational changes in the intrinsic properties of pyramidal neurons and their possible significance for epileptogenesis. In: *Molecular and cellular targets for anti-epileptic drugs*, eds. G. Avanzini, G. Regesta, P. Tanganelli & M. Avoli, pp. 79–87. London: John Libbey.

Franceschetti, S., Sancini, G., Panzica, F., Radici, C. & Avanzini, G. (1998): Postnatal differentiation of firing properties and morphological characteristics in layer V pyramidal neurons of the sensorimotor cortex. *Neurosci.* **83 (4)**, 1013–1024.

Fukuda, A., Mody, I. & Prince, D.A. (1992): Postnatal development of electrogenic sodium pump acivity in rat hippocampal pyramidal neurons. *Dev. Brain Res.* **65**, 101–114.

Gastaut, H., Roger, J., Soulayrol, R., Tassinari, C., Régis, H., Dravet, C., Bernard, R., Pinsard, N. & Saint-Jean, M. (1966): Childhood epileptic encephalopathy with diffuse slow spike-waves (otherwise known as petit mal variant) or Lennox syndrome. *Epilepsia* **7**, 139–179.

Hauser, W.A., Annegers, J.F. & Kurland, L.T. (1993): Incidence of epilepsy and unprovoked seizures in Rochester, Minnesota: 1935–1984. *Epilepsia* **34 (3)**, 453–468.

Holmes, G.L. (1997): Epilepsy in the developing brain: lessons from the laboratory and clinic. *Epilepsia* **38 (1)**, 12–30.

Huguenard, J.R., Hamill, O.P. & Prince, D.A. (1988): Developmental changes in Na^+ conductances in rat neocortical neurons: appearance of a slowly inactivating component. *J. Neurophysiol.* **59**, 778–795.

Innocenti, G.M. (1986): General organization of callosal connections in the cerebral cortex. In: *Sensory-motor areas and aspects of cortical connectivity.* Cerebral cortex, Vol. 5, eds. E.G. Jones & A. Peters, pp. 291–353. New York: Plenum Press.

Isokawa, M. & Levesque, M.F. (1991): Increased NMDA responses and dendritic degeneration in human epiteptic hippocampal neurons in slices. *Neurosci. Lett.* **132**, 212–216.

Kang, J., Huguenard, R. & Prince, A. (1996): Development of BK channels in neocortical pyramidal neurons. *J. Neurophysiol.* **76**, 188–198.

Klee, R., Ficher, E. & Heinemann, U. (1995): Comparison of voltage-dependent potassium currents in rat pyramidal neurons acutely isolated from hippocampal regions CA1 and CA2. *J. Neurophysiol.* **74**, 1982–1995.

Kriegstein, A.R., Suppes, T. & Prince, D.A. (1987): Cellular and synaptic physiology and epileptogenesis of developing rat neocortical neurons in vitro. *Dev. Brain Res.* **34**, 161–171.

Lorenzon, N.M. & Foehring, R.C. (1995): Characterization of pharmacologically identified voltage-gated calcium channel currents in acutely isolated rat neocortical neurons. II. Postnatal development. *J. Neurophysiol.* **73**, 1443–1451.

Lorenzon, N.M. & Foehring, R.C. (1993): The ontogeny of repetitive firing and its modulation by norepinephrine in rat neocortical neurons. *Dev. Brain Res.* **73**, 213–223.

Luhman, H.J., & Prince, D.A. (1991): Postnatal maturation of the GABAergic system in rat neocortex. *J. Neurophysiol.* **65**, 247–263.

Mares, P. (1991): Epileptic phenomena in the immature brain. *Physiol. Res.* **40**, 577–584.

Mathern, G.W., Cifuentes, F., Leite, J.P., Pretorius, J.K. & Babb, T.L. (1993): Hippocampal EEG excitability and chronic spontaneous seizures are associated with aberrant synaptic reorganization in the rat intrahippocampal kainate model. *Electroencephalogr. Clin. Neurophysiol.* **87**, 326–339.

Mattia, D., Hwa, G.G.C. & Avoli, M. (1993): Membrane properties of rat subicular neurons in vitro. *J. Neurophysiol.* **70**, 1244–1248.

McCormick, D.A. & Prince D.A. (1987): Post-natal development of electrophysiological properties of rat cerebral cortical pyramidal neurons. *J. Physiol.* **393**, 743–762.

Miller, M. (1981): Maturation of rat visual cortex. III. Postnatal morphogenesis and synaptogenesis of local circuit neurons. *Dev. Brain Res.* **25**, 271–285.

Miller, M.W. (1988): Development of projection and local circuit neurons in neocortex. In: *Cerebral cortex, Vol. 7, Development and maturation of cerebral cortex*, eds. A. Peters & E.G. Jones, pp. 133–175. New York: Plenum Press.

Miller, M. & Peters, A. (1981): Maturation of rat visual cortex. II. A combined Golgi-electron microscope study of pyramidal neurons. *J. Comp. Neurol.* **203**, 555–573.

Mulle, C., Madariaga, A. & Deschines, M. (1986): Morphology and electrophysiological properties of reticularis thalamai neurons in cat: in vivo study of a thalamic pacemaker. *J. Neurosci.* **6**, 2134–2145.

Ohtahara, S. (1978): Clinico-electrical delineation of epileptic encephalopathies in childhood. *Asian Med. J.* **21**, 7–17.

Ohtahara, S., Ishida, T., Oka, E., Yamatogi, Y., Inique, H., Ohtsuka, Y. & Kanda, S. (1976): On the age-dependent epileptic syndromes: the early infantile encephalopathies with suppression-bursts. *Brain Dev.* **8**, 270–288.

Parnavelas, J.G., Bradford, R., Mounty, E.J. & Lieberman, A.R. (1978): The development of non-pyramidal neurons in the visual cortex of the rat. *Anat. Embryol.* **155**, 1–14.

Peters, A. & Feldman, M. (1973): The cortical plate and molecular layer of the late rat foetus. *Z. Anat. Entwicklungsgesch.* **141**, 3–37.

Rice, F.L., Gomez, C., Barstow, C., Burnet, A. & Sands, P. (1985): A comparative analysis of the development of the primary somatosensory cortex: interspecies similarities during barrel and laminar development. *J. Comp. Neurol.* **236**, 477–495.

Sloviter, R.S. (1991): Permanently altered hippocampal structure, excitability and inhibition after experimental status epilepticus in the rat "dormant basket cell" hypothesis and its possible relevance to temporal lobe epilepsy. *Hippocampus* **1**, 41–66.

Sloviter, R.S. (1994): The functional organisation of the hippocampal dentate gyrus and its relevance to the pathogenesis of temporal lobe epilepsy. *Ann. Neurol.* **35**, 640–654.

Spreafico, R., Angelini, L., Binelli, S., Granata, T., Rumi, V., Rosti, D., Runza, L. & Bugiani, O. (1993): Burst suppression and impairment of neocortical ontogenesis: Electroclinical and neuropathologic findings in two infants with early myoclonic encephalopathy. *Epilepsia* **24**, 800–808.

Stafstrom, C.E., Schwindt, P.C., Chubb, M.C. & Crill, W.E. (1985): Properties of persistent sodium conductance and calcium conductance of layer V neurons from cat sensorimotor cortex in vitro. *J. Neurophysiol.* **53**, 153–170.

Steriade, M., Amzica, F. & Contreras, D. (1994): Cortical and thalamic cellular correlates of electroencephalographic burst suppression. *Electroencephalogr. Clin. Neurophysiol.* **90**, 1–16.

Tauck, D. & Nadler, J.V. (1985): Evidence of functional mossy fiber sprouting in hippocampal formation of kainic acid-treated rats. *J. Neurosci.* **5**, 1016–1022.

Tsakiridou, E., Bertollini, L., De Curtis, M., Avanzini, G. & Pape, H.C. (1995): Selective increase in T-type calcium conductance of reticular thalamic neurons in a rat model of absence epilepsy. *J. Neurosci.* **15**(4), 3110–3117.

Volpe, J.J. (1995): Neonatal seizures. In: *Neurology of the newborn*. pp. 172–202. New York: Saunders.

Wise, S.P. & Jones, E.G. (1976): The organisation and postnatal development of the commissural projection to the somatic sensory cortex of the rat. *J. Comp. Neurol.* **168**, 313–344.

Wise, S.P. & Jones, E.G. (1978): Developmental studies of thalamocortical and commissural connections in the rat somatic sensory cortex. *J. Comp. Neurol.* **178**, 187–208.

Zona, C., Pirrone, G., Avoli, M. & Dichter, M. (1988): Delayed and fast transient potassium currents in rat neocortical neurons in cell cultures. *Neurosci. Lett.* **94**, 285–290.

Chapter 6

Mechanisms of corticogenesis: cell proliferation and death in the developing human central nervous system

Alessandro Simonati, Cinzia Tosati, Elena Piazzola* and Nicolò Rizzuto

Dipartimento di Scienze Neurologiche e della Visione – Sezione di Neurologia Clinica, Ospedale Policlinico Borgo Roma, 37134 Verona, Italy
*Servizio di Anatomia Patologica, Università di Verona, Verona, Italy

Summary

Growth and maturation of the cerebral cortex is a complex event which is under the control of several genes, some of them showing specific morphogenetic functions. Key steps of corticogenesis occur in the pseudostratified epithelium of the ventricular zone, such as the molecular control of cell proliferation and number, cell commitment and timing of cell type specification; even more after the last mitotic round neurons leave the ventricular zone and migrate to the cortical plate along radial glia guides. Cell proliferation and death are the morphogenetic events that determine the number of neurones in the cortical plate. Epigenetic mechanisms seem to modulate them in the ventricular zone, whereas the selective mechanisms that control the number of neurones by regulating cell proliferation and death during the later stages of corticogenesis are not yet fully defined. In humans a sharp decline of cell proliferation in the ventricular zone is observed by the 15th week of gestation corresponding to the end of the second neuronal migratory wave. Cell proliferation is completed in the ventricular zone soon after mid-gestation, whereas lower numbers of mitotic cells are detected in the intermediate zone and the subplate until its end. Apoptotic cell death is recognized in the transient compartments of the telencephalic wall during the same periods. The amount of genetic events related to CNS morphogenesis accounts for the increasing evidence of a genetic origin of several conditions associated with disturbances of corticogenesis. Moreover the prolonged duration of these processes during gestation in humans is related to the vulnerability of the developing brain to extrinsic noxious agents. The effects of these insults can be either destructive lesions, or cytoarchitectonic disturbances related to an epigenetic negative effect on the deployment of the genetic programmes necessary for corticogenesis to occur properly.

General principles of CNS development

Development of the vertebrate Central Nervous System (CNS) occurs through an ordered sequence of temporally and spatially related morphogenetic events. Following neural induction, neural tube expansion occurs along its antero-posterior axis, forming the spinal cord posteriorly. From its expanded anterior end the different vesicles originate, which are the anlagen for the forebrain, midbrain and hindbrain. These early steps of CNS organogenesis are under the control of genes which show position-specific expression, and predict the regional specialization (Davis & Joyner, 1988; Gruss & Walther, 1992; Simeone *et al.*, 1992; Shimamura *et al.*, 1995). Thus, early development of the CNS occurs according to region-specific patterning, such as segmentation in the transverse domain in the hindbrain and spinal cord (Lumsden & Krumlauf, 1996). Regionalization of the most anterior parts of the forebrain (from which the telencephalon takes origin) is still a matter of discussion. According to some authors a segmental compartmentalization in metameric units (prosomeres) is suggested, as the result of patterning along the anterior-posterior and medial-dorsal axes, which generate longitudinally aligned domains (Rubenstein *et al.*, 1994; Shimamura & Rubenstein, 1997). On the other hand, it is suggested that the telencephalon is a single field, subdivided longitudinally into two subregions, the anlagen of the cortex and striatum, which express different regulatory genes, located either in the dorsal or in the ventral domains (Xuan *et al.*, 1995; Lumsden & Krumlauf, 1996). Patterning of the developing CNS is also associated with the histogenetic specification of distinct neuroanatomical primordia, which is a crucial process for the later acquisition of anatomical and functional identities by the CNS regions. The specification of histogenetic primordia is a necessary step to the deployment of the genetic programmes which regulate the morphogenetic events underlying the anatomical and functional growth of the CNS compartments. That occurs by regulating the duration of region-specific cell proliferation and death, by determining the lineage specification and cell differentiation, and eventually regulating the migratory steps which are necessary for the cytoarchitectonic organization of the distinct neuroanatomical regions (Fig. 1). Later on, target-recognition by the ingrowing axons is the fundamental event that leads to the establishment of the connections among CNS structures, the framework through which the different grey nuclear components and the cortical compartments can dialogue to fulfil the functional requirements of the nervous system.

Each of the above mentioned morphogenetic steps occurs within a species-related time span during embryonic and foetal development, and its duration is somehow related to the length of gestation. In humans most of them take place and are concluded by the end of the sixth gestational month, whereas in other mammalian species they are concluded after birth.

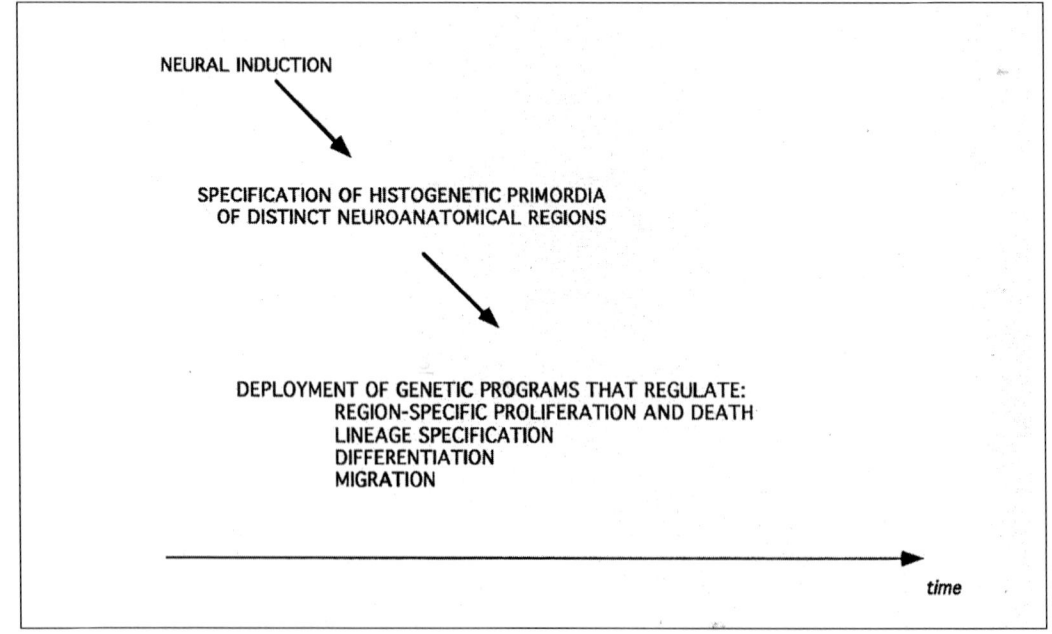

Fig. 1. Sequence of major morphogenetic events during the early stages of CNS development

Table 1. List of known genetically determined cortical malformations in humans and rodents, as well as of transgenic animals bearing disturbances of corticogenesis

Chromosome	Gene	Protein product	Function	Pathology	References	
Human						
7q36	Sonic Hedgehog	Secretory protein	CNS patterning	Holoprosencephaly	Roessler et al.	(1996)
???	EMX-2 (homeobox)	???	CNS patterning	Schizencephaly	Brunelli et al.	(1996)
17p13	LIS-1	PAF-Acetylhydrolase (G-Protein-like)	Neuronal differentiation; axonal guidance	Lissencephaly	Renier et al.	(1993)
Xq22	???	???	???	"Double cortex" Lissencephaly	Eksioglu et al.	(1996)
Xq28	???	???	???	Periventricular nodular heterotopia	Dobyns et al.	(1996)
Rodent						
Mutant						
Small Eye (mouse) 2	PAX-6	Transcription factor (homeobox)	CNS Patterning	Cortical malformation	Schmahl et al.	(1993)
Scrambled (mouse) 4	mDab-1	Cytoplasmic protein	Protein–protein interactions	Abnormal lamination	Ware et al.	(1997)
Reeler (mouse) 5	Reeler	Extracellular matrix glycoprotein	Neuronal migration; axonal growth	Abnormal lamination	D'Arcangelo et al.	(1995)
Tish (rat) ???	???	???	???	Neuronal heterotopia	Lee et al.	(1997)
'Knock out'						
—	p35	???	Cdk5 activation	Abnormal lamination	Chae et al.	(1997)
—	OTX-1 (homeobox)	???	CNS patterning	Abnormal lamination	Acampora et al.	(1996)
—	DLX-1 DLX-2	Transcription factors (homeobox)	Phenotypic specification?	Striatal abnormalities	Anderson et al.	(1997a)
—	BF-1	Transcription factor	Control of cell proliferation	Telencephalon size reduction	Xuan et al.	(1995)
—	CPP32	ICE-Protease	Apoptosis	Abnormal lamination	Kuida et al.	(1996)

A second round of morphogenetic processes during CNS development, however, is concluded after birth even in higher mammalian species, including humans. It deals with the events which lead to the acquisition of the phenotypic properties of mature neuronal and glial cells, to the ensheathing of axonal tracts by the myelin (myelination), to the establishment of the appropriate number of synapses, and to refine the definite number of neurones and axons. It was shown that in humans (Huttenlocher & de Courten, 1987) and in monkeys synaptic density is higher in infancy than in adulthood, and that in Rhesus monkey synaptogenesis takes place synchronously in different cortical areas until puberty, before declining (Rakic et al., 1986). On the contrary, myelination occurs asynchronously in the different fibre tracts during both pre-natal and post-natal development (Yakovlev & Lecours, 1967). That is in accordance with the temporal gradient of expression of the different neurofunctional competences, which indeed reflects the full maturation of the related axonal tracts.

Implications on morphogenetic disturbances of the human CNS

The complexity of cellular events occurring during prenatal CNS development makes it particularly vulnerable to a large number of adverse conditions during its ontogenesis. The high number of genetically related developmental steps explains why gene alterations represent a frequent cause of abnormalities during CNS growth. The outcome of this condition might be a null result, implying such a destructive effect that it is not compatible with the survival of the embryo (spontaneous abortion and/or stillbirth). On the other hand the outcome can be a vital foetus (or newborn) with a brain malformation. The genetic basis of several conditions related to specific patterns of CNS developmental abnormalities has been recently demonstrated both in rodents and humans (Table 1). This can help elucidate the pathogenetic mechanisms leading to the developmental abnormalities of the CNS, and moreover it has obvious implications for genetic counselling on these diseases. Extrinsic factors (either of maternal origin, or from the outer environment) may also interfere with the deployment of the genetic programme, and therefore abnormal morphogenesis of the developing CNS may be the result of altered gene functions by an epigenetic mechanism. A dramatic example was observed in humans, following *in utero* exposure to atomic blasts in Japan. One of the effects of exposure of pregnant women (during the first trimester of gestation) to atomic radiation was the birth of a microcephalic baby whose brain showed thinned cortex and massive neuronal ectopia in the periventricular region. This was ascribed to both the death of radiation-sensitive proliferating cells and to the impaired migration of those that survived (Yokota et al., 1961). Steps of brain development are characterized by a highly intense cellular activity, requiring a large energy consumption. It follows that impairment of the main energy source, such as oxidative metabolism, or of other metabolic pathways, can give origin to cellular dysfunctions which can affect important processes of brain maturation, as seen in some inherited metabolic disorders (Bohm, et al., 1982; Powers et al., 1989; Michotte et al., 1993). That is particularly true for proliferating cells, which need high oxygen consumption, and which therefore are particularly vulnerable to hypoxia and/or ischemia. And it has been known for a long time that hypoxic-ischemic insults can account for cytoarchitectonic abnormalities, such as polymicrogyria, if foetal CNS is affected when neuronal migration and cortical lamination are still in progress. Recent evidence has shown that hypoxia is a powerful agent to diverge proliferating cells to the apoptotic cycle (Jacks & Weinberg, 1996). It may therefore follow that hypoxic-ischemic insults can lead to tissue necrosis as a result of the impaired perfusion and oxygen deprivation; furthermore this same condition may also drive proliferating cells to die by the apoptotic pathway, leading to the reduction in size of the developing brain.

Advances in the knowledge of the molecular and cellular mechanisms leading to brain morphogenesis have recently found a tremendous counterpart in high resolution, neuroimaging techniques, such as Magnetic Resonance Imaging. The acquisition of precise neuroradiological images (and their correlations with detailed clinical findings) has revealed that neocortical malformations are much more common than expected. Taken together, advances in cell biology and *in vivo* imaging of brain development have allowed the formulation of a new classification of malformations of cortical development, according to the recognized disturbance of a corticogenetic event (Barkovich et al., 1996). This has also provided new insights into the knowledge of the relationship between disturbances of corticogenesis and epilepsy.

Cell proliferation, migration and death during corticogenesis

Over the last decade, several experimental papers have been published that have detailed out the process of cortical mantle development at molecular and cellular levels. Our attention will focus on the issues of cell proliferation and death, and precursor cell differentiation during corticogenesis, reviewing recent data on this subject and presenting results from observations performed on CNS specimens of human foetuses. In vertebrate CNS, the main site where proliferation occurs is the pseudostratified epithelium lining the lumen of the ventricular cavities (ventricular zone). A further transient structure of the telencephalic wall where relevant amounts of cell proliferation take place is the adjacent subventricular zone. The ventricular epithelium contains a mosaic of proliferating cells whose fate is somehow determined by their genetic programme; in this region key steps in neurogenesis occur, such as molecular control of cell number, cell commitment and cell type specification (Rakic, 1988; McConnell, 1995).

Autoradiographic studies have been utilized to track the movements of the progenitor cells during the cell cycle. Replication of DNA during the S-phase is accomplished in the outer (basal) third of the ventricular zone; in the G2-phase, nuclei translocate to the luminal (apical) surface, where they divide. Prior to the onset of neurogenesis, mitoses occur symmetrically: both daughter cells re-enter the cell cycle, replenishing the pool of progenitor cells. Later on, asymmetric divisions are observed: one of the daughter cells re-enters the cycle, whereas the post-mitotic cell migrates away from the proliferative zone. The orientation of the mitotic cleavage is then suggested to predict the behaviour of the progenitor cells. Recently, refined experiments using time-lapse confocal microscopy of fluorescent-labelled cortical progenitors have demonstrated that cleavage planes of the mitotic cells actually predict the kind of cell division (Chenn & McConnell, 1995). Horizontal cleavage was related to asymmetric division, the basal cell daughter being committed to migrate and differentiate into a neuron. On the other hand, cells dividing along the vertical plane give origin to two daughter cells which remain attached to the ventricular surface, probably continuing to proliferate. Recent studies of the proliferative events in the ventricular zone have examined the parameters which predict the total number of neurones to be generated and the rate at which they are formed (Caviness et al., 1995; Takahashi et al., 1996). Results from these investigations have shown that the proliferative activity is changing over time. Early in neurogenesis the number of cells that leave the proliferative cycle is relatively low, whereas the number of cells that continue to proliferate remains high: that is, associated with the rapid expansion of the proliferative epithelium. It was also shown that the duration of the cell cycle, and therefore the output of daughter cells, seems regulated by the progression in the length of the G1-phase of the cycle. Different functional classes of molecules, which control the pattern of division and the fate of cortical precursors in the proliferative epithelium, have been described, such as a membrane-associated protein (*Numb*), and a trans-membrane receptor which mediates cell-cell interactions (*Notch-1*; Chenn & McConnell, 1995; Zhong et al., 1997). Differential distribution of both *Notch-1* (to the basal daughter cell) and *Numb* (to the apical daughter cell) during a horizontal asymmetric division seems to determine the fate of each daughter cell (see Fig. 2). Therefore epigenetic influences in the ventricular epithelium modulate both progenitor cell proliferation and neuronal differentiation during mammalian corticogenesis.

After the final cell division, postmitotic neurones leave the ventricular zone and migrate outwards through the telencephalic wall toward the pial surface and form the cortical plate. The time of origin of the progenitor cells and the clone to which they belong will predict the laminar location in the cortical mantle where post-mitotic neurones will migrate along the radial glia guides. That is carried out according to an inside-out gradient, the first generated cells being committed to locate the deepest cortical layers (Kornack & Rakic, 1995; Rakic et al., 1996). The duration of this pro-

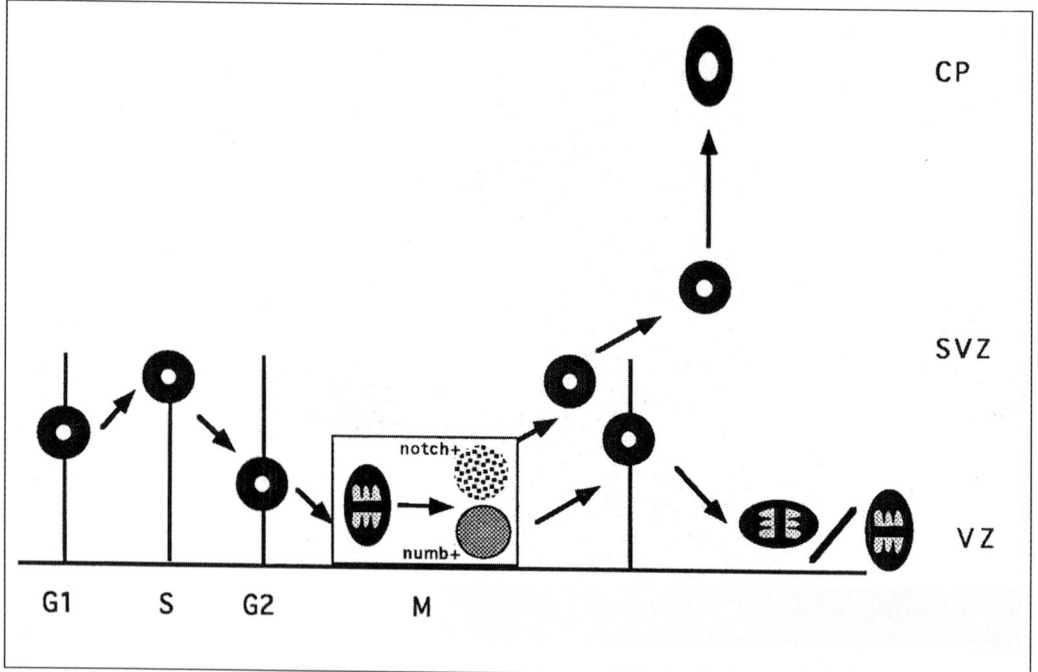

Fig. 2. *Molecular influences on the pattern of cell division in the proliferative epithelium. Ventricular cell nuclei undergo interkinetic migration during the cell cycle. Asymmetric cell division occurs (M) when differential distribution of Notch-1 and numb occurs between the daugter cells. Inheritance of Notch-1 leads the basal cell to migrate to the cortical plate (CP), whereas the apical cell which has high numb activity remains as a progenitor in the ventricular zone (VZ) and re-enters the cycle. The opposite occurs during symmetric division when both daughter cells inherit high levels of numb, inhibiting Notch-1 activity, and therefore they re-enter the mitotic cycle. (Modified by Chenn & McConnell, 1995 and Zhong et al., 1997.)*

cess varies according to the different species, and it is longer in higher mammals. Neuronal migration occurs asynchronously in different cytoarchitectonic areas, which implies that simultaneously generated neurones occupy different cortical layers, probably due to the specific cues they meet along their way to the cortical plate (Rakic, 1974). Neuronal migration and commitment to reach the proper location are modulated in the subplate, a transient structure of the telencephalic wall, which is prominent in primates and humans. It consists of neurones and of a dense network of cell processes, such as axons and dendrites. Based on its developing stages, it has been suggested that the subplate plays a role in the specification of the cortical plate, by providing local cues to the ingrowing axons from subcortical nuclei, before they reach the specific layer (Kostovic & Rakic, 1990). As suggested by the tangential dispersion of clonally related cells by retroviral lineage studies (Walsh & Cepko, 1992), and confirmed by direct observations *in vivo* as well as on *in vitro* preparations, post-mitotic neurones can migrate tangentially (Rakic, 1995; O'Rourke et al., 1997). Even if the precise significance of this pattern of migration has not been fully defined yet, there is some evidence that this mechanism can be used by distinct neuronal population in several CNS regions (Anderson et al., 1997b).

The number of post-mitotic cells during CNS development is refined by a genetically determined regressive process, the naturally occurring cell death, which is recognized as a prominent developmental event of the vertebrate neurogenesis (Cowan et al., 1984). Morphologically it is characterized by specific features of the nuclei, such as chromatine condensation, membrane blebbing and apoptotic bodies formation; it is also named apoptosis (Clarke, 1990). Based on its time of occurrence during the stages of CNS maturation, two functionally distinct types of cell death have been indicated, which share however similar morphological and biochemical features (Thomaidou *et al.*, 1997). 'Proliferative'cell death is observed in the ventricular epithelium, during the early stages of development, and the simultaneous occurrence of both proliferation and apoptosis in some cell populations has suggested that the two processes may be related. Indeed, evidence has been provided that cell death occurs soon after the phase of DNA replication during the S-phase, in the G1-phase of the cycle (Thomaidou *et al.*, 1997); furthermore it was shown that some molecules act at key points during the cascade of events leading to either processes (Ross, 1996). It was also suggested that signals by the interstitial environment may play an epigenetic role on the fate of precursor cells, either to proliferate or to die. Results from *in vitro* studies have shown that extrinsic factors from the extra-cellular environment may regulate cellular proliferation, and they can drive replicating cells to either differentiate or to the apoptotic pathway (Howard *et al.*, 1993).

Later in development, cell death has been observed in well established anatomical areas: in these cases it has been related to the lack of availability of trophic factors or of functional inputs (such as synaptic activity) which are necessary to the survival of post-mitotic, mature elements ('target-related' cell death; Oppenheim, 1991). Apoptotic cells have been observed both in transient structures of the developing nervous system (such as the proliferative ventricular and subventricular zones), or to a lesser extent in the cortical plate by the end of foetal growth (Ferrer *et al.*, 1992). The number of dying cells in the proliferating epithelium, as evidenced by classical and histochemical (such as the TUNEL method, see below) techniques is always low, probably due to the rapid course of the apoptotic cycle. To have a good estimate of the extent of the process it is therefore necessary to compare the figures of dying cells with the number of cells which are in the particular phases of the mitotic cycle, given the known duration of each phase. Recent data have shown that during the early stages of the proliferative activity in the ventricular epithelium low percentages of dying cells (as compared to the dividing progenitors) are seen, whereas these numbers are increasing at the later stages, when the actual number of proliferating cells is decreasing (Thomaidou *et al.*, 1997). The early occurrence of programmed cell death during corticogenesis suggests that by this mechanism the post-mitotic cells in the ventricular zone that are uncommitted to differentiate and/or migrate are eliminated. The presence of apoptotic cells in the more dorsally located transient structures of the telencephalic wall also suggests that post-mitotic cells can be eliminated by programmed cell death, either as neurones uncommitted to reach the cortical plate or as glial cell precursors unselected to further differentiate.

Cell proliferation and death during corticogenesis in human foetal CNS

Studies on corticogenesis in the human brain are relatively rare for practical reasons, such as the difficulties of obtaining human tissue suitable to be processed for molecular and cellular studies. Moreover, ethical arguments prevent *in vitro* studies on living foetal samples of CNS, to study the cellular events during corticogenesis. Classical papers, however, are available which analysed large collections of human embryos utilizing anatomical techniques and described the main maturative events of the developing CNS (Lemire *et al.*, 1975; Marín-Padilla, 1988; Sidman & Rakic, 1982; O'Rahilly & Muller, 1994). More recently the availability of specific probes has allowed further information to be gained on cellular differentiation and specification during CNS maturation, even on fixed tissue.

In higher mammals, including primates and humans, cell proliferation is completed at about mid-gestation; it mainly occurs in the ventricular zone, where precursor cells divide asynchronously from the 6th week of gestation in humans (Rakic & Sidman, 1968). Following symmetric division both daughter cells re-enter the cell cycle, whereas after asymmetric division one of the cells gets out and can either differentiate or start to migrate. Cell differentiation has been demonstrated in the ventricular zone of the cerebral hemispheres and by the 9/10th week of gestation markers for glial cells can be recognized (Choi, 1986; Wilkinson *et al.*, 1990). Another transient structure where intense proliferative activity is recognized is the subventricular zone; it has been proposed that it generates late-born, local circuit neurones, and at later stage, glial cells (Rakic, 1982). Cell proliferation is also present in the intermediate zone and in the subplate, two transient structures of the telencephalic wall. In these regions mitotic cells are observed until the end of gestation, and the proliferating elements are suggested to be glial cell precursors, committed either to astrocyte differentiation or to oligodendrocyte formation (Kendler & Golden, 1996).

Due to the scarce number of pyknotic and apoptotic cells detectable with classic histological methods, there were few studies on the topographic distribution of the process of cell death during CNS development in humans. After the introduction of a combined method that allows the recognition of the early stages of the apoptosis morphologically (TUNEL method; Gavrieli et al., 1992), it was possible to better examine this process on fixed tissue. In a recent study on developing human brain, the topography of cell death was examined in the telencephalic wall of the human CNS, and it was confirmed that 'proliferative' cell death occurs in the same transient structures where cell proliferation is observed, sparing however the cortical plate (Simonati et al., 1997).

To obtain an estimate of the amount of cell proliferation in the developing human CNS, we have performed a quantitative study of selected anatomical specimens (full thickness of the dorsal telencephalic wall from both the anterior and the posterior regions of the cerebral hemispheres) from human foetuses, obtained either following therapeutic abortions or as stillborns. The gestational age of foetuses ranged between the 10th and the 24th week. Inclusion criteria were the absence of cerebral malformations as well as the lack of evidence of any CNS lesion following neuropathological examination. Proliferating cells were examined by combining histological analysis (to evaluate the M-phase of the cell cycle) with PCNA (a marker of the S-phase of the cell cycle) immunohistochemistry. It was confirmed that cell proliferation is markedly evident in both ventricular and subventricular zones. In the ventricular zone mitotic elements are lined along the ventricular wall, showing different orientation of the mitotic spindle (Fig. 3). Quantitative analysis revealed that the highest density PCNA positive cells, i.e. labelled during the longest stage of the mitosis, is observed by the 15th week of gestation, followed by a sharp decline of their number. Positive elements, however, can be still observed at later observations. The decline of PCNA labelled cells occurs synchronously in both frontal and occipital germinal zones. These events are accompanied by a progressive reduction of the volume of both proliferative regions, along with an increasing thickness of the cortical plate and the subplate. A steady increase of proliferating cells is observed in both the intermediate zone and the subplate. The number of proliferating cells, however, is always relatively low and its peak of density is about 13% of the labelled nuclei in the proliferative ventricular zones. The origin of these precursor cells is still debated. Recent evidence, however, has shown that in the intermediate zone, cells can re-enter the mitotic activity following a stand-by period in the G0-phase of the cycle. It can be therefore assumed that cells which have ceased to proliferate in the ventricular zone can stop during their migration at their definite location and re-enter the cycle before differentiating. The topography of these late proliferating elements suggests that at least some of these cells differentiate into glial lineages, to give origin either to astrocytes or to oligodendrocytes, and then to participate in the process of myelination, which at these ages is in progress in the hemispheric white matter (Yakovlev & Lecours, 1967). It is not known by which mechanisms precursor cells reach the transient structures of the telencephalic wall where they start proliferating, but several lines of evidence suggest that they do not move along radial guides. It would be interesting to see whether neurones, leaving the ventricular zone tangentially, and therefore without radial glia guidance, can re-enter the cycle along their route to the definite location (Rakic, 1995; O'Rourke et al., 1997). No evidence has been provided of PCNA labelled in the cortical plate at any examined age. In our opinion these data confirm that post-mitotic neurones only reach the cortical plate, and that once the fate of a neuron has been determined and the proper location in the cortical layer of progenitor cells specified, it cannot re-enter the cycle.

The process of cell death was also examined in the same regions at the same developmental ages, utilizing histological techniques and the TUNEL method. The number of labelled cells was also low, as compared to the PCNA positive ones (Fig. 4). At the earliest stages they were observed in

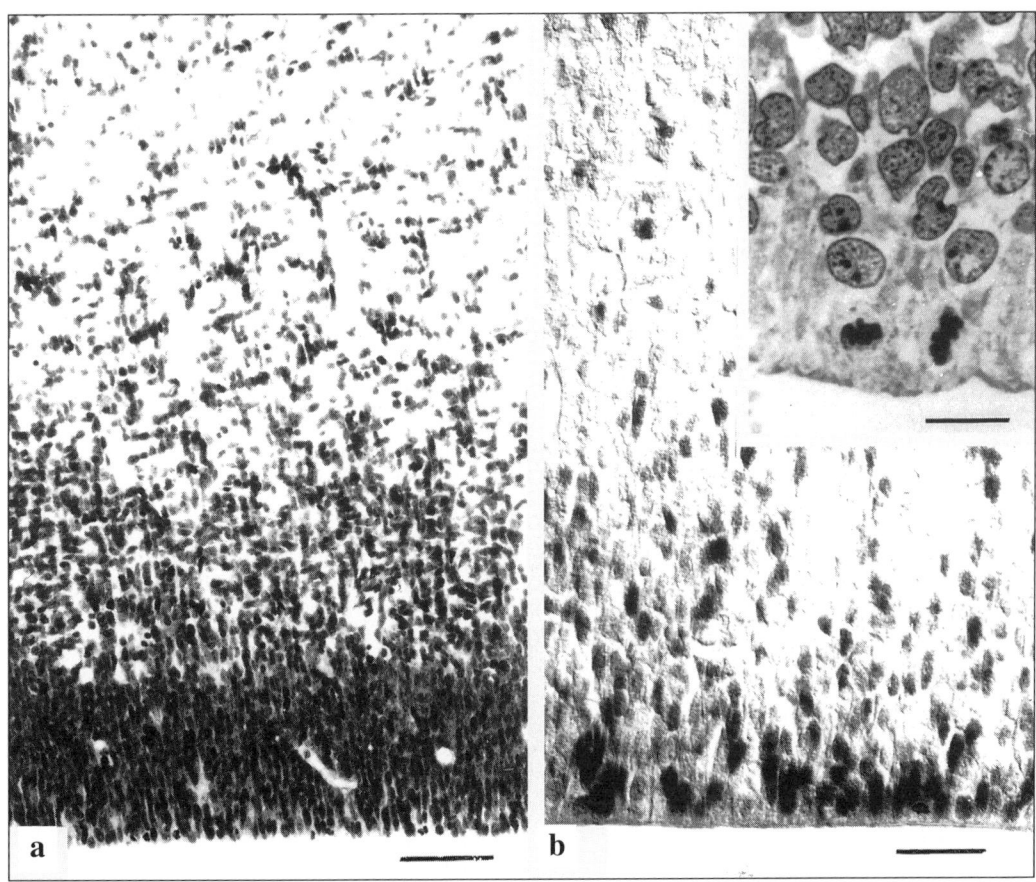

Fig. 3. Patterns of cell proliferation in the telencephalic wall of the human CNS. (a) Anterior region: densely packed cells of the ventricular zone; several mitoses can be recognized on the luminal surface; decreased cell density in the more dorsal subventricular zone; spare cells nuclei in the intermediate zone/subplate (upper half of the figure). 12 week foetus; Nissl stain. Bar=50 µm. (b) Posterior region: labelling of proliferating cells (S-phase) in both apical and basal portions of the ventricular zone, as well as in the subventricular zone. 12 week foetus; PCNA immunohistochemistry. Bar=20 µm. Inset: mitotic fuse arranged according to either parallel or vertical planes of cleavage in two proliferating cells of the ventricular zone. 18 week foetus; Toluidine blue stain (resin embedded sections). Bar=10 µm.

the ventricular epithelium, and later sparse labelled cells could be detected also in the intermediate zone and subplate; no labelled cells were seen in the cortical plate. Thus, cell death occurs through the transient structures of the developing telencephalic wall, and the topography of the apoptotic cells appears to be related to the changing distribution of the mitotic ones. This confirms previous experimental data that mitosis and cell death can be considered as two opposite processes during the proliferative stages of the corticogenesis. These results are also in accordance with experimental studies which showed low absolute figures of cells undergoing the process (Ferrer *et al.*, 1992; Thomaidou *et al.*, 1997). Labelling was observed in the post-mitotic cells of the ventricular and subventricular zones, as recognized by their histological appearance. We cannot rule out, however, that even proliferating cells can leave the mitotic cycle, and enter the death pathway. Indeed, the concurrent thickening of the more dorsal portions of the telencephalic wall, particularly of the subplate and cortical plate, and the progressive reduction in size of the ventricular neuroepithelium suggest that most of the cells which have left the proliferation have migrated away, and that they have not died by programmed cell death. The significance of apoptotic cells in the intermediate zone and in the subplate is still obscure, but a few hypotheses can be put forward. It may represent a mecha-

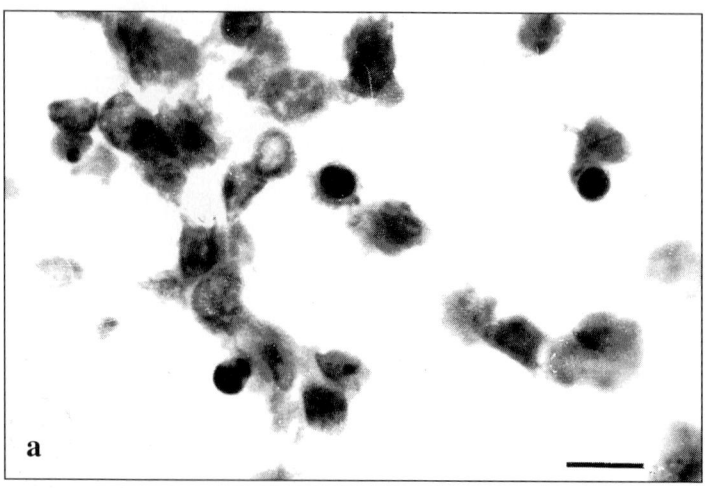
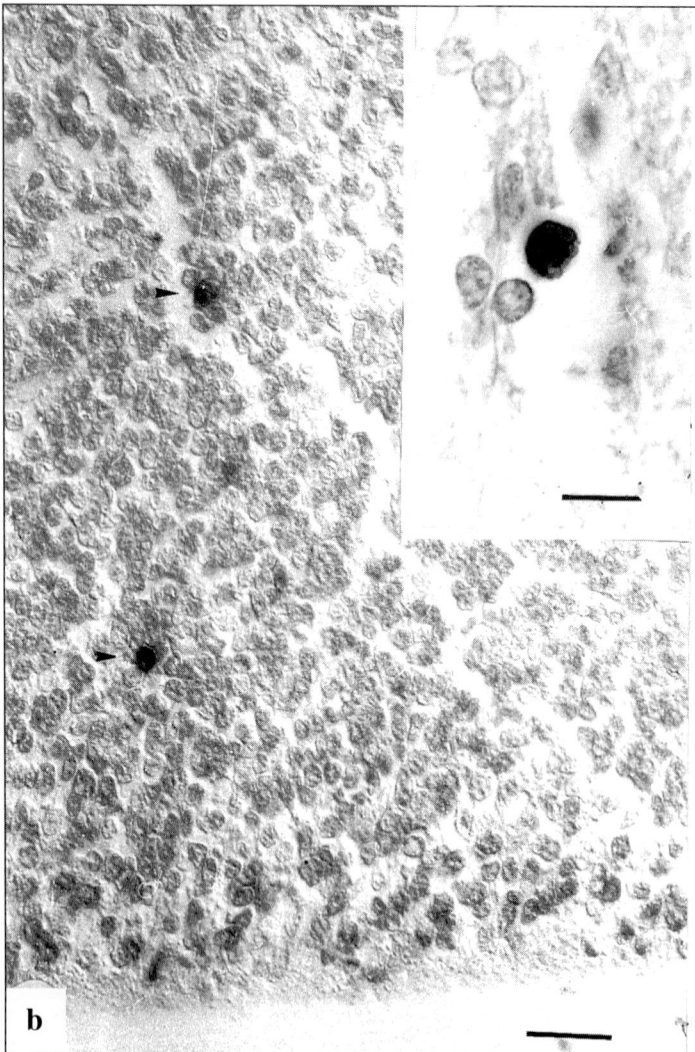

Fig. 4. Patterns of cell death in the telencephalic wall of the human CNS. (a) Chromatine condensation and apoptotic bodies in the ventricular zone. 10 week foetus; HE stain. Bar=10 μm. (b) Posterior region: two apoptotic nuclei in the ventricular zone (arrowheads). 13 week foetus; TUNEL method. Bar=20 μm. Insert: DNA fragmentation (condensed chromatine stage) in the intermediate zone. 21 week foetus; TUNEL method. Bar=10 μm.

nism to select the number of cells which are committed to differentiate into glial lineages, or to refine the number of neurones which will definitively settle in the cortical plate. This probably occurs in the subplate during the long stationary stage (20-35th week of gestation), when it reaches the largest size and ingrowing axons seem to stand by to be 'instructed' before reaching the proper target. If laminar position and cortical specificity of differentiated neurones are indeed determined very early during development, still in the ventricular zone (Rakic, 1988; McConnell, 1995), mechanisms of selection can exist along the pathway for post-mitotic neurones to reach their appropriate location in the cortex.

Concluding remarks

In developing human CNS the decline in the density of proliferating cells by the 15th week of gestation occurs synchronously in both the anterior and posterior ventricular zones. Accordingly, the simultaneous shrinkage of the ventricular epithelium and increasing thickness of subplate and cortical plate may be ascribed to the migration of the post-mitotic neurones, which is completed by this age (Sidman & Rakic, 1982). These findings are in agreement with the suggestion that genetic mechanisms which control the timing and number of cell divisions work synchronously all over the ventricular zone. In fact, homogeneous and diffuse reduction in size of the forebrain growth is observed in mouse-carrying homozygous null mutation for BF-1, a gene which codes for a transcription factor expressed specifically in telencephalic neuroepithelium, where it seems to regulate the rate of cell proliferation and the timing of neuronal differentiation (Xuan *et al.*, 1995). Furthermore, the length of the cell cycle of proliferating cells is overlapping in the ventricular zones of distinct telencephalic compartments, which again outlines the homogeneity of cell proliferation all over the proliferative neuroepithelium (Cai *et al.*, 1997). Increasing density of PCNA positive cells in both the intermediate zone and subplate, even at the latest observation (24th week of gestation), indicates that in these compartments the proliferation of presumed precursors of glial cells lasts longer than in the ventricular epithelium. The presence of apoptotic cells in the telencephalic wall during the stages of cell proliferation accounts for the importance of cell death to refine the number of cells committed to further differentiation. The relevance of this mechanism, possibly underestimated in human post-mortem fixed tissue (Blaschke *et al.*, 1996), in the pathogenesis of CNS malformations is however confirmed by the evidence that impairment of normally occurring cell death by homologous recombination in mice leads to major abnormalities of the structural organization over all the brain (Kuida *et al.*, 1996).

In this paper, features of the genetic control during CNS development, namely corticogenesis, have been reviewed. Either gene coding for transcription factors, and acting as regulatory molecules of DNA expression, or gene coding for protein involved in specific cell functions during development have been recognized to be affected in human CNS malformations as well as in mutant animals (Table 1). Moreover the evidence of prolonged duration of maturative events during human gestation accounts for the protracted risk of exposure to several noxae, such as hypoxia-ischemia, radiation, drugs and toxic agents. These elements can either cause destructive lesions to the foetal tissue, or exert adverse influence by an epigenetic mechanism, thus interfering with the deployment of the genetic programme involved in CNS development. When the processes of cell proliferation and/or death are affected, severe malformations can result, such as microcephaly or microlissencephaly. In general, however, the outcome is a disturbance of corticogenesis, namely of cytoarchitectonic organization, often associated with severe neurological symptoms in humans, such as seizures, mental retardation and motor function impairment.

Acknowledgement

This work was partly supported by MURST 1997.

References

Acampora, D., Mazan, S., Avantaggiato, V., Barone, P., Tuorto, F., Lallemand, Y., Brulet, P. & Simeone, A. (1996): Epilepsy and brain abnormalities in mice lacking Otx1 gene. *Nature Gen.* **14**, 218–222.

Anderson, S.A., Qiu, M., Bulfone, A., Eisenstat, D.D., Meneses, J., Pedersen, R. & Rubenstein, J.L.R. (1997a): Mutations of the homeobox genes *Dlx-1* and *Dlx-2* disrupt the striatal subventricular zone and differentiation of late born striatal neurones. *Neuron* **19**, 27–37.

Anderson, S.A., Eisenstat, D.D., Shi, L. & Rubenstein, J.L.R. (1997b): Interneuron migration from basal forebrain to neocortex: dependence on *Dlx* genes. *Science* **278**, 474–476.

Barkovich, A.J., Kuzniecky, R.I., Dobyns, W.B., Jackson, G.D., Becker, L.E. & Evrard, P. (1996): A classification scheme for malformations of cortical development. *Neuropediatrics* **27**, 59–63.

Blaschke, A.J., Staley, K. & Chun, J. (1996): Widespread programmed cell death in proliferative and postmitotic regions of the foetal cerebral cortex. *Development* **122**, 1165–1174.

Bohm, N.U., Uy, J., Kiessling, M. & Lehnert, W. (1982): Multiple acylCoA dehydrogenase deficiency (glutaric aciduria type II), congenital polycystic kidneys and symmetric warty dysplasia of the cerebral cortex in two newborn brothers. II. Morphology and pathogenesis. *Eur. J. Pediatr.* **139**, 60–65.

Brunelli, S., Faiella, A., Capra, V., Nigro, V., Simeone., A., Cama, A. & Boncinelli, E. (1996): Germline mutations in the homeobox gene EMX2 in patients with severe schizencephaly. *Nature Genet.* **12**, 94–96.

Cai, L., Hayes, N.L. & Nowakowski, R.S. (1997): Local homogeneity of cell cycle length in developing mouse cortex. *J Neurosci.* **17**, 2079–2087.

Caviness Jr, V.S., Takahashi, T. & Nowakowski, R.S. (1995): Numbers, time and neocortical neuronogenesis: a general developmental and evolutionary model. *Trends Neurosci.* **18**, 379–383.

Chae, T., Kwon, Y.T., Bronson, R., Dikkes, O., Li, E. & Tsai, L.-H. (1997): Mice lacking p35, a neuronal specific activator of Cdk5, display cortical lamination defects, seizures, and adult lethality. *Neuron* **18**, 29–42.

Chenn, A. & McConnell, S.K. (1995): Cleavage orientation and the asymmetric inheritance of Notch-1 immunoreactivity in mammalian neurogenesis. *Cell* **82**, 631–641.

Choi, B.H. (1986): Glial Fibrillary Acidic Protein in radial glia of human foetal cerebrum: a light and electron microscopic immunoperoxidase study. *J. Neuropath. Exp. Neurol.* **45**, 408–418.

Clarke, P.G.H. (1990): Developmental cell death: morphological diversity and multiple mechanisms. *Anat. Embryol.* **181**, 195–213.

Cowan, W.M., Fawcett, J.W., O'Leary, D.D.M. & Stanfield, B.B. (1984): Regressive events in neurogenesis. *Science* **225**, 1258–1265.

D'Arcangelo, G., Miao, G.G., Chen, S.-C., Soares, H.D., Morgan, J.I. & Curran, T. (1995): A protein related to extracellular matrix proteins deleted in the mouse reeler. *Nature* **374**, 719–723.

Davis, C. A. & Joyner, A.L. (1988): Expression paterns of the homeobox-containing gene En1 and En2 and the protooncogene int-1 during mouse development. *Genes Dev.* **2**, 1736–1744.

Dobyns, W.B., Andermann, E., Andermann, F., Czapansky-Beilman, D., Dubeau, F., Dulac, O., Guerrini, R., Hirsch, B., Ledbetter, D.H., Lee, N.S., Motte, J., Pinard, J.-M., Radtke, R.A., Ross, M.E., Tampieri, D., Walsh, C.A. & Truwit, C.L. (1996): X-linked malformations of neuronal migration. *Neurology* **47**, 331–339.

Eksioglu, Y.Z., Scheffer, I.E., Cardenas, P., Knoll, J., Di Mario, F., Ramsby, G., Berg, M., Kamuro, K., Berkovic, S.F., Duyk, M., Parisi, J., Huttenlocher, P.R. & Walsh, C.A. (1996): Periventricular heterotopia: an X-linked dominant epilepsy locus causing aberrant cerebral cortical development. *Neuron* **16**, 77–87.

Ferrer, I., Soriano, E., Del Rio, J.A., Alcantara, S. & Auladell, C. (1992): Cell death and removal in the cerebral cortex during development. *Prog. Neurobiol.* **39**, 1–43.

Gavrieli, Y., Sherman, Y. & Ben-Sasson, S.A. (1992): Identification of programmed cell death in situ via specific labelling of nuclear DNA fragmentation. *J. Cell. Biol.* **119**, 493–501.

Gruss, P. & Walther, C. (1992): Pax in development. *Cell* **69**, 719–722.

Howard, M.K., Linksey, C.B., Mailhos, C., Pizzey, A., Gilbert, C.S., Lawson, W.D., Colling, M.K.L., Thomas, N.S.B. & Latchman, D. (1993): Cell cycle arrest of proliferating neuronal cells by serum deprivation can result in either apoptosis or differentiation. *J. Neurochem.* **60**, 1783–1791.

Huttenlocher, P.R. & deCourten, C. (1987): The development of synapses in striate cortex of man. *Hum. Neurobiol.* **6**, 1–9.

Jacks, T. & Weinberg, R.A. (1996): Cell-cycle control and its watchman. *Nature* **381**, 643–644.

Kendler, A. & Golden, J.A. (1996): Progenitor cell proliferation outside the ventricular and subventricular zones during human brain development. *J. Neuropath. Exp. Neurol.* **55**, 1253–1258.

Kornack, D.R. & Rakic, P. (1995): Radial and horizontal deployment of clonally related cells in the primate neocortex: relationship to distinct mitotic lineage. *Neuron* **15**, 311–321.

Kostovic, I. & Rakic, P. (1990): Developmental history of the transient subplate zone in the visual and somatosensory cortex of the macaque monkey and human brain. *J. Comp. Neurol.* **297**, 441–470.

Kuida, K., Zheng, T.S., Na, S., Kuan, C., Yang, D., Karasuyama, H., Rakic, P. & Flavell, R.A. (1996): Decreased apoptosis in the brain and premature lethality in CPP32-deficient mice. *Nature* **384**, 368–372.

Lee, K.S., Schottler, F., Collins, J.L., Lanzino, G., Couture, D., Rao, A., Hiramatsu, K-I, Goto, Y, Hong, S.-C., Caner, H., Yamamoto, H., Chen, Z.-F., Bertram, E., Berr, S., Omary, R., Scrable, H., Jackson, T., Goble, J. & Eisenman, L. (1997): A genetic animal model of human neocortical heterotopia associated with seizures. *J. Neurosci.* **17**, 6236–6242.

Lemire, R.J., Loeser, J.D., Leech, R.W. & Alvord Jr., E.C. (1975): *Normal and Abnormal Development of the Human Nervous System.* New York: Harper & Row.

Lumsden, A. & Krumlauf, R. (1996): Patterning the vertebrate neuraxis. *Science* **274**, 1109–1115.

Marín-Padilla, M. (1988): Early ontogenesis of the human cerebral cortex. In: *Cerebral cortex, Vol. 7, Development and maturation of the cerebral cortex*, eds. A. Peters and E.G. Jones, pp. 1–34. New York: Plenum Press.

McConnell, S.K. (1995): Constructing the cerebral cortex: Neurogenesis and fate determination. *Neuron* **15**, 761–768.

Michotte, A., De Meirleir, L., Lissens, W., Denis, R., Wayenberg, J.L., Liebaers, I. & Brucher, J.M. (1993): Neuropathological findings of a patient with pyruvate dehydrogenase E1 alpha deficiency presenting as a cerebral lactic acidosis. *Acta Neuropathol.* **85**, 674–678.

Oppenheim, R.W. (1991): Cell death during development of the nervous system. *Ann. Rev. Neurosci.* **14**, 453–501.

O'Rahilly, R. & Muller, F. (1994): *The embryonic human brain. An atlas of developmental stages.* New York: Wiley.

O'Rourke, N.A., Chenn, A. & McConnell, S.K. (1997): Postmitotic neurones migrate tangentially in the cortical ventricular zone. *Development* **124**, 997–1005.

Powers, J.M., Tummons, R.C., Caviness Jr., V.S., Moser, A.B. & Moser, H.W. (1989): Structural and chemical alterations in the cerebral maldevelopment of foetal cerebro-hepato-renal (Zellweger) syndrome. *J. Neuropathol. Exp. Neurol.* **48**, 270–289.

Rakic, P. (1974): Neurones in the monkey visual cortex: systemic relation between time of origin and eventual disposition. *Science* **183**, 425–427.

Rakic, P. (1982): Early developmental events: cell lineages, acquisition of neuronal positions, and areal and laminar development. *Neurosci. Res. Prog. Bull.* **20**, 439–445.

Rakic, P. (1988): Specification of cerebral cortical areas. *Science* **241**, 170–176.

Rakic, P (1995): Radial versus tangential migration of neuronal clones in the developing cerebral cortex. *Proc. Natl. Acad. Sci. USA* **92**, 11323–11327.

Rakic, P. and Sidman R.L. (1968): Supravital DNA synthesis in developing human and mouse brain. *J. Neuropathol. Exp. Neurol.* **27**, 246–276.

Rakic, P., Bourgeois, J.-P., Eckenhoff, M.E., Zecevic, N. & Goldman-Rakic, P. (1986): Concurrent overproduction of synapses in diverse regions of the primate cerebral cortex. *Science* **232**, 232–235.

Rakic, P., Cameron, R.S. & Komuro H. (1994): Recognition, adhesion and transmembrane signalling in guided neuronal cell migration. *Curr. Opin. Neurobiol.* **4**, 63–69.

Renier, O., Carrozzo, R., Shen, Y., Wehnert, M., Faustinella, F., Dobyns, W.B., Caskey, C.T. & Ledbetter, D.H. (1993): Isolation of a Miller-Dieker lissencephaly gene containing G protein-subunit-like repeats. *Nature* **364**, 717–721.

Roessler, E., Belloni, E., Gaudenz, K., Jay, P., Berta, P., Scherer, S.W., Tsui, L.C. & Muenke, M. (1996): Mutations in the human Sonic Hedgehog gene cause holoprosencephaly. *Nature Genet.* **14,** 357–360.

Ross, M. (1996): Cell division and the nervous system: regulating the cycle from neural differentiation to death. *Trends Neurosci.* **19,** 62–68.

Schmahl, W., Knoedlseder, M., Favor, J. & Davidson, D. (1993): Defects of neuronal migration in the pathogenesis of cortical malformations are associated with Small eye (Sey) in the mouse, a point mutation at the Pax-6-locus. *Acta Neuropathol.* **86,** 126–135.

Shimamura, K. & Rubenstein, J.L.R. (1997): Inductive interactions direct early regionalization of the mouse forebrain. *Development* **124,** 2709–2718.

Shimamura, K., Hartigan, D.J., Martinez, S., Puelles, L. & Rubenstein, J.L.R. (1995): Longitudinal organization of the anterior neural plate and neural tube. *Development* **121,** 3923–3933.

Sidman, R.L. & Rakic, P. (1982): Development of the human central nervous system. In: *Histology and histopathology of the nervous system,* eds. W. Haymaker & R.D. Adams. pp. 3–145 Springfield, IL: Charles C. Thomas.

Simeone, A., Acampora, D., Gulisano, M., Stornaiuolo, A. & Boncinelli E. (1992): Nested expression domains of four homeobox genes in developing rostral brain. *Nature* **358,** 687–690.

Simonati, A., Rosso, T. & Rizzuto, N. (1997): DNA fragmentation in normal development of the human central nervous system: a morphological study during corticogenesis. *Neuropathol. Appl. Neurobiol.* **23,** 203–211.

Takahashi, T., Nowakowski, R.S. & Caviness Jr., V.S. (1996): The leaving or Q fraction of the murine cerebral proliferative epithelium: a general model of neocortical neuronogenesis. *J. Neurosci.* **16,** 6183–6196.

Thomaidou, D., Mione, M.C., Cavanagh, J.F.R. & Parnavelas, J.G. (1997): Apoptosis and its relation to the cell cycle in the developing cerebral cortex. *J. Neurosci.* **17,** 1075–1085.

Yakovlev, P.I. & Lecours, A.R. (1967): The myelogentic cycles of regional maturation of the brain. In: *Regional development of the brain in early life,* ed. A. Minkowski, pp. 3–70. Oxford: Blackwell.

Yokota, S., Tagowa, D., Tsura, S.O., Nakayama, K., Neriishi, S., Namiki, H. & Hirose, K. (1961): Microcephaly in an *in vitro* survivor: an autopsy case. *Nagasaki Tgaki Zushi* **38,** 92–95.

Walsh, C. & Cepko, C.L. (1992): Widespread dispersion of neuronal clones across functional regions of the cerebral cortex. *Science* **255,** 434–440.

Ware, M.L., Fox, J.W., Gonzalez, J.L., Davis, N.M., Lambert de Rouvroit, C., Russo, C.J., Chua, S.C. Jr., Goffinet, A.M. & Walsh, C.A. (1997): Aberrant splicing of a mouse disabled homolog, mdab1, in the scrambler mouse. *Neuron* **19,** 239–249.

Wilkinson, M., Hume, R., Strange, R. & Bell, J.E. (1990): Glial and neuronal differentiation in the human foetal brain 9–23 weeks of gestation. *Neuropathol. Appl. Neurobiol.* **16,** 193–204.

Xuan, S., Baptista, C.A., Balas, G., Tao, W., Soares, V.C. & Lai, E. (1995): Winged helix transcription factor BF-1 is essential for the development of the cerebral hemispheres. *Neuron* **14,** 1141–1152.

Zhong, W. Ming-Ming, J., Weinmaster, G., Jan, L.Y. & Jan, Y.N. (1997): Differential expression of mammalian Numb, Numblike and Notch1 suggests distinct roles during mouse cortical neurogenesis. *Development* **124,** 1887–1897.

Chapter 7

Preferential impairment of motor and somatosensory cortices in two murine models of human diseases: the ethanol-exposed rat and the dystrophic mdx mouse

Diego Minciacchi, Maria Laura Santarelli, Donatella Carretta, Riccardo Carrai, Alberto Granato[1] and Francesco Pinto

Dipartimento di Scienze Neurologiche e Psichiatriche, Università di Firenze, Viale Morgagni 85, 50134 Florence, Italy and [1]Istituto di Anatomia, Università Cattolica di Roma, Largo Francesco Vito 1, 10168 Rome, Italy.

Summary

The cortices of two rodents in which the development of central nervous structures is altered by completely different injuries are described and compared. In the first experimental paradigm on rats, the abnormal development is achieved by prenatal administration of ethanol to reproduce a situation mimicking the human Foetal Alcohol Syndrome. Adult animals received thalamic injections of an axonal tracer to study the corticothalamic circuitry. The second experimental paradigm is represented by the mutant mdx mice which lack dystrophin expression and are the acknowledged model for the human Duchenne Muscular Dystrophy. Brains of adult mdx mice were processed immunohistochemically to characterize the cortical expression of selected calcium-binding proteins.

The study of the cortices in these two rodents reveals important similarities, in spite of the different nature of the primary damage. The cortical response to an abnormal development appears not uniformly distributed through the cortical mantle, but rather involves some fields and spares some others. Furthermore, in both animals the impairment is evident on motor and somatosensory cortices whereas the other areas are less or not involved. The conclusion can be drawn that motor and somatosensory fields appear more susceptible than non-sensori-motor areas to insults that occur during the process of developmental modelling.

Introduction

The structural and functional maturation of the cerebral cortex is realized through a series of stages which follow each other in precise sequential order during prenatal and early postnatal life. Milestones of this delicate operation are the distinct gradients of cortical neurogenesis, the intermittent invasion of the cortical plate by ingrowing afferent fibres, and the fine tuning of early established circuits (Bayer & Altman, 1991; McConnell, 1995). The intricate progression of events leading to mature subcortico-cortical, cortico-cortical, and cortico-fugal connections necessarily implies intermediate phases of reshaping. These temporary structural configurations appear to express developmental frames of transient functional significance (Minciacchi & Granato, 1988, 1989; McConnell et al., 1989; Antonini & Shatz, 1990; Friauf et al., 1990; Meinecke & Rakic, 1992).

Most of the dynamic changes occurring in the cortical circuits during maturation can be affected by a wide range of factors. With this in mind, several experimental protocols have been realized and studied in the search for information on normal development and pathological key events of brain teratology (Hicks et al., 1959; Altman & Anderson, 1972; Jones et al., 1982).

Here we describe and compare the cortical alterations of two rodents in which brain development is impaired as a result of completely different injuries. In one case, the rats are exposed to ethanol during prenatal life to mimic the human Foetal Alcohol Syndrome (Clarren & Smith, 1978). In the other case, mdx mice, as consequence of spontaneous mutation, lack expression of dystrophin and are model for human Duchenne Muscular Dystrophy (Bulfield et al., 1984; Torres & Duchen, 1987; Sicinski et al., 1989).

The first experimental paradigm we refer to is represented by the rat prenatally exposed to ethanol. Previous investigations on ethanol-exposed rats have demonstrated specific damages of several nervous structures including, in particular, the cerebral cortex (see, for review, Jones, 1988; West & Goodlett, 1990). Changes involve the distribution of cortico-spinal cells, the arrangement of cortical synapses and the morphology of pyramidal neurones (Inomata et al., 1987; Miller, 1987b; Miller et al., 1990). We focused on the thalamo-cortical and cortico-thalamic circuits of adult rats exposed to ethanol during the last week of gestation, a critical period for cortical and thalamic neurogenesis, and for the shaping of thalamo-cortical connections (Wise & Jones, 1978; Altman & Bayer, 1979; Van Eden, 1986; Minciacchi & Granato, 1988, 1989). We found specific contraction and aberrant location of the thalamic recipient region in the cortex and reduction of neuropil staining in the thalamus. These structural alterations led us to affirm that the damage is predominantly localized on terminal arborizations of thalamo-cortical and cortico-thalamic axons (Minciacchi et al., 1993; Granato et al., 1995).

The second experimental model we discuss is the mutant mdx mouse. This animal actually represents the most investigated model of Duchenne Muscular Dystrophy since it possesses an analogous X-linked genetic alteration preventing dystrophin expression in muscle fibres and central nervous system neurones (Hoffman et al., 1987; Torelli et al., 1992; Lidov et al., 1993; Uchino et al., 1994). We analyzed extensively the brain of these animals and we found evident but localized structural alterations of central motor pathways. The cortico-spinal neurones are reduced in number by about 50 per cent and appear morphologically altered, as are the rubro-spinal projecting neurones; conversely, the motor neurone populations in the spinal cord are apparently normal (Carretta et al., 1995; Minciacchi et al., 1995; Sbriccoli et al., 1995). To further investigate the cortical damage in mdx mice we studied the distribution of cell populations marked by selected calcium-binding proteins (CBPs). CBPs are low molecular weight acid proteins that buffer Ca^{2+} ions or trigger the activity of various enzymes upon binding Ca^{2+}. These proteins have often been used as markers for specific neuronal subsets and are known to modify their expression pattern as a result of developmental perturbations (Braun, 1990; Celio, 1990; Cellerino et al., 1992). We present here preliminary results from the study of the cortical expression of calbindin-D28k (CB) and parvalbumin (PV) (Santarelli et al., 1995).

During the different steps of analyses performed in our laboratory, we were intrigued by certain relevant similarities of data obtained from experiments on the above two animal models. The impression that a differential structure-dependent ability interacts with various prenatal insults to result in a preferential topographic involvement, prompted us to further compare and analyze our findings. The present report is thus concentrated on the description and comparison of some cortical fields in ethanol-exposed rats and mutant mdx mice.

Materials and methods

Tract tracing experiments on ethanol-exposed rats

To obtain accurate evaluation of gestational period, nulligravid rats were mated at night and the presence of vaginal plug on next day indicated conception (gestational day one). From gestational day 14 to 19, pregnant rats were given intragastric boles of a 20 per cent w/v aqueous solution of ethanol by acute gavage. The total daily amount (2.4 g/kg) was subdivided into four administrations (8:00 and 11:00 a.m., 2:00 and 5:00 p.m.). From gestational day 17 to 19, before the early morning administration, and on gestational day 20, fourteen hours after the last administration, animals were observed for signs of withdrawal syndrome according to the criteria of Majchrowicz (1975); animals not fulfilling withdrawal criteria were discarded. A second group of control rats received, during the same gestational period and with the same schedule of administration, equal volumes of an isocaloric solution containing sucrose. These animals served as control for nutritional deficits and for stress associated with intubation. Rats exposed to ethanol were fed a diet of rat chow and water *ad libitum*; control rats were fed the average volume of water and weight of chow consumed by ethanol-fed rats of corresponding gestational age. After delivery, offspring of ethanol-exposed and control rats were allowed to be suckled by their own mothers.

When 2 months old, both ethanol-exposed and control animals received injections of a 7.5 per cent aqueous solution of wheat germ agglutinin-horseradish peroxidase (Sigma). To label the cell body of cortico-thalamic neurones and the fibres and terminals of thalamo-cortical axons the animals were anaesthetized with Nembutal (40 mg/kg) and the tracer injections were performed stereotaxically in the thalamus (injected volume 0.05 µl; Bregma co-ordinates: A-P = -2.3 mm, D-V = 6.5 mm, Lat = 1.6 mm; according to atlas by Paxinos & Watson, 1986). Forty-eight hours later, injected animals were perfused with phosphate buffered saline followed by 2.5 per cent buffered glutaraldehyde; brains were then dissected out and soaked overnight in 30 per cent buffered sucrose. Forty µm thick coronal sections were cut on freezing microtome from frontal pole to mesencephalon. For the study of labelling in the cortex, every third section was incubated with tetramethylbenzidine, according to the procedure by Mesulam (1978). Adjacent sections were counterstained with thionin for cytoarchitectonic analysis. Some thalamic sections containing the needle track were incubated with diaminobenzidine for evaluation of injection areas (Graham & Karnowsky, 1966). Sections were mounted on slides, dehydrated, and coverslipped. Material was studied under light- and dark-field illumination.

Immunohistochemical experiments on mdx mice

In order to study the CBPs expression in the cortex, mdx and control C57 BL/6 mice were anaesthetized with Nembutal (40 mg/kg) and perfused transcardially with phosphate buffered saline, followed by buffered fixative solution containing four per cent paraformaldheyde. Brains were dissected out, placed in the same fixative solution for two hours, and immersed overnight in 30 per cent buffered sucrose at 4°C. Brains were then cut on freezing microtome into 40 µm thick coronal sections which were subdivided into three series and stored free-floating in buffered saline. Two series were immunohistochemically reacted for expression of PV and CB. To suppress non-specific binding, sections designated for immunohistochemical reaction were incubated with three per cent normal serum in phosphate buffered saline containing 0.3 per cent Triton X-100. The two series of sections were incubated with two different primary antibodies solutions at 4°C for 48 hours. Primary antibodies were used as follows: mouse anti-CB (Sigma) 1:1000 and mouse anti-PV (Sigma) 1:10000. Immunoreagents were diluted in three per cent normal serum in phosphate buffered saline containing 0.3 per cent Triton X-100. After incubation with primary antibodies the sections were washed in phosphate buffered saline. This was followed by sequential incubations with goat anti-mouse 1:200 for one to two hours and with ABC standard Kit (Vector) 1:100 for 2 hours. Tissue bound peroxidase was visualized with 0.03 per cent 3',3-diaminobenzidine tetrahydrochloride and 0.01 per cent H_2O_2 for 10 to 15 minutes. The third series of sections was counterstained with thionin for cytoarchitectonic control. Sections were mounted on slides, dehydrated and coverslipped. Material was studied under light- and dark-field illumination.

Quantitative evaluations

We studied the agranular and granular motor and somatosensory, the anterior and posterior cingulate, and the visual cortices, according to the subdivisions proposed by Krettek & Price (1977), Donoghue & Wise (1982) and Miller (1987a), for the rat, and by Caviness (1975) and Wree et al. (1983), for the mouse. Digital images of selected sections were captured by a CCD video camera module (SONY XC-77 CE/Camera Adaptor DC-777 CE) coupled to the microscope stage and entered on a PowerMacintosh 7300/200 computer through a Scion LG3 PCI frame grabber card. Analyses on the digital images were performed using the public domain NIH Image program (US National Institutes of Health).

In experiments on ethanol-exposed rats two parameters were evaluated. First, the areal numeric density of cortical labelled cells was calculated by counting positive neurones falling into squared samples of 19,600 μm^2. Second, the ratio between thickness of the region containing packed grains anterogradely labelled and thickness of the entire cortex, from pial surface to white matter, was calculated. The upper and lower edges of the anterogradely labelled region, the pial surface, and the border between cortex and white matter were charted. On each chart, lines through the cortex normal to the pial surface were drawn, and thicknesses of the region labelled anterogradely and of the entire cortex were measured on these lines.

In experiments on mutant mdx mice digital images were captured as described above, and the cortical immuno-positive neurones were then charted and studied in terms of spatial distribution. Voronoi diagrams, which assign to each neurone the free area surrounding it and represent an advanced tool for topographic parametrization, were used to evaluate the spatial relationships between cells (see Minciacchi & Granato, 1997). All quantitative analyses were performed blind with respect to experimental groups. Cell counts, cortical measures and Voronoi polygon areas were evaluated, as differences between experimental groups, by ANOVA for nested designs (using the Systat software package for Macintosh).

Results

Ethanol-exposed rats

Relatively large injections were performed in the thalamus and involved primarily the ventral lateral, central lateral and mediodorsal nuclei, the ventrobasal complex, and the lateral part of ventral medial and midline nuclei. As result of the considerable extent of the thalamic injection sites, peroxidase reaction products were present in several regions of the ipsilateral cortex. Labelled terminals and cells were consistently observed in the motor and somatosensory fields AGl, and G, in AGm and in the more medial prefrontal areas. Sparse labelled cells and terminals were also observed in auditory and visual fields. In the motor and somatosensory regions, the tangential distribution of labelling was similar for normal and ethanol-exposed animals whereas the radial distribution of anterograde labelling was remarkably different (Fig. 1). In AGl and G of normal animals the bulk of labelled grains was located in layer IV and lower part of layer III. On the contrary, in the same fields of ethanol-exposed rats labelled grains were concentrated in the lower part of layer IV and the upper part of layer V. Labelling of layer Va often extended deeply into the region containing retrogradely labelled neurones of layer Vb. No anterograde labelling was detectable in the upper part of layer IV and lower part of layer III. Finally, no differences between experimental groups were observed for the laminar location of terminals in AGm; in this latter field the grains were always aggregated into layer III.

Quantitative evaluations show that the ratio between thickness of region of dense anterograde labelling and thickness of entire cortex was variously but significantly altered (Fig. 2). In the motor

Chapter 7 Impairment of sensorimotor cortex in two animal models

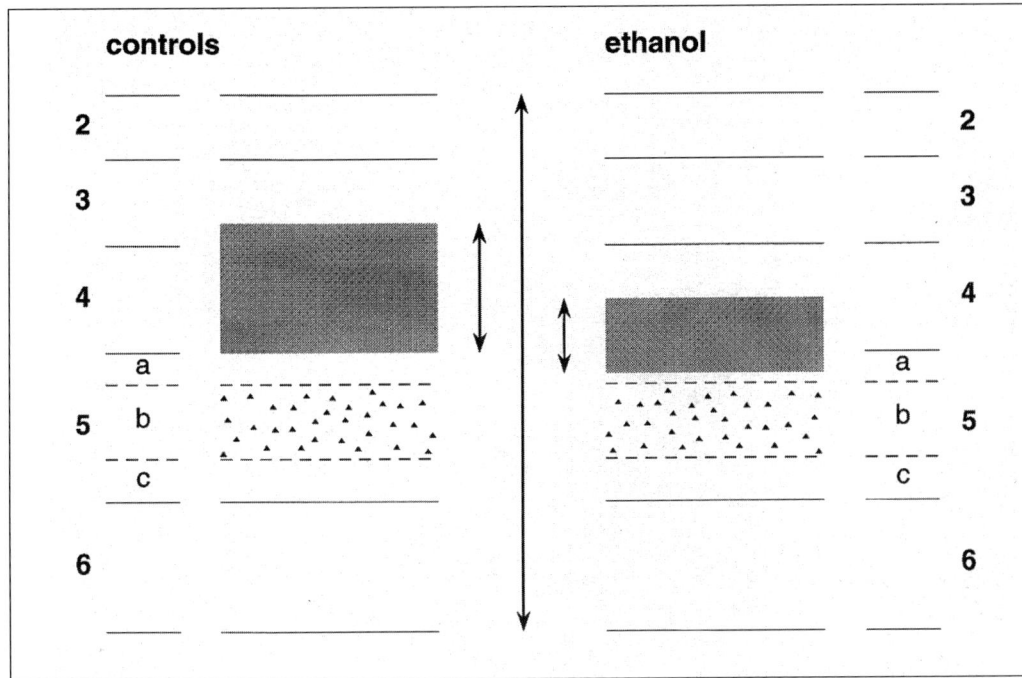

Fig. 1. Diagram showing the labelling in the cortex of control and ethanol-exposed rats after thalamic injection of wheat germ agglutinin-horseradish peroxidase. The anterograde labelling (shaded areas) in ethanol-exposed animals is narrower and abnormally located. Small triangles represent retrogradely labelled pyramidal neurones of layer Va. Neurones in layer VI (not represented) are retrogradely labelled as well.

and somatosensory fields AGl and G the relative thickness of the terminal recipient zone was shrunk by about 35 per cent and 47 per cent, respectively. In AGm, however, the shrinkage of the terminal recipient zone accounted for only seven per cent, whereas no differences between groups were observed in more medial cortical regions. The reductions of the cortical zones recipient of thalamic terminals were thus unevenly distributed and were more conspicuous in the motor and somatosensory fields, i.e. AGl and G, than in others. Populations of large layer Vb pyramidal neurones and smaller layer VI neurones were retrogradely labelled in normal and ethanol-exposed animals. Comparisons of areal density values of layer V labelled neurones displayed no differences between groups. A statistically significant difference was found only for AGl, where the areal numeric density of layer VI neurones was reduced by about 24 per cent in ethanol-exposed animals.

Mdx mice

In mice we analyzed the motor, somatosensory, visual, and cingulate cortices. No apparent differences between normal and mdx mice were evident in the relative proportions and cytoarchitectonic characteristics of the investigated cortices. On immunoreacted material we analyzed in detail the distribution and number of CB and PV immuno-positive neurones. CB and PV positive neurones were evident in all cortices though their amount and laminar distribution varied across the different fields.

In normal and mdx mice CB positive neurones were present in all layers except layer I. They were mostly concentrated in the upper layers II-III and the lower layers V-VI. In the supragranular layers CB positive neurones were either bipolar (double 'bouquet') or multipolar cells whereas in the infragranular layers multipolar neurones largely prevailed. The main difference between normal and mdx mice was represented by the number of CB positive cells (Fig. 3). Counts revealed that the number of CB positive neurones was increased of about 40 per cent in the motor cortex and about 35 per cent in the somatosensory cortex of mdx animals.

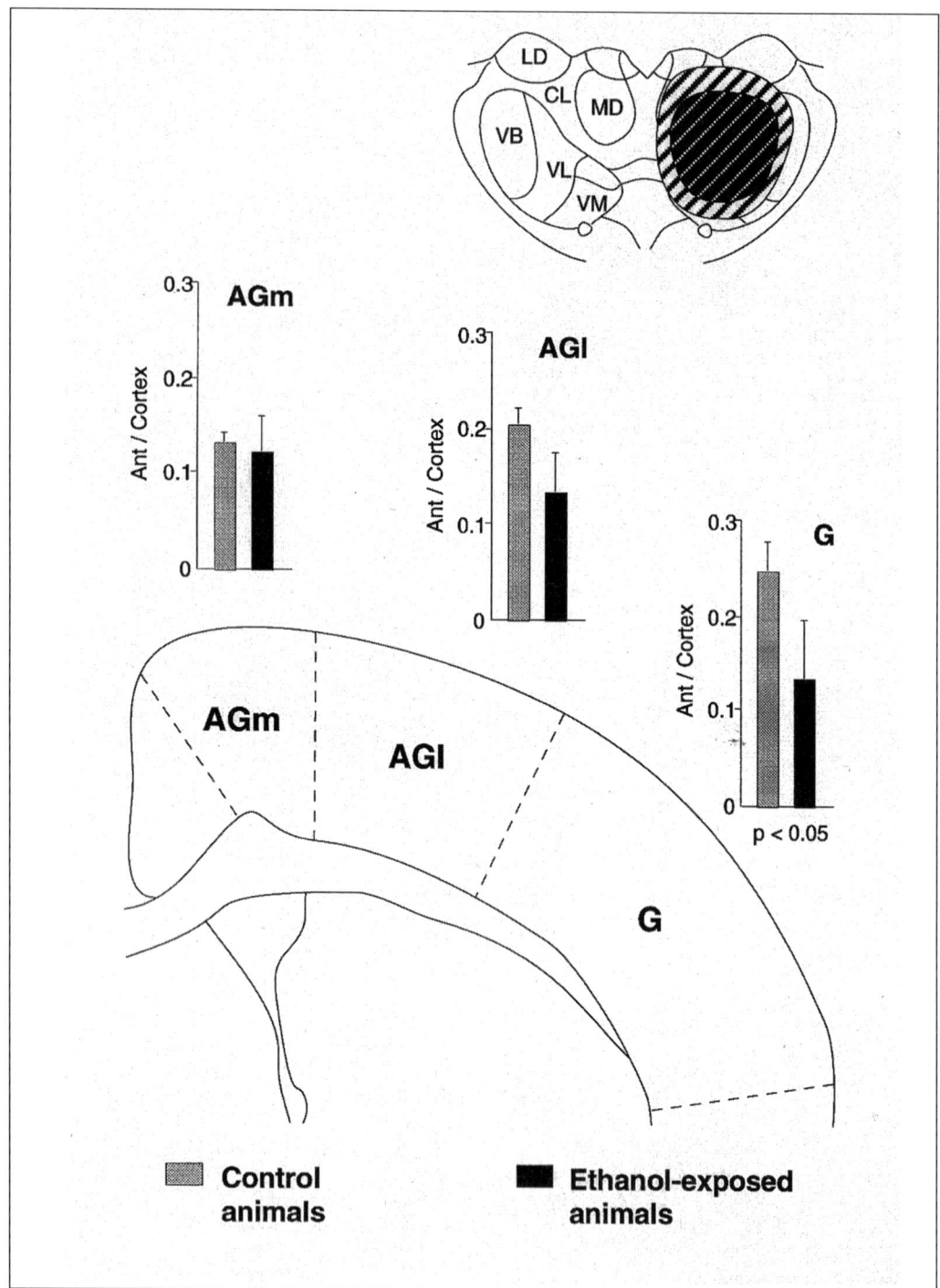

Fig. 2. Summary diagram showing the ratio between the height of the anterogradely labelled zone and that of the entire cortex (Ant/Cortex) for different fields of the sensori-motor cortex. This parameter was significantly lower in area G of ethanol-exposed animals, whereas AGm was not affected by ethanol exposure. The extent of thalamic injection of wheat germ agglutinin-horseradish peroxidase is shown at upper right.

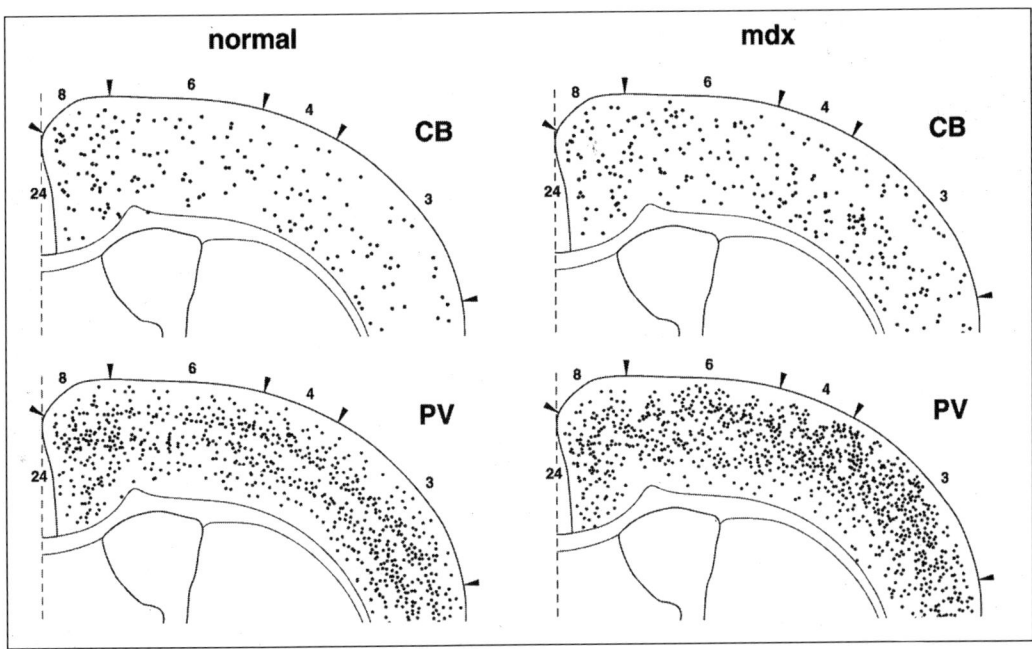

Fig. 3. Distribution of calbindin (CB) and parvalbumin (PV) immunoreactive cells in the cortex of normal and mdx mice. Note that changes in distribution of positive cells are only evident on somatosensory and motor cortices (3, 4 and partially 6). Note also the quasi-even radial distribution of PV positive cells in mdx mice, as opposed to the layered pattern observed in normal animals. Each dot represents a labelled neurone.

In normal mice PV positive neurones were present in all cortical layers except layer I. The majority of positive neurones pertained to multipolar basket or chandelier type cells. In the motor cortex PV positive neurones appeared concentrated in the upper layers II-III and in layer VI. In layer IV and the upper part of layer V PV positive neurones were consistently less numerous. In the somatosensory cortex PV positive neurones were concentrated in layer IV and were less numerous in layers VI and III. Sparse positive cells were also found in layers II and V. Again, a major difference between normal and mdx mice was represented by the number of PV positive cells, which is increased of about 20 per cent in the motor cortex and about 17 per cent in the somatosensory cortex of mdx animals (Fig. 3). Furthermore, in mdx mice PV positive neurones of the motor and somatosensory cortices displayed an altered lamination and were more numerous in layers IV and V (Fig. 4).

As for the other investigated fields, namely the visual and the cingulate cortices, we found no differences between normal and mdx mice in either the laminar distribution or in the number of CB and PV positive neurones. In conclusion, the overall pattern of immunoreactivity is similar in the different cortices of normal and mdx mice with two main exceptions. The CB and PV positive neurones of the motor cortex appeared more numerous in mdx animals. Secondly, in both motor and somatosensory cortices PV positive neurones lost their normal laminar distribution.

We analyzed the spatial distribution of CB and PV positive neurones by performing Voronoi diagrams. Results are described only for the motor and somatosensory cortices where differences between normal and mdx animals were encountered. Voronoi diagrams performed on sampled regions of the motor and somatosensory cortices showed that, in normal animals, CB and PV positive neurones were concentrated in two preferential bands as described above. For the CB positive neurones, although the number of cells was increased in mdx animals, the laminar location was maintained. This was not the case for the PV positive neurones, since their number increased in mdx animals but they also lost the normal laminar distribution (Fig. 5).

Discussion

Ethanol-exposed rats

Our study of the cortex in ethanol-exposed animals led to the following conclusions: (a) prenatal exposure to ethanol is able to induce permanent structural modifications of the cerebral cortex; (b) evident alterations reside on the terminal field of thalamo-cortical axons; (c) individual cortical fields display different sensitivity to ethanol intoxication; (d) the cell populations of cortico-thalamic neurones are not greatly affected.

Modifications of cortical staining in ethanol-exposed animals are mostly evident as a specific reduction of preterminal and terminal arborization of thalamo-cortical axons labelled anterogradely from the thalamic injections. In this specific case, since findings are obtained with the use of an axonal tracer, the possibility of false negative results due to impairment of axonal transport mechanisms should be considered. Although this issue has not been addressed directly in previous studies, McLane *et al.* (1992) observed normal rates of fast axonal transport in adult ethanol-fed rats. Additionally, the abatement of cortical anterograde labelling in ethanol-exposed animals could be explained either by a diminished number of thalamo-cortical axons or by a contraction of their terminal arbor. Our data favour the latter hypothesis: following injections of wheat germ agglutinin-horseradish peroxidase in the cortex, we observed that thalamo-cortical projecting neurones are not

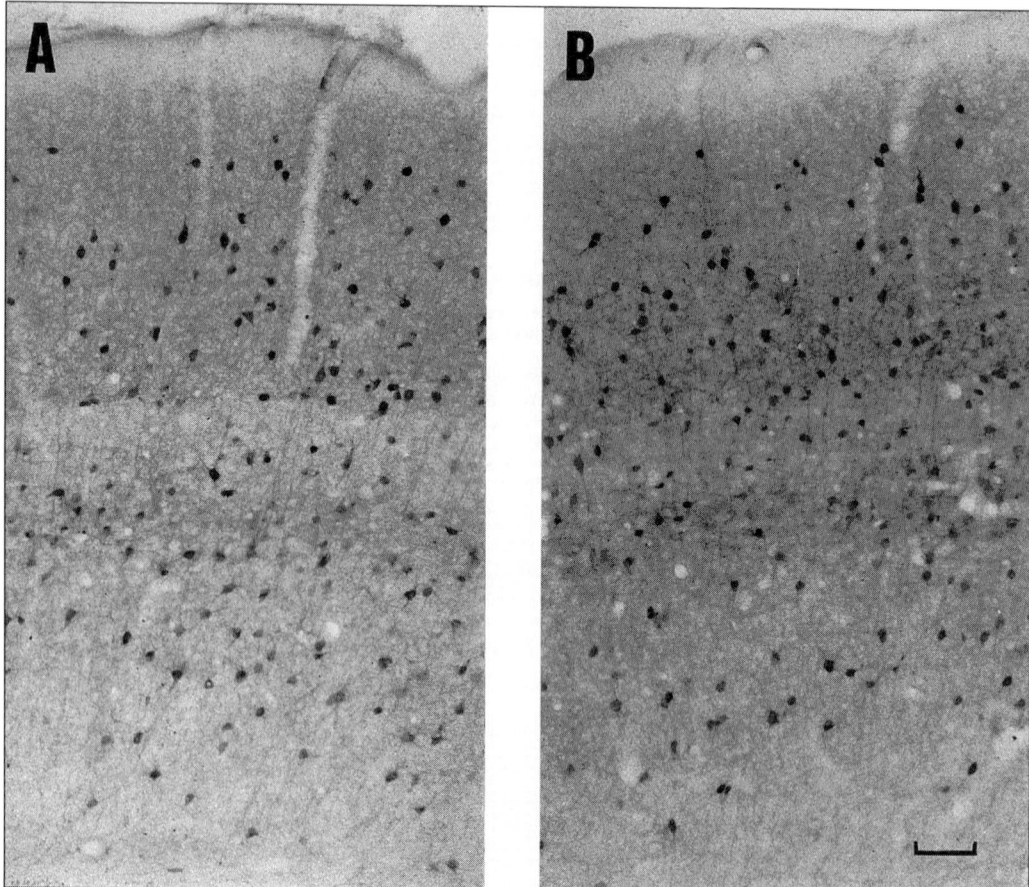

Fig. 4. Microphotographs of parvalbumin reacted coronal sections in the cortical area 3. (A) normal and (B) mdx mouse. Note the increase in number and the aberrant layer location of immuno-positive cells in mdx mice. Scale bar is 50 μm.

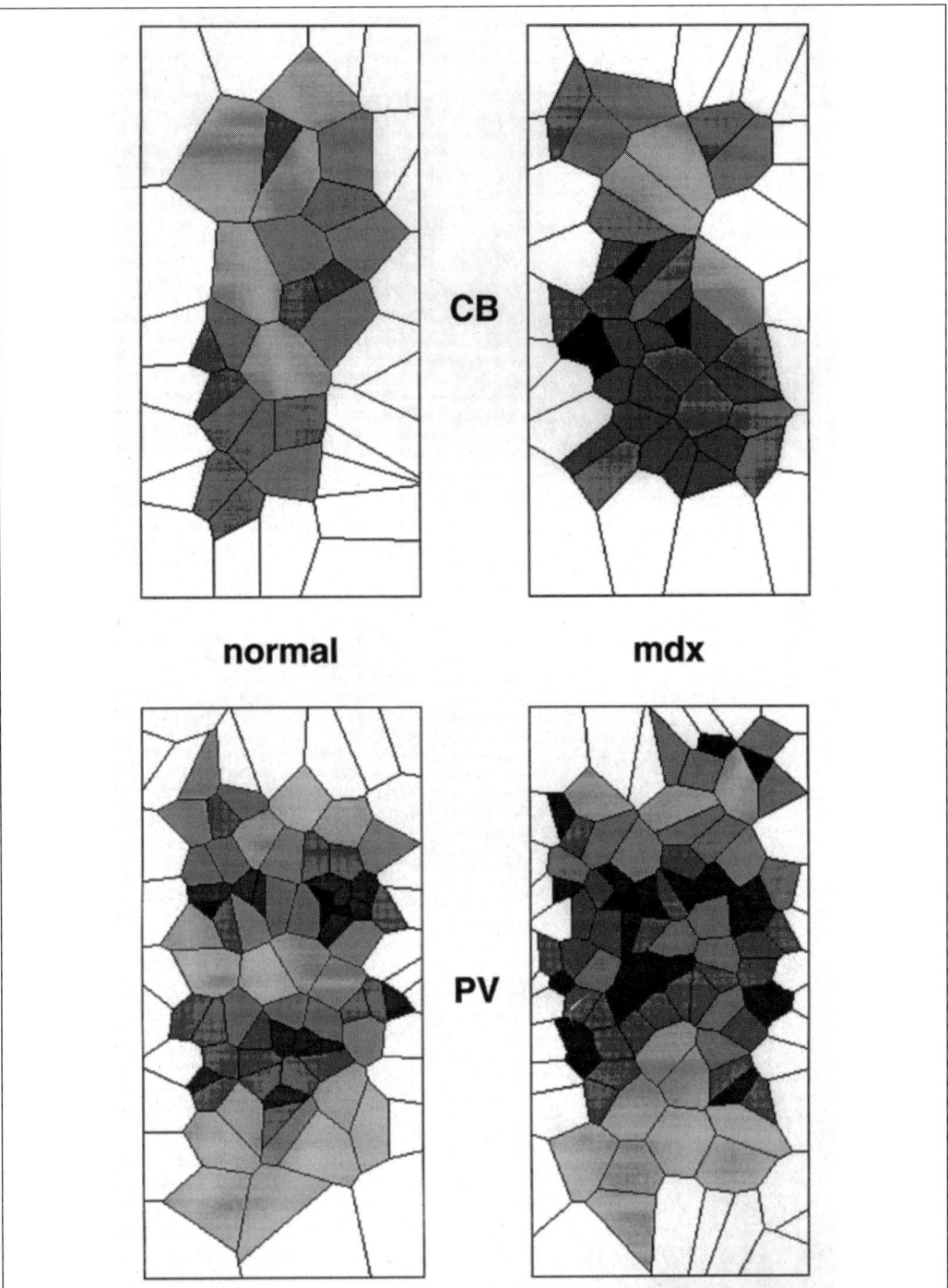

Fig. 5. Spatial tessellation performed by Voronoi diagrams on samples of somatosensory cortex immunostained for calbindin (CB) and parvalbumin (PV) in normal and mdx mice. Each polygon contains one labelled cell (not shown). The areas of polygons are coded by intensity of shading with smaller areas more heavily shaded. In the CB samples the number of cells, i.e. the number of polygons with small areas, is increased for mdx animals. In the PV samples the number of polygons with small areas is increased for mdx animals but the loss of normal laminar distribution is also evident.

reduced in number and thus ethanol-exposed animals possess a normal amount of thalamic axons reaching the cortex and contributing to anterograde labelling of the thalamic-recipient zone (data not presented here, Granato et al., 1995).

We demonstrated that the radial distribution of thalamic fibres and terminals to sensori-motor cortices is aberrant. In ethanol-exposed animals the thalamo-cortical fibres are distributed in layer Va and the deeper part of layer IV, and the thalamic recipient zone of the cortex is considerably narrower (Minciacchi et al., 1993, Granato et al., 1995). Alterations of terminals of thalamo-cortical connections are unevenly distributed through the cortical fields of ethanol-exposed animals. This is evident by observing collectively the fronto-parietal cortices where a medio-lateral gradient of severity is clearly recognizable. The thalamic recipient zone of AGm in ethanol-exposed animals displays only negligible reductions; in G the same zone is reduced by approximately 50 per cent. Previous reports indicate that layer IV of G cortex in ethanol-exposed animals is normal in terms of relative thickness and cell packing density (Miller & Dow-Edwards, 1988; Miller & Potempa, 1990) although a reduction of absolute cortical thickness has been described, especially for lateral fronto-parietal cortical regions (Miller & Dow-Edwards, 1988). Since cortical layer IV is the main recipient of thalamic input (Wise & Jones, 1978; Frost & Caviness, 1980), the population of neurones receiving thalamic information seems to be maintained. This is in line with our conclusion that prenatal exposure to ethanol affects predominantly terminal arborizations but relatively spares cell populations in the central nervous system (Minciacchi et al., 1993; Granato et al., 1995). Conversely, it is conceivable that more subtle alterations are operating within the thalamic recipient zone of the cortex, especially in cortices where an organized layer IV is present. Decrease of glucose utilization, possibly related to biochemical changes, has been observed specifically in layer IV of ethanol-exposed animals (Miller & Dow-Edwards, 1988). Furthermore AGm, which lacks a clearly recognizable layer IV (Donoghue & Wise, 1982), is relatively spared by ethanol intoxication.

Mdx mice

We found that mdx mice display a normal pattern of CBPs expression in the visual and cingulate cortices, whereas in the motor and somatosensory cortices the number of CB positive neurones is increased, with respect to normal mice, as is the number of PV positive neurones which also exhibit aberrant laminar location.

We can attempt to explain the increased number of CB and PV positive neurones in the motor and somatosensory cortices by considering the relations between dystrophin and the intracellular metabolism of Ca^{2+} (Matsumura & Campbell, 1994). In dystrophic muscles, alterations of intracellular Ca^{2+} regulation are described and an increased number of Ca^{2+} channels has been hypothesized (Mongini et al., 1988; Turner et al., 1988, 1991). Variations of intracellular Ca^{2+} metabolism are also described in mdx neuronal populations. In cell cultures of mdx cerebellar granule cells the levels of free Ca^{2+} are significantly higher than in cultures of granule cells from normal mice (Hopf & Steinhardt, 1992). On the other hand, there is some evidence to indicate that CBPs are involved in the regulation of intracellular Ca^{2+} (Braun, 1990; Heizmann & Hunziker, 1991; Baimbridge et al., 1992) and that they possibly have a protective effect on specific cell populations exposed to stimuli leading to cell death through an increase of intracellular Ca^{2+} (Malenka et al., 1988; Baimbridge et al., 1992; Geloso et al., 1996). CBPs could have a similar role in specific cell populations of the cerebral cortex. In this view, the increase of intracellular Ca^{2+} due to lack of dystrophin expression would start a process of cell decline and thus a reaction to expand calcium binding capabilities including increased expression of CBPs (Hopf & Steinhardt, 1992).

Alternatively, the increase of CB and PV positive neurones in motor and somatosensory cortices could be explained as a result of a modification in the activity of neurones involved in sensori-motor integration. The levels of several intracellular proteins are in fact under the influence of cell activity both in the peripheral and central nervous system (Tigges & Tigges, 1991; Rausell *et al.*, 1992; Caicedo *et al.*, 1997). We have previously described major alterations of the cortico-spinal system in mdx mice (Sbriccoli *et al.*, 1995). These alterations include a dramatic reduction of cortico-spinal neurones and visible changes of their morphology. It is thus possible that the changes of the cortico-spinal cell population lead to a rearrangement of intrinsic cortical circuits and consequently to a change in the activity of interneurones, which are known to be marked by CB and PV (Hendry *et al.*, 1989; Celio, 1990; Hendry & Jones, 1991).

Concluding remarks

Very different mechanisms for the establishment of cortical damages operate in the two described experimental animals. In one case, i.e. the ethanol-exposed rat, the contraction and aberrant location of the thalamic recipient region, for the different motor and somatosensory fields, clearly suggest that prenatal exposure to ethanol selectively affects terminal arborization of axons involved in thalamo-cortical communications. In the other case, i.e. the mutant mdx mouse, the changes observed in the pattern of CBPs expression can be the result of either an altered ability to handle the intracellular metabolism of Ca^{2+} or an altered functional state of intracortical circuitry.

These two examples of altered development however, in spite of the different nature of the primary damage, reveal some remarkable similarities. In both cases the damage appears concentrated in the motor and somatosensory areas (Fig. 6). It appears that, at least for the two models we describe

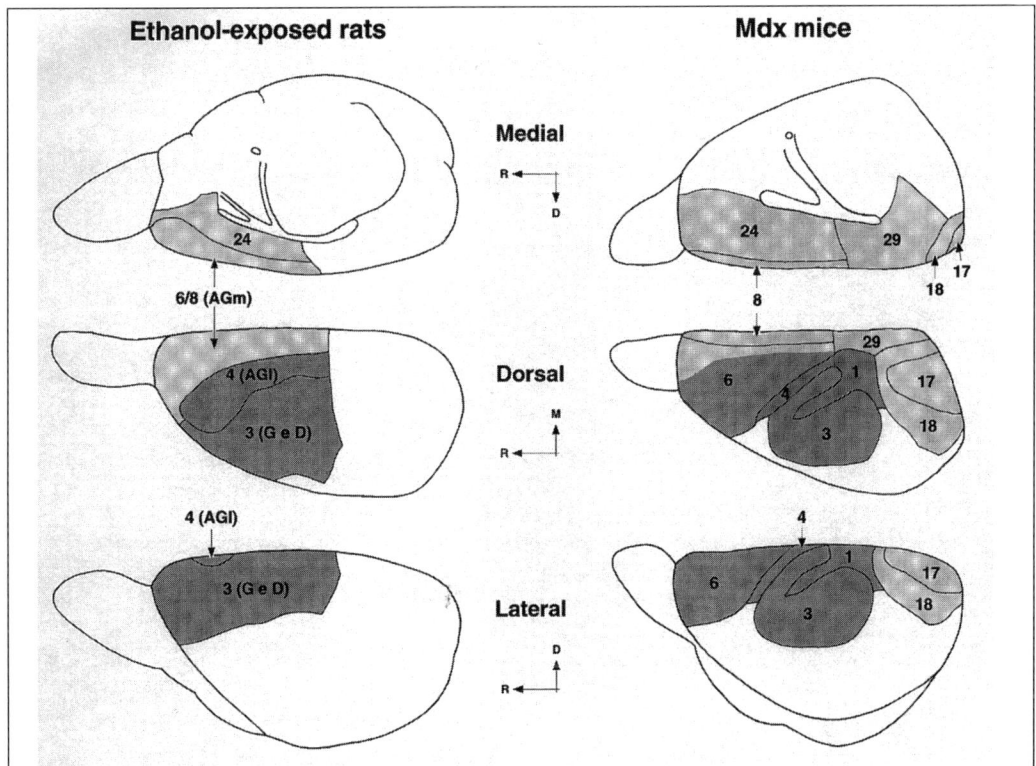

Fig. 6. Diagram summarizing the different involvement of cortical fields in the two models considered in the present study (investigated regions are shaded). Both in ethanol-exposed rats and in mdx mice, the highest degree of impairment is found in motor and somatosensory fields (heavily shaded areas). For the rat maps, areas are named and illustrated according to subdivisions by Donoghue & Wise (1982) and Miller (1987a); for the mouse maps, areas are named and illustrated according to subdivisions by Caviness (1975). In the cartesian axes, R = rostral, D = dorsal and M = medial.

here, the cortical response to a disturbed development is not uniformly distributed through the cortical mantle but rather involves some functionally homogeneous fields and spares some others. Even more relevant is the fact that in both animals the impairment is evident on the motor and somatosensory cortices. Our observation is not unique; it has been in fact reported that cortical alterations of glucose metabolism are specific to motor and somatosensory fields, in rats prenatally exposed to cocaine (Dow-Edwards *et al.*, 1990), and that abnormalities in dendritic spines of pyramidal neurones are selectively present in the somatosensory cortex of rats prenatally exposed to methylmercury (Stoltenburg Didinger & Markwort, 1990).

At present we do not have a conclusive explanation to account for these facts. We can only assume that motor and somatosensory cortices appear more susceptible than non-sensori-motor areas to insults which occur during the process of developmental modelling. In this case the main questions that arise are: Can this specific susceptibility be explained in terms of the intrinsic properties of sensori-motor machinery or as a consequence of some time-dependent developmental characteristics? Or even as a result of the particular functional role of sensori-motor cortices in massive elaboration of input-output operations? Elucidating these aspects is obviously open to future research; in our opinion, however, this issue appears of primary importance for a better understanding of the developmental processes and the operational handling of the highest centres for integration in the nervous system.

References

Altman, J. & Anderson, W.J. (1972): Experimental reorganization of the cerebellar cortex. I. Morphological effects of elimination of all microneurones with prolonged X-irradiation started at birth. *J. Comp. Neurol.* **146**, 355–406.

Altman, J. & Bayer, S.A. (1979): Development of the diencephalon in the rat. IV. Quantitative study of the time of origin of neurones and the internuclear chronological gradients in the thalamus. *J. Comp. Neurol.* **188**, 455–472.

Antonini, A. & Shatz, C.J. (1990): Relation between putative transmitter phenotypes and connectivity of subplate neurones during cerebral cortical development. *Eur. J. Neurosci.* **2**, 744–761.

Baimbridge, K.G., Celio, M.R. & Rogers, J.H. (1992): Calcium-binding proteins in nervous system. *Trends Neurosci.* **15**, 303–308.

Bayer, S.A. & Altman, J. (1991): *Neocortical development.* New York: Raven Press.

Braun, K. (1990): CaBPs in avian and mammalian central nervous system: localization, development and possible functions. *Prog. Histochem. Cytochem* **21**, 1–62.

Bulfield, G., Siller, W.G., Wight, P.A. & Moore, K.J. (1984): X chromosome-linked muscular dystrophy (*mdx*) in the mouse. *Proc. Natl. Acad. Sci. USA* **81**, 1189–1192.

Caicedo, A., D'Aldin, C., Eybalin, M. & Puel, J.-L. (1997): Temporary sensory deprivation changes calcium-binding proteins levels in the auditory brainstem. *J. Comp. Neurol.* **378**, 1–15.

Carretta, D., Santarelli, M., Carrai, R., Pinto, F., Granato, A., Sbriccoli, A. & Minciacchi, D. (1995): Motor neuronal arrays in the spinal cord of mutant *mdx* and *mnd* mice. *Eur. Neurosci. Ass. Abstr.* **68.16**, 173.

Caviness, V.S. (1975): Architectonic map of the neocortex of the normal mouse. *J. Comp. Neurol.* **164**, 247–264.

Celio, M.R. (1990): Calbindin-D28k and parvalbumin in the rat nervous system. *Neuroscience* **35**, 375–475.

Cellerino, A., Siciliano, R., Domenici, L. & Maffei, L. (1992): Parvalbumin immunoreactivity: a reliable marker for the effects of monocular deprivation in the rat visual cortex. *Neuroscience* **51**, 749–753.

Clarren, S.K. & Smith, D.W. (1978): The fetal alcohol syndrome. *N. Engl. J. Med.* **298**, 1063–1067.

Donoghue, J.P. & Wise, S.P. (1982): The motor cortex of the rat: cytoarchitecture and microstimulation mapping. *J. Comp. Neurol.* **212**, 76–88.

Dow-Edwards, D.L., Freed, L.A. & Fico, T.A. (1990): Structural and functional effects of prenatal cocaine exposure in adult rat brain. *Dev. Brain Res.* **57**, 263–268.

Friauf, E., McConnell, S.K. & Shatz, C.J. (1990): Functional synaptic circuits in the subplate during fetal and early postnatal development of cat visual cortex. *J. Neurosci.* **10,** 2601–2613.

Frost, D.O. & Caviness Jr, V.S. (1980): Radial organization of thalamic projections to the neocortex in the mouse. *J. Comp. Neurol.* **194,** 369–393.

Geloso, M.C., Paola, V. & Michetti, F. (1996): Parvalbumin-immunoreactive neurones are not affected by trimethyltin-induced neurodegeneration in the rat hippocampus. *Exp. Neurol.* **139,** 269–277.

Graham, R.C. & Karnowsky, M.J. (1966): The early stages of absorption of injected horseradish peroxidase in the proximal tubules of mouse kidney in ultrastructural cytochemistry by a new technique. *J. Histochem. Cytochem.* **14,** 291–302.

Granato, A., Minciacchi, D., Santarelli, M. & Sbriccoli, A. (1995): Multifaceted alterations of the thalamo-cortico-thalamic loop in adult rats prenatally exposed to ethanol. *Anat. Embryol.* **191,** 11–23.

Heizmann, C.W. & Hunziker, W. (1991): Intracellular calcium binding proteins: more sites than insights. *Trends Biochem. Sci.* **16,** 98–101.

Hendry, S.H. & Jones, E.G. (1991): GABA neuronal subpopulations in cat primary auditory cortex: co-localization with calcium binding proteins. *Brain Res.* **543,** 45–55.

Hendry, S.H., Jones, E.G., Emson, P.C., Lawson, D.E., Heizmann, C.W. & Streit, P. (1989): Two classes of cortical GABA neurones defined by differential calcium binding protein immunoreactivities. *Exp. Brain Res.* **76,** 467–472.

Hicks, S.P., D'Amato, C.J. & Lowe, M.J. (1959): The development of the mammalian nervous system. I. Malformation of the brain, especially the cerebral cortex, induced in rats by radiation. II. Some mechanisms of the malformation of the cortex. *J. Comp. Neurol.* **113,** 435–469.

Hoffman, E.P., Brown Jr, R.H. & Kunkel, L.M. (1987): Dystrophin: the protein product of the Duchenne muscular dystrophy locus. *Cell* **51,** 919–1128.

Hopf, F.W. & Steinhardt, R.A. (1992): Regulation of intracellular free calcium in normal and dystrophic mouse cerebellar neurones. *Brain Res.* **578,** 49–54.

Inomata, K., Nasu, F. & Tanaka, H. (1987): Decreased density of synaptic formation in the frontal cortex of neonatal rats exposed to ethanol in utero. *Int. J. Dev. Neurosci.* **5,** 455–460.

Jones, D.G. (1988): Influence of ethanol on neuronal and synaptic maturation in the central nervous system - Morphological investigations. *Prog. Neurobiol.* **31,** 171–197.

Jones, E.G., Valentino, K.L. & Fleshman Jr, J.W. (1982): Adjustment of connectivity in rat neocortex after prenatal destruction of precursor cells of layers II-IV. *Dev. Brain Res.* **2,** 425–431.

Krettek, J.E. & Price, J.L. (1977): The cortical projection of the mediodorsal nucleus and adjacent thalamic nuclei in the rat. *J. Comp. Neurol.* **171,** 157–192.

Lidov, H.J.W., Byers, T.J. & Kunkel, L.M. (1993): The distribution of dystrophin in the murine central nervous system: an immunocytochemical study. *Neuroscience* **54,** 167–187.

Majchrowicz, E. (1975): Induction of physical dependence upon ethanol and the associated behavioral changes in rats. *Psychopharmacologia (Berl.)* **43,** 245–254.

Malenka, R.C., Kauer, J.A., Zucker, R.S. & Nicoll, R.A. (1988): Postsynaptic calcium is sufficient for potentiation of hippocampal synaptic trasmission. *Science* **242,** 81–84.

Matsumura, K. & Campbell, K.P. (1994): Dystrophin-glycoprotein complex: its role in the molecular pathogenesis of muscular dystrophies. *Muscle Nerve* **17,** 2–15.

McConnell, S.K. (1995): Constructing the cerebral cortex: neurogenesis and fate determination. *Neuron* **15,** 761–768.

McConnell, S.K., Ghosh, A. & Shatz, C.J. (1989): Subplate neurones pioneer the first axon pathway from the cerebral cortex. *Science* **245,** 978–982.

McLane, J.A., Atkinson, M.B., McNulty, J. & Breuer, A.C. (1992): Direct measurement of fast axonal organelle transport in chronic ethanol-fed rats. *Alcohol Clin. Exp. Res.* **16,** 30–37.

Meinecke, D.L. & Rakic, P. (1992): Expression of GABA and GABA_A receptors by neurones of the subplate zone in developing primate occipital cortex: evidence for transient local circuits. *J. Comp. Neurol.* **317,** 91–101.

Mesulam, M.M. (1978): Tetramethyl benzidine for horseradish peroxidase neurohistochemistry. A non-carcinogenic blue reaction product with superior sensitivity for visualizing neural afferents and efferents. *J. Histochem. Cytochem.* **25**, 106–117.

Miller, M.W. (1987a): The origin of corticospinal projection neurones in rat. *Exp. Brain Res.* **67**, 339–351.

Miller, M.W. (1987b): Effect of prenatal exposure to alcohol on the distribution and time of origin of cortico-spinal neurones in the rat. *J. Comp. Neurol.* **257**, 372–382.

Miller, M.W. & Dow-Edwards, D.L. (1988): Structural and metabolic alterations in rat cerebral cortex induced by prenatal exposure to ethanol. *Brain Res.* **474**, 316–326.

Miller, M.W. & Potempa, G. (1990): Numbers of neurones and glia in mature rat somatosensory cortex: effects of prenatal exposure to ethanol. *J. Comp. Neurol.* **293**, 92–102.

Miller, M.W., Chiaia, N.L. & Rhoades, R.W. (1990): Intracellular recording and injection study of corticospinal neurones in rat somatosensory cortex: effect of prenatal exposure to ethanol. *J. Comp. Neurol.* **297**, 91–105.

Minciacchi, D. & Granato, A. (1988): Developmental remodeling of thalamic projections to the frontal cortex in rats. In: *Cellular thalamic mechanisms*, eds. M. Bentivoglio & R. Spreafico, pp. 501–516, Amsterdam: Elsevier/North-Holland.

Minciacchi, D. & Granato, A. (1989): Development of the thalamocortical system: transient-crossed projections to the frontal cortex in neonatal rats. *J. Comp. Neurol.* **281**, 1–12.

Minciacchi, D. & Granato, A. (1997): How relevant are subcortical maps for the cortical machinery? A hypothesis based on parametric study of extra-relay afferents to primary sensory areas. In: *Self-organization, computational maps and motor control*, eds. P. Morasso & V. Sanguineti, pp. 149–168, Amsterdam: Elsevier/North-Holland.

Minciacchi, D., Granato, A., Santarelli, M. & Sbriccoli, A. (1993): Modifications of thalamo-cortical circuitry in rats prenatally exposed to ethanol. *NeuroReport* **4**, 415–418.

Minciacchi, D., Carretta, D., Santarelli, M., Carrai, R., Pinto, F., Sbriccoli, A. & Granato, A. (1995): Rubral, vestibular, and reticular projections to spinal cord in the mutant mdx mouse. *Soc. Neurosci. Abstr.* **21**, p1489.

Mongini, T., Ghigo, D. & Doriguzzi, C. (1988): Free cytoplasmic Ca^{2+} at rest and after cholinergic stimulus is increased in cultured muscle cells from Duchenne muscular dystrophy patients. *Neurology* **38**, 476–480.

Paxinos, G., & Watson, C. (1986): *The Rat brain in stereotaxic coordinates*. Second Edition. North Ride, Australia: Academic Press.

Rausell, E., Cusick, C.G., Taub, E. & Jones, E.G. (1992): Chronic deafferentation in monkeys differentially affects nociceptive and non-nociceptive pathways distinguished by specific calcium-binding proteins and down-regulates y-amminobutyrric acid type A receptors at thalamic levels. *Proc. Natl. Acad. Sci. USA* **89**, 2571–2575.

Santarelli, M., Dell'Anna, M.E., Carretta, D., Pinto, F., Zito, G., Granato, A. & Minciacchi, D. (1995): Differential immunoreactivity to parvalbumin, calbindin-d28k, and calretinin, in the somatosensory cortex of normal c57bl/6 and mutant *mdx* mice. *Europ. Neurosci. Ass. Abstr.* **50.04**, p. 123.

Sbriccoli, A., Santarelli, M., Carretta, D., Pinto, F., Granato, A. & Minciacchi, D. (1995): Architectural changes of the cortico-spinal system in the dystrophin defective mdx mouse. *Neurosci. Lett.* **200**, 53–56.

Sicinski, P., Geng, Y., Ryder-Cook, A.S., Barnard, E.A., Darlison, M.G. & Barnard, P.J. (1989): The molecular basis of muscular dystrophy in the mdx mouse: a point mutation. *Science* **244**, 1578-1580.

Stoltenburg Didinger, G. & Markwort, S. (1990): Prenatal methylmercury exposure results in dendritic spine dysgenesis in rats. *Neurotoxicol. Teratol.* **12**, 573–576.

Tigges, M. & Tigges, J. (1991): Parvalbumin immunoreactivity of the lateral geniculate in adult rhesus monkeys after monocular eye enucleation. *Vis. Neurosci.* **6**, 375–382.

Torelli, S., Sogos, V., Ennas, M.G., Muntoni, F., Clerk, A., Strong, P.N. & Gremo, F. (1992): Dystrophin immunoreactivity in normal and Duchenne human fetal neurones in culture. *J. Neurosci. Res.* **32**, 116–125.

Torres, L.F.B. & Duchen, L.W. (1987): The mutant mdx: inherited myopathy in the mouse. *Brain* **110**, 269–299.

Turner, P.R., Westwood, T., Regan, C.M. & Steinhardt, R.A. (1988): Increased protein degradation results from elevated free calcium levels found in muscle from mdx mice. *Nature* **335**, 735–738.

Turner, P.R., Fong, P., Denetclaw, W.F. & Steinhardt, R.A. (1991): Increased calcium influx in dystrophic mice. *J. Cell Biol.* **115,** 1701–1712.

Uchino, M., Yoshioka, K., Miike, T., Tokunaga, M., Uyama, E., Teramoto, H., Naoe, H. & Ando, M. (1994): Dystrophin and dystrophin-related protein in the brains of normal and mdx mice. *Muscle Nerve* **17,** 533–538.

Van Eden, C.G. (1986): Development of connections between the mediodorsal nucleus of the thalamus and the prefrontal cortex in the rat. *J. Comp. Neurol.* **244,** 349–359.

West, J.R. & Goodlett, C.R. (1990): Teratogenic effects of alcohol on brain development. *Ann. Med.* **22,** 319–325.

Wise, S.P. & Jones, E.G. (1978): Developmental studies of thalamocortical and commissural connections in the rat somatic sensory cortex. *J. Comp. Neurol.* **178,** 187–208.

Wree A., Zilles, K. & Schleicher, A. (1983): A quantitative approach to cytoarchitectonics. VIII. The areal pattern of the cortex of the albino mouse. *Anat. Embryol.* **166,** 333–353.

PART III

ANIMAL MODELS

Chapter 8

The methylazoxymethanol (MAM) treated rat as an animal model for human development brain dysgeneses: morphological features

Claudia Colacitti[1], Giulio Sancini[1], Silvana Franceschetti[1], Flaminio Cattabeni[2], Roberto Spreafico[1], Monica Di Luca[2], and Giorgio Battaglia[1]

[1]*Divisione di Neurofisiologia Sperimentale ed Epilettologia, Istituto Nazionale Neurologico 'C. Besta', Via Celoria 11, 20133 Milan, Italy;*
[2]*Istituto di Scienze Farmacologiche, Università di Milano, via Balzaretti 9, 20133 Milan, Italy.*

Summary

A double intraperitoneal injection of the cytotoxic agent methylazoxymethanol acetate (MAM) was prenatally administered to pregnant rats on gestational day 15 to induce developmental brain dysgeneses. The offspring of treated dams were characterized by extensive cortical layering abnormalities, subpial bands of heterotopic neurones in layer I, and subcortical nodules of heterotopic neurones extending from the periventricular region to the hippocampus and neocortex. The anatomical connections of these heterotopia were investigated by means of anterograde and retrograde tract tracing techniques. The tract tracing data demonstrated the existence of reciprocal connections between the neuronal heterotopia and the ipsilateral and contralateral cortical areas. On the basis of the anatomical features and connectivity patterns, it may be speculated that the subcortical heterotopias were formed by neurones originally committed to the neocortex. The subcortical heterotopias were characterized by morphological features similar to those found in human periventricular nodular heterotopias. The present study demonstrates that double MAM treatment at gestational day 15 induces in rats developmental brain abnormalities with anatomical features similar to those observed in human brain dysgeneses associated with intractable epilepsy. MAM treated rats could be therefore considered as useful tools in investigating the pathogenetic mechanisms by which human brain dysgeneses develop in human patients.

Introduction

Developmental brain abnormalities are frequently associated with mental and neurological impairment in human patients. These abnormalities have been reported since the second half of the last century, in neuropathological studies based on autoptic specimens from severely retarded or disabled patients (Friede, 1989). Thanks to the recent improvement of neuroimaging techniques, it is now possible to diagnose *in vivo* an increasing number of developmental brain abnormalities (Barkovich *et al.*, 1992), in patients affected by dyslexia, motor and language deficits, and medically intractable epilepsy (Galaburda *et al.*, 1985; Kuzniecky *et al.*, 1993; Barkovich *et al.*,

1994; Battaglia et al., 1997). Different etiologic factors – genetic, vascular, toxic – have been proposed for the different types of human brain dysgeneses, but the pathogenetic mechanisms that eventually lead to the development of these brain malformations and the related clinical phenotype are still largely unknown.

A useful approach to understanding the mechanism underlying developmental neurological disorders is to produce appropriate animal models with acquired or genetically determined structural brain abnormalities. Many animal models have been so far described (Ferrer et al., 1993; D'Arcangelo et al., 1995; Roper et al., 1995; Jacobs et al., 1996; Lee et al., 1996). Among the acquired models, one based on the administration of methylazoxymethanol acetate (MAM) has been used by different groups interested in producing developmental brain dysfunction in rodents (Cattabeni & Di Luca, 1997). MAM is an antiproliferative agent, selective for neuroepithelial cells during their S phase (Cattaneo et al., 1995). MAM exerts its effect by methylating guanine and other pyrimidine bases in a time window of two to 24 hours, with maximal activity at 12 hours after administration. If intraperitoneally administered to pregnant rats, MAM produces structural brain abnormalities in the offsprings, related to the time and dose of administration. Single MAM exposures (25 mg per kg of maternal body weight) on embryonic day 15 (E15), corresponding in rodents to the neurogenetic peak of the neocortex, produce hippocampal heterotopias primarily involving the CA1 and CA2 regions (Singh, 1977), reduction of the neocortical thickness (Johnston & Coyle, 1979), and subcortical neuronal heterotopia (Dambska et al., 1982; Collier & Ashwell, 1993). The treated animals develop with normal spontaneous locomotor activity and reflexes; however, in adulthood they show impairment in several tests of learning and memory, and at cellular and subcellular level they exhibit alterations of electrophysiological and biochemical parameters related to synaptic plasticity (Ramakers et al., 1993; Di Luca et al., 1995). Moreover, hippocampal neurones in MAM rats are characterized by hyperexcitable responses if maintained in elevated extracellular potassium, and MAM-rats are associated with increased susceptibility to flurothyl- and hyperthermia-induced seizures (Baraban & Schwartzkroin, 1995, 1996; Germano et al., 1996).

In order to induce in rats structural brain abnormalities similar to those observed in human cortical dysgeneses (Barkovich et al., 1992; Battaglia et al., 1996), we administered a double MAM intraperitoneal injection to pregnant rats at E15. We describe in the present study the morphological features of the brain abnormalities induced by this treatment by means of a combined cytoarchitectural and immunocytochemical analysis. In addition, we report the anatomical connections of the MAM-induced heterotopic structures, investigated by means of anterograde and retrograde tract tracing techniques.

Materials and methods

MAM administration

Pregnant Sprague-Dawley rats received two MAM (Sigma Chemical Co., St. Louis, MO, USA) intraperitoneal doses (15 mg/kg maternal body weight, in sterile saline) on E15, the first injection at 12.00 a.m. and the second at 12.00 p.m. On the same day, control pregnant rats were sham injected with the vehicle alone. The day after conception (as determined by vaginal smear) was designated embryonic day one. Litters were born on day 22 or 23 of gestation. No differences in gestational parameters, pups' weight and litters' size were observed. The pups were weaned at three weeks of age and housed under standard conditions with water and food ad libitum.

Morphological analysis

Twelve adult rats (1 to 15 months of age) that had been exposed to MAM *in utero* ('MAM rats') and four adult sham operated control rats (one to six months of age) were employed for the morphological analysis. The rats were deeply anesthetized with chloral hydrate (1 ml/100 g body weight of a four per cent solution) and perfused with one per cent paraformaldehyde followed by four per cent paraformaldehyde and 0.5 per cent glutaraldehyde in 0.1 M phosphate buffer at pH 7.2 (PB). Brains were removed from the skull, postfixed overnight in four per cent paraformaldehyde, and cut with a vibratome into 50 µm thick coronal sections. Sections were collected in phosphate buffered saline (PBS: 0.01 M, pH 7.5) in serial order.

For immunocytochemistry, sections were pretreated with three per cent hydrogen peroxide (H_2O_2) in PBS for 10 min, to neutralize endogenous peroxidase activity, and incubated in 10 per cent normal serum and 0.2 per cent Triton X-100 in PBS for 60 min to mask non-specific absorption sites and to increase the penetration of the reagents. The sections were then incubated overnight at room temperature with the primary antibodies (Table 1). On the following day, the sections were rinsed for 60 min in PBS, incubated either with biotinylated goat anti-rabbit IgGs (Vector Inc; diluted 1:200; for polyclonal primary antisera) or anti-mouse IgGs (Vector Inc; diluted 1:200; for monoclonal primary antibodies) for 75 min, and then washed for 60 min in PBS. The sections were then incubated for 60 min with the avidin-biotin complex (ABC, Vector; 10 µl avidin-DH and 10 µl biotinylated horseradish peroxidase in 1 ml of 50 mM Tris-buffered saline). All immunoreagents were diluted in two per cent normal serum (NHS for monoclonal antibodies, NGS for polyclonal antisera: Vector), 0.2 per cent Triton X-100, one per cent Bovine Serum Albumin (Sigma) in PBS.

Table 1. Primary antibodies employed in the morphological analysis.

Type	Name	Antigen	Source	Producer	Dilution
Neuronal marker	Monoclonal	MAP2	Microtubule-associate protein-2	Mouse	Boehringer Mannheim	1:800
Neuronal marker	Monoclonal	SMI 311	Non-phosphorylated neurofilaments	Mouse	Sternberger Monoclonals Inc.	1:2000
Glial marker	Monoclonal	GFAP	Glial fibrillary acid protein	Mouse	Boehringer Mannheim	1:1500
Glial marker	Monoclonal	VIM	57 KDa intermediate filament protein vimentin	Mouse	DAKO	1:200
Calcium binding protein	Monoclonal	Calbindin	Calbindin D-28 $_K$Da	Mouse	SWant	1:10000
Calcium binding protein	Monoclonal	Parvalbumin	Parvalbumin 12 $_K$Da	Mouse	SWant	1:10000
Calcium binding protein	Polyclonal	Calretinin	Calretinin	Rabbit	SWant	1:10000
GABA	Polyclonal	GABA (γ-Aminobutyric acid)	GABA	Rabbit	Sigma Immunochemicals	1:10000
AMPA-type glutamate receptors	Polyclonal	GLUR1	Subunit 1 AMPA-type glutamate receptor	Rabbit	Kindly supplied by Dr. R.J. Wenthold*	1:2000
AMPA-type glutamate receptors	Polyclonal	GLUR2-3	Subunits 2-3 AMPA-type glutamate receptor	Rabbit	Kindly supplied by Dr. R.J. Wenthold*	1:750

The table reports the specifications of the primary antibodies used in the present study.
*Petralia & Wenthold (1992).

Peroxidase staining was obtained by reacting the sections in a solution containing 3-3'-diaminobenzidine (DAB, Sigma; 0.075 per cent) and H_2O_2 (0.002 per cent) in 50 mM Tris-HCl buffer at pH 7.6. Sections were mounted on gelatin-coated glass slides, air-dried, dehydrated, and coverslipped with DPX. Selected sections were charted with a computerized X-Y plotter connected with a Leitz Diaplan microscope and matched with the adjacent thionin counterstained sections for cytoarchitectural analysis (Zilles, 1985).

Tract tracing experiments

Eight adult (seven weeks to six months of age) MAM rats were deeply anesthetized (as specified above) and mounted on a stereotaxic device. Iontophoretic injections of the anterograde tracer biotinylated dextran amine (BDA; Molecular Probes, Inc., Eugene, OR, USA; 10 per cent in 10 mM phosphate buffer, pH 7.4) or of the retrograde tracer Fluorogold (FG; Fluorochrome, Inc., Englewood, CO, USA; one per cent in Na-Acetate 0.1 M, pH 3.3) were placed in the motor cortex. The injections were placed at a rostrocaudal level slightly anterior (0.2 mm) to the skull bregma, corresponding in the microcephalic MAM rats to the level of the anterior commissure. Five rats were injected with BDA, and three rats with FG. The injections were made through glass microelectrodes (tip diameter: 30-40 μm) by using positive current pulses of 5 μA (7 sec on/ 7 sec off) for 10-15 minutes. The pipette was left *in situ* for an additional five minutes to minimize the diffusion of the tracer during pipette removal.

After a survival time of 5-15 days, the rats were re-anesthetized and perfused as specified above. The brains were then removed from the skull, postfixed overnight in four per cent paraformaldehyde, and cut with a vibratome into 50 μm thick coronal sections. The sections were collected in phosphate buffered saline (PBS: 0.01 M, pH 7.5) in groups of two. For BDA experiments, one series of sections waspretreated with three per cent H_2O_2 in PBS for 10 min, then incubated in ABC and 0.4 per cent Triton X 100 for 4 h. Peroxidase staining was obtained as indicated above. After washing in PBS, the sections were mounted on gelatin-coated slides and counterstained with 0.1 per cent thionin. The adjacent series of sections was pretreated with 10 per cent methanol and one per cent H_2O_2 in PBS for 10 min, and then incubated with 10 per cent NRS and 0.75 per cent Triton-X 100 for 45 min. The sections were then subsequently incubated with affinity-purified antibiotin antiserum (Vector) for 24 h at 4 °C, with biotinylated rabbit anti-goat IgG (Vector, diluted 1:200) for 75 min, and with the ABC complex for 2 h at 4 °C. Peroxidase staining was obtained as indicated above. The BDA injection sites and the anterogradely labelled axons were charted at 100X with a computerized X-Y plotting system attached via transducers to a Leitz microscope stage.

For FG experiments, one series of sections was immediately mounted on gelatin-coated slides, air-dried, coverslipped with DPX, and examined with a Nikon FXA fluorescence microscope. Selected sections were photographed, and the FG injections sites and the retrogradely labelled neurones were charted as above. The adjacent series of sections were stained with 0.1 per cent thionin for cytoarchitectonic analysis.

Results

Morphological analysis

In contrast to sham operated rats, the double MAM treatment consistently produced a severe reduction of cortical thickness in regions caudal to the anterior commissure and lateral to the cingulate cortex, with a relative thickness increase of layer VI and decrease of layer V (Fig. 1A). In these regions, all cortical layers were severely disorganized, with appearance of superficial and deep clusters of heterotopic neurons (Figs. 1A-B). The superficial clusters were made up of densely packed neurones, separated by cell free areas (Fig. 1A). The neuropil and small perikarya within the clusters were calbindin immunoreactive (ir), as in the superficial cortical layers of normal rats. The apical dendrites of layer V pyramidal neurones, immunopositive for anti-MAP2 and anti- SMI 311, were located in the cell free areas thus surrounding the calbindin-ir clusters.

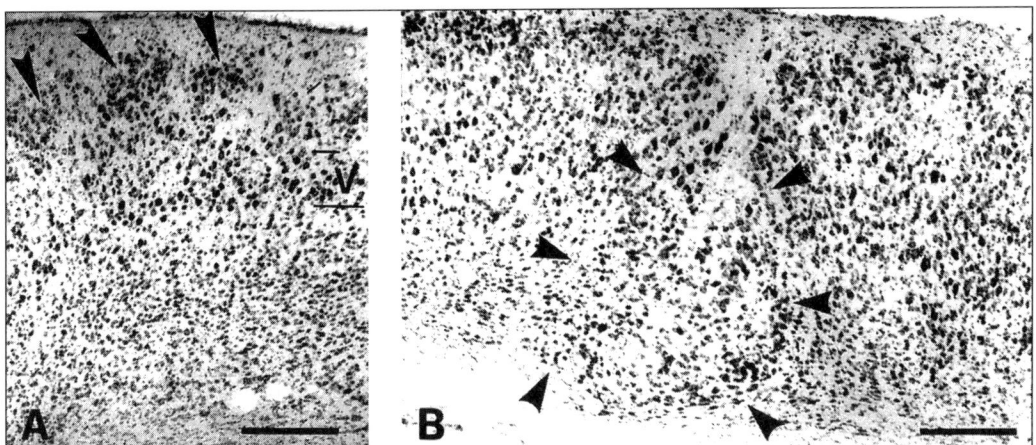

Fig. 1. Cortical layering abnormalities and heterotopic clusters in MAM rats. Photomicrographs from coronal sections through the somatosensory cortex stained with thionin. (A) After double MAM injections on E15 the cortical thickness is reduced and the layering abnormalities are severe. Note the heterotopic clusters (arrows) in the superficial layers and the superficial position of layer V neurones. (B) A large round heterotopic cluster (arrowheads) is evident in the deep cortical layers. Intensely thionin stained neurones are located at the cluster borders. Scale bars: 250 μm.

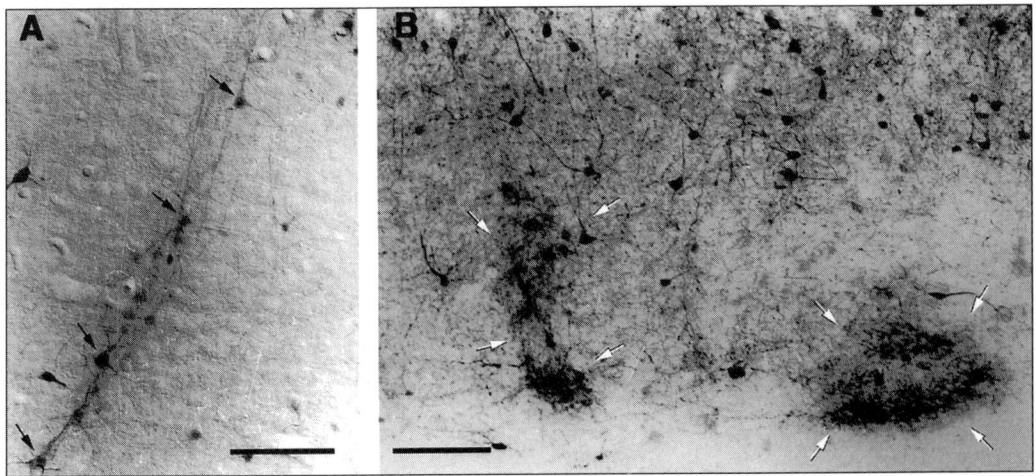

Fig. 2. Cortical heterotopia in deep layers of MAM rats. Photomicrographs from coronal sections through the somatosensory cortex immunoreacted with anti-calbindin (A) or anti-parvalbumin (B) antibodies. (A) Closely associated pyramidal neurones, immunopositive for calbindin (arrows) organized in radial columns. (B) Two clusters of heterotopic neurones (white arrows) intensely immunoreactive for parvalbumin. Scale bars: 100 μm in A, 250 μm in B.

In the same cortical areas, clusters of heterotopic neurones were evident also in deep cortical layers (Figs. 1B, 2 and 3). These round or elongated clusters of different size were characterized by densely packed, intensely thionin-stained neurones, preferentially located at the clusters edges (Fig. 1B). In most cases these cells showed pyramidal morphology with distorted apical dendrites. They could be also organized in radial columns of densely packed cells, immunopositive for AMPA receptors GluR2-3 and calbindin (Fig. 2A). The clusters were also characterized by intense parvalbumin and GABAergic immunoreactivity of both neuropil and perikarya (Figs. 2B and 3). Neurones at the borders of the clusters were frequently surrounded by GABA-ir puncta (Fig. 3B).

Another striking feature was the presence of a thick subpial band of heterotopic neurones in layer I, separated from the underlying neocortex by a band of white matter (Fig. 4A). The heterotopic

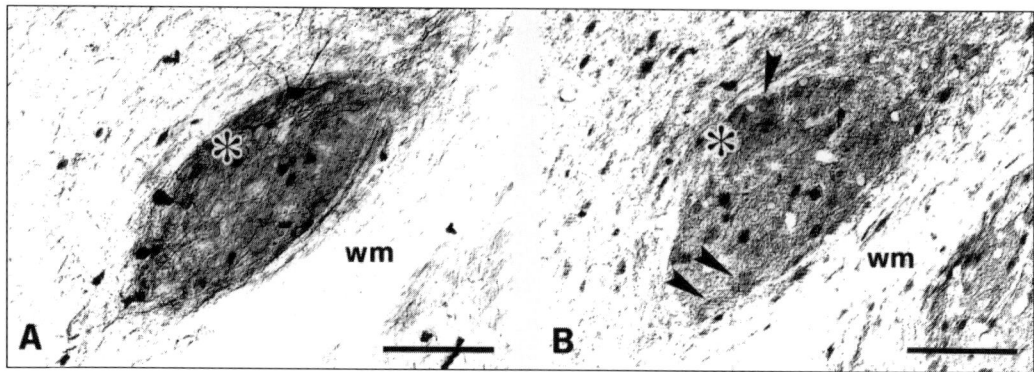

Fig. 3. Cortical heterotopia in deep layers of MAM rats. High-power photomicrographs from adjacent coronal sections immunoreacted with anti-parvalbumin (A) or anti-GABA (B) antibodies. Many parvalbumin-ir (A) or GABA-ir (B) interneurones are located in a small heterotopic cluster. Note the dense parvalbumin-ir neuropil (A) and the neurones outlined by GABA-ir terminals (arrowheads in B) at the borders of the cluster. Asterisks mark cortical vessels as reference; wm: white matter. Scale bars: 100 μm.

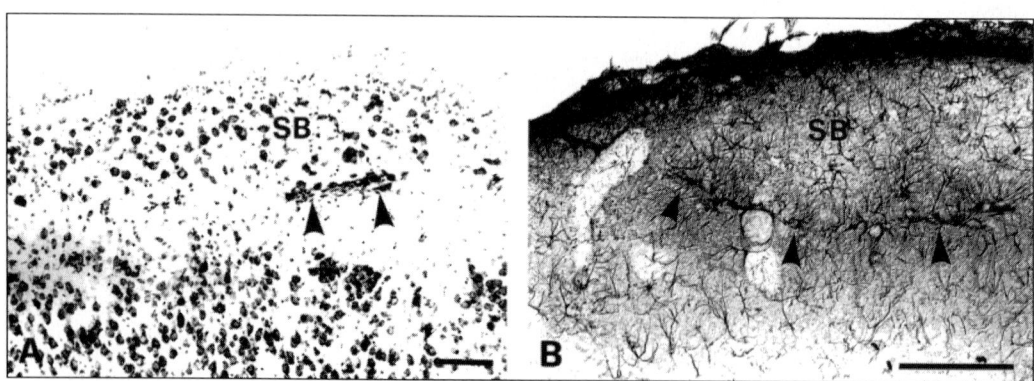

Fig. 4. Subpial band (SB) of heterotopic neurones in layer I. Photomicrographs from coronal sections through the lateral somatosensory cortex stained with thionin (A) or immunoreacted with anti-GFAP (B) antibody. Tangential vessels (arrowheads in A and B), better revealed by the GFAP immunoreactivity (B), divide the heterotopic band from the underlying white matter. Scale bars: 100 μm in A, 170 μm in B.

band was more evident in caudal sections dorsal to the rhinal sulcus. It was thicker ventrally (approximately 300 μm), and it became thinner dorsally, where it merged with the superficial heterotopic clusters described above. At the ventral border of the heterotopic band tangentially oriented vascular structures were present, associated with a thin rim of GFAP immunoreactivity (Fig. 4B).

In subcortical regions close to the septum and anterior caudate nuclei, periventricular nodules of heterotopic neurones were evident at the ventricle laterodorsal borders (Fig. 5A). Several periventricular nodules could be present, isolated or in anatomical continuity with each another. The core of the nodules was made up by round and pyramidal neurones of normal size, with randomly oriented apical dendrites. At the borders of the nodules, fusiform and pyramidal neurones, intensely MAP2- and SMI-ir, were frequently observed in a marginal position, with the major axis oriented parallel to the edge of the nodule (Fig. 5B). In the same position, glial processes were immunopositive for vimentin, a marker for radial glial fascicles. In some MAM rats, the periventricular nodules were in anatomical continuity with the overlying neocortex.

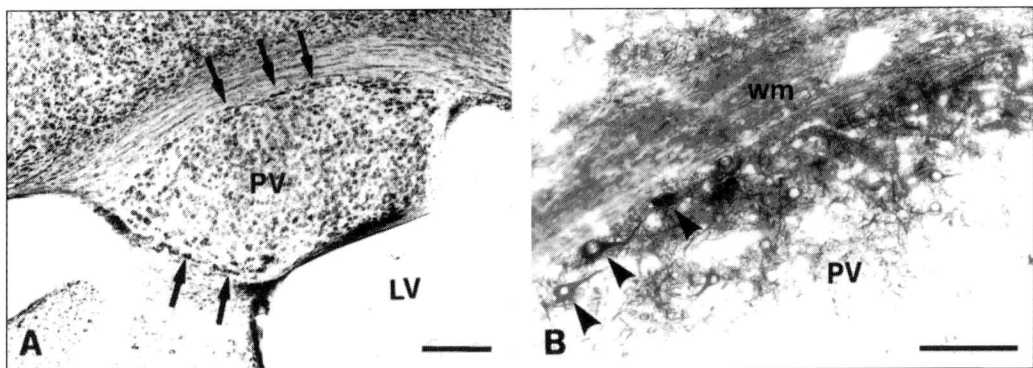

Fig. 5. Periventricular (PV) heterotopic nodules in MAM rats. Photomicrographs from coronal sections through the rostral lateral ventricle (LV), stained with thionin (A), or immunoreacted with anti-SMI 311 (B) antibody. The marginal neurones oriented parallel to the edge of the PV nodules (arrows in A) are intensely SMI 311-immunoreactive (arrowheads in B). wm: white matter. Scale bars: 250 μm in A, 75 μm in B.

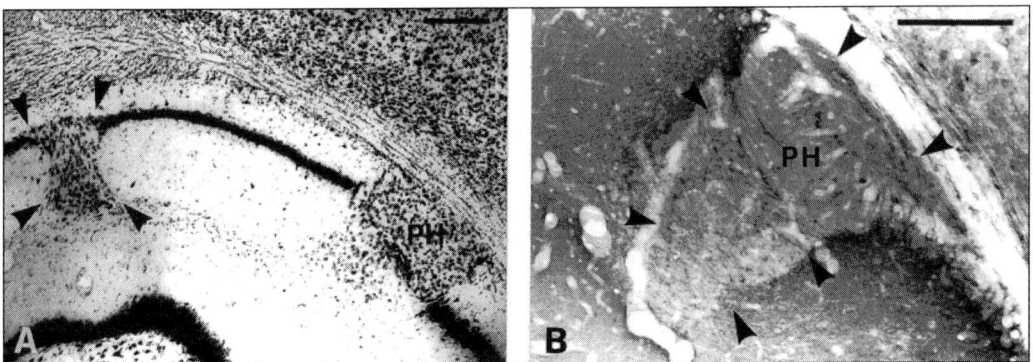

Fig. 6. Perihippocampal (PH) heterotopic nodules in MAM rats. Photomicrographs from coronal sections through the hippocampus stained with thionin (A), or immunoreacted with anti-GluR1 (B) antibody. (A) A perihippocampal nodule (right) extends into the CA2 pyramidal cell layer; heterotopic neurones (arrowheads) are also present more medially, disrupting the CA1 layering and extending into stratum radiatum and lacunosum-molecularis. (B) A perihippocampal nodule (arrowheads) with neuropil and perikaryal GluR1 immunoreactivity similar to the neocortical rather than hippocampal staining pattern. Scale bars: 250 μm.

At more posterior rostro-caudal levels, multiple ovoid nodules were present at the latero-dorsal border of the hippocampus, close to the CA2 region. More caudally, the perihippocampal nodules extended into the hippocampus, disrupting the normal CA1 and CA2 layering (Fig. 6A). In contrast to the normal hippocampus, the perihippocampal nodules were characterized by patterns of neuropil and perikaryal immunoreactivity similar to that of the neocortex, for all employed anatomical markers (Fig. 6B). The border of the nodules was characterized by dense parvalbumin and GABA immunoreactivity, suggesting a particularly abundant GABAergic innervation of this marginal region.

Tract tracing experiments

To ascertain whether the altered cortical areas were connected with the periventricular and perihippocampal heterotopic nodules, injections of anterograde and retrograde tracers were performed in neocortical areas close to the heterotopic subcortical structures, approximately at the rostrocaudal level of the anterior commissure.

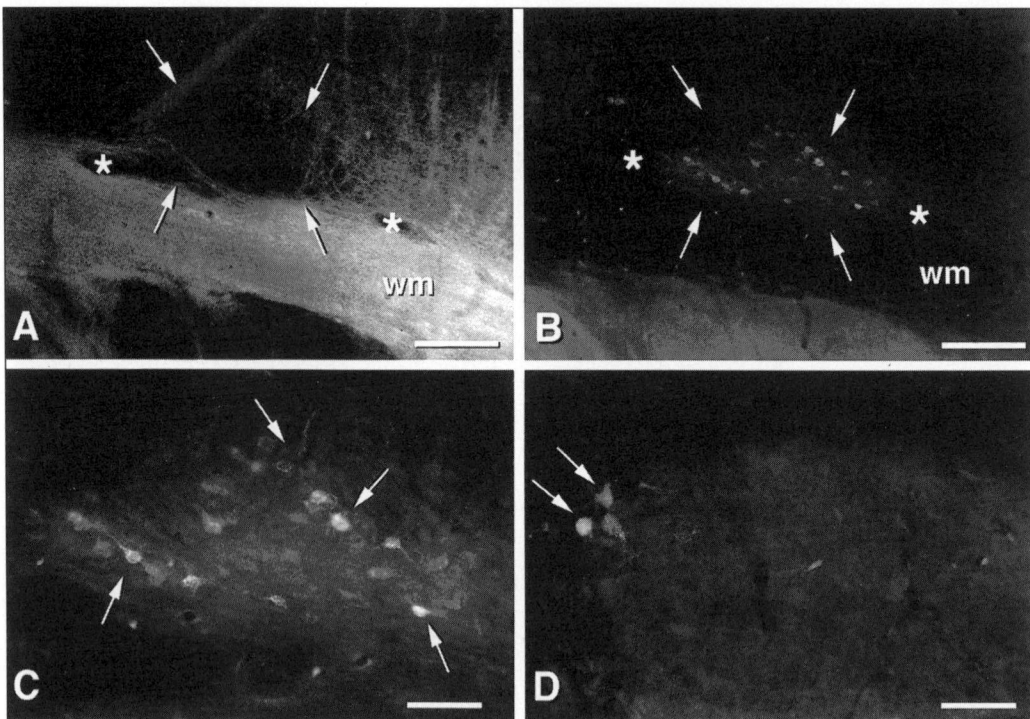

Fig. 7. Dark-field (A) and fluorescence (B-D) photomicrographs of retrogradely labelled neurones in cortical areas (A-C) and periventricular heterotopia (D) contralateral to an FG injection in deep motor cortex. (A-C) The photomicrographs are taken from the same cortical field to show the location of retrogradely labelled neurones in a deep heterotopic clusters, that is outlined by arrows (A and B) and appears darker in dark-field illumination (A). At higher magnification (C), pyramidal and fusiform commissural neurones are mainly located at the border of the heterotopic cluster. Asterisks in A and B mark cortical vessels as reference. wm: white matter. (D) Retrogradely labelled neurones are marginally located at the edge of a periventricular nodule contralateral to the injection site. Calibration bars: 250 μm (A-B), 100 μm (C and D).

After iontophoretic injections of the anterograde tracer BDA in superficial and deep motor cortical areas, anterogradely labelled fibres were found in both periventricular and perihippocampal heterotopic nodules, both ipsilaterally and contralaterally. Dense clusters of nerve fibres and terminals were distributed within the nodules. In addition, beaded fibres of small caliber surrounded some periventricular nodules, running along their edges, in close contact with the marginal fusiform neurones described above. Anterogradely labelled fibres penetrated also into the perihippocampal nodules, and extended more caudally through the nodule into the hippocampus to innervate a restricted region in the stratum lacunosum-moleculare, possibly contacting the apical dendrites of pyramidal neurones.

After iontophoretic injections of the retrograde tracer Fluorogold in motor cortical areas, retrogradely labelled neurones were consistently found in the neocortex contralateral to the injection site (Fig. 7A-C). Many contralaterally labelled neurones were located in the deep cortical heterotopic clusters, characterized by fusiform or pyramidal perikarya (Fig. 7B and C). Many labelled commissural cells were located at the marginal edge of the heterotopic clusters (Fig. 7C).

Retrogradely labelled neurones were also found in the periventricular and perihippocampal nodules, both ipsilaterally and contralaterally (Fig. 7D). The labelled neurones were very similar for location and morphology in both heterotopic nodules. They were particularly numerous on the side ipsilateral to the injection site. Some intensely labelled neurones were located, both ipsilaterally and contralaterally, in a marginal position within the nodules (Fig. 7 D). Labelled neurones were also found within the hippocampus, where the perihippocampal nodules extended into the hippocampus to disrupt the CA1 and CA2 pyramidal cell layer.

Discussion

In previous studies it has been demonstrated that single MAM exposures on E15 produced neocortical hypoplasia and neuronal heterotopia primarily involving the hippocampal CA1 and CA2 regions (Singh, 1977; Johnston & Coyle, 1979; Dambska et al., 1982; Collier & Ashwell, 1993).

The double MAM administration in the range of 15 to 16 embryonic day probably increased the antimitotic effect of MAM on dividing neuroblasts. Indeed the double MAM treatment determined not only more severe cortical hypoplasia when compared to single MAM administration (Colacitti et al., 1998), but it also induced previously unreported dramatic abnormalities of the cortical cytoarchitecture, and more pronounced subcortical neuronal heterotopia. From the laterodorsal periventricular region the heterotopic nodules extended not only to the hippocampal formation but also to the overlying neocortical areas. These more pronounced brain abnormalities were responsible for functional impairments which might bear resemblance to those observed in human neurological diseases (Sancini et al., 1998; see below).

The pathogenesis of MAM-induced neuronal heterotopia is not completely understood. It has been clearly demonstrated that MAM is capable of methylating purine and pyrimidine bases of nucleic acid, thus determining the blockade of neuroblast proliferation (Matsumoto et al., 1972; Cattaneo et al., 1995). However, despite the intensive use of different doses and time-schedules of administration, the exact mechanisms by which MAM produces *in vivo* alterations of the normal brain structuring and neuronal heterotopia have been differently interpreted in previous papers dealing with this subject (Singh, 1977; Collier and Ashwell, 1993; Zhang et al., 1995; Chevassus-au-Louis et al., 1998).

The present experiments suggest that cortical and subcortical heterotopia share common morphological features. For instance, marginal neurones and dense parvalbumin and GABAergic marginal staining of the neuropil are present in all MAM-induced heterotopia. In some rats, moreover, an anatomical continuity between these heterotopias was observed. In addition, all heterotopias were characterized by neocortical, rather than hippocampal, pattern of staining with all the different antibodies used. For these reasons, it may be speculated that the different heterotopias are formed, through the same pathogenic mechanism, by neurones originally committed to the neocortex. This hypothesis is supported by two lines of evidence: (i) the firing properties of neurones within the heterotopias, similar to those of supra- and infra-granular pyramidal cortical neurones (Sancini et al., 1998); (ii) the tract tracing data here reported, which demonstrate the existence of reciprocal anatomical connections between neocortical areas and the subcortical heterotopias. It should be remembered that no hippocampal projections from or to dorsal neocortical areas, similar to those reported in the present study, have ever been described in normal rats. The heterotopic neurones could have maintained the potential for connecting with the cortical areas to which they were presumably committed; their altered location could explain the establishment of the abnormal connections here reported.

The relevant number of heterotopic neurones forming the subcortical heterotopia, the columns of densely packed pyramidal neurones in deep cortical layers, and the subpial band of heterotopic neurones in layer I, all clearly suggest a disturbance of migration from the germinative periventricular layer to the developing neocortex. In addition, vimentin immunopositive processes are still present in the adult rat at the nodules' border, suggesting a migratory pathway around the periventricular heterotopia. The MAM-induced ablation of a selected population of precursor cells within the germinative layer could have produced a lack of soluble factors defining and permitting the appropriate environment for the migration of further waves of young post-mitotic neurones. It is therefore possible that periventricular heterotopias (and cortical and hippocampal heterotopia as well) are formed by neurones proliferating in the periventricular zone and committed to the cortex which do not find a normally permissive environment for a correct migration to their final cortical destination (McKay, 1989).

Developmental dysgeneses in human patients are characterized by varying neuropathologic features, presumably related to the type and timing of the involved causative factor (Mischel *et al.*, 1995; Battaglia *et al.*, 1996). The present data demonstrated that macroscopical and microscopical similarities exist between MAM rats and human patients affected by unilateral periventricular nodular heterotopia (PNH; Raymond *et al.*, 1995; Battaglia *et al.*, 1997). In human PNH multiple coalescent nodules of heterotopic gray matter extend from the paratrigonal region of the lateral ventricles to the overlying neocortex and along the temporal horns to the hippocampus (Raymond *et al.*, 1995; Battaglia *et al.*, 1997), as the subcortical nodules of MAM rats. In human PNH, however, neurones are present at the borders of the nodules with the same morphological and immunocytochemical features of marginal neurones in the subcortical nodules of MAM rats (Battaglia *et al.*, 1996). In addition, the subcortical nodules are characterized by dense GABAergic innervation, particularly at their borders, in both human PNH and MAM rats (Battaglia *et al.*, in preparation). Furthermore, the heterotopic structures in MAM rats are reciprocally connected with the neocortex, and connections between periventricular nodules and neocortex have been suggested also in human PNH by the presence of fibres radiating from the nodules (Spreafico *et al.*, 1998). Finally, periventricular nodules in human PNH can be the site of onset of epileptic discharges (Dubeau *et al.*, 1995), and a substantial fraction of heterotopic neurones in MAM rats are prone to abnormal burst firing (Sancini *et al.*, 1998). An increased susceptibility to epileptogenic agents has been previously demonstrated in single-treated MAM rats (De Feo *et al.*, 1995; Baraban and Schwartzkroin, 1995, 1996; Germano *et al.*, 1996). Our excessively bursting neurones, inserted in an aberrant cortico-subcortical circuitry, are likely to increase the susceptibility of MAM rats to extrinsic epileptogenic factors as well, even if spontaneous behavioural seizures have not been demonstrated.

In summary, the double MAM administration on E15 produces anatomical and physiological brain abnormalities that bear resemblance to those observed in human PNH, which are frequently associated with intractable epilepsy. We therefore propose that double-treated MAM rats could serve as an useful model not only to study the normal cortical development but also to investigate the pathogenetic mechanisms involved in the development of human brain dysgeneses and associated neuronal hyperexcitability.

Acknowledgements

The authors wish to thank Dr A. Caputi and Ms F. Cacciatore for their help in the early part of this study, Dr. R.J. Wenthold for the gift of the polyclonal anti-GLUR1 and -GLUR2-3 antisera, and Ms M. De Negri for editing the manuscript. This study was supported by grants from the Italian Ministry of Health (ICS 030.3RF95/223) and the Mariani Foundation for Paediatric Neurology, Milan.

References

Baraban, S.C. & Schwartzkroin, P.A. (1995): Electrophysiology of CA1 pyramidal neurones in an animal model of neuronal migration disorders: prenatal methylazoxymethanol treatment. *Epilepsy Res.* **22,** 145-56.

Baraban, S.C. & Schwartzkroin, P.A. (1996): Fluorothyl seizure susceptibility in rats following prenatal methylazoxymethanol treatment. *Epilepsy Res.* **23,** 189-94.

Barkovich, A.J., Gressens, P. & Evrard, P. (1992): Formation, maturation, and disorders of brain neocortex. *Am. J. Neuradiol.* **13,** 423-46.

Barkovich, A.J., Guerrini, R., Battaglia, G., Kalifa, G., N'Guyen, T., Parmeggiani, A., Santucci, M., Giovanardi-Rossi, P., Granata, T. & D'Incerti, L. (1994): Band heterotopia: correlation of outcome with Magnetic Resonance Imaging parameters. *Ann. Neurol.* **36,** 609-17.

Battaglia, G., Arcelli, P., Granata, T., Selvaggio, M.T., Andermann, F., Dubeau, F., Olivier, A., Tampieri, D., Villemure, J.G., Avoli, M., Avanzini, G. & Spreafico, R. (1996): Neuronal migration disorders and epilepsy: a morphological analysis of three surgically treated patients. *Epilepsy Res.* **26,** 49-58.

Battaglia, G., Granata, T., Farina, L., D'Incerti, L., Franceschetti, S. & Avanzini, G. (1997): Periventricular Nodular Heterotopia: epileptogenic findings. *Epilepsia* **38,** 1173-82.

Cattabeni, F. & Di Luca, M. (1997): Developmental models of brain dysfunctions induced by targeted cellular ablations with methylazoxymethanol. *Physiol. Rev.* **77,** 199-215.

Cattaneo, E., Reinach, B., Caputi, A., Cattabeni, F. & Di Luca, M. (1995): Selective in vitro blockade of neuroepithelial cells proliferation by methylazoxymethanol, a molecule capable of inducing long lasting functional impaiments. *J. Neurosci. Res.* **41,** 640-47.

Chevassus-Au-Louis, N., Rafiki, A., Jorquera, I., Ben-Ari, Y. & Represa, A. (1998): Neocortex in the hippocampus: an anatomical and functional study of CA1 heterotopias after prenatal treatment with methylazoxymethanol in rats. *J. Comp. Neurol.* **394,** 520-36.

Colacitti, C., Sancini, G., Franceschetti, S., Cattabeni, F., Avanzini, G., Spreafico, R., Di Luca, M. & Battaglia, G. (1998): Altered connections between neocortical and heterotopic areas in methylazoxymethanol-treated rats. *Epilepsy Res.* **32,** 49–62.

Collier, P.A. & Ashwell, K.W. (1993): Distribution of neuronal heterotopiae following prenatal exposure to methylazoxymethanol. *Neurotoxicol. Teratol.* **15,** 439-44.

Dambska, M., Haddad, R., Kozlowski, P.B., Lee, M.H. & Shek, J. (1982): Telencephalic cytoarchitectonics in the brains of rats with graded degrees of microencephaly. *Acta Neuropathol.* **58,** 203-09.

D'arcangelo, G., Miao, G.G., Chen, S.C., Soares, H.D., Morgan, J.I. & Curran, T. (1995): A protein related to extracellular matrix proteins deleted in the mouse mutant reeler. *Nature* **374,** 719-23.

De Feo, M.R., Mecarelli, O. & Ricci, G.F. (1995): Seizure susceptibility in immature rats with microencephaly induced by prenatal exposure to methylazoxymethanol acetate. *Pharmaco. Res.* **31,** 109-14.

Di Luca, M., Caputi, A., Cinquanta, M., Cimino, M., Marini, P., Princivalle, A., De Graan, P.N.E., Gispen, W.H. & Cattabeni, F. (1995): Changes in protein kinase C and in its presynaptic substrate B-50/GAP-43 after intrauterine exposure to methylazoxymethanol, a treatment inducing cortical and hippocampal damage and cognitive deficit in rats. *Eur. J. Neurosci.* **7,** 899-906.

Dubeau, F., Tampieri, D., Lee, N., Andermann, E., Carpenter, S., Leblanc, R., Olivier, A., Radtke, R., Villemure, J.G. & Andermann, F. (1995): Periventricular and subcortical nodular heterotopia. A study of 33 patients. *Brain* **118,** 1273-87.

Ferrer, I., Alcántara, S., Zújar, M.J. & Cinós, C. (1993): Structure and pathogenesis of cortical nodules induced by prenatal X-irradiation in the rat. *Acta Neuropathol.* **85,** 205-12.

Friede, R.L. (1989): *Developmental Neuropathology.* 2nd edition. New York: Springer Verlag.

Galaburda, A.M., Sherman, G.F., Rosen, G.D., Aboitz, F. & Geschwind N. (1985): Developmental dyslexia: four consecutive cases with cortical anomalies. *Ann. Neurol.* **18,** 222-33.

Germano, I.M., Zhang, Y.F., Sperber, E.F. & Moshé, S.L. (1996): Neuronal migration disorders increase susceptibility to hyperthermia-induced seizures in developing rats. *Epilepsia* **37,** 902-10.

Jacobs, K.M., Gutnick, M.J. & Prince, D.A. (1996): Hyperexcitability in a model of cortical maldevelopment. *Cerebral Cortex* **6,** 514-23.

Johnston, M.V. & Coyle, J.T. (1979): Histological and neurochemical effects of foetal treatment with methylazoxymethanol on rat neocortex in adulthood. *Brain Res.* **170,** 135-55.

Kuzniecky, R., Andermann, F. & Guerrini R. (1993): Congenital bilateral perisylvian syndrome: study of 31 patients. *Lancet* **341,** 608-12

Lee, K.S., Schottler, F., Collins, J.L., Lanzino, G., Couture Rao, A., Hiramatsu, K., Goto, Y., Hong, S.C., Caner, H., Yamamoto, H., Chen, Z.F., Bertram, E., Berr, S., Omary, R., Scrable, H., Jackson, T., Goble, J. & Eisenman, L. (1997): A genetic animal model of human neocortical heterotopia associated with seizures. *J. Neurosci.* **17,** 6236-42.

Matsumoto, H., Spatz, M. & Laqueur, GL. (1972): Quantitative changes with age in the DNA content of MAM-induced microencephalic rat brain. *J. Neurochem.* **19,** 297-306.

McKay, R.D.G. (1989): The origin of cellular diversity in the mammalian central nervous system. *Cell* **58,** 815–21.

Mischel, P.S., Nguyen, L.P. & Vinters, H.V. (1995): Cerebral cortical dysplasia associated with pediatric epilepsy. Review of neuropathologic features and proposal for a grading system. *J. Neuropathol. Exp. Neurol.* **54,** 137-153.

Petralia, R.S. & Wenthold, R.J. (1992): Light and electron immunocytochemical localization of AMPA-selective glutamate receptors in the rat brain. *J. Comp. Neurol..* **318,** 329-54.

Ramakers, M.J., Urban, I.J.A., De Graan, P.N.E., Di Luca, M., Cattabeni, F. & Gispen, W.H. (1993): The impaired long-term potentiation in the CA1 field of the hippocampus of cognitive deficient microencephalic rats is restored by D-serine. *Neuroscience* **54,** 49-60.

Raymond, A.A., Fish, D.R., Sisodiya, S.M., Alsanjari, N., Stevens, J.M. & Shorvon, S.D. (1995): Abnormalities of gyration, heterotopias, tuberous sclerosis, focal cortical dysplasia, microdysgenesis, dysembrioplastic neuroepithelial tumour and dysgenesis of the archicortex in epilepsy. Clinical, EEG and neuroimaging features in 100 adult patients. *Brain* **118,** 629-60.

Roper, S.N., Gilmore, R.L. & Houser, C.R. (1995): Experimentally induced disorders of neuronal migration produce an increased propensity for electrographic seizures in rats. *Epilepsy Res.***21,** 205-19.

Sancini, G., Franceschetti, S., Battaglia, G., Colacitti, C., Di Luca, M., Spreafico, R. & Avanzini, G. (1998): Dysplastic neocortex and subcortical heterotopias in methylazoxymethanol-treated rats: an intracellular study of identified pyramidal neurones. *Neurosci Lett.* **246,** 181-185.

Singh, S.C. (1977): Ectopic neurones in the hippocampus of the postnatal rat exposed *in utero* to methylazoxymethanol during foetal development. *Acta Neuropathol.* **40,** 111-16.

Spreafico, R., Pasquier, B., Minotti, L., Garbelli, R., Kahane, P., Grand, S., Benabid, A.L., Tassi, L., Avanzini, G., Battaglia, G., & Munari, C. (1998): Immunocytochemical investigation on dysplastic human tissue from epileptic patients. *Epilepsy Res.* **32,** 34–48.

Zhang, L.L., Collier, P.A. & Ashwell, K.W.S. (1995): Mechanisms in the induction of neuronal heterotopias following prenatal cytotoxic brain damage. *Neurotoxicol. Teratol.* **17,** 297-311.

Zilles, K. (1985): *The cortex of the rat. A stereotaxic atlas.* Berlin: Springer-Verlag

Chapter 9

The methylazoxymethanol (MAM) treated rat as an animal model for the neuronal migration disorders: electrophysiological findings in identified pyramidal neurones

Silvana Franceschetti[1], Giulio Sancini[1], Claudia Colacitti[1], Monica Di Luca[2], Tatiana Lavazza[1], Ferruccio Panzica[1], Roberto Spreafico[1], Giorgio Battaglia and Giuliano Avanzini[1]

[1]*Divisione di Neurofisiologia Sperimentale ed Epilettologia, Istituto Nazionale Neurologico 'C. Besta', Via Celoria 11, 20133 Milan, Italy*
[2]*Istituto di Scienze Farmacologiche, Università degli Studi di Milano, Via Balzaretti 9, 20133 Milan, Italy*

Summary

The congenital defects of neuronal migration occurring in humans consistently give rise to severe epilepsies; the study of animal models of neuronal migration disorders (NMD) may be considered a suitable approach to the understanding of the pathophysiological mechanisms underlying the epileptogenic propensity of maldeveloped cortical structures, and much interesting evidence, collected in recent years, suggests that different hyperexcitability phenomena can occur depending on the characteristics of different NMD models. We report here the results of an electrophysiological investigation performed in a NMD model obtained by a double transplacental treatment with the teratogenic agent MAM and resulting in both hippocampal and neocortical cytoarchitectonic derangement, associated with ectopic periventricular and parahippocampal aggregates of grey matter. One hundred and eleven pyramidal neurones were recorded in neocortex and in subcortical heterotopic aggregates, 53 of which were successfully labelled with biocytin.

Most neurones recorded in dysplastic neocortical areas as well as in the subcortical neuronal aggregates displayed normal firing characteristics; both regular spiking and intrinsically bursting pyramidal neurones were found in all of the examined structures. In about 1/5 of the neuronal population located either in neocortex or in subcortical heterotopic aggregates, the injection of depolarising current pulses elicited an aberrant firing pattern, characterised by the appearance of long-lasting repeated bursts of high-frequency action potentials, progressively increasing in duration and leading to 'tonic' discharge often outlasting the pulse depolarisation; the gradual development of this 'excessive' bursting behaviour suggests a progressive run-down of the slow components of the hyperpolarising after-potential. White matter stimulation was found to evoke physiological response in neurones located either in dysplastic neocortex or in subcortical heterotopias, moreover biocytin labelled neurones were found to send efferent axons travelling outside the dysplastic areas. Such evidence suggests that, in the MAM-induced NMD model, the heterotopic neurones (including those showing a hyperexcitable firing behaviour) could participate to an aberrant, potentially epileptogenic, circuitry.

Introduction

Developmental brain defects, usually defined as neuronal migration disorders (NMDs), can result in humans with either genetic determinants (Eksioglu et al., 1996; DesPortes et al., 1998) or pathogenic factors impairing the ordered sequence of the maturative events occurring during foetal life. The NMDs giving rise to macroscopic structural malformations, well recognisable by neuroimaging examination, are known to be often associated with severe epilepsies (Palmini et al., 1991; Dubeau et al., 1995; Battaglia et al., 1997). The powerful epileptogenic endowment of the maldeveloped nervous structures is further testified by the frequent neuropathological finding of microscopic neuronal heterotopias in patients presenting with nominally cryptogenic epilepsies, surgically treated for medically intractable seizures (Plate et al., 1993; Emery et al., 1997). The understanding of the specific pathophysiological mechanisms sustaining the high epileptogenic propensity of human NMDs is still at the initial stages, however the particular aptitude of dysplastic human neocortex in generating epileptogenic events has been demonstrated by the electrophysiological data obtained by Mattia et al. (1995) on surgically removed human specimens; in fact these authors found that the bath application of the convulsant 4-aminopyridine is capable of consistently inducing seizure-like discharges in slices prepared from dysplastic neocortex but not in those prepared from normal neocortex removed from patients operated on for limbic epilepsies.

Animal NMD models and increased neuronal excitability

Several animal models of NMDs can be obtained by exposure, during the embryonic life, to physical (i.e. X-ray) or chemical (e.g. ethanol, methylazoxymethanol) teratogenic agents capable of killing the neuroblasts and/or disarranging the neuro–glial relationship. In addition, genetically determined developmental brain abnormalities have been found in spontaneous mutant rodents, such as dreher (Falconer 1951; Sekiguchi et al., 1994) or reeler mice (Caviness, 1976), and local neuronal heterotopias have been detected in some special strain of genetically epilepsy prone rodents (Amano et al., 1996). Among them, an interesting mutant rat, presenting with bilateral subcortical heterotopias and spontaneous seizures, has been discovered and recently described by Lee et al. (1997) - also see Chapter 11 in this volume. Finally, targeted genetic manipulations can result in a selective impairment of cortical development which may associate with spontaneous seizures, as demonstrated by Acampora et al. (1996) in a mouse model lacking the Otx 1 gene. It must be noted, however, that most of both genetic and induced NMD animal models do not present with obvious spontaneous epileptic seizures, or alternatively recurrent seizures may occur in only a limited subpopulation of the affected individuals (Lee et al., 1997).

To clarify the physiopathological changes resulting from the migrational defects, several NMD animal models have recently been deeply investigated using both *in vivo* and *in vitro* preparations. Most of the *in vivo* experiments have been carried out to ascertain the presence, in the affected animals, of an increased propensity to develop seizures; *in vitro* studies have been primarily aimed at characterising the basic mechanisms capable of sustaining an increased excitability of maldeveloped structures.

In NMD models obtained by chemical or physical manipulations, much evidence clearly indicates that behavioural or electrographic seizures can be induced by 'pro-convulsant' manipulation which are not effective (or significantly less effective) in control animals. A peculiar propensity to develop seizures in response to sedating agents has been reported in rats with irradiation-induced NMDs (Roper et al., 1995, 1997) and a lower threshold for hyperthermia (Germano et al., 1996) or kainate-induced seizures (De Feo et al., 1995; Germano & Sperber, 1997, 1998) has been demonstrated in rats with neocortical and hippocampal NMDs induced by the exposition *in utero* to the alkylating agent methylazoxymethanol (MAM). In the same MAM model, Baraban & Schwartzkroin (1996) demonstrated a significant decrease in latency to develop fluorothyl-induced seizures in comparison to the controls and, interestingly, an inverse correlation between the seizure latency and the number of heterotopic neurones in the hippocampal CA1–CA2 region.

The basic mechanisms supporting the increased seizure susceptibility have been investigated in *in vitro* slices obtained from both maldeveloped neocortex and hippocampus. Electrophysiological evidence of a decreased synaptic inhibition, leading to local multiphasic epileptiform activity, has been obtained by Jakobs *et al.*, (1996) and Prince *et al.* (see Chapter 10 in this volume) in a NMD model induced by local cortical freezing. In this model, mimicking human polymicrogyria, an inbalance between synaptically driven excitation and inhibition is also supported by the data of Luhmann & Raabe, 1996), indicating an increased aminoacid-mediated hyperexcitability in neocortical areas closely surrounding the microgyri.

In those NMD models in which a migration defect is induced at early embryonic stages, when the differentiation processes are still ongoing, a rearrangement in the intrinsic cell properties may also be hypothesised. This assumption is especially supported by the evidence obtained by Baraban & Schwartzkroin (1995) in the MAM model of NMD, revealing remarkable changes in neuronal firing behaviour and the occurrence of hyperexcitability phenomena attributable to changes in the intrinsic cellular properties (possibly due to a defective K^+ channel expression) rather than to a synaptic malfunction.

The NMD model induced in rat by transplacental MAM treatment

Adult rats treated with MAM during the embryonic stages of cortical development display different neuronal arrangement abnormalities, depending on the time of the exposure to the neurotoxic agent (Gillies & Price, 1993; Zhang *et al.*, 1995; Cattabeni & Di Luca, 1997). The ability of MAM to kill neuroblasts in their mitotic phase (Cattaneo et al., 1995) is the primary mechanism on which the narrowing and disarrangement of the neocortical mantle is based. In addition, MAM-induced structural abnormalities of the radial glia (Zhang *et al.*, 1995) may lead to an obstructed and misdirected migration of the neocortical precursors (Gillies & Price, 1993) and have been considered as the main mechanism giving rise to subcortical heterotopias. Moreover, residual migratory events occurring during early post-natal life may concur in the induction of the final NMD picture that can be found in mature animals (Sing, 1977; Chevassus-au-Louis, 1998a).

The MAM model of NMD submitted to neurophysiological evaluations until now (De Feo *et al.*, 1995; Baraban & Schwartzkroin, 1995, 1996; Germano *et al.*, 1996; Germano & Sperber, 1997, 1998; Chevassus-au-Louis *et al.*, 1998a) has been obtained by a single transplacental treatment with the teratogenic agent MAM at the 15th embryonic day (E15). This treatment, performed in pregnant rats, regularly induces hippocampal heterotopias in the offspring (Sing, 1977; Collier & Ashwell, 1993; Chevassus-au-Louis *et al.*, 1998a) involving the CA1–2 regions and small periventricular heterotopias associated with microcephaly and altered neocortical lamination. Recently, Chevassus-au-Louis *et al.* (1998a), using both morphological and electrophysiological evaluation, demonstrated that pyramidal neurones located in peri-hippocampal heterotopias share with supra-granular pyramidal neurones some physiological phenotypic characteristics and a similar migrational and neurogenetic profile, thus suggesting that the heterotopic aggregates predominantly originate from neuroblasts fated to neocortical mantle rather than to hippocampal formation.

The NMD model on which we performed our electrophysiological and morpho-functional study has been obtained by a double transplacental administration of MAM (15 mg/kg in the morning and the same dose 12 hours later intraperitoneally injected in the pregnant mother) performed on E15. This procedure was found to induce in the offspring microcephaly and hippocampal heterotopias similar to those found with the single E15 MAM treatment and, in addition, it caused large heterotopic aggregates surrounding the ventricular floor (in continuity with hippocampal heterotopia) and the appearance of large irregular neuronal clusters in the sensorimotor cortical area (Battaglia *et al.*, 1996; Colacitti *et al.*, 1998a, b; see also Chapter 8 in this volume).

The NMD model induced by double MAM treatment: experimental results

Electrophysiological evidences

The results of the electrophysiological experiments that we reported here have been aimed at evaluating the firing characteristics and the synaptic excitability of pyramidal neurones located in dysplastic neocortex and in the periventricular heterotopic aggregates which characterise the NMD model based on double MAM treatment.

Most of the evidence obtained has been previously reported by Sancini *et al.* (1998) and is supplemented here with the results of experiments carried out more recently in our laboratory. The electrophysiological recordings were made in brain slices obtained from adult (45–60 days old) MAM-treated rats. Coronal slices (400 µm thick) were cut by means of a vibratome from a tissue block containing both the dorsal fronto-parietal cortex and subcortical (periventricular) structures, including the dorsal hippocampus in the most caudal sections; the typical features found in two representative thionin stained slices are displayed in Fig. 1. The subcortical neuronal aggregates appeared to be ordinary, separated from the neocortical mantle by the subcortical white matter, and the most caudal nodular heterotopias, neighbouring the hippocampal formation, appeared to be separated from the CA1-2 area by a macroscopically preserved stratum oriens (Fig. 1A).

Intracellular recordings were performed in neurones located 350-550 µm below the surface of the dysplastic sensorimotor cortex and in neurones located in the periventricular heterotopic aggregates. A few recordings were performed in the disarranged CA1–CA2 areas close to the heterotopic neuronal aggregates, but are not included in this report. Biocytin-filled glass microelectrodes (2-4 per cent biocytin in 0.5-1 M K-acetate, buffered with Tris HCl at pH 7.3; resistance 80-150 MΩ) were used to identify the physiological characterised neurones and their morphological features.

The firing characteristics were evaluated by means of the injection of square current pulses with a duration of 10-600 ms. Post-synaptic potentials were evoked by means of electrical stimulation of the subcortical white matter close to the recording site. At the end of the electrophysiological experiments the biocytin-injected slices were fixed by immersion in 4 per cent paraformaldehyde, embedded in agarose (6 per cent in distilled H_2O) and cut by a vibratome into 50-80 µm sections. The sections were then incubated for 2-4 hours in avidin-biotin complex, reacted with 3-3' diaminobenzidine, mounted on slides, and counterstained with 0.1 per cent thionin.

One hundred and eleven neurones were selected for analysis, 53 of which were successfully labelled by biocytin and identified as pyramidal neurones; 66 neurones were recorded in the sensorimotor cortex, 45 in the periventricular aggregates.

On the basis of their firing behaviour in response to the injection of just supra-threshold depolarising current pulses, the neurones were classified as intrinsically bursting (IB) or regular spiking (RS) (Connors *et al.*, 1982). Fast spiking neurones (putative GABAergic interneurones) were also occasionally recorded but are excluded from the present report. Of the 66 neocortical neurones, 36 (55 per cent) were classified as IB and 18 as RS (27 per cent, all but four showing spike frequency adaptation). Different neuronal subtypes could be encountered, spread about the dysplastic neocortical areas, independently of the depth of the recording site.

Of the 45 neurones recorded in the subcortical heterotopic aggregates, 30 (66 per cent) were classified as RS (A_1 in Fig. 2), all showing spike frequency adaptation, and eight as IB (18 per cent) (B_1 in Fig. 2).

The remaining 12 neurones recorded in the neocortex (18 per cent) and the seven recorded in the heterotopic subcortical neuronal aggregates (16 per cent) revealed the peculiar firing behaviour shown in Fig. $2A_{1-2}$ and Fig. 3. Shortly after the impalement, these neurones fired with long-

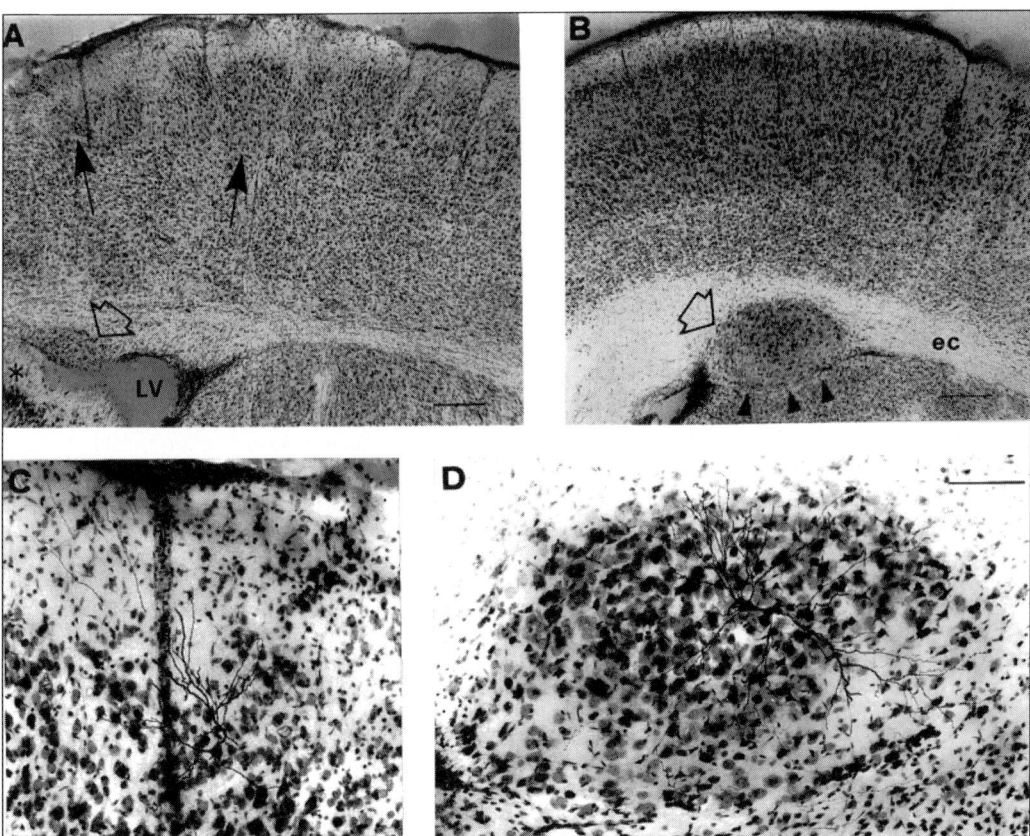

Fig. 1. These microphotographs respectively display the irregular clusters of densely packaged neurones (arrows) found in sensorimotor cortex (A) and the heterotopic neuronal aggregates found close to the ventricular floor (A and B, open arrow). The large heterotopic periventricular aggregate (B, open arrow) appears to be segregated from both neocortex and basal ganglia (arrowheads); (A and B, calibration bar 500 μm). In panels C and D, two biocytin injected neurones are displayed, respectively located in dysplastic neocortex (C) and in a heterotopic subcortical aggregate (D): note the distorted arborisation of the apical dendrite in the neocortical neurone (C and D, calibration bar 200 μm).

lasting repetitive bursts of APs in response to the low-amplitude depolarising current pulses (200-600 ms duration) ordinarily used to evaluate the qualitative firing behaviour of the recorded cells; at the beginning each burst included four to seven fast APs but, during the subsequently delivered supra-threshold depolarising current pulses, progressively increased in duration merging into long trains of high-frequency APs (A_4 in Fig. 3), often outlasting the duration of the depolarising pulse. In parallel with the increasing duration of burst discharge, the post-burst after hyperpolarisation progressively shortened and tended to diminish (Fig. 3). If left unstimulated for a few minutes, all these neurones recovered to their original firing behaviour but reproduced the same firing sequence during the injection of a new series of depolarising current pulses (Sancini et al., 1998). The APs generated by these 'excessively bursting neurones' had a slightly slower rise time than the other IB neurones, whereas the repolarising phase was quite fast and did not show any significant impairment during the recurrent bursting behaviour.

No significant differences were found in resting membrane potential, membrane input resistance or time constant on comparing the neurones recorded in the neocortex and those recorded in the heterotopic aggregates. In both structures the average input resistance value of RS neurones was higher than that of the bursting neurones, but the difference did not reach statistical significance (Sancini et al., 1998).

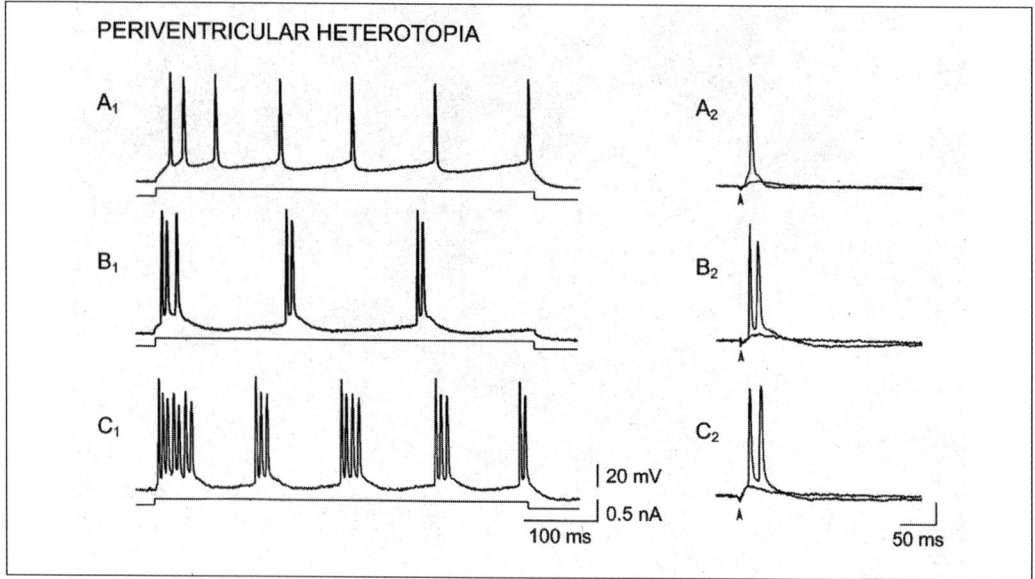

Fig. 2. Firing characteristics found in three representative neurones recorded in the heterotopic aggregates. The neurones in A1 and B1 were respectively classified as RS and IB. The neurone discharging with long repetitive burst of action potentials displayed in C1 was defined as 'excessively' bursting. The response to white matter stimulation of the three neurones are displayed in A2, B2, and C2.

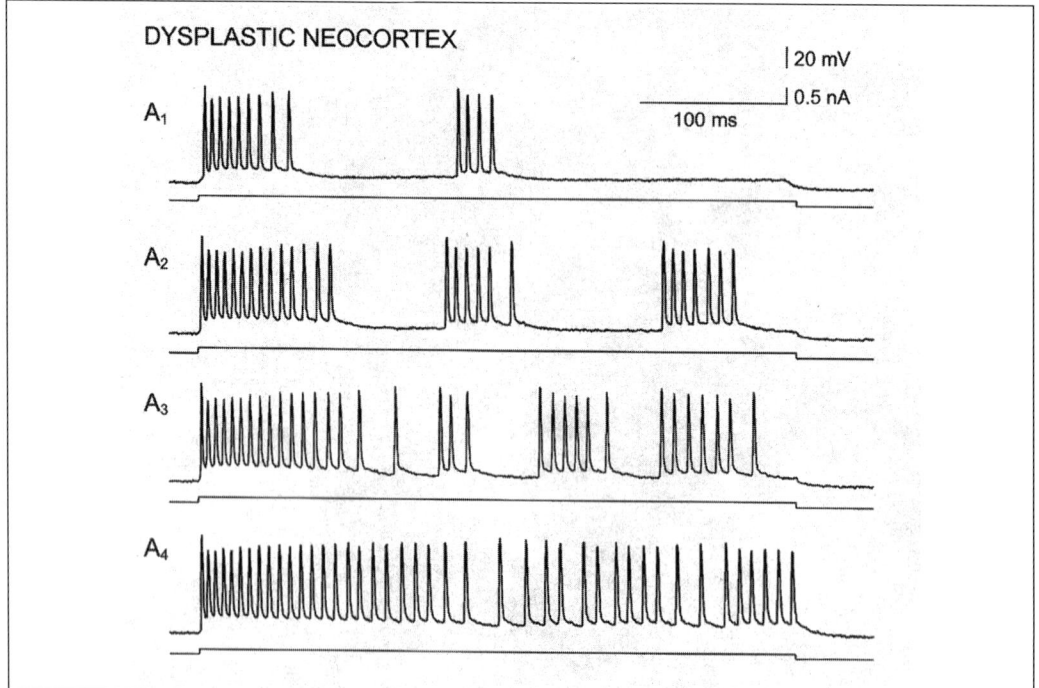

Fig. 3. The typical firing behaviour of the neurones categorised as 'excessively bursting' is exemplified. Note the long burst of AP recorded shortly after the cell impalement (A1) and the progressive increase in burst duration (A2) (corresponding to a progressive post-burst after-hyperpolarisation shortening), leading to a long lasting train of high-frequency AP discharge.

In all of the neocortical and subcortical heterotopic neurones, excitatory post-synaptic potentials (EPSPs) could be consistently elicited by means of the electrical stimulation of the white matter. Threshold stimuli for orthodromic AP generation evoked a single AP in RS neurones (A_2 in Fig. 2) and a short burst of two or three APs (or a single AP followed by a depolarising afterpotential) in both IB and 'excessively bursting' neurones (B_2 and C_2 in Fig. 2). The synaptically evoked response of 'excessively bursting neurones' did not show any particular characteristic under baseline conditions, but its duration appeared slightly increased only when the stimulus was delivered after long-lasting burst discharges had been elicited (Sancini et al., 1998). Individual antidromic APs could be evoked, by slightly increasing the strength of the stimulus, in both neocortical neurones and in those recorded in the heterotopic aggregate (Fig. 4C). Inhibitory post-synaptic potentials (IPSPs) were consistently elicited in all the neurones; pronounced long-lasting biphasic IPSPs were more commonly recorded in a subpopulation of RS neurones (41 per cent) located in the heterotopic aggregates (Sancini et al., 1998).

Morphological features

As exemplified in Fig. 1, sensorimotor cortex exhibited a marked derangement of cortical layering, including many clusters of densely packaged neurones. In half of the neocortical biocytin-labelled pyramidal neurones that were reconstructed by camera lucida drawing, the apical dendrites showed various aberrant arborisation patterns consisting of a proximal split (at less than 150 µm from the soma) into two or three main branches or in an abnormal orientation. The primary axon of all labelled neocortical neurones regularly entered the white matter, whereas the extension of the axon collaterals varied depending on the completeness of the biocytin filling.

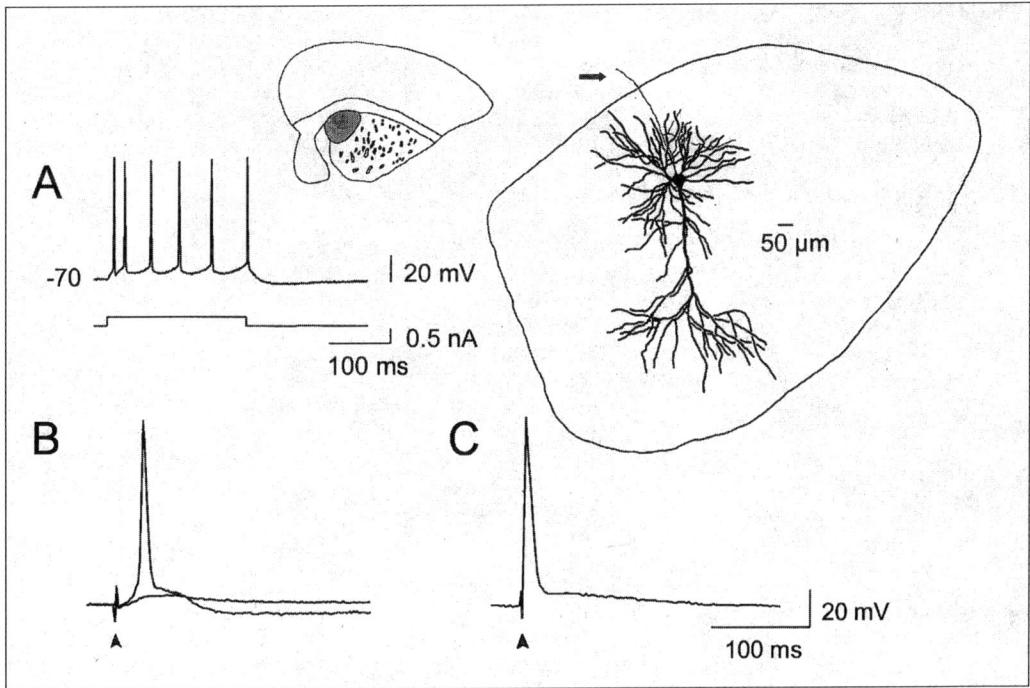

Fig. 4. Pyramidal neurone recorded in a heterotopic aggregate (marked by a shadowed area in the schematic slice representation) defined as regular spiking, according to its firing characteristics in response to the injection of a depolarising current pulse (A). The neurone responded to white matter stimulation with an EPSP or, at threshold, with an individual AP followed by an IPSP (B). The axon of the neurone crossed the border of the periventricular heterotopia (arrow) reaching the white matter; accordingly, an antidromic action potential (C) could be elicited by slightly increasing over threshold the intensity of the white matter stimuli.

Sixteen of the 27 biocytin-labelled pyramidal neurones recorded in the heterotopic subcortical aggregates were drawn in camera lucida: the main axis of the 12 neurones located within the central area of the nodular aggregates had a radial orientation, with their apical dendrites being directed toward the external border of the heterotopia (Fig. 1D); the four neurones located at the border of the heterotopia had their main axis parallel to the border of the neuronal aggregate, with an asymmetric disposition of their dendritic arborisation that was exclusively expanded toward the inner part of the aggregate. In seven of these 16 neurones, the primary axon and/or a variable number of axon collaterals clearly crossed the border of the heterotopic aggregate (Fig. 4), reaching the subcortical white matter. In the remaining labelled neurones, the partial filling of the axon branching did not allow any conclusion to be drawn concerning their efferent projections.

Out of six successfully labelled 'excessively bursting neurones', only two showed a clearly distorted apical dendritic arborisation similar to those observed in neurones not showing any aberrant discharge behaviour.

Comments

The MAM treatment based on a double MAM injection given at E15 resulted in a disruption of neuronal cortical layering associated with intracortical clusters of densely packed neurones and in the formation of subcortical nodular aggregates neighbouring both the hippocampus and the lateral ventricular floor. These features mimic NMD pictures that can be frequently seen in spontaneous human NMDs characterised by extensive periventricular nodular heterotopic aggregates (Palmini et al., 1991; Battaglia et al., 1997). The results of anatomical and immunocytochemical studies of this model have been recently reported by Battaglia et al. (1996) and by Colacitti et al. (1998a, b; see also Chapter 8 in this volume).

The present data, based on the electrophysiological characterisation of a population of pyramidal neurones, indicated that considerable excitability changes occur in a neuronal subpopulation located in the heterotopic subcortical aggregates as well as in the dysplastic neocortex. This hyperexcitability is testified by the appearance of prolonged burst of APs in response to the injection of just supra-threshold depolarising current pulses. The analysis of the electrophysiological data, in association with the information provided by the anatomical investigation (Battaglia et al., 1996; Colacitti et al., 1998a; see also Chapter 8 in this volume), allows some hypothesis about the functional consequences of the neuronal heterotopias with particular regard to the hyperexcitability phenomena found in individual neurones.

Pyramidal neurone phenotypes and connectivity

The majority of the neurones recorded in dysplastic neocortex showed physiological properties that were not different from those reported for neocortical neurones of normal sensorimotor cortex in rodents (Connors et al., 1982, 1990). They included a quite large percentage of IB neurones that in rats are known to be confined to the deep layers (mainly in layer V), thus suggesting that many neurones fated to neocortical layer V actually escape the killing ability of MAM and largely participate in the organisation of intracortical neuronal clusters. Unlike neocortex, the neurones recorded in the subcortical heterotopias were found to fire as RS. This difference could be due to a different origin and/or commitment of most of the neurones making up the periventricular heterotopic aggregates with respect to those making up the dysplastic neocortical areas (i.e. neurones fated to Cornu Ammonis or to the superficial cortical layers) (Sing, 1977; Collier & Ashwell, 1993; Zhang et al., 1995). Our observation agrees well with the evidence obtained by Chevassus-au-Louis et al. (1998a) in the NMD model obtained by a single MAM treatment performed at E15, indicating that hippocampal heterotopic neurones share many physiological and neurogenetic characteristics with neocortical pyramidal neurones pertaining to the supra-granular layers, where all the pyramidal neurones are known to discharge with an RS firing (Connors et al., 1982). Accordingly, in our NMD model, obtained by double MAM treatment, much immunocytochemical and anatomical evidence (i.e. presence of ipsilateral and contralateral connections between periventricular aggregates and neocortical structures) strongly indicates a neocortical rather than hippocampal commitment of the periventricular heterotopic neurones (Colacitti *et al.*, 1998a; see also Chapter 8 in this volume). Our finding of a small percentage of IB neurones participating in the formation of periventricular heterotopias could suggest that more than one neuronal phenotype (presumably fated to different cortical layers) cooperate to the formation of extensive heterotopic aggregates induced by the double E15 MAM treatment.

The finding of an effective synaptic activation, in most of the recorded neurones, in response to the electrical stimulation of the subcortical white matter, supports the possibility that the neurones located both in dysplastic neocortical areas and in periventricular or parahippocampal aggregates can be influenced by incoming inputs. At the same time, both physiological results and morphological reconstructions of the labelled neurones indicate that either neocortical or periventricular heterotopic neurones send their efferent projections to the white matter from which they also receive synaptic influences. Therefore, these neurones must be considered capable of influencing downstream structures giving rise to an aberrant circuitry. The data obtained by recording and labelling individual pyramidal neurones are substantially supported by the anatomical results obtained by Colacitti *et al.* (1998a; see also Chapter 8 in this volume) in the same model of NMD, indicating the presence of reciprocal connections between the subcortical heterotopic aggregates and the ipsilateral and contralateral dysplastic neocortex; moreover, they substantially agree with the evidence obtained by Chevassus-au-Louis *et al.* (1998) on single E15 MAM-treated rat, demonstrating a functioning connectivity between hippocampal heterotopias and neocortex.

Excessively bursting behaviour

Both in dysplastic neocortex and in the subcortical neuronal aggregates a subpopulation (16-18 per cent) of pyramidal neurones showed hyperexcitability phenomena leading to an aberrant firing pattern that we defined as an 'excessively bursting' behaviour, thus suggesting that the mechanisms supporting these firing characteristics are widely expressed. A defective control of intrinsic membrane excitability appears to be the more appropriate mechanism to account for the observed aberrant firing behaviour, as direct membrane depolarisation was found to be necessary and sufficient to induce it and no evidence of any primary synaptic hyperexcitability was detectable.

A defect in the K^+-mediated control of membrane excitability has been previously hypothesised by Baraban & Schwartzkroin (1995) to account for the increased neuronal excitability that these authors found in a subpopulation of pyramidal neurones recorded in dysplastic CA1 area of rats submitted to a single E15 MAM treatment. In fact, a slight increase in extracellular K^+ concentration (6 µM) has been found to lead these neurones to an epileptiform activity which cannot be obtained in control animals. In our observation, the 'excessive bursting' behaviour, consisting of an unusual long burst of APs followed by a rather weak post-burst after-hyperpolarisation, was detectable early after cell impalement. The burst length was found to progressively increase in response to long-lasting repeated depolarisations leading to repetitive cell firing, and to recover to basal condition after stimulus discontinuation, suggesting that this firing behaviour is due to a use-dependent run-down of a hyperpolarising current. However, in our cell population, a low increase of extracellular K^+ concentration was not found effective in inducing a significant increase in neuronal excitability in comparison to controls (personal observations). Different local conditions (in terms of neuro-glial interactions, cell geometry or channel distribution in different neuronal phenotype) may perhaps account for the difference between our observation and the observation of Baraban & Schwartzkroin (1995) on CA1 pyramidal neurones. Further experimental examinations are needed to understand the observed hyperexcitability phenomena; however our results, suggesting a progressive reduction in post-burst hyperpolarisation and a parallel increase in burst duration (Sancini *et al.*, 1998), lead us to hypothesise the occurrence of a progressive decline in the Ca^{2+}-activated K^+ current that is primary involved in hyperpolarising after-potential generation and in firing control in neocortical pyramidal neurones (Schwindt *et al.*, 1988). A dysfunction of an intracellular metabolic pathway involving protein kinases has been described in rats treated at E15 with a single MAM injection (Caputi *et al.*, 1996); an impairment in protein-kinase regulation of the Ca^{2+} activated K^+ currents (Reinhart & Levitan, 1995; Sah, 1996) may at least partially explain the observed membrane excitability disorder. Furthermore, the aminergic hyperinnervation of dysplastic tissue that has been demonstrated in MAM-treated rats by Johnston *et al.* (1981) and by Jonsson & Hallman (1982) may contribute towards modifying the function of Ca^{2+} dependent K^+ channels, which are known to be modulated by aminergic agonists (Nicoll, 1988).

Conclusions

The electrophysiological evidence obtained in rats exposed *in utero* to the teratogenic agent MAM indicates that a consistent subpopulation of pyramidal neurones located in both dysplastic neocortex and heterotopic aggregates exhibits an abnormal membrane excitability.

The presence of effective synaptic responses to the white matter stimulation, together with the evidence of efferent axon projections travelling outside the dysplastic areas (either cortical or subcortical), suggest that virtually all the neurones, and particularly those showing a hyperexcitable behaviour, may participate in an aberrant, potentially epileptogenic, circuitry.

Our results, together with those of Baraban & Schwartzkroin (1995), suggest that intrinsic neuronal properties can be impaired in early induced NMDs, and concur with a circuitry rearrangement to allow epileptic discharge generation and spread. The observed excitability changes do not appear, on the contrary, to be linked to obvious distortion of the dendritic tree that was observed in a large number of the biocytin-filled cells.

In spite of neuronal hyperexcitability and permissive circuitry suitable for generating epileptic phenomena, our MAM-induced NMD model (like most of the other NMD models) did not present with obvious spontaneous seizures. This evidence suggests that the complex neuronal organisation in which the maldeveloped structures are included significantly influences the final epileptogenic aptitude, so that a further disinhibition (e.g. proconvulsant manipulation) is required for generating true ictal discharges. The apparently lower aptitude for presenting with spontaneous seizures found in rodents compared to humans, could simply derive from the different complexity of cortical organisation between the two species. However, also in humans, a complex relationship between the predisposing factors (e.g. maldeveloped cortical structures) and the appearance of epileptic fits is not an unexpected finding, since epilepsies associated with NMDs often begin only in late childhood or in adult age (Battaglia *et al.*, 1997), and could present with variable clinical pictures in spite of a similar congenital structural disruption.

Acknowledgement

Supported by a grant ICS 030.3/RF95/223 from the Italian Ministry of Health and by the Mariani Foundation for Paediatric Neurology, Milan.

References

Acampora, D., Mazan, S., Avantaggiato, V., Barone, P., Tuorto, F., Lallemand, Y., Brulet, P. & Simeone, A. (1996): Epilepsy and brain abnormalities in mice lacking the Otx1 gene. *Nature Genetics* **14**, 218–222.

Amano, S., Ihara, N., Uemura, S., Yokoama, M., Ikeda, M. & Hazama, M. (1996): Microdysgenesis in the hippocampal formation in a newly developed Ihara's genetically epileptic rat (IGER). *Epilepsia* **37**, S3, 100–101.

Baraban, S.C. & Schwartzkroin, P.A. (1995): Electrophysiology of CA1 pyramidal neurons in an animal model of neuronal migration disorders: prenatal methylazoxymethanol treatment. *Epilepsy Res* **22**, 145–156.

Baraban, S.C. & Schwartzkroin, P.A. (1996): Fluorothyl seizure susceptibility in rats following prenatal methylazoxymethanol treatment. *Epilepsy Res* **23**, 189–194.

Battaglia, G., Colacitti, C., Di Luca, M., Frassoni, C., Cattabeni, F. & Spreafico, R. (1996): The methylazoxymethanol-treated rat: an animal model for human developmental dysgeneses. *Epilepsia* **37 (Suppl. 5)**, 3.75 (Abstract).

Battaglia, G., Granata, T., Farina, L., D'Incerti, L., Franceschetti, S. & Avanzini G. (1997): Periventricular nodular heterotopia: epileptogenic findings. *Epilepsia* **38**, 1173–1182.

Caputi, A., Rurale, S., Pastorino, L., Cimino, M., Cattabeni, F. & Di Luca, M. (1996): Differential translocation of protein kinase C isoenzymes in rats characterized by a chronic lack of LTP induction and cognitive impairment. *FEBS Lett.* **393**, 121–123.

Cattabeni, F. & Di Luca, M. (1997): Developmental models of brain dysfunction induced by targeted cellular ablations with methylazoxymethanol. *Physiol. Rev.* **77**, 199–215.

Cattaneo, E., Reinach, B., Caputi, A., Cattabeni, F. & Di Luca, M. (1995): Selective *in vitro* blockade of neuroepithelial cells by methylazoxymethanol, a molecule capable of inducing long lasting functional impairments. *J. Neurosci. Res.* **41**, 640–647.

Caviness Jr, V.S. (1976): Patterns of cells and fiber distribution in the neocortex of reeler mutant mouse. *J. Comp. Neurol.* **170**, 435–448.

Chevassus-au-Louis, N., Rafiki, A., Jorquera, I., Ben-Ari, Y. & Represa, A. (1998a): Neocortex in the hippocampus: an anatomical and functional study of CA1 heterotopias after prenatal treatment with methylazoxymethanol in rats. *J. Comp. Neurol.* **394**, 520–536.

Chevassus-au-Louis, N., Congar, P., Represa, P., Ben-Ari, Y. & Gaiarsa, J.L. (1998b): Neuronal migration disorders: heterotopic neocortical neurons in CA1 provide a bridge between the hippocampus and the neocortex. *Proc. Natl. Acad. Sci.* **95 (17)**, 10263–10268.

Colacitti, C., Sancini, G., Franceschetti, S., Cattabeni, F., Avanzini, G., Spreafico, R., Di Luca, M. & Battaglia, G. (1998a): Altered connections between neocortical and heterotopic areas in methylazoxymethanol-treated rat. *Epilepsy Res.* **32**, 49–62.

Colacitti, C., Sancini, G., De Biasi, S., Franceschetti, S., Caputi, A., Frassoni, C., Cattabeni, F., Avanzini, G., Spreafico, R., Di Luca, M. & Battaglia, G. (1998b): Prenatal methylazoxymethanol treatment in rats produces brain abnormalities with morphological similarities to human developmental brain dysgeneses. *J. Neuropathol. Exp. Neurol.* **58**, 92–106.

Collier, P.A. & Ashwell, K.W. (1993): Distribution of neuronal heterotopiae following prenatal exposure to methylazoxymethanol. *Neurotoxicol. Teratol.* **15**, 439–444.

Connors, B.W. & Gutnick, M.J. (1990): Intrinsic firing patterns of diverse neocortical neurones. *TINS* **13**, No 3, 99–104.

Connors, B.W., Gutnick, M.J. & Prince, D.A. (1982): Electrophysiological properties of neocortical neurons *in vitro*. *J. Neurophysiol.* **48**, 1302–1320.

De Feo, M.R., Mecarelli, O. & Ricci, G.F. (1995): Seizure susceptibility in immature rats with microencephaly induced by prenatal exposure to methylazoxymethanol acetate. *Pharmacol. Res.* **31**, 109–114.

DesPortes, V., Pinard, J.M., Billuart, P., Vinet, M.C., Koulakoff, A., Carrié, A., Gélot, A., Dupuis, A., Motte, J., Berwald-Netter, Y., Catala, M., Khan, A., Beidjourd, C. & Kelly, J. (1998): Identification of a novel CNS gene required for neuronal migration and involved in X-linked subcortical heterotopias and lissencephaly syndrome. *Cell* **92**, 51–61.

Dubeau, F., Tampieri, D., Lee, N., Andermann, E., Carpenter, S., Leblanc, R., Olivier, A., Radtke, R., Villemure, J.G. & Andermann F. (1995): Periventricular and subcortical nodular heterotopia. A study of 33 patients. *Brain* **118**, 1273–1287.

Eksioglu, Y.Z., Scheffer, I.E., Cardenas, P., Knol, J., DiMario, F., Ramsby, G., Berg, M., Kamuro, K., Berkovic, S.F., Duyk, G.M., Parisi, J., Huttenlocher, P.R. & Walsh, C.A. (1996): Periventricular heterotopia: an X-linked dominant epilepsy locus causing aberrant cerebral cortical development. *Neuron* **16**, 77–87

Emery, J.A., Roper, S.N. & Rojiani, A.M.(1997): White matter neuronal heterotopia in temporal lobe epilepsy: a morphometric and immunohistochemical study. *J. Neuropathol. Exp. Neurol.* **56**, 1276–82.

Falconer, D.S. (1951): Two mutants, 'trembler' and 'reeler', with neurological actions in the house mouse (Mus musculus L.). *J. Genet.* **50**, 192–201.

Germano, I. & Sperber, E.F. (1997): Increased seizure susceptibility in adult rats with neuronal migration disorders. *Brain Res.* **777**, 219–222

Germano, I. & Sperber, E.F. (1998): Transplacentally induced neuronal migration disorders: an animal model for the study of the epilepsies. *J. Neurosci. Res.* **51**, 473–488.

Germano, I.M., Zhang, Y.F., Sperber, E.F. & Solomon, L.M. (1996): Neuronal migration disorders increase susceptibility to hyperthermia-induced seizures in developing rats. *Epilepsia* **37**, 902–910.

Gillies, K. & Price, D.J. (1993): The fates of cells in developing cerebral cortex of normal and methylazoxymethanol acetate-lesioned mice. *Eur. J. Neurosci.* **3**, 73–84.

Jacobs, K.M., Gutnick, M.J. & Prince, D.A. (1996): Hyperexcitability in a model of cortical maldevelopment. *Cerebral Cortex* **6**, 514–523.

Johnston, M.V., Carman, A.B. & Coyle, J.T. (1981): Effect of foetal treatment with methylazoxymethanol acetate at various gestational dates on the neurochemistry of the adult neocortex of the rat. *J. Neurochemistry* **366**, 124–128.

Jonsson, G. (Hallman, H. (1982): Effects of prenatal methylazoxymethanol treatment on the development of central monoamine neurons. *Dev. Brain Res.* **2**, 513–530.

Lee, S.K., Schottler, F., Collins, J.L., Lanzino, G., Couture, D., Rao, A., Hiramatsu, K., Goto, Y., Hong, S., Caner, H., Yamamoto, Y., Chen, Z., Bertram, E., Berr, S., Omary, R., Scrable, H., Jackson, T., Goble, J. & Eisenman, L. (1997): A genetic animal model of human neocortical heterotopia associated with seizures. *J. Neurosci.* **17**, 6236–6242.

Luhmann, H.J. & Raabe, K. (1996): Characterization of neuronal migration disorders in neocortical structures. I. Expression of epileptiform activity in an animal model. *Epilepsy Res.* **26**, 67–74.

Mattia, D., Olivier, A. & Avoli, M. (1995): Seizure-like discharges recorded in human dysplastic neocortex maintained *in vitro*. *Neurology* **45**, 1391–1395.

Nicoll, R.A. (1988): The coupling of neurotransmitter receptors to ion channels in the brain. *Science* **241**, 545–551.

Palmini, A., Andermann, F., Olivier, A., Tampieri, D., Robitaille, Y., Andermann, E. & Wright, G. (1991): Focal neuronal migration disorders and intractable partial epilepsy: a study of 30 patients. *Annal Neurol.* **30**, 741–749.

Plate, K.H., Wieser, H.G., Yasargil, M.G. & Wiestler, O.D. (1993): Neuropathological findings in 224 patients with temporal lobe epilepsy. *Acta Neuropathol.* **86**, 433–438.

Reinhart, P.H. & Levitan, I.B. (1995): Kinase and phosphatase activities associated with a reconstituted calcium-dependent potassium channel. *J. Neurosci.* **15**, 4572–4679.

Roper, S.N., Gilmore, R.L. & Houser, C.R. (1995): Experimentally induced disorders of neuronal migration produce an increased propensity for electrographic seizures in rats. *Epilepsy Res.* **21**, 205–219.

Roper, S.N., King, M.A., Abraham, L.A. & Boillot, M.A. (1997): Disinhibited *in vitro* neocortical slices containing experimentally induced cortical dysplasia demonstrate hyperexcitability. *Epilepsy Res.* **26**, 443–449.

Sah, P. (1996): Ca^{2+}-activated K^+ channels in neurones: types, physiological role and modulation. *TINS* **19**, 150–154.

Sancini, G., Franceschetti, S., Battaglia, G., Colacitti, C., Di Luca, M., Spreafico, R. & Avanzini, G. (1998): Dysplastic neocortex and subcortical heterotopias in methylazoxymethanol-treated rats: an intracellular study of identified pyramidal neurones. *Neurosci. Lett.* **246**, 181–185.

Schwindt, P.C., Spain, W.J., Foehring, R.C., Chubb, M.C. & Crill, W.E. (1988): Slow conductances in neurons from cat sensorimotor cortex *in vitro* and their role in slow excitability changes. *J. Neurophysiol.* **50**, 450–467.

Sekiguchi, M., Abe, H., Shimai, K., Huang, G., Inoue, T. & Nowakowski, R.S. (1994): Disruption of neuronal migration in the neocortex of the dreher mutant mouse. *Dev. Brain Res.* **77**, 37–43.

Sing, S.C. (1977): Ectopic neurones in hippocampus of the postnatal rat exposed to methylazoxymethanol during foetal development. *Acta Neuropathol.* **40**, 111–116.

Zhang, L.L., Collier, P.A. & Ashwell, K.W.S. (1995): Mechanisms in the induction of neuronal heterotopia following prenatal cytotoxic brain damage. *Neurotoxicol. Teratol.* **3**, 297–311.

Chapter 10

Epileptogenesis in the freeze model of cortical microgyria

David A. Prince and Kimberle M. Jacobs

Department of Neurology & Neurological Sciences, Stanford University School of Medicine, Stanford, California 94305, USA

Summary

The mechanisms by which cortical developmental malformations give rise to partial epilepsy are unknown. We studied rats with transcranial freeze lesions made on P0 or P1 that result in formation of layered microgyri closely resembling those found in human polymicrogyria. Beginning at P12, epileptiform field potentials were evoked in neocortical slices cut through the experimental microgyri. The epileptogenic area surrounded the microgyrus ('paramicrogyral zone'), extending about two millimetres across the cortex. Epileptiform activities in the paramicrogyral zone persisted after transcortical cuts that removed the microgyrus from the circuit. Enhanced immunoreactivity for neurofilaments and misoriented pyramidal cells in the paramicrogyral zone suggested that structural reorganization of cortical circuits takes place during development of the microgyrus. Cytochrome oxidase (CO) staining showed that even small microgyral lesions in the whisker barrelfield of somatosensory cortex produced substantial cortical reorganization. Areas of distorted and intense CO staining extended over regions larger than the microgyrus and corresponded to the zone in which epileptiform field potentials could be evoked. The ratio of the frequency of spontaneous excitatory to inhibitory post-synaptic currents (sEPSCs/sIPSCs) in layer V pyramidal cells adjacent to the microgyrus was increased in these neurons. Spontaneous and evoked IPSCs were larger in pyramidal neurones that participated in the epileptogenesis than in controls, and IPSCs were more dependent on glutamatergic excitation of interneurons in the epileptogenic cortex. Findings support the hypothesis that formation of aberrant and excessive excitatory connectivity in the cortex adjacent to the microgyrus is an important mechanism underlying epileptogenesis.

Introduction

Application of magnetic resonance imaging techniques and careful evaluation of pathological material removed at surgery for intractable epilepsy have shown that various types of developmental cortical malformations are a common cause of mental retardation and seizure disorders in man (Palmini *et al.*,1991). The seizures are often refractory to anti–epileptic drugs and can lead to status epilepticus (Palmini *et al.*,1991, 1994). A number of important issues are raised by clinical and neuropathological observations. It is not clear how the anatomic rearrangements found in malformations of various types get translated into functional abnormalities. For example, the mechanisms underlying hyperexcitability of neuronal aggregates in these lesions are unknown. Are the cellular mechanisms different in different clinical–anatomic subclasses of malformation? There is controversy about whether a malformation itself, or adjacent abnormal cortex is the generator of epileptogenic activity. It is also not clear why some malformations are so refractory to anti-epileptic drugs – is it some specific cellular or circuit abnormality, or merely an indication of the extent of the abnormal tissue?

In order to begin to address these and other questions, we selected a model of one type of cortical malformation found in the human brain, polymicrogyria. By using a technique first described by Dvorak et al. (1978) and Dvorak and colleagues (1988), we have been able to produce isolated microgyri in the rat whose pathology closely resembles that of layered human polymicrogyria. Advantages of this preparation include the ability to produce stereotyped focal lesions surrounded by normal brain, and the robust epileptogenesis that occurs in the area of such lesions and persists within in vitro neocortical slices cut through the lesion, making it possible to do detailed electrophysiological and anatomic experiments. A number of important findings have emerged to date including: (1) dynamic changes in epileptogenesis that occur over time following a neonatal lesion; (2) important differences in development of epileptic discharges that are dependent on the age of the animal at the time the lesion occurs; (3) evidence suggesting that the cortex surrounding the microgyrus is the generator of epileptogenic discharge; and (4) evidence for structural abnormalities in excitatory afferents to the cortex surrounding the microgyrus suggesting that this area becomes hyperinnervated, leading to hyperexcitability.

Methods

Focal freeze lesions were made in P0 or P1 rats according to techniques previously described (Dvorak & Feit, 1977, 1988; Rosen et al., 1992; Jacobs et al.,1996a). Pups were anesthetized with hypothermia, the skull exposed and either a round (2–3 mm diameter) or rectangular (2 mm x 5 mm) freezing probe was touched to the skull for 3–7 sec (see Jacobs et al., 1996a for details). The scalp was sutured and animals were allowed to recover for varying periods of time before a final slice experiment or transcardiac perfusion under deep Nembutal anesthesia for histological studies was done. At various recovery times extending from nine to 171 days, animals were re-anesthetized with Nembutal (55 mg/kg.) and standard techniques used to prepare and maintain neocortical slices taken through the area of the microgyrus, seen as a small dimple on the pial surface, or from control somatosensory cortex of littermates. Other experimental details can be found in Jacob et al., (1996a, 1999)

Neocortical slices through the area of the microgyrus are epileptogenic

Nissl stained sections through the area of the freeze lesion revealed a typical four-layered microgyrus in each experimental animal (Fig. 1). Stimulation of slices in the white matter or layer VI in the area adjacent to the microgyrus could evoke field potential epileptiform events that had properties similar to those previously reported in slices from chronic models of epileptogenesis (Prince & Tseng, 1993). A schematic diagram of a slice containing a microgyrus and the placement of recording and stimulating electrodes, as well as representative field potentials, are shown in Fig. 2. A short latency evoked field potential similar to that seen in control slices was present in the region of the microgyrus (Fig. 2A,B), however this was typically followed by a long and shifting latency polyphasic event that occurred in an all-or-none manner (Fig. 2B). Increases in stimulus intensity and/or stimulus frequency to more than about 0.2 Hz caused failures in evoked epileptiform events (not shown; see also Prince & Tseng, 1993; Jacobs et al., 1996a). It was possible to evoke epileptiform activities in slices from both adult (>P40) and juvenile (P12–P20) animals, suggesting that the events in the microgyral area were not merely due to the enhanced cortical excitability that occurs in juvenile rats under normal circumstances (Luhmann & Prince, 1990). The focal nature of the abnormality (see below) also eliminated this possibility. Intracellular recordings with sharp electrodes showed that the field potential epileptiform events were associated with polyphasic synaptic potentials and burst discharges in layer V pyramidal neurones (Fig. 3).

Chapter 10   Freeze model of cortical microgyria

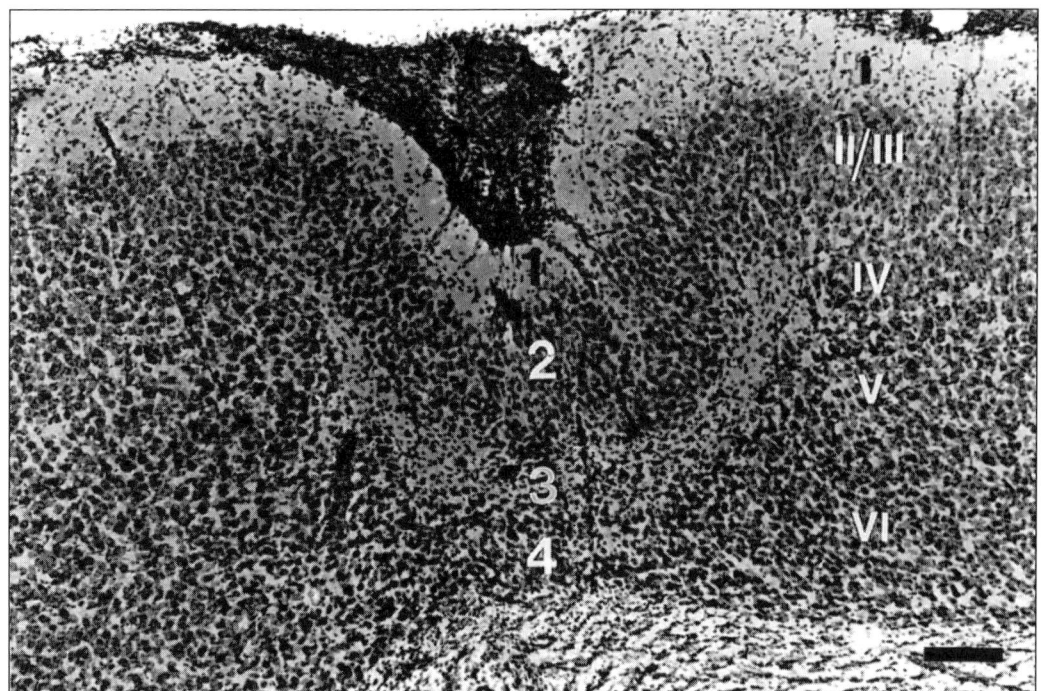

Fig. 1. Nissl–stained section containing a microgyrus. Roman numerals indicate cortical laminae and Arabic numbers indicate layers of the microgyrus. Scale bar: 200 µm.

Several findings suggested that the interaction between the lesion and developing cortex was a dynamic one in terms of epileptogenesis. There was a remarkable change in the incidence of epileptogenesis over time. Evoked epileptiform events rarely occurred before about P12, but the incidence abruptly increased so that almost 100 % of P1 lesioned animals had at least one epileptogenic slice on P12 or thereafter. There was also a significant tendency for lesions made at P0 to be less epileptogenic than those made at P1 when slices were evaluated at longer survival times (Jacobs et al., 1999). Thus there was a tendency for epileptogenesis to appear and then resolve in P0 lesioned slices, whereas lesions at P1 still produced a relatively high incidence at P40.

Site of origin of epileptogenic discharge

To determine the sites at which epileptiform events could be evoked, slices were surveyed systematically using pairs of stimulating and recording electrodes placed in the same cortical column, or arrays of multiple extracellular electrodes. Results of a typical experiment are shown in Fig. 4. Stimuli within or beneath the microgyrus did not evoke epileptiform events within the microgyrus proper (Fig. 4, trace one). There was a zone beginning about 0.5 mm from the microgyrus and extending about two mm in which epileptiform events could be evoked (Fig. 4, traces two and three). Beyond about two mm from the edge of the microgyrus it was not possible to evoke abnormal activities (Fig. 4, trace four). In another series of experiments, we separated the microgyrus from surrounding cortex and found that the paramicrogyral zone could still generate epileptiform activities when stimulated (Jacobs et al., 1999). Thus, the microgyrus itself has a role in inducing epileptogenesis but it is not the generator of abnormal activities.

Reorganization of excitatory connectivity within the paramicrogyral zone

Results of experiments focused on the mechanisms of epileptogenesis in this model are incomplete. One could picture hyperexcitability developing because of depression in inhibitory electrogenesis,

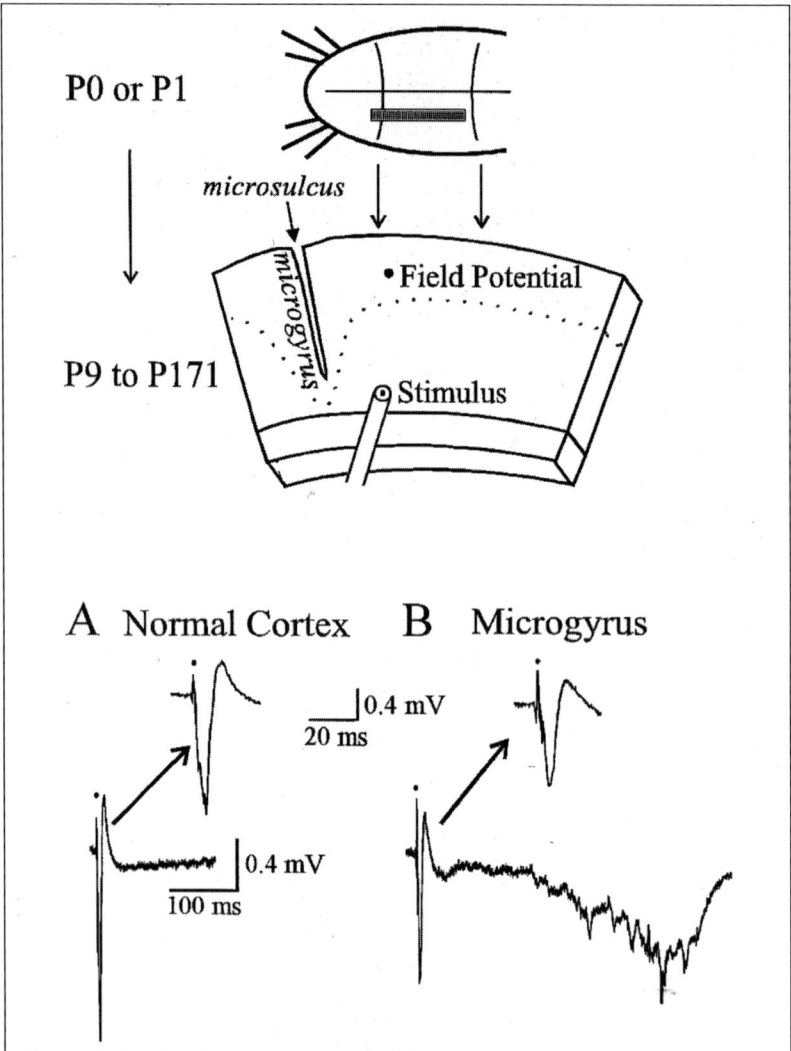

Fig. 2. Upper: Schematic of rat skull showing area of transcranial freeze lesion as a gray bar. Diagram of brain slice containing a microgyrus shown below with the position of the stimulus and field potential recording electrodes. A: Normal evoked short latency negative–positive field potential in a cortical slice from control rat. Arrow points to inset showing averaged evoked event (n=9) at a faster sweep speed and lower gain. B: A similar stimulus in a slice with microgyrus evokes a normal short latency event in the region adjacent to the microgyrus, followed by a late polyphasic epileptiform negativity. Inset shows averaged early event (n=9). Upper calibration is for expanded sweeps in A and B and lower calibration is for sweeps below. Stimulating electrode located 500 μm lateral to the microgyrus in layer 6 in A and B. Modified from Jacobs et al., 1996, with permission.

enhancement of excitatory synaptic coupling through some mechanism, and/or changes in the intrinsic properties of the membranes of involved neurons. The latter have not been examined in detail to this point. However, there are several lines of evidence suggesting abnormalities in the development of excitatory connectivity in the area surrounding the microgyrus that coincides with the epileptogenic zone. Immunoreactivity for neurofilament proteins is enhanced at the margins of the microgyrus extending into the paramicrogyral zone (Humphreys *et al.*, 1991; K.M. Jacobs, I. Parada & D.A. Prince, unpublished observations), suggesting that a structural reorganization of afferents in this area has taken place. Other studies (Humphreys *et al.*, 1991) have shown disorga-

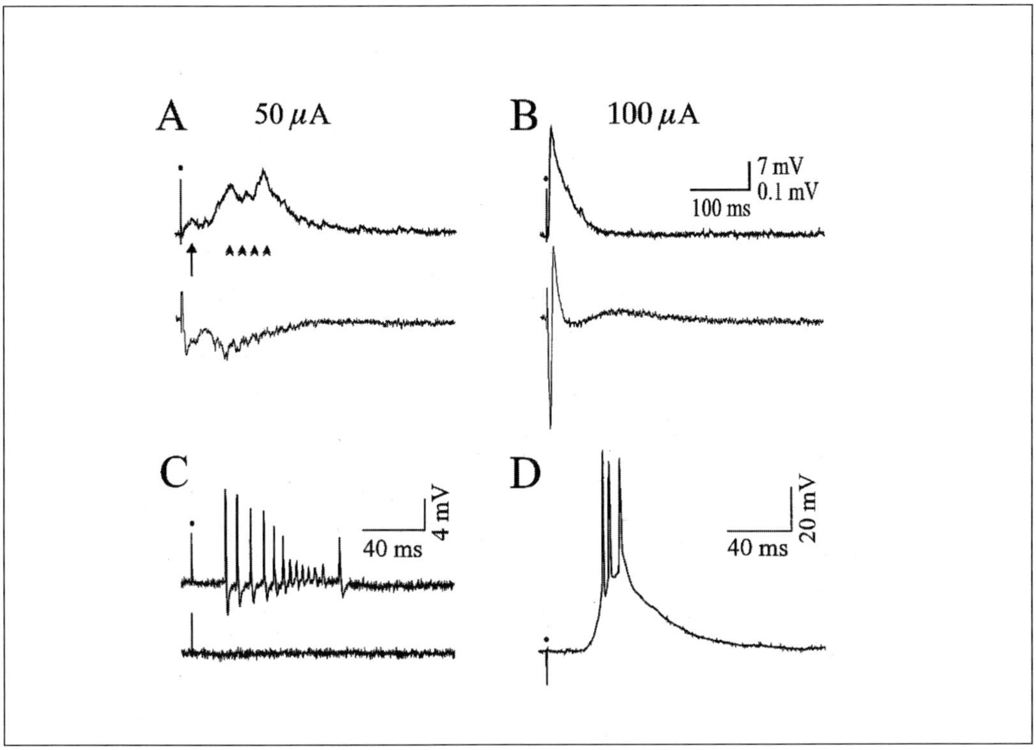

Fig. 3. Examples of intracellular (A, B, D) and extracellular (C) evoked events in epileptogenic slices containing microgyri. (A) Extracellular stimulus at 50 μA evokes a short latency EPSP in neuron (upper trace, arrow) followed by polyphasic excitatory synaptic potentials (arrowheads). Lower trace: extracellular field potential. (B) Same neuron (upper) and field potential recording (lower) with response evoked by 100 μA stimulus. Note that polyphasic excitatory responses are blocked and replaced by a large EPSP, probably associated with a depolarizing IPSP on its falling phase. (C) Upper and lower traces: Two consecutive responses obtained from microelectrode located extracellularly, showing all-or-none burst response of this neuron. (D) recording of large EPSP with burst response coincident with epileptiform field (not shown). Intracellular recordings obtained with sharp electrodes. Calibrations in B for A and B. Modified from Jacobs et al., 1996, with permission.

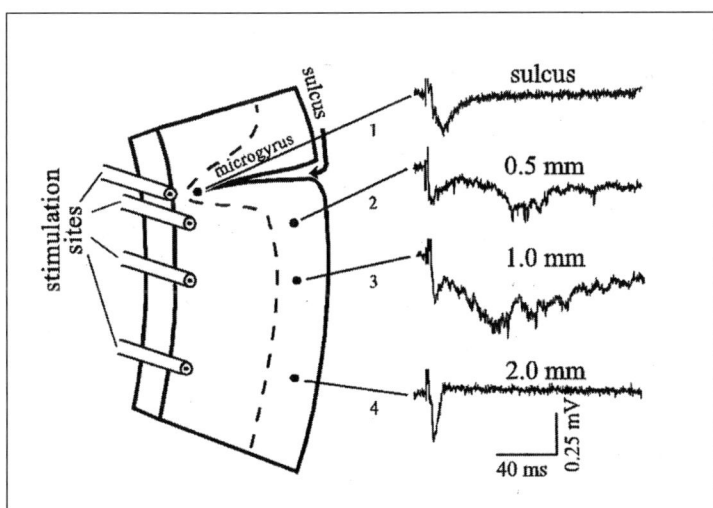

Fig. 4. Field potential responses evoked at different distances from the microsulcus. Recordings from superficial layers directly above the stimulating electrode at each point (1–4). Long latency polyphasic activity is only evoked by stimulation within 2 mm of the microsulcus (traces 2 and 3). Modified from Jacobs et al., 1996, with permission.

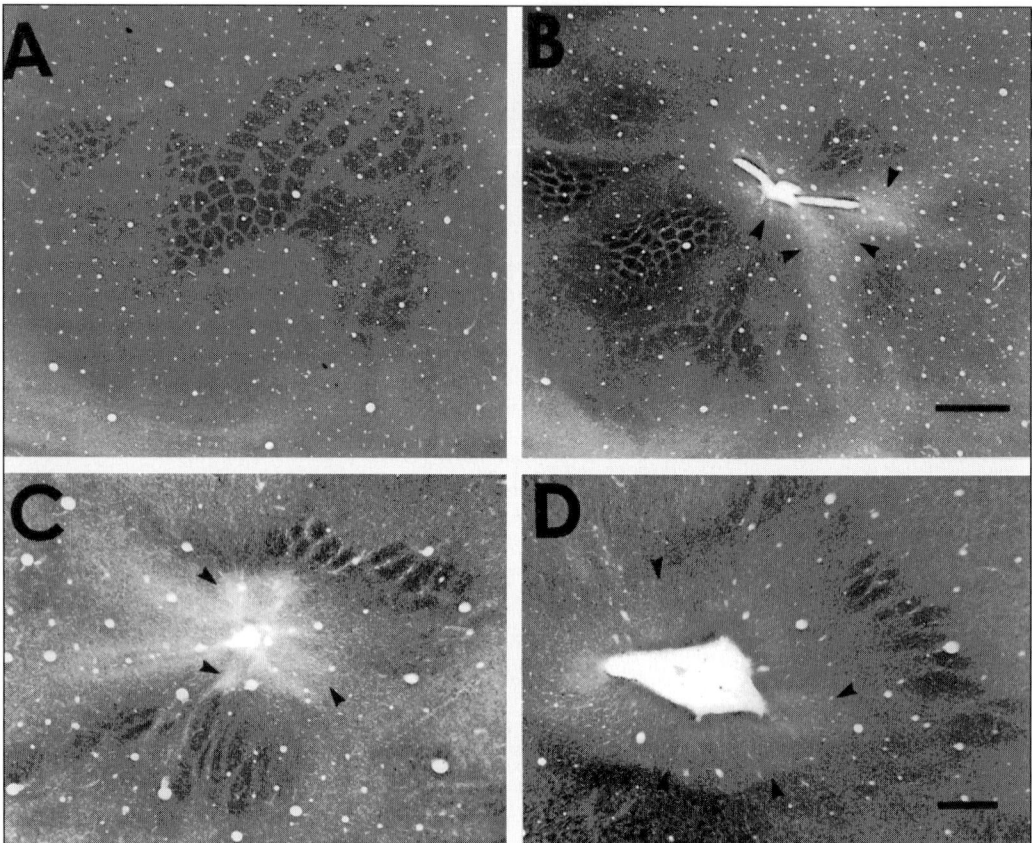

Fig. 5. Tangential sections through layer IV of control somatosensory cortex (A) and area of a microgyrus from three different rats (B, C, D) stained with cytochrome oxidase to reveal the structure of the somatosensory barrelfield. Note pale staining in microgyrus (area surrounding slit-like microsulcus). Arrows (B, C, D) point to boundary of pale stained microgyrus with heavily stained surrounding zone. Abnormally shaped barrels and regions of undifferentiated dark CO staining shown in C and D. Scale bar in B: 800 μm for A and B. Scale bar in D: 400 μm for C and D.

nization of glutamatergic fibres in this same area. We have hypothesized that the loss of normal lamina IV, V and upper VI in the area beneath the microgyrus removes normal targets for afferents from intracortical, callosal and thalamic sources. Such afferents might then find their normal laminar targets in the area adjacent to the microgyrus resulting in hyperinnervation with excitatory axons. To test this possibility, we have done neuroanatomic studies of the organization of the whisker barrelfields in rat somatosensory cortex and the effects of cortical microgyri made by placing freeze lesions in the developing barrel field on P1 (Jacobs et al., 1997). The whisker barrelfield afforded a sensitive anatomic index of changes in cortical organization in the area of a microgyrus. Ordinarily, this system is organized with each whisker represented by a cluster of cells and fibres called a 'barrel' (Van der Loos & Woolsey, 1973). This stereotyped anatomic representation can be visualized by staining tangentially cut sections through layer IV with cytochrome oxidase (CO; Wong-Riley & Welt, 1980). A typical photomicrograph of such a section is shown in Fig. 5A. Normally, within the whisker area there are 36 barrels arranged in five rows. Several important changes in this pattern were found in the region of the microgyrus and its surround. The microgyrus proper was stained relatively lightly compared to surrounding cortex (Fig. 5B). In the zone surrounding the microgyrus, individual barrels were often distorted so that these structures became elongated, thinner than usual, indistinct, or even absent from their expected locations (Fig. 5B–D). There were also zones of hyperintense CO staining (Fig. 5C, D). These changes were not related to loss of neurones in the cortex surrounding the microgyrus, because Nissl stains showed that the density of cells in surrounding areas was similar to that in control barrel cortex. CO staining revealed that ventrobasal thalamic barreloids, structures analogous to cortical barrels (Land *et al.*,1995), were still present in animals with major disruptions in the cortical barrel field. Nissl staining of the ventrobasal thalamus showed no obvious paucity of thalamocortical cells even in animals in which there were few whisker barrels remaining. Processing of sections for acetylcholinesterase, which stains thalamocortical axons (De Carlos *et al.*, 1995), showed alterations that were similar to those for CO staining, suggesting that there had been a reorientation of thalamocortical axons in the disrupted area. These findings provide clear evidence for a reorganization of the thalamocortical somatosensory system, and support the hypothesis that the paramicrogyral epileptogenic zone may be hyperinnervated.

Patch-clamp techniques have been used to measure synaptic currents in layer V neurones in the paramicrogyral zone to detect potential abnormalities in excitatory or inhibitory circuits. Disinhibition might be one mechanism that could underlie epileptogenesis (see Prince *et al.*, 1997; Prince, 1999 for reviews). Although studies are incomplete, thus far data suggest that there is not a loss of inhibitory control among layer V pyramidal neurones in the epileptogenic zone (Jacobs *et al.*, 1996b). In fact, both spontaneous and evoked IPSCs in cells that participate in the late polysynaptic discharge are increased in amplitude at threshold, compared to control cortex (Fig. 6, A–C). The mechanism for this change might be enhanced connectivity from interneurones onto pyramidal cells, an increased excitatory drive onto the interneurones and/or changes in post-synaptic receptor responsiveness to GABA. The timing of the electrophysiological experiment in relation to the lesion may significantly influence the assessment of functional inhibition, since we have found that parvalbumin staining of cohorts of GABAergic interneurones within the microgyrus is decreased when sections from P13 animals are examined (Jacobs *et al.*, 1996a), but appears normal if studies are done at P21 or older (Rosen *et al.,* 1998). To test for the possibility that interneurones might be hyperinnervated by glutamatergic fibres, we recorded the frequency of spontaneous IPSCs in pyramidal neurones under control conditions and during perfusion of slice solutions containing blockers of ionotropic glutamatergic neurotransmission D, L-2-amino-5-phosphono valeric acid (AP5, 50 µM) and 6,7-dinitroquinoxaline-2-3 dione (DNQX, 20 µM). When cells in control slices were compared to those in the paramicrogyral zone, it was found that there was a much larger decrease in frequency among neurones participating in epileptogenesis, suggesting that there was indeed an increased glutamatergic innervation of GABAergic interneurones (Fig. 6D., Jacobs *et al.,* 1996b). The role of this enhanced functional inhibition is unclear at this time. It might be looked upon as a compensatory change that decreases the intensity of excitatory events in the epileptogenic paramicrogyral zone. It is also possible that inhibition has a significant role in synchronizing activities of large groups of pyramidal cells and is an important component of abnormal discharge.

Thus far, the excitatory input onto pyramidal cells in the paramicrogyral zone has not been thoroughly examined. One result, however, does suggest a disturbance in the balance between excitation and inhibition for these cells. When the frequency of spontaneous EPSCs and IPSCs was examined in these neurons, it was found that the ratio of EPSCs to IPSCs was significantly higher in the epileptogenic neuronal population than in controls. As in the case of some other forms of epileptogenic discharge, the polysynaptic events in the microgyrus model were reversibly eliminated when solutions containing the NMDA receptor blocker AP5 (50 µM) were added to the slice solution (Jacobs *et al.*,1996a). This suggests that activation of NMDA receptors plays an important role in generating the abnormalities, but does not necessarily mean that there is a functional abnormality of glutamatergic neurotransmission at these receptors.

Conclusions

The freeze microgyrus model is a useful one in which to assess relationships between abnormalities in cortical development and epileptogenesis, and is a reasonable model for polymicrogyria in

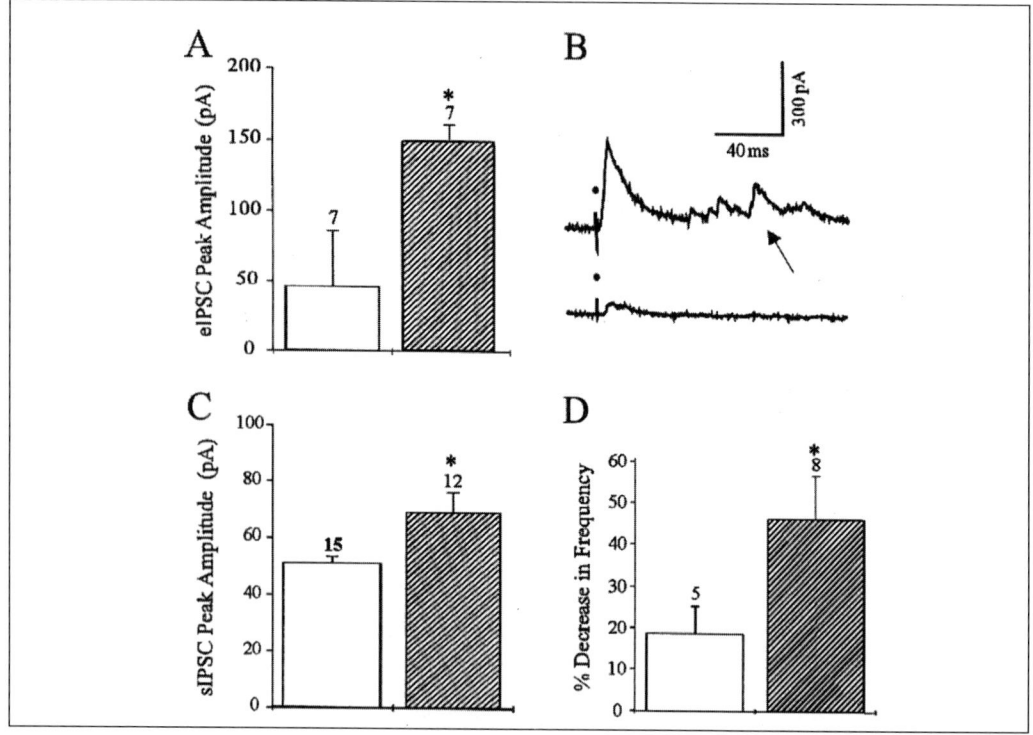

Fig. 6. Bar graphs showing peak amplitude of threshold evoked IPSCs in control (open bar) and epileptogenic microgyral cortex (hatched bar). B: Sample traces showing inhibitory currents evoked in response to threshold stimuli in epileptogenic tissue (upper trace) and control cortex (lower trace). Arrow under upper trace shows polyphasic inhibitory currents coincident with the field potential epileptiform event. Dots: Stimuli in white matter in paramicrogyral zone, beneath the patch clamp electrode located in layer V. C: Bar graph showing amplitude of spontaneous IPSCs in control (open bar) and epileptogenic slices (hatched bar). D: Percentage decrease in frequency of spontaneous IPSCs following blockade of ionotropic glutamatergic synaptic transmission with AP5 and DNQX for control layer five neurones (open bar) and layer five neurones of the epileptogenic zone adjacent to a microgyrus (hatched bar). *: $P < 0.05$ t-test. All recordings obtained under voltage clamp with patch electrodes. eIPSC: Evoked inhibitory post-synaptic current; sIPSC: Spontaneous inhibitory post-synaptic current. Numbers of neurones given above each bar in A, C and D.

man. We have not monitored the EEG or behavioural seizures in microgyric rats. Casual observation suggests that seizures are not common, perhaps because of the limited nature of the pathology. Also, single microgyri in the rat affect a more limited cortical area than polymicrogyria in man. With these limitations in mind, results provide insights into some of the issues important to our understanding of epileptogenesis in human cortical dysgenesis.

The lesions are dynamic in that the incidence of abnormality changes over time. This is probably due to interactions between the evolving neuropathological consequences of the perinatal lesion and normal or lesioned-altered developmental events. The rather abrupt emergence of epileptogenesis at P12 following a P0 or P1 lesion is one example of a functional consequence of these dynamic changes, although the precise structural–functional events underlying this emergence of epileptogenesis are at present unknown. Other evidence for ongoing changes within the injured developing cortex is a tendency for epileptogenesis to resolve in older animals, particularly those lesioned at P0 (Jacobs et al., 1999). This loss of epileptogenicity could be a consequence of increases in the efficacy of cortical inhibitory networks, perhaps evidenced by changes in parvalbumin IR and/or glutamatergic innervation of interneurones that are mentioned above. Quantitative evaluation of inhibitory and excitatory events within microgyri of different aged animals may provide an answer to this important question.

The maturational status of the cortex at the time of the lesion influences the subsequent outcome. There is a striking difference between the epileptogenesis elicited by lesions at P1 versus P0, suggesting that timing of a given insult during brain maturation in man will be a critical factor in determining whether seizures develop and their severity. We speculate that the freeze lesions at P1 produce more extensive neuronal damage because more cells have migrated into place at that time, however there are other possible explanations and additional data are necessary to resolve this question.

Evidence to date suggests that epileptogenesis is the result of hyperinnervation of the zone surrounding the microgyrus that occurs when developing axons have lost their targets in laminae beneath the microgyrus that are destroyed by the freeze lesion. Our studies do not eliminate decreases in inhibition as a contributing factor at early stages in the development of the microgyrus when parvalbumin IR is decreased. Luhmann and colleagues have noted decreased IPSPs in neurones of the microgyrus proper (Luhmann et al., 1997), and Hablitz has reported changes in $GABA_A$ post-synaptic receptors on pyramidal neurones in the region of the microgyrus that could result in decreased inhibitory efficacy (DeFazio & Hablitz, 1997). However, our data do show that polysynaptic inhibition is robust in the epileptogenic paramicrogyral zone after P12.

There are obviously a large number of subtypes of cortical malformation that can be associated with neurological defects and epilepsy in man. As in other models of chronic epileptogenesis, it seems likely that more than one underlying pathophysiologic mechanism will turn out to be present in each instance, although this may be different in different types of cortical dysgenesis. For example, neurones of unusual morphology and location are found in the MAM model of brain maldevelopment and there is some evidence that ectopic neurones in this model may have acquired abnormal burst–generating capacities because of alterations in intrinsic properties (see Baraban & Schwartzkroin, 1995; Franceschetti et al., 1996; also see Chapter 5 in this volume). Abnormalities in cell properties would be particularly likely to occur when the genetic or another underlying etiology affects neurones around the time of their birth and differentiation. The freeze microgyrus model is not one of abnormal neuronal migration since layer two neurones in the microgyrus appear to find their usual laminar positions (Dvorak & Feit, 1977; Rosen et al., 1996). Rather, the abnormalities of structure in the microgyrus are a consequence of loss of particular subsets of neurones in the deeper lamina, as a result of the presumably ischemic (Dvorak & Feit, 1977) lesion. The major pathophysiological mechanism appears to be an aberrant reorganization of cortical connectivity that leads to hyperactive circuits.

Surgical treatment of a focal cortical dysgenesis requires some strategy to eliminate the generator of epileptiform events. In the experimental microgyrus, it is very clear that removal of the microgyric cortex per se without adequate resection of the surrounding zone would not eliminate the source of epileptogenesis. This finding may be rather specific for the type of lesion we have induced. Evidence from clinical electrophysiological recordings of cortical malformations in man has suggested that the malformed cortex in some instances may itself generate epileptiform activities (Palmini et al., 1995), however removal of surrounding cortex improves outcome in other cases (Palmini et al., 1996).

Finally, results of our study on abnormalities in somatosensory cortical organization in areas of microgyri, together with other studies cited above indicate that critically timed lesions during cortical development can produce disorganization of connectivity that is significantly more widespread than the gross anatomic extent of the lesion per se. These findings may explain apparently widespread functional defects in animals with microgyri (Fitch et al., 1994; Rosen et al., 1995) and cortical dysgenic lesions in man.

References

Baraban, S.C. & Schwartzkroin, P.A. (1995): Electrophysiology of CA1 pyramidal neurones in an animal model of neuronal migration disorders: prenatal methylazoxymethanol treatment. *Epilepsy Res.* **22,** 145–156.

De Carlos, J.A., Schlaggar, B.L. & O'Leary, D.D.M. (1995): Development of acetylcholinesterase-positive thalamic and basal forebrain afferents to embryonic rat neocortex. *Exp. Brain Res.* **104,** 385–401.

DeFazio, T. & Hablitz, J.J. (1997): Loss of high affinity zolpidem-induced enhancement of GABAergic post-synaptic currents in a freeze-induced microgyria model of epilepsy. *Epilepsia* **38,** 17 (Abstract).

Dvorak, K. & Feit, J. (1977): Migration of neuroblasts through partial necrosis of the cerebral cortex in newborn rats – contribution to the problems of morphological development and developmental period of cerebral microgyria. Histological and autoradiographical study. *Acta Neuropathol. (Berl.)* **38,** 203–212.

Dvorak, K., Feit, J. & Jurankova, Z. (1978): Experimentally induced focal microgyria and status verrucosus deformis in rats – pathogenesis and interrelation. Histological and autoradiographical study. *Acta Neuropathol. (Berl.)* **44,** 121–129.

Fitch, R.H., Tallal, P., Brown, C.P., Galaburda, A.M. & Rosen, G.D. (1994): Induced microgyria and auditory temporal processing in rats: a model for language impairment? *Cereb. Cortex* **4,** 260–270.

Franceschetti, S., Sancini, G., Battaglia, G., Spreafico, R., Di Luca, M. & Avanzini, G. (1996): Aberrant firing patterns of neocortical neurones from methylazoxymethanol (MAM)-treated rats *in utero. Epilepsia* 37 **(Suppl. 5)**, 72 (Abstract).

Humphreys, P., Rosen, G.D., Press, D.M., Sherman, G.F. & Galaburda, A.M. (1991): Freezing lesions of the developing rat brain: a model for cerebrocortical microgyria. *J. Neuropathol. Exp. Neurol.* **50,** 145–160.

Jacobs, K.M., Gutnick, M.J. & Prince, D.A. (1996a): Hyperexcitability in a model of cortical maldevelopment. *Cereb. Cortex* **6,** 514–523.

Jacobs, K.M., Huguenard, J.R. & Prince, D.A. (1996b): Inhibitory currents in a developmental model of epilepsy. *Soc. Neurosci. Abstr.* **22,** 2102 (Abstract).

Jacobs, K.M., Mogensen, M., Warren, L., & Prince, D.A. (1997): Experimental microgyri disrupt cytochrome oxidase–identified barrel formation in rat somatosensory cortex. *Soc. Neurosci. Abstr.* **23,** 811 (Abstract).

Jacobs, K.M., Hwang, B.J. & Prince, D.A. (1999): Focal epileptogenesis in a rat model of polymicrogyria. *J. Neurophysiol.* [in press].

Land, P.W., Buffer Jr, S.A., & Yaskosky, J.D. (1995): Barreloids in adult rat thalamus: three-dimensional architecture and relationship to somatosensory cortical barrels. *J. Comp. Neurol.* **355,** 573–588.

Luhmann, H.J. & Prince, D.A. (1990): Transient expression of polysynaptic NMDA receptor-mediated activity during neocortical development. *Neurosci. Lett.* **111,** 109–115.

Luhmann, H.J., Karpuk, N., Qu, M.& Zilles, K. (1997): Neuronal migration disorders in rat cerebral cortex: electrophysiological and anatomical characterization. *Soc. Neurosci. Abstr.* **23,** 807, #316.6 (Abstract).

Palmini, A., Andermann, F., Olivier, A., Tampieri, D., Robitaille, Y., Andermann, E. & Wright, G. (1991): Focal neuronal migration disorders and intractable partial epilepsy: a study of 30 patients. *Ann. Neurol.* **30,** 741–749.

Palmini, A., Gambardella, A., Andermann, F., Dubeau, F., da Costa, J.C., Olivier, A., Tampieri, D., Robitaille, Y., Paglioli, E. & Paglioli Neto, E. (1994): Operative strategies for patients with cortical dysplastic lesions and intractable epilepsy. *Epilepsia* 35 **(Suppl. 6)**, S57–S71.

Palmini, A., Gambardella, A., Andermann, F., Dubeau, F., da Costa, J.C., Olivier, A., Tampieri, D., Gloor, P., Quesney, F., Andermann, E., Paglioli, E., Paglioli-Neto, E., Coutinho, L., Leblanc, R. & Kim, H.-I. (1995): Intrinsic epileptogenicity of human dysplastic cortex as suggested by corticography and surgical results. *Ann. Neurol.* **37,** 476–487.

Palmini, A., Gambardella, A., Andermann, F., Olivier, A., Costa da Costa, J. *et al.*, (1996): Outcome of surgical treatment in patients with localized cortical dysplasia and intractable epilepsy. In: *Dysplasias of cerebral cortex and epilepsy,* eds. R. Guerrini, F. Andermann, R. Canapicchi, J. Roger, B.G. Zifkin & P. Pfanner, pp. 367–374. New York: Lippincott-Raven.

Prince, D.A. (1999): Epileptogenic neurones and circuits. In: *Jasper's basic mechanisms of the epilepsies,* eds. A.V. Delgado-Esqueta, W. Wilson, R. Olsen, & R.J. Porter. Philadelphia: Lippincott-Raven. [in press].

Prince, D.A., Jacobs, K.M., Salin, P.A., Hoffman, S. & Parada, I. (1997): Chronic focal neocortical epileptogenesis: does disinhibition play a role? *Can. J. Physiol. Pharmacol.* **75,** 500–507.

Prince, D.A. & Tseng, G.-F. (1993): Epileptogenesis in chronically injured cortex: *in vitro* studies. *J. Neurophysiol.* **69,** 1276–1291.

Rosen, G.D., Jacobs, K.M., & Prince, D.A. (1998): Effects of neonatal freeze lesions on expression of parvalbumin in rat neocortex. *Cerebral Cortex* **8,** 753–761.

Rosen, G.D., Press, D.M., Sherman, G.F. & Galaburda, A.M. (1992): The development of induced cerebrocortical microgyria in the rat. *J. Neuropathol. Exp. Neurol.* **51,** 601–611.

Rosen, G.D., Sherman, G.F. & Galaburda, A.M. (1996): Birthdates of neurones in induced microgyria. *Brain Res.* **727,** 71–78.

Rosen, G.D., Waters, N.S., Galaburda, A.M. & Denenberg, V.H. (1995): Behavioral consequences of neonatal injury of the neocortex. *Brain Res.* **681,** 177–189.

Van der Loos, H. & Woolsey, T.A. (1973): Somatosensory cortex: structural alterations following early injury to sense organs. *Science* **179,** 395–398.

Wong-Riley, M.T. & Welt, C. (1980): Histochemical changes in cytochrome oxidase of cortical barrels after vibrissal removal in neonatal and adult mice. *Proc. Natl. Acad. Sci. USA* **77,** 2333–2337.

Chapter 11

Neuronal development in an epileptic rat with cortical heterotopia

Kevin S. Lee, Frank Schottler, Matthew J. Anzivino,
Jennifer L. Collins, Eric A. Frankel, Zong-Fu Chen,
Edward Bertram and Laila Zai

*Departments of Neuroscience, Neurological Surgery and Neurology, Health Sciences Center,
University of Virginia, Box 420 HSC, Charlottesville, Virginia 22908, USA*

Summary

Malformations of the cerebral cortex are present in over one per cent of the general human population and approximately 20–40 per cent of intractable epileptics. Increasing evidence implicates misplaced (heterotopic) cortical neurones in the etiology of many of the early-onset epilepsies and certain forms of mental retardation. The lack of appropriate animal models for studying the natural development of human-like heterotopia associated with epilepsy represents a major impediment to understanding: (1) the roles of heterotopic neurones in epilepsy, and (2) the developmental mechanisms responsible for generating heterotopic neurones. Recently a novel mutant animal (the tish rat) was discovered that exhibits bilateral, subcortical band heterotopia. Interestingly, some tish rats display recurrent spontaneous seizures that persist over a considerable part of their life span. The tish rat thus represents a unique animal for investigating the developmental and functional characteristics of heterotopic neurones in an epileptic brain. Initial studies indicate that heterotopic neurones in the tish cortex establish characteristic and topographic axonal connections with cortical and subcortical targets. Unlike the neurones in the overlying normotopic cortex, heterotopic neurones do not exhibit characteristic lamination or radial orientation. Heterotopic neurogenesis is a novel early event in the developing tish cortex, suggesting that misplaced cellular proliferation, in addition to disturbed neuronal migration, contributes to the formation of cortical heterotopia. Studies characterizing this animal are underway with the ultimate goal of understanding mechanisms underlying epilepsy associated with misplaced cortical neurones.

Cortical malformations and epilepsy

A major advance in the field of epilepsy during the last decade has been the growing recognition that structural errors are a common feature of many epileptic brains (Guerrini *et al.*, 1992; Prayson *et al.*, 1993). The widespread use of magnetic resonance imaging in recent years has revealed a high incidence of cortical malformations in patients with developmental epilepsies and cognitive impairment (Barkovich *et al.*, 1989, 1992, 1994, 1996; Palmini *et al.*, 1991; Kuzniecky *et al.*, 1993; Dobyns *et al.*, 1996; Harding, 1996). Complementary findings from histological studies of surgical and post-mortem material have also demonstrated a high incidence of cortical malformations in individuals with intractable epilepsy (Meencke & Janz, 1984;

Hardiman et al., 1988; Meencke & Veith, 1992). It is estimated that malformations of the human neocortex are present in over one per cent of the general population and in approximately 20–40 per cent of intractable epileptics (Meencke & Janz, 1984; Hardiman et al., 1988; Farrell et al., 1992; Meencke & Veith, 1992; Mischel et al., 1995). A common feature of many of these malformations is the presence of heterotopic neurones in the cerebral cortex. However, the central issue of how heterotopic neurones participate in recurrent seizures is, at best, poorly understood. In addition, the developmental mechanisms responsible for the formation of many human cortical heterotopia are unknown. It is therefore of substantial clinical importance to determine how cortical heterotopias are formed and how they contribute to epilepsy.

Cortical malformations range in severity from minor displacements of a few neurones to massive rearrangements of cortical structure. Although many human neocortical malformations are classified as neuronal migration disorders (Barkovich et al., 1989, 1992; Palmini et al., 1993), the etiologies of most of these anomalies remain unknown (Barkovich et al., 1996). It has become increasingly evident that disturbances in other developmental events, such as cellular proliferation and programmed cell death, also contribute to cortical malformations (Rakic, 1988; Evrard et al., 1989; Barkovich et al., 1992, 1996; Rorke, 1994; Eksioglu et al., 1996; Kuida et al., 1996; Brunstrom et al., 1997). Among the most profound types of human cortical malformation are subcortical band heterotopias (SBH), which are sometimes termed double cortex. Subcortical band heterotopias are characterized by a large collection of heterotopic neurones located in the white matter below a relatively normal appearing neocortex (Matell, 1893; Jacob, 1936; Barkovich et al., 1989). Individuals affected with this disorder are prone to intractable epilepsy and mental retardation (Barkovich et al., 1989; Livingston & Aicardi, 1990; Vahldiek et al., 1990; Palmini et al., 1991; Ricci et al., 1992; Soucek et al., 1992; Hashimoto et al., 1993; Iannetti et al., 1993; Granata et al., 1994). As is the case for most human cortical malformations, the mechanisms responsible for forming SBH, and the role of heterotopic neurones in the associated epilepsy, are unknown. An important advance in the effort to understand the etiology of SBH was the recent mapping and cloning of a gene (doublecortin) that is affected in cases of human SBH (Ross et al., 1997; des Portes et al., 1997, 1998; Gleeson et al., 1998). Identification of this gene should allow the generation of specific doublecortin knock-out animals, and will facilitate cellular and molecular analyses of SBH formation.

The tish rat as an animal model for cortical heterotopia and epilepsy

The paucity of appropriate animal models for studying human cortical malformations associated with epilepsy has made it difficult to investigate the role of heterotopic neurones in epilepsy. The recent discovery of a novel neurologically mutant rat (tish) may prove to be of value in this effort (Lee et al., 1997). The tish rat displays inherited heterotopia (Fig. 1) resembling the human malformation of SBH (Lee et al., 1997). These animals are seizure-prone, with some animals exhibiting spontaneous, recurrent seizures that persist for a substantial portion of the animals' life span. The tish rat therefore appears to be a promising animal model for evaluating developmental mechanisms involved in the formation of cortical heterotopia, and for characterizing the role(s) of heterotopic neurones in epileptogenesis. Initial studies on the tish rat have shown that the heterotopic neurones are cortical in nature. Heterotopic neurones exhibit typical features of cortical neurones including cellular morphology, afferent connectivity and efferent connectivity (Lee et al., 1997; Schottler et al., 1998). However, the heterotopic neurones do not display characteristic neocortical patterns of lamination and radial orientation. Based on the general cortical phenotypes of the misplaced neurones, these cells are collectively termed the *heterotopic cortex*, while the overlying laminated cortex is termed the *normotopic cortex* (Fig 1). The issue of whether the heterotopic cortex should be considered 'neocortex' is arguable because of the lack of typical lamination. In fact, it is conceivable that the organization of the heterotopic cortex is atavistic, representing a more primitive form of cortical organization. Despite these intriguing issues, the heterotopic neurones will be considered here as part of the neocortex.

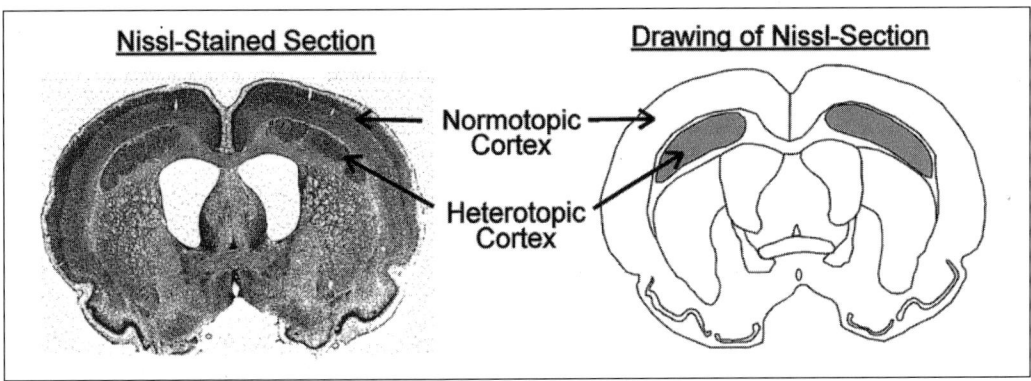

Fig. 1. Cortical heterotopia in the tish brain. The left frame shows a coronal section of the tish brain at the level of the decussation of the anterior commissure. The right frame is a drawing of the same section with the heterotopia (heterotopic cortex) shaded. The heterotopic cortex is present bilaterally in the white matter underlying a normotopic cortex. The heterotopic cortex typically extends from the frontal cortex to the rostral portion of the occipital cortex. The heterotopic cortex varies somewhat in size from animal to animal, and mild-to-moderate ventriculomegaly is typically observed.

Connectivity of cortical neurones in the tish brain

Neurones in both the heterotopic and normotopic cortices establish topographic connections with typical subcortical targets (Lee et al., 1997; Schottler et al., 1998). These sets of neurones exhibit characteristic morphologies of cortical projection neurons. For instance, large pyramidal cells in layer V of the normotopic sensory/motor cortex project to the spinal cord in the tish rat. In the heterotopic cortex, similar appearing, large pyramidal cells also project to the spinal cord. In general, neighbouring areas of the normotopic and heterotopic cortices project topographically to the same subcortical targets in the tish brain. These findings indicate that the same types of projection neurons are located in both the heterotopic and normotopic cortices, and that these cells establish similar patterns of topographic connectivity.

Another hallmark of normal cortical organization is topographic bidirectional connectivity with the thalamus. For instance, corticothalamic neurones located in layer VI of somatosensory cortex project to restricted portions of the ipsilateral ventrobasal complex. Neurones in the ventrobasal complex, in turn, project to topographically restricted portions of layer IV of the somatosensory cortex. In the tish brain, corticothalamic neurones are found in both the heterotopic and normotopic cortices (Lee et al., 1997; Schottler et al., 1998). The somata of these cells are concentrated in layer VI of the normotopic cortex. In contrast to the normotopic neurones, the somata of heterotopic corticothalamic neurones do not exhibit a typical pattern of lamination. As described in detail in Schottler et al. (1998), the axons of heterotopic and normotopic corticothalamic neurones project topographically to multiple thalamic nuclei. Thalamocortical axons also project topographically to both the heterotopic and normotopic cortices of the tish brain. For instance, projections from the ventroposterolateral thalamus (VPL) terminate predominantly in layer IV of the medial normotopic sensory cortex, and in a broad column in the underlying medial portion of the heterotopic cortex. In the case of projections from the ventroposteromedial thalamus (VPM) to the cortex, terminal fields are found in barrel-like complexes in layer IV of the lateral portions of the normotopic somatosensory cortex. Patch-like terminal fields are observed for the projection from VPM to the lateral aspects of the heterotopic cortex. Taken together, these observations indicate that topographic, bidirectional connectivity with the thalamus is established in both the normotopic and heterotopic cortices of the tish brain.

Corticocortical projections in the tish brain also exhibit typical features of regional connectivity; however, these connections are somewhat more elaborate than normal (Schottler et al., unpublished). Neurones in both the normotopic and heterotopic cortices establish commissural connections with corresponding (homotopic) areas of the contralateral cortex. Commissural connections emanating from the normotopic cortex appear to be sparser than those arising from the heterotopic region. Ipsilateral cortical projections of the tish brain also exhibit typical features of associational connectivity. For instance, neurones in the normotopic somatosensory cortex project to characteristic ipsilateral cortical targets including motor areas, secondary somatosensory cortex, and ventral parietal areas. In addition to projecting to normotopic sites, neurones in the normotopic cortex send axons to the contralateral and ipsilateral heterotopic cortices. These projections to the heterotopia follow the same basic pattern of topography as the connections with the normotopic targets. In general, a given area of the normotopic cortex projects to both its homotopic contralateral area, and to the subjacent heterotopic cortex.

Corticocortical neurones with their somata in somatosensory portions of the heterotopic cortex exhibit a similar pattern of connectivity, sending commissural projections to corresponding (homotopic) areas of the contralateral heterotopic cortex and to the adjacent normotopic cortex. A similar topographic organization is seen for the associational projections of neurones in somatosensory portions of the heterotopia. Thus, bidirectional topographic connections characterize the interactions between normotopic and heterotopic cortices. These findings are consistent with the broader principle that both normotopic and heterotopic neurones establish typical connectivity with cortical as well as subcortical targets.

Is there more cortex in the tish brain?

It is conceivable that the formation of large cortical heterotopia increases the overall size of the cortex in the tish brain. Alternatively, a compensatory loss of normotopic cortex could accompany the development of cortical heterotopia. Qualitative observations of histological sections suggest that the normotopic cortex of the tish brain is thinner than the corresponding cortex in control animals. This finding is consistent with the concept that the heterotopic cortex is constructed at the expense of the normotopic cortex. The issue of whether the total amount of cortex is conserved between control and tish animals was examined quantitatively by measuring the size of the neocortex in heterozygous (normal phenotype) and homozygous (tish phenotype) littermates. As shown in Figure 2, the total volume of neocortex in the tish brain (i.e. normotopic cortex plus heterotopic cortex) is almost identical to the volume of corresponding neocortex in control animals. Area measurements at several anterior-posterior levels of the cortex indicate that the addition of heterotopic cortex in a given region is accompanied by a loss of normotopic cortex (Fig. 2). In the occipital cortex of the tish brain, where the heterotopic cortex is small or absent, there is also a tendency for the normotopic cortex to be somewhat reduced in size. In general, these findings indicate that the addition of heterotopic cortex is offset by a reduction in the size of normotopic cortex. However, several issues remain to be resolved regarding the equivalency of cortical size in control and tish animals. Differences in cell packing and/or size could exist between the normotopic and heterotopic cortices. Such differences would affect the overall number of cells present in a given volume of cortex. In this way, the cortices of control and tish animals could exhibit similar total volumes, but could differ in terms of the numbers of cells present. It is also possible that the absolute levels of cellular proliferation and death could differ considerably between control and tish rats. For example, cortical size and cell numbers could be similar in the tish and control brains, even though the events responsible for producing this parity could differ substantially. Despite these caveats, the observation that the overall amount of neocortex is similar in control and tish rats is parsimonious with the concept that a normal balance of cellular proliferation and death is preserved during development of the tish cortex.

Development of the tish cortex

The complex organization of the adult neocortex derives from a carefully choreographed series of developmental events (for recent reviews, see Allendoerfer & Shatz, 1994; McConnell, 1995; Reid

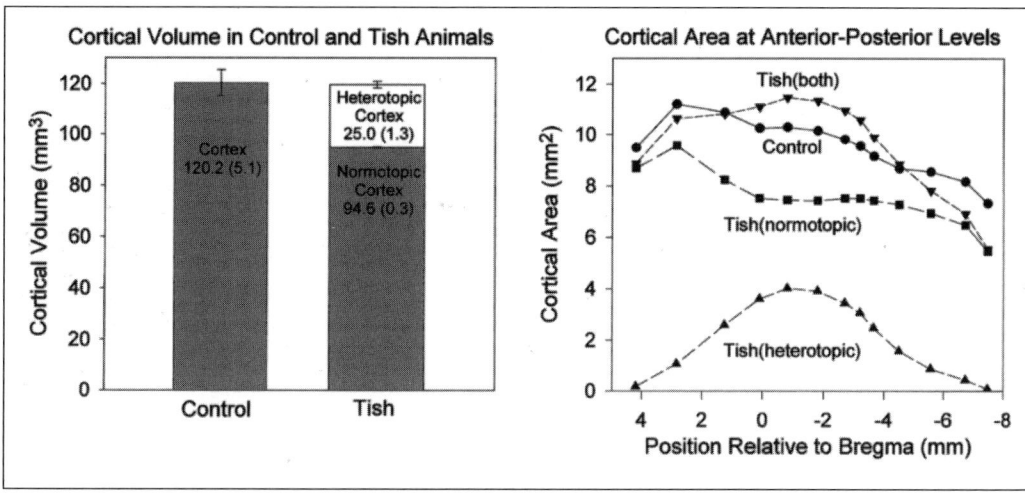

Fig. 2. Neocortical size in tish and control animals. The total volume of neocortex is nearly identical in tish and control animals (left frame). Area measurements of individual sections at different anterior-posterior levels of the tish brain show that the parts of the brain containing the heterotopic cortex exhibit reductions in the size of the normotopic cortex (right frame). In this study, the area of neocortex was measured bilaterally in coronal sections from the brains of 30-day-old littermates exhibiting either the tish or normal phenotype. In control animals (n = 2), the area of neocortex located dorsal to the rhinal fissure was measured at anterior-posterior (A-P) intervals in semi-serial coronal sections stained with cresyl violet. The A-P intervals were matched to the rat brain atlas of Paxinos & Watson (1986) and expressed relative to Bregma (right frame). In tish animals (n = 2), similar measurements were made except that the areas of normotopic cortex and heterotopic cortex were measured separately. Cortical volumes were calculated by multiplying the individual area measurements by the A-P interval and summing the individual values for each brain.

& Walsh, 1996). Precisely timed phases of proliferation, elaborate paths of migration, intricate patterns of differentiation and selective cell loss are all essential for the proper construction of the neocortex. Although subcortical band heterotopias are generally considered to be neuronal migration disorders (e.g. Barkovich *et al.*, 1996), disturbances in any of the aforementioned developmental events could conceivably contribute to the formation of cortical heterotopia. We have therefore initiated a series of studies investigating the cellular and molecular events participating in the formation of the tish cortex.

During normal development, the earliest generated neurones in the neocortex (Cajal–Retzius and subplate cells) occupy a superficial position termed the cortical *preplate* (Marín-Padilla, 1978). These two classes of neurone are then separated by the later-arriving cells of the cortical plate: the Cajal–Retzius cells remain in a superficial position in the marginal zone, while the subplate cells take up progressively deeper positions. In this manner, the cortical plate cells, which will ultimately comprise layers II-VI of the adult cortex, are intercalated between the early-generated preplate cells. Preplate cells are thought to play critical roles in organizing the neocortex by influencing the positioning of cortical plate neurones, and by guiding the formation of afferent and efferent connections (McConnell *et al.*, 1989, 1994; DeCarlos & O'Leary, 1992; O'Leary & Koester, 1993; Allendoerfer & Shatz, 1994; D'Arcangelo *et al.*, 1995; Ogawa *et al.*, 1995).

In the tish cortex, a single *preplate* forms in a normal position in the superficial aspect of the developing cortex (Lee *et al.*, 1998). These cells are generated around embryonic days (E) 13–14, which is the typical period of cortical preplate neurogenesis in the rat (Bayer & Altman, 1990). Molecular markers for preplate neurones exhibit typical patterns of distribution during development of the tish cortex. In particular, a marker for Cajal–Retzius cells (CR50; Ogawa *et al.*, 1995) is restricted to the preplate, and subsequently to the marginal zone, during prenatal development

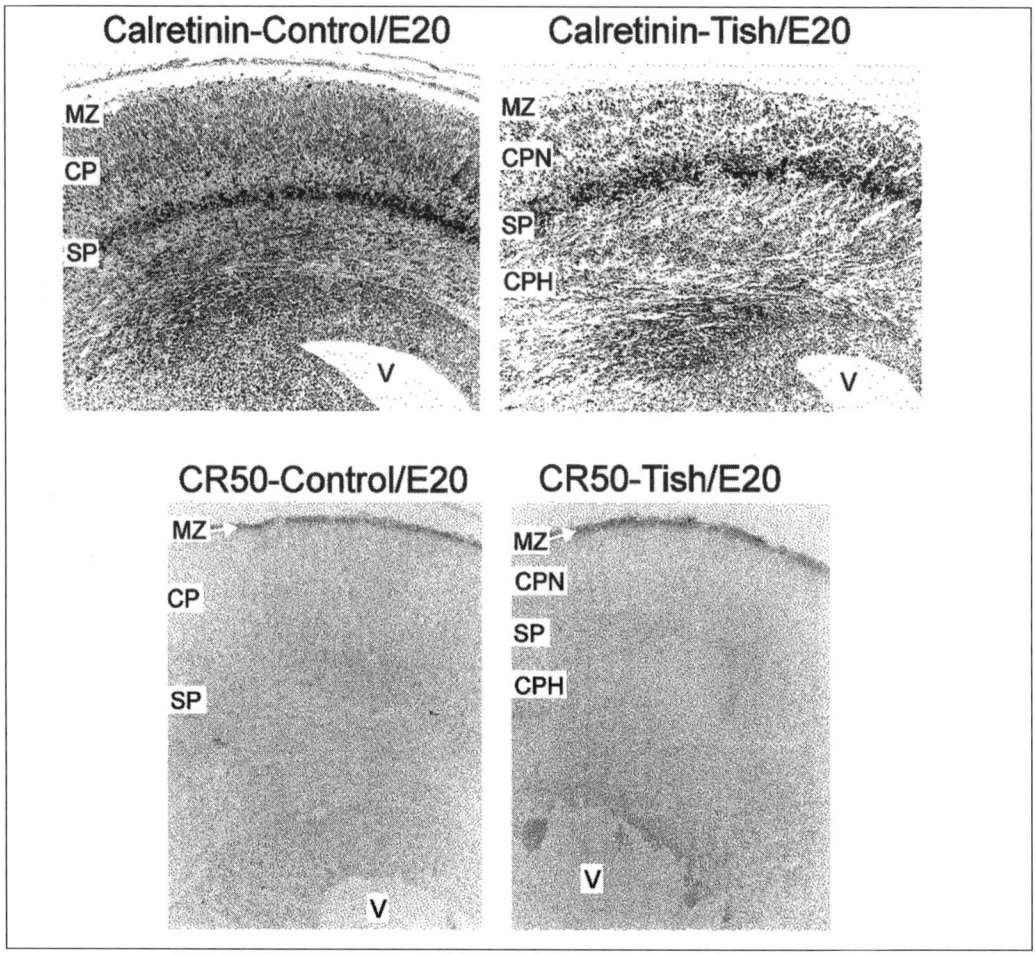

Fig. 3. The distribution of subplate and Cajal–Retzius cells in the developing cortex of E20 control and tish rats. During later stages of prenatal cortical development, subplate cells are selectively immunopositive for the calcium-binding protein, calretinin (Fonseca et al., 1995). The upper frames show calretinin-immunopositive neurones in the subplate of control and tish rats. In both cases, a single layer of labelled cells is observed at the base of a normotopic cortical plate. The normotopic cortical plate in the tish rat (CPN) is thinner than that in the control animal (CP). The lower frames show the distribution of CR50 in the cortex of control and tish rats. CR50 is an antibody that recognizes the protein reelin, which is selectively localized to Cajal–Retzius cells (Ogawa et al., 1995). A single band of CR50 immunoreactivity (arrow) is observed in the marginal zone (i.e. the normal position of Cajal–Retzius cells) of both control and tish animals. The calretinin-stained sections were counterstained with methyl green while the CR50-stained sections were not counterstained. Abbreviations: MZ = marginal zone; CP = cortical plate; SP = subplate; V = ventricle; CPN = normotopic cortical plate; CPH = heterotopic cortical plate.

(Fig. 3). This pattern of distribution is similar to that observed in control animals (see also Ogawa et al., 1995). Previous studies have shown that both subplate cells and Cajal–Retzius cells are immunopositive for the calcium binding protein calretinin during early cortical development (Fonseca et al., 1995). However, at later stages of embryonic cortical development, calretinin immunoreactivity is concentrated in the subplate cells (Fonseca et al., 1995). We have confirmed this pattern of calretinin immunoreactivity in control rats (Fig. 3). Moreover, a similar pattern of calretinin immunoreactivity is observed in tish rats (Lee et al., 1998) (Fig. 3). At later stages of embryonic cortical development, a single band of calretinin-positive cells is found in the subplate located at the base of the normotopic cortical plate of the tish rat. There does not appear to be a secondary subplate associated with the heterotopic cortex. It is important to recognize that the absence of staining for reelin and calretinin in the heterotopic cortex could indicate that the preplate cells are not present, or that the preplate cells are present but simply lack immunoreactivity for CR50 and calretinin. However, cell birthdating studies during early cortical development argue against the latter possibility (Lee et al., 1998). In particular, cells generated during the typical period of preplate neurogenesis (E13.5 and E14) are found in the marginal zone and at the base of the normotopic cortex in tish rats on postnatal day one, but not in the heterotopic cortex. Taken together, these findings indicate that a single preplate is formed in a normotopic position in the tish rat.

In contrast to the presence of a single cortical preplate, two cortical *plates* are observed in the developing tish brain (Lee et al., 1998). A normotopic cortical plate (CPN in Fig. 3) develops in a typical superficial position between the Cajal–Retzius and subplate cells, while a heterotopic cortical plate (CPH in Fig. 3) develops in the upper part of the intermediate zone. Cells occupying both cortical plates are generated during the normal phase of cortical plate neurogenesis in the rat (approximately E14–E21; Bayer and Altman, 1991). The cells in the normotopic cortical plate exhibit a typical 'inside-out' pattern of neurogenesis (Fig. 4), with older cells positioned deeper than later developing cells (Lee et al., 1997). In contrast, the heterotopic cortical plate displays a 'rim-to-core' gradient of neurogenesis (Fig. 4). Thus, the neurogenetic patterns differ substantially between the normotopic and heterotopic cortices. For further discussion of this issue see Lee et al. (1998).

One consequence of having a single preplate and two cortical plates is that cells in the heterotopic cortical plate do not appear to be directly associated with preplate cells. This contrasts with the situation of the neurones in the normotopic cortex which are intercalated between preplate cells in a normal manner. It is possible that the absence of a dedicated preplate for the heterotopic

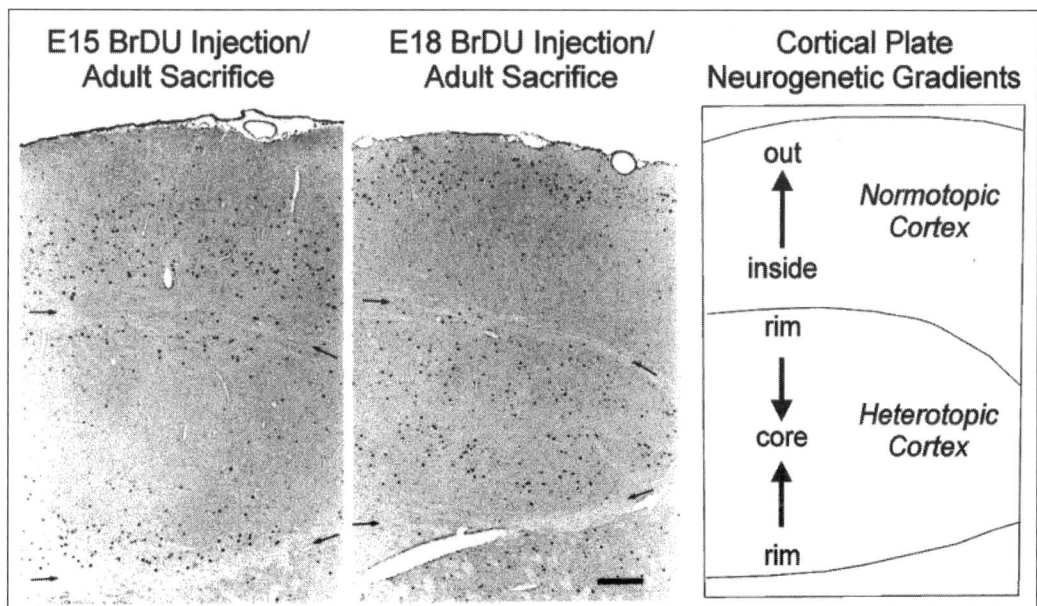

Fig. 4. Neurogenetic gradients of cortical plate neurones in the tish brain. BrDU-labelled cells (dark dots) are shown in coronal sections of the tish cortex from adult animals that were injected on embryonic day 15 (E15; left frame) or embryonic day 18 (E18; centre frame). Cells generated on E15 are located in the deep aspect of the normotopic cortex and along the rim of the heterotopic cortex. In contrast, cells generated on E18 are located in the superficial aspect of the normotopic cortex and the core of the heterotopic cortex. The inside-out and rim-to-core neurogenetic gradients of the normotopic and heterotopic cortices, respectively, are illustrated in the drawing shown in the right frame. Abbreviation: BrDU = bromodeoxyuridine.

cortex contributes to the failure of heterotopic neurones to laminate and orient properly. However, despite the absence of normal interactions with the preplate, the heterotopic neurones retain their ability to establish topographic afferent and efferent connections with appropriate synaptic targets (Lee et al., 1997; Schottler et al., 1998). These observations reinforce findings from the reeler mouse and prenatally-irradiated rats indicating that substantial misplacements of cortical neurones do not severely impair their ability to identify appropriate synaptic partners (Caviness & Yorke, 1976; Steindler & Colwell, 1976; Simmons et al., 1982; Caviness & Frost, 1983; Terashima et al., 1983; Jensen & Killackey, 1984; Frost et al., 1986; Caviness et al., 1988).

Heterotopic neurogenesis in the tish cortex

As discussed earlier, subcortical band heterotopias are generally assumed to develop as a result of an error in neuronal migration. However, when experiments were undertaken to evaluate this concept in the tish rat, a rather unexpected outcome was obtained. A heterotopic zone of cellular proliferation was discovered in the upper aspect of the intermediate zone (Lee et al., 1998). In these experiments, proliferating cells were labelled during S-phase using bromodeoxyuridine (BrDU) and survival times ranging from two hours to two days were examined to determine the location of proliferating cells and their routes of migration. Normally, cortical neurogenesis takes place in a proliferative zone restricted to the vicinity of the cerebral ventricle (e.g. Bayer & Altman, 1991). The same pattern is observed in our control animals (Fig. 5). In the developing tish cortex, cellular proliferation also occurs in the ventricular zone; however, an additional, heterotopic zone of proliferating cells is observed in a position superficial to the normal ventricular proliferative zone. Heterotopic proliferating cells are observed as early as E15, which is the earliest time point we have examined to date. This is a time point at which the majority of cortical plate cells have not begun to migrate. In fact, many of the cortical plate neurones are yet to be generated by this time. The distribution of labelled cells in animals that survived for 24 hours after a BrDU injection on E18 suggests that the heterotopic proliferative zone contributes cells to both the normotopic and heterotopic cortical plates. Unfortunately, cellular migration in animals surviving more than 24 hours post-injection is difficult to analyse because of the apparent convergence of cells from the ventricular and heterotopic proliferative zones. In other words, it is not possible to identify the zone of origin of a given cell at longer survival times. The results of this study suggest that heterotopic neurogenesis is a key early event in the development of the tish cortex.

An alternative explanation for the heterotopic placement of BrDU-labelled cells in the preceding study is that some cells undergo rapid cellular migration from the ventricular proliferative zone into the intermediate zone of the tish brain. If this were to occur, then the BrDU-labelled cells in the intermediate zone could represent a subset of cells that proliferates in the ventricular zone but rapidly migrates (within two hours) into the intermediate zone. To further evaluate the issue of heterotopic cellular proliferation, two additional indices of cellular proliferation were examined. In the first series of experiments, the distribution of mitotic profiles was investigated in toluidine-stained semi-thin sections of the developing tish cortex. Mitotic profiles are present in both the ventricular proliferative zone and in the superficial aspect of the intermediate zone (Lee et al., 1998). The heterotopic mitotic profiles are thus located in the same general area as the BrDU-labelled cells following short survival periods. In another series of experiments, the distribution of proliferating cell nuclear antigen (PCNA) was examined in the tish brain. Antibodies against PCNA recognize mitotically competent cells and label cells in S-phase most prominently (Morris & Mathews, 1989; Waseem & Lane, 1990). In control animals, PCNA-immunoreactivity is restricted to the ventricular proliferative zone, consistent with a single zone of cellular proliferation during normal development (Fig. 5). In contrast, the developing tish cortex exhibits PCNA-immunoreactive cells in both the ventricular proliferative zone and in the superficial aspect of the intermediate zone (Lee et al., 1998). Again, the superficial intermediate zone is the same area of the developing tish brain exhibiting mitotic profiles and BrDU-labelled cells in the preceding experiments. Taken

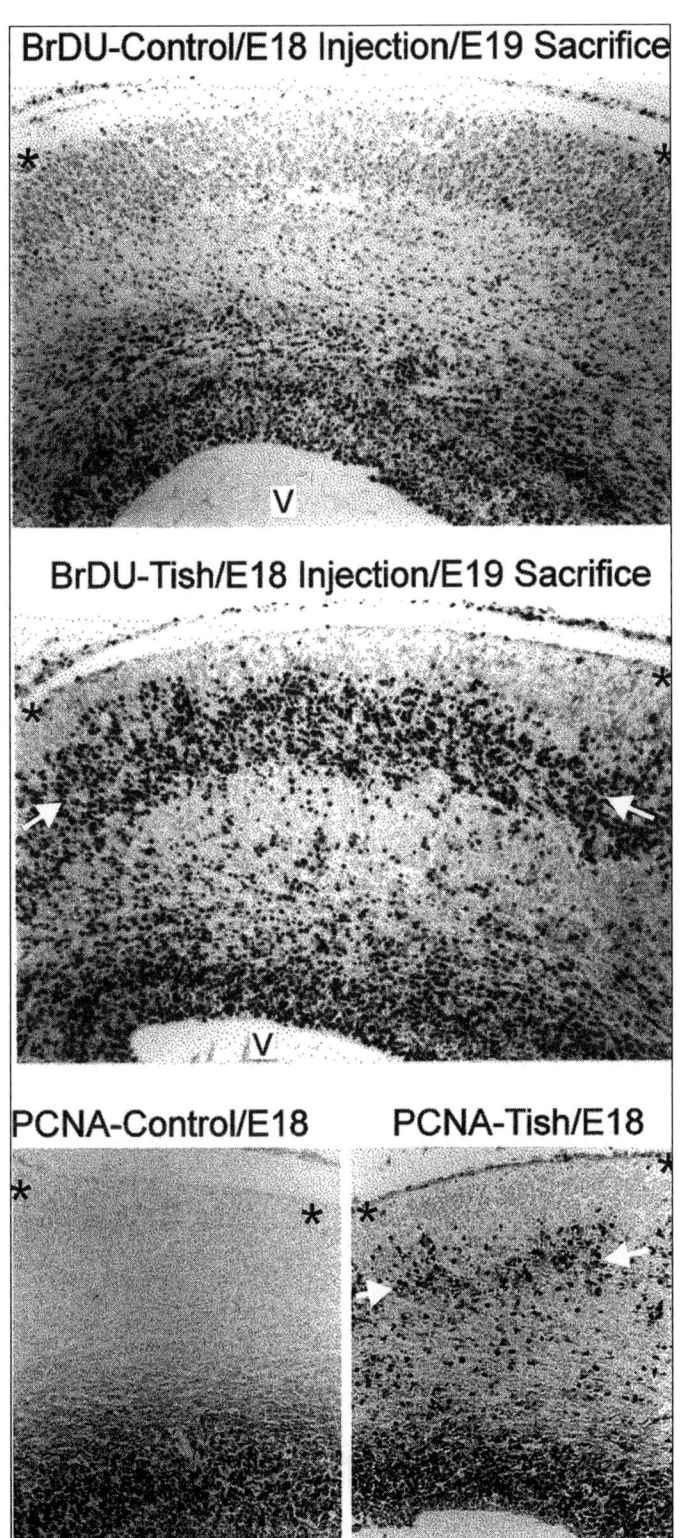

Fig. 5. Heterotopic neurogenesis in the tish rat. In the upper two frames, the distribution of BrDU-positive neurones (black dots) is shown for control and tish rats. An in utero injection of BrDU was given on E18 and the embryos survived until E19 (i.e. 24 hours). In the cortex of the control embryo, labelled cells are present in the ventricular and subventricular zones, with some cells having migrated into the deep intermediate zone. In the cortex of the tish embryo, a similar distribution of labelled cells is seen in the ventricular, subventricular and deep intermediate zones. However, an additional thick band of labelled cells is observed in the superficial intermediate zone (white arrows). Some labelled cells are also found in the deep aspect of the normotopic cortical plate. The lower two frames show proliferating cell nuclear antigen (PCNA)-positive cells in the cortices of control and tish embryos at E18. In the control cortex, cells are concentrated in the ventricular zone, with virtually no cell staining in the intermediate zone or cortical plate. The tish cortex also exhibited PCNA-positive cells in the vicinity of the ventricle. However, an additional band of labelled cells is present in the superficial intermediate zone. A few labelled cells are also scattered in the deep aspect of the intermediate zone. Abbreviations: V = ventricle; asterisks = marginal zone; BrDU = bromodeoxyuridine.

together, these results support the presence of a secondary, heterotopic zone of cellular genesis in the superficial intermediate zone of the developing tish cortex. Although it is likely that an error in neuronal migration also contributes to the formation of cortical heterotopia in the tish brain, heterotopic neurogenesis is a key early event that is already well established prior to the migration of most cortical plate neurones.

Epilepsy in the tish rat

Inasmuch as subcortical band heterotopias are associated with epilepsy in some humans, we sought to determine if tish animals are similarly afflicted. During the establishment of our breeding colony of tish animals, spontaneous seizures were serendipitously observed in some animals. The affected animals typically exhibited partial seizures with variable secondary generalization (Lee et al., 1997); all of the affected animals possessed the tish phenotype. These observations were of considerable interest because they suggested that some of the tish animals exhibit a form of epilepsy similar to that observed in human patients with SBH. However, it is important to recognize that a *seizure* represents a sudden alteration of electrical activity in the brain of sufficient magnitude to alter motor or sensory function, behaviour, or consciousness (e.g. Freeman, 1995). In contrast, *epilepsy* is a chronic disorder characterized by recurrent seizures over a sustained period of time. Electrophysiological recordings with implanted depth electrodes and simultaneous video monitoring have therefore been initiated to characterize the nature and course of seizures in the tish rat. These studies are still in progress; however, spontaneous, recurrent seizures have already been monitored in individual tish animals for a period of up to six months (i.e. the longest period examined). The presence of spontaneous, recurrent seizure activity for a substantial portion of the life span of the tish rat indicates that the affected animals are epileptic. Although these observations do not provide quantitative information regarding possible longitudinal changes in the rate and/or intensity of the seizures, they demonstrate that seizures are a chronic feature of the affected tish rats.

Conclusions

A novel mutant rat (tish) has been identified that displays structural and functional features of human epilepsy associated with cortical heterotopia. A colony of tish animals was established and is being used to characterize the structure, function and development of band heterotopia. Although heterotopic neurones fail to laminate and orient properly in the tish brain, several features of cortical connectivity appear to be normal in these neurones. A novel developmental error involving misplaced cellular proliferation (heterotopic neurogenesis) is an early event in the development of the tish cortex. This finding suggests that errors in cellular proliferation may play a key role in the formation of certain types of cortical heterotopia, and that these malformations do not result exclusively from neuronal migration disorders. Similar to the human disorder of band heterotopia, some of the affected animals exhibit a form of partial epilepsy that persists for a significant portion of the animal's life span. The tish rat thus represents a unique resource for investigating the roles of cortical heterotopia in epilepsy, and for elucidating the developmental mechanisms contributing to the formation of heterotopia.

Acknowledgement

This work was supported by NIH Grant NS 34124. We thank Natalie Harrison for excellent technical assistance, and Masaharu Ogawa for providing the CR50 antibody.

References

Allendoerfer, K.L. & Shatz, C.J. (1994): The subplate, a transient neocortical structure: its role in the development of connections between thalamus and cortex. *Annu. Rev. Neurosci.* **17**, 185–218.

Barkovich, A.J., Jackson, D.E. & Boyer, R.S. (1989): Band heterotopias: a newly recognized neuronal migration anomaly. *Radiol.* **171**, 455–458.

Barkovich, A.J., Gressens, P. & Evrard, P. (1992): Formation, maturation, and disorders of brain neocortex. *AJNR* **13**, 423-446.

Barkovich, A.J., Guerrini, R., Battaglia, G., Kalifa, G., N'Guyen, T., Parmeggiani, A., Santucci, M., Giovanardi-Rossi, P., Granata, T. & D'Incerti, L. (1994): Band heterotopia: correlation of outcome with magnetic resonance imaging parameters. *Ann. Neurol.* **36**, 609–617.

Barkovich, A.J., Kuzniecky, R.I., Dobyns, W.B., Jackson, G.D., Becker, L.E. & Evrard, P. (1996): A classification scheme for malformations of cortical development. *Neuropediatrics* **27**, 59–63.

Bayer, S.A. & Altman, J. (1990): Development of layer I and the subplate in the rat neocortex. *Exp. Neurol.* **107**, 48–62.

Bayer, S.A. & Altman, J. (1991): *Neocortical development.* New York: Raven Press.

Brunstrom, J.E., Gray-Swain, M.R., Osborne, P.A. & Pearlman, A.L. (1997): Neuronal heterotopias in the developing cerebral cortex produced by neurotophin-4. *Neuron* **18**, 505-517.

Caviness Jr, V.S. & Yorke Jr, C.H. (1976): Interhemispheric neocortical connections of the corpus callosum in the reeler mutant mouse: a study based on anterograde and retrograde methods. *J. Comp Neurol.* **170**, 449–460.

Caviness Jr, V.S., Crandall, J.E. & Edwards, M.A. (1988): The reeler malformation: implications for neocortical histogenesis. In: *Cerebral Cortex, Vol. 7,* eds. A. Peters & E. Jones, pp. 59–89. New York: Plenum Press.

Caviness Jr, V.S. & Frost, D.O. (1983): Thalamocortical projections in the reeler mutant mouse. *J. Comp. Neurol.* **219**, 182–202.

D'Arcangelo, G., Miao, G.G., Chen, S.C., Soares, H.D., Morgan, J.I. & Curran, T. (1995): A protein related to extracellular matrix proteins deleted in the mouse mutant reeler. *Nature* **374**, 719–723.

De Carlos, J.A. & O'Leary, D.D.M. (1992): Growth and targeting of subplate axons and establishment of major cortical pathways. *J. Neurosci.* **12**, 1194–1211.

des Portes, V., Pinard, J.M., Smadja, D., Motte, J., Boespflug-Tanguy, O., Moutard, M.L., Desguerre, I., Billuart, P., Carrie, A., Bienvenu, T., Vinet, M.C., Bachner, L., Beldjord, C., Dulac, O., Kahn, A., Ponsot, G. & Chelly, J. (1997): Dominant X-linked subcortical laminar heterotopia and lissencephaly syndrome (X-SCLH/LIS): evidence for the occurrence of mutation in male and mapping of a potential locus in Xq22. *J. Med. Genet.* **34**, 177–183.

des Portes, V., Pinard, J.M., Billuart, P., Vinet, M.C., Koulakoff, A., Carrie, A., Gelot, A., Dupuis, E., Motte, J., Berwald-Netter, Y., Catala, M., Kahn, A., Beldjord, C. & Chelly, J. (1998): A novel CNS gene required for neuronal migration and involved in X-linked subcortical laminar heterotopia and lissencephaly syndrome. *Cell* **92**, 51–61.

Dobyns, W., Andermann, E., Andermann, F., Czapansky-Beilman, D., Dubeau, F., Dulac, O., Guerrini, R., Hirsch, B., Ledbetter, D., Lee, N.S., Motte, J., Pinard, J.M., Radtke, R.A., Ross, M.E., Tampieri, D., Walsh, C.A. & Truwit, C.L., (1996): X-linked malformations of neuronal migration. *Neurology* **47**, 331–339.

Eksioglu, Y.Z., Scheffer, I.E., Cardenas, P., Knoll, J., DiMario, F., Ramsby, G., Berg, M., Kamuro, K., Berkovic, S.F., Duyk, G.M., Parisi, J., Huttenlocher, P.R., & Walsh, C.A. (1996): Periventricular heterotopia: an X-linked dominant epilepsy locus causing aberrant cerebral cortical development. *Neuron* **16**, 77–87.

Evrard, P., de Saint-Georges, P., Kadhim, H., J-F. (1989): Pathology of prenatal encephalopathies. In: *Child neurology and developmental disabilities,* ed. J. French. pp. 153–176. Baltimore: Paul H. Brookes.

Farrell, M.A., De Rosa, M.J., Curran, J.G., Secor, D.L., Cornford, M.E., Comair, Y.G., Peacock, W.J., Shields, W.D. & Vinters, H.V. (1992): Neuropathologic findings in cortical resections (including hemispherectomies) performed for the treatment of intractable childhood epilepsy. *Acta Neuropathol.* **83**, 246–259.

Fonseca, M., del Rio, J.A., Martinez, A., Gomez, S. & Soriano, E. (1995): Development of calretinin immunoreactivity in the neocortex of the rat. *J. Comp. Neurol.* **361**, 177–192.

Freeman, J. (1995): A clinician's look at the developmental neurobiology of epilepsy. In: *Brain development and epilepsy*, eds. P. Schwartzkroin *et al.*, pp. 10–33. Oxford, Oxford University Press.

Frost, D.O., Edwards, M.A., Sachs, G.M. & Caviness Jr, V.S. (1986): Retinotectal projection in reeler mutant mice: relationships among axon trajectories, arborization patterns and cytoarchitecture. *Dev. Brain Res.* **28**, 109–120.

Gleeson, J.G., Allen, K.M., Fox, J.W., Lamperti, E.D., Berkovic, S., Scheffer, I., Cooper, E.C., Dobyns, W.B., Minnerath, S.R., Ross, M.E., & Walsh, C.A. (1998): Doublecortin, a brain-specific gene mutated in human X-linked lissencephaly and double cortex syndrome, encodes a putative signaling protein. *Cell* **92**, 63–72.

Granata, T., Battaglia, G.T., D'Incerti, G., Franceschetti, S., Zucca, C., Savoiardo, M. & Avanzini, G. (1994): Double cortex syndrome: electroclinical study of three cases. *Ital. J. Neurol. Sci.* **15**, 15–23.

Guerrini, R., Dravet, C., Raybaud, C. *et al.* (1992): Epilepsy and focal gyral anomalies detected by MRI: electro-clinico-morphological correlations and follow-up. *Dev. Med. Child Neurol.* **34**, 706–718.

Hardiman, O., Burke, T., Phillips, J., Murphy, S., O'Moore, B., Staunton, H. & Farrell, M.A. (1988): Microdysgenesis in resected temporal neocortex: incidence and clinical significance in focal epilepsy. *Neurology* **38**, 1041–1047.

Harding, B. (1996): Gray matter heterotopia. In: *Dysplasias of cerebral cortex and epilepsy*, eds. R. Guerrini, F. Andermann, R. Canapicchi, J. Roger, B. Zilfkin & P. Pfanner, pp. 81–88. Philadelphia: Lippincott-Raven.

Hashimoto, R., Seki, T., Takuma, Y. & Suzuki, N. (1993): The 'double cortex' syndrome on MRI. *Brain and Devel.* **15**, 57–59.

Iannetti, P., Raucci, U., Basile, L.A., Spalice, A., DiBiasi, C., Trasimeni, G. & Gualdi, G.F. (1993): Neuronal migrational disorders: diffuse cortical dysplasia or the 'double cortex' syndrome. *Acta Paediatr.* **82**, 501–503.

Jacob, H. (1936): Faktoren bei der Entstehung der normalen und entwicklungsgestörten Hirnrinde. *Ztschrf. dges Neurol. Psych.* **155**, 1–39.

Jensen, K.F. & Killackey, H.P. (1984): Subcortical projections form ectopic neocortical neurones. *Proc. Natl. Acad. Sci. USA* **81**, 964–968.

Kuida, K., Zheng, T.S., Na, S., Kuan, C., Yang, D., Karasyuama, H., Rakic, P. & Flavell, R.A. (1996): Decreased apoptosis in the brain and premature lethality in CPP32-deficient mice. *Nature* **384**, 368–372.

Kuzniecky, R., Murro, A., King, D., Morawetz, R., Smith, J., Powers, R., Yaghmai, F., Faught, E., Gallagher, B. & Snead, O.C.. (1993): Magnetic resonance imaging in childhood intractable partial epilepsy: pathologic correlations. *Neurology* **43**, 681–687.

Lee, K.S., Schottler, F., Collins, J.L., Lanzino, G., Couture, D., Rao, A., Hiramatsu, K.I., Goto, Y., Hong, S.-C., Caner, H., Yamamoto, H., Chen, Z.-F., Bertram, E., Berr, S., Omary, R., Scrable, H., Jackson, T., Goble, J. & Eisenman, L. (1997): A genetic animal model of human neocortical heterotopia associated with seizures. *J. Neurosci.* **17**, 6236–6242.

Livingston, J. & Aicardi, J. (1990): Unusual MRI appearance of diffuse subcortical heterotopia or 'double cortex' in two children. *J. Neurol. Neurosurg. Psychiat.* **53**, 617–620.

Marín-Padilla, M. (1978): Dual origin of the mammalian neocortex and evolution of the cortical plate. *Anat. Embryol.* **152**, 109–126.

Matell, M. (1893): Ein Fall von Heterotopie der grauen Substanz in den beiden Hemispheren des Grosshirns. *Arch. Psychiatr. Nervenkr.* **25**, 124–136.

McConnell, S.K. (1995): Strategies for the generation of neuronal diversity in the developing central nervous system. *J. Neurosci.* **15**, 6987–6998.

McConnell, S.K., Ghosh, A. & Shatz, C.J. (1989): Subplate neurones pioneer the first axon pathway from the cerebral cortex. *Science* **245**, 978–982.

McConnell, S.K., Ghosh, A. & Shatz, C.J. (1994): Subplate pioneers and the formation of descending connections from cerebral cortex. *J. Neurosci.* **14**, 1892–1907.

Meencke, H.-J. & Janz, D. (1984): Neuropathological findings in primary generalized epilepsy: a study of eight cases. *Epilepsia* **25**, 8–21.

Meencke, H.-J. & Veith, G. (1992): Migration disturbances in epilepsy. *Epilepsy Res.* **Suppl. 9,** 31-40.

Mischel, P.S., Nguyen, L.P. & Vinters, H.V. (1995): Cerebral cortical dysplasia associated with pediatric epilepsy. Review of neuropathologic features and proposal for a grading system. *J. Neuropathol. Exp. Neurol.* **54,** 137–153.

Morris, G.F. & Mathews, M.B. (1989): Regulation of proliferating cell nuclear antigen during the cell cycle. *J. Biol. Chem.* **264,** 13856–13864.

Ogawa, M., Miyata, T., Nakajima, K., Yagyu, K., Seike, M., Ikenaka, K., Yamamoto, H. & Mikoshiba, K. (1995): The reeler gene-associated antigen on Cajal–Retzius neurones is a crucial molecule for laminar organization of cortical neurones. *Neuron* **14,** 899–912.

O'Leary, D.D.M. & Koester, S.E. (1993): Development of projection neurone types, axon pathways, and patterned connections of the mammalian cortex. *Neuron* **10,** 991–1006.

Palmini, A., Andermann, F., Aicardi, J., Dulac, O., Chaves, F., Ponsot, G., Pinard, J., Goutieres, F., Livingston, J., Tampieri, D., Andermann, E. & Robitaille, Y. (1991): Diffuse cortical dysplasia, or the 'double cortex' syndrome: the clinical and epileptic spectrum in 10 patients. *Neurology* **41,** 1656–1662.

Palmini, A., Andermann, F., de Grissac, H., Tampieri, D., Robaitaille, Y., Langevin, P., Desbiens, R. & Andermann, E. (1993): Stages and patterns of centrifugal arrest of diffuse neuronal migration disorders, *Dev. Med. Child Neurol.* **35,** 331–339.

Paxinos, G. & Watson, C. (1986): *The rat brain in sterotaxic coordinates.* Academic Press (Florida).

Prayson, R.A., Estes, M.L. & Morris, H.H. (1993): Coexistence of neoplasia and cortical dysplasia in patients presenting with seizures. *Epilepsia* **34,** 609–615.

Rakic, P. (1988): Defects of neuronal migration and the pathogenesis of cortical malformations. *Prog. Brain Res.* **73,** 15–37.

Reid, C.B. & Walsh, C.A. (1996): Early development of the cerebral cortex. *Prog. Brain Res.* **108,** 17–30.

Ricci, S., Cusmai, R., Fariello, G., Fusco, L. & Vigevano, F. (1992): Double cortex. A neuronal migration anomaly as a possible cause of Lennox-Gastaut syndrome. *Arch. Neurol* **49,** 61–64.

Rorke, L.B. (1994): A perspective: the role of disordered genetic control of neurogenesis in the pathogenesis of migration disorders. *J. Neuropathol. Exp. Neurol.* **53,** 105–117.

Ross, M.E., Allen, K., Srivastava, A., Featherstone, T., Gleeson, J., Hirsch, B., Harding, B., Andermann, E., Abdullah, R., Berg, M. *et al.* (1997): Linkage and physical mapping of X-linked lissencephaly/SBH (XLIS): a gene causing neuronal migration defects in human brain. *Hum. Mol. Genet.* **6,** 555–562.

Schottler, F., Couture, D., Rao, A., Kahn, H. & Lee, K.S. (1998): Subcortical connections of normotopic and heterotopic neurones in sensory and motor cortices of the tish mutant rat. *J. Comp. Neurol.* **395,** 29–42.

Simmons, P.A., Lemmon, B., & Pearlman, A.L. (1982): Afferent and efferent connections of the striate and extrastriate visual cortex of the normal and reeler mouse. *J. Comp. Neurol.* **211,** 295–308.

Soucek, D., Birbamer, G., Luef, G., Felber, S., Kristmann, E. & Bauer, G. (1992): Laminar heterotopic grey matter (double cortex) in a patient with late onset Lennox-Gastaut syndrome. *Wien Klin. Wochenschr.* **104,** 607–608.

Steindler, D.A. & Colwell, S.A. (1976): Reeler mutant mouse: maintenance of appropriate and reciprocal connections in the cerebral cortex and thalamus. *Brain Res.* **105,** 386–393.

Terashima, T., Inoue, K., Inoue, Y., Mikoshiba, K. & Tsukada, Y. (1983): Distribution and morphology of corticospinal tract neurones in reeler mouse by the retrograde HRP method. *J. Comp. Neurol.* **218,** 314–326.

Vahldiek, G., Terwey, B., Hanefeld, F. & Sperner, J. (1990): Magnetic resonance tomography of laminar heterotopia. *Fortschr. Roentgenstr.* **152,** 378–383.

Waseem, N.H. & Lane, D.P. (1990): Monoclonal antibody analysis of the proliferating cell nuclear antigen (PCNA): structural conservation and the detection of nucleolar form. *J. Cell. Sci.* **96,** 121–129

PART IV

ELECTROCLINICAL, IMAGING AND NEUROPATHOLOGICAL STUDIES

Chapter 12

Neuroradiology of malformations of cortical development: band heterotopia, hemimegalencephaly, and polymicrogyria

A. James Barkovich

*Department of Paediatric Neuroradiology, University of California San Francisco,
Parnassus Avenue, San Francisco, California 94143-0628, USA*

Introduction

Malformations of cortical development are a group of disorders that result from abnormal proliferation, migration, or organization of neurons destined for the cerebral cortex (Barkovich *et al.*, 1996). As a result of a greater awareness of their presence and of steadily improving imaging techniques, malformations of cerebral cortical development are being discovered with increasingly greater frequency on imaging examinations of children with developmental delay and, especially, patients with partial epilepsies. In this chapter, the imaging characteristics of band heterotopia, hemimegalencephaly and polymicrogyria are discussed.

Band heterotopia

Band heterotopia, also known as the double cortex syndrome, is a malformation in which a relatively normal gyral pattern is maintained despite a significant arrest of migration of neurons within the intermediate zone. (Barkovich *et al.*, 1989, 1994; Livingston & Arcardi, 1990; Palmini *et al.*, 1991a). Therefore, it is classified as a malformation resulting from impaired neuronal migration. (Barkovich *et al.*, 1996). Affected patients typically present with either epilepsy or developmental delay; associated neurologic signs and symptoms may be present as well. Patients have a variable clinical course, ranging from mildly impaired to severely retarded. (Palmini *et al.*, 1991; Barkovich *et al.*, 1994; Oinard *et al.*, 1994). The overwhelming majority of female patients (> 90 per cent) is consistent with the report of a genetic locus on chromosome Xq22.3-q23 (Ross *et al.*, 1997). Rarely, male patients with band heterotopia have been described (Barkovich *et al.*, 1994; Ono *et al.*, 1997).

A correlation of imaging findings with outcome has shown that patients with more severe cortical anomalies (shallower sulci) and more severe ventricular enlargement have significantly earlier onset of seizure disorders than patients with less severe pachygyria and smaller ventricles (Barkovich *et al.*, 1994). Moreover, those with early seizure onset, more severe pachygyria and greater ventricular enlargement have significantly worse prognoses for intelligence (at least so far

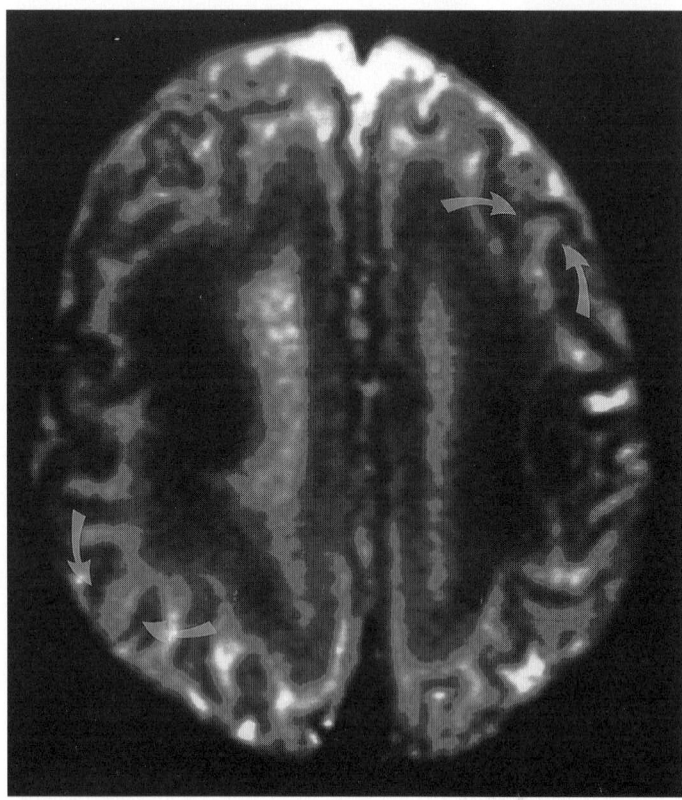

Fig.1. Band heterotopia. Axial T2 weighted image shows that the size of the gyri (arrows) are relatively normal in spite of the thick band of heterotopic gray matter lying central to the cortex. This helps to differentiate band heterotopia from classical lissencephaly.

as can be determined by testing) and normal neurologic development (Palmini *et al.*, 1991a; Barkovich *et al.*, 1994).

On imaging studies, band heterotopia can be identified by the characteristic layer of gray matter that is deep to the cerebral cortex and separated from the cortex by a layer of normal-appearing white matter. The overlying cortex typically has normal thickness with shallow sulci. Interestingly, the size (transverse width) of the gyri always seems to be smaller in band heterotopia than in classical lissencephaly (Fig. 1), a feature that may aid in differentiation between the two conditions. Band heterotopia may completely or partially surround the central white matter (Pinard *et al.*, 1994; Frangoni *et al.*, 1995); when partial (Fig. 2), the frontal lobes seem to be preferentially involved (Pinard *et al.*, 1994; Frangoni *et al.*, 1995). The greater the anomaly of the cortex, the worse the clinical prognosis for epilepsy. Foci of T2 prolongation may be seen in the cerebral white matter; the presence of these foci is associated with a poor motor outcome (Barkovich *et al.*, 1994).

When studied by PET using (^{18}F)-fluorodeoxyglucose, band heterotopias are found to have a glucose uptake that is similar to (Falconer *et al.*, 1990; Miura *et al.*, 1993) or greater than (De Volder *et al.*, 1994) normal cortex. This finding contrasts with the hypometabolism found in cortical dysplasias and in most epileptogenic foci. Morell *et al.* (1992) have found epileptiform discharges emanating from the band, suggesting that it is the source of the seizure activity in some affected patients.

Hemimegalencephaly

Hemimegalencephaly was first described by Sims in 1835. The name is the given to a hamartomatous overgrowth of all or part of a cerebral hemisphere with abnormalities of neurons, neuronal

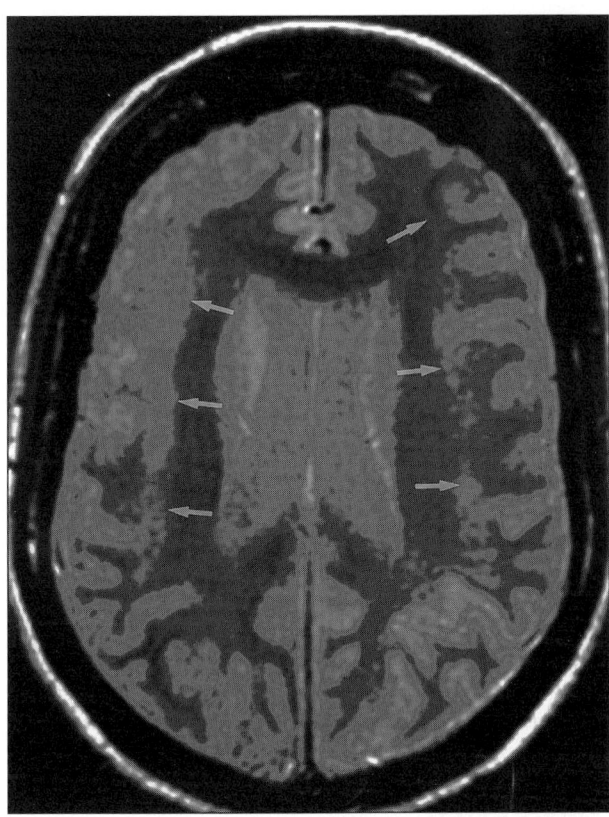

Fig. 2. Partial band heterotopia. Axial first echo of a T2 weighted image shows a thin band heterotopia in the frontal white matter (arrows). Note that the band on the right side is larger than that on the left.

migration, and neuronal organization in the affected hemisphere (Townsend *et al.*, 1975; Fitz *et al.*, 1978; Barkovich *et al.*, 1987; Kalifa *et al.*, 1987; Barkovich & Chuang, 1990). It is therefore classified as a malformation resulting from abnormal stem cell formation (Barkovich *et al.*, 1996). The many different radiologic (Kalifa *et al.*, 1987; Barkovich & Chuang, 1990; Revionden & Squer, 1994) and pathologic (Townsend *et al.*, 1975; Manz *et al.*, 1979; Bosman *et al.*, 1996) appearances suggest that hemimegalencephaly is not a single entity; disorders with several different causes may be included under this heading. The brain can be affected in isolation or can be associated with hemihypertrophy of part or all of the ipsilateral body. Affected patients typically present with an intractable seizure disorder that begins at a very early age (usually before the first birthday), hemiplegia, and severe developmental delay (Townsend *et al.*, 1975; Manz *et al.*, 1979; Kalifa *et al.*, 1987; Barkovich & Chuang, 1990). Hemimegalencephaly has been described in association with the epidermal nevus syndrome (Sawar & Schafer, 1988; Hager *et al.*, 1991; Parsone *et al.*, 1991), Proteus syndrome [sometimes (Happle, 1991) considered a form of epidermal nevus syndrome] (Griffiths *et al.*, 1994), unilateral hypomelanosis of Ito (Peserico *et al.*, 1988) and neurofibromatosis type I (Cusmai *et al.*, 1990).

On neuroimaging studies, the affected regions of the brain are always abnormal from the ventricular margin to the cortex. The involved hemisphere is moderately to markedly enlarged. The hemispheric white matter is typically too massive and shows abnormally low signal on CT and usually shows diffusely mottled areas of prolonged T1 and T2 relaxation times on MR studies (Fig. 3). The cortex most commonly has an appearance of broad gyri, shallow sulci and cortical thickening with irregularity of the cortical–white matter junction; however, in some cases, the gyral pattern may appear grossly normal or may be frankly agyric. In severely affected patients, the usually sharp border between the cortex and the subcortical white matter may blur or disappear altogether (Kalifa *et al.*, 1987; Barkovich & Chuang, 1990). The ipsilateral lateral ventricle is typically enlarged,

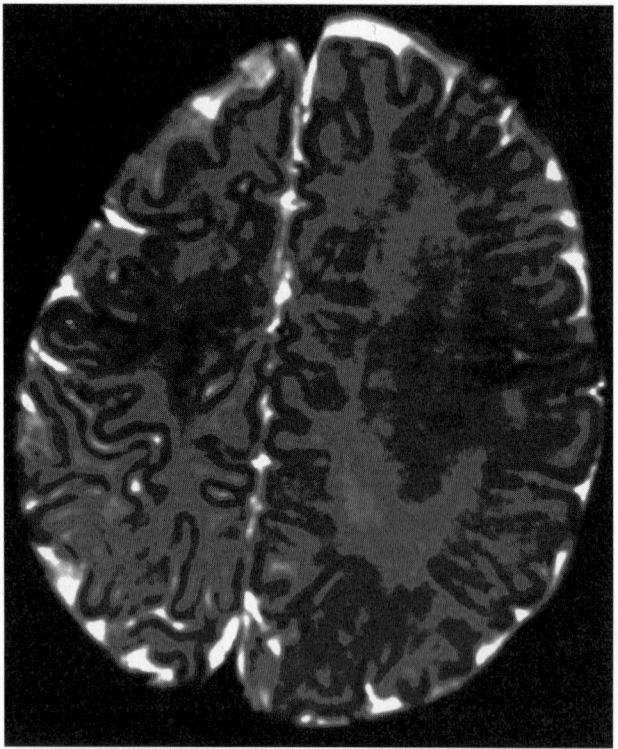

Fig. 3. Hemimegalencephaly. Axial T2 weighted images shows that the involved hemisphere is moderately to markedly enlarged with too much white matter and that shows diffusely mottled areas of abnormal T2 signal.

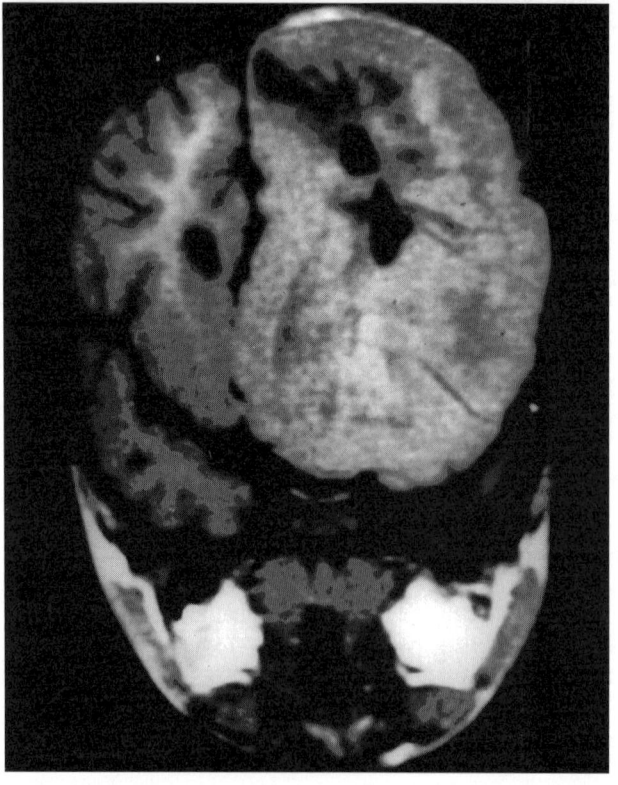

Fig. 4. Hemimegalencephaly. Axial T2 weighted image shows bizarre enlargement of the left hemisphere.

usually in proportion to the enlargement of the affected hemisphere, with an abnormal straightening of the frontal horn. In occasional patients, however, the ipsilateral ventricle is small (Renowden & Squier, 1994). Rarely, the affected portion of the brain has a bizarre, hamartomatous appearance (Kalifa et al., 1987; Barkovich & Chuang, 1990) (Fig. 4); in this situation, the malformation is recognized by the characteristic enlargement of the affected white matter and ipsilateral ventricle.

Wolpert et al. reported a patient in whom the affected hemisphere atrophied during the first year of life and was smaller than the contralateral (normal) hemisphere when imaged at age 1 year. An analogous change was seen on SPECT imaging, where the tracer uptake in the affected hemisphere diminished over time (Tagawa et al., 1994). We have also seen changes in the brains of affected patients, particularly after episodes of status epilepticus. Thus, the affected hemisphere may not be enlarged at the time of imaging.

Polymicrogyria

Polymicrogyria is an anomaly in which the neurons reach the cortex but distribute abnormally, resulting in the formation of multiple small gyri; thus, it is a disorder of neuronal organization (Barkovich et al., 1996). Polymicrogyria has a range of histologic appearances, all having in common a derangement of the normal six-layered lamination of the cortex (Barkovich et al., 1992). Thus, as with hemimegalencephaly, it is a category that contains a number of malformations that have different causes.

Patients with polymicrogyria have variable clinical presentations, depending upon the portion(s) of brain involved. They may present at almost any age with developmental delay, focal neurologic signs and symptoms, or epilepsy. The severity of the clinical presentation depends upon the extent of cortical involvement; bilateral involvement and involvement of more than half of a single hemisphere are poor prognostic indicators, portending moderate to severe developmental delay and significant motor dysfunction (Barkovich & Kjos, 1992a). Causes include congenital cytomegalovirus infection, in utero ischemia (Hallervorden, 1949; Barkovich et al., 1995), or, probably, chromosomal mutations (Kuzniecky, 1994). No difference in neurologic manifestations can be detected in patients who have congenital infections compared with those who have cortical dysplasia from other causes (Barkovich et al., 1992a; Guerrini et al., 1992a; Barkovich & Linden, 1994).

Polymicrogyria may involve small or large portions of the brain. The malformation may be focal, multifocal, or diffuse; it may be unilateral, bilateral and asymmetric, or bilateral and symmetric. The most common location is around the Sylvian fissure, particularly the posterior aspect of the fissure; however, any area, including the frontal, occipital, and temporal lobes, can be affected (Palmini et al., 1991b, c; Barkovich & Kjos, 1992a, b; Guerrini et al., 1992a).

Several clinical syndromes are associated with cerebral polymicrogyria. Kuzniecky et al. have described a syndrome of bilateral opercular cortical dysplasia (*Congenital bilateral perisylvian syndrome*) in which patients present with a syndrome of developmental pseudobulbar palsy (oropharyngeal dysfunction and dysarthria, 100 per cent), epilepsy (80–90 per cent), mental retardation (50–80 per cent) and sometimes congenital arthrogryposis (Becker et al., 1989; Kuzniecky et al., 1989; Guerrini et al., 1992b; Kuzniecky et al., 1993; Gropman et al., 1998). Some patients present in infancy or early childhood with developmental delay (60 per cent), poor palatal function (40 per cent), hypotonia (30 per cent), arthrogryposis (30 per cent), motor deficits (25 per cent). Seizures (many clinical types) are shown in 40–60 per cent of cases (Rolland et al., 1995; Gropman et al., 1998). Guerrini et al. (1994, 1997) have described patients with bilateral medial parietal-occipital polymicrogyria. I have seen a number of patients with bilateral symmetrical frontal polymicrogyria, bilateral anterior parietal polymicrogyria, bilateral posterior parietal polymicrogyria (Fig. 5), and bilateral occipital polymicrogyria. Therefore, it seems that bilateral symmetrical polymicrogyria can occur in nearly any location in the brain.

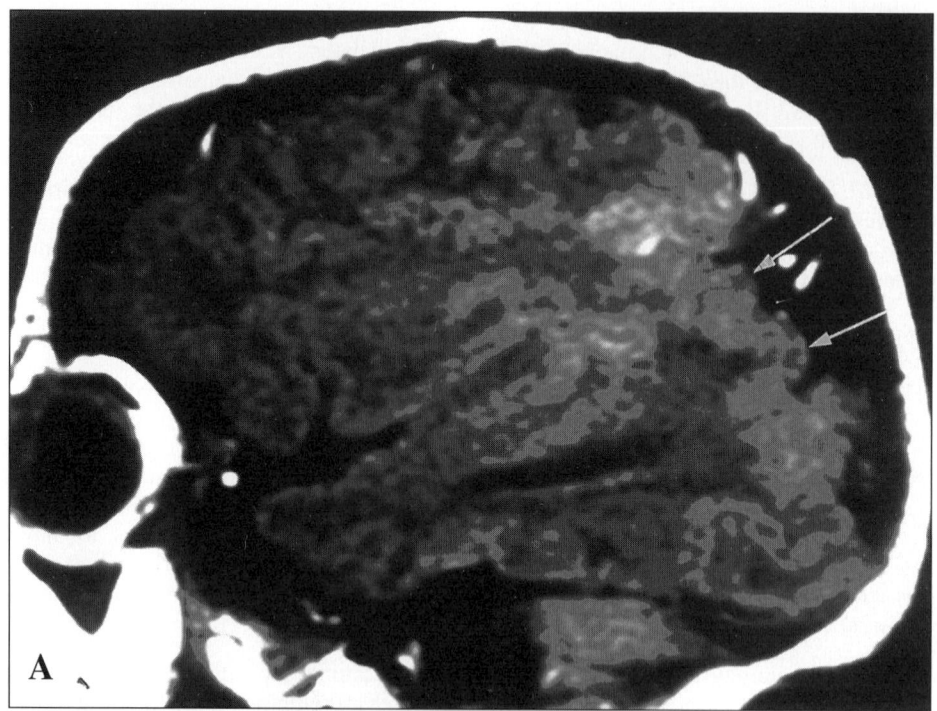

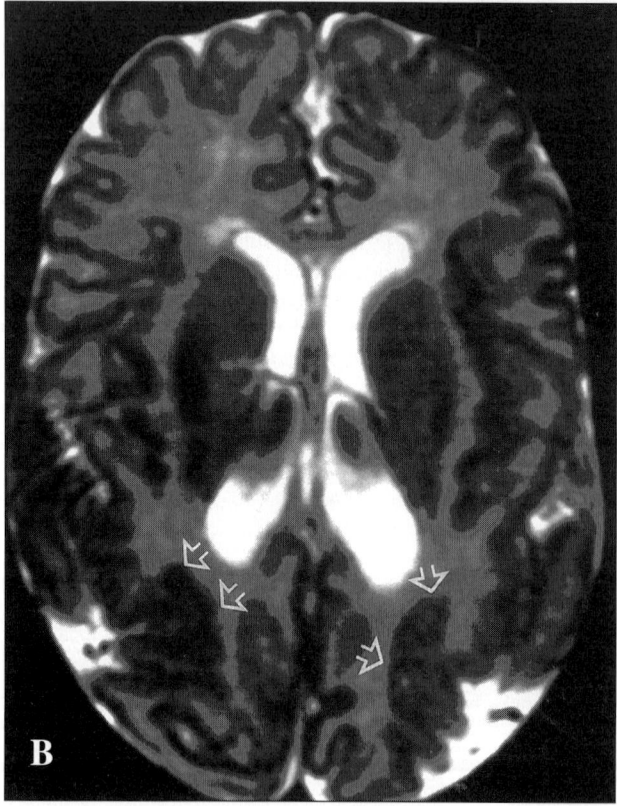

Fig. 5. Bilateral posterior parietal polymicrogyria. Bilateral symmetrical polymicrogyria can be seen in nearly any portion of the cerebral hemispheres. In this case, sagittal (A) and axial (B) images show polymicrogyria (arrows) in the posterior parietal lobes.

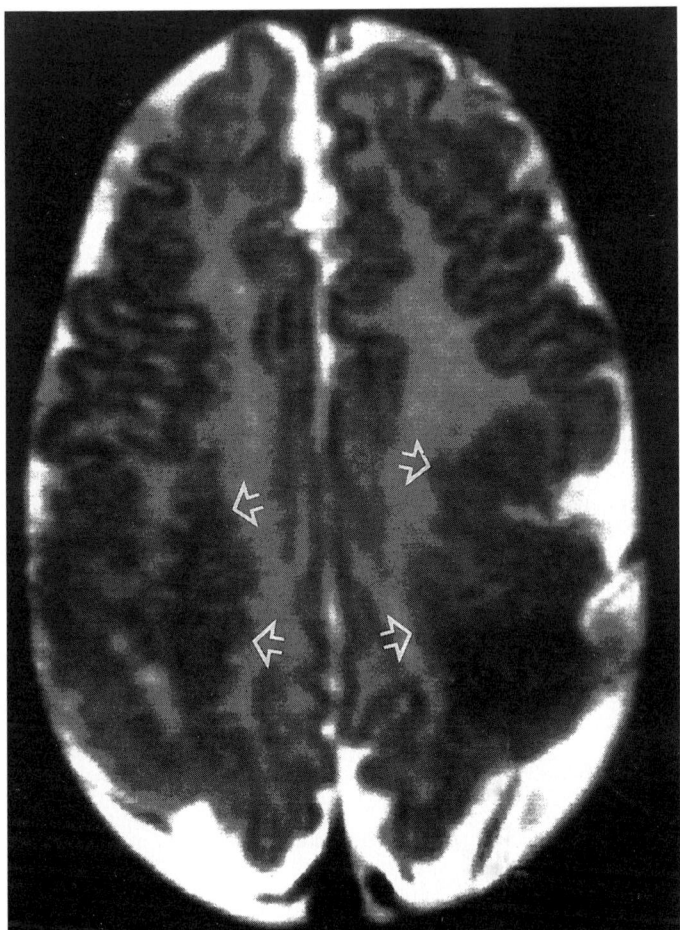

Fig. 6. Bilateral perisylvian/perirolandic polymicrogyria. Thin sections, show the multiple small gyri (arrows) and the irregularity of the cortical-white matter junction in these patients.

The imaging appearance of polymicrogyria depends, to some degree, on the technique used. If sections with large (5 mm or larger) thickness are acquired, areas of polymicrogyria may be missed or misdiagnosed as pachygyria on routine spin echo images. Images with thin sections and optimal gray matter-white matter contrast (we use volume spoiled gradient 3D acquisition with ⩽1.5 mm partition size and 2–3 mm sections on fast spin echo T2 weighted images, Fig. 6) and evaluation in three planes is often necessary to detect irregularities of the gray matter–white matter junction, often the only evidence of dysplastic brain (Raybaud et al., 1996).

Regions of polymicrogyria can be superficial or may extend centripetally, pointing inward. The infolding of cortex may be small or large; the character of the cortex in these regions of infolding is similar to that in superficial cortical dysplasia, with bumpy, irregular inner and outer cortical surfaces (Barkovich & Kuzniecky, 1996).

Typically, polymicrogyria is isointense to normal cortex on both CT and MR. Occasionally, however, prolonged T2 relaxation time is present in the white matter underlying the dysplastic cortex [20 per cent of affected patients (Palmini et al., 1991b, c; Barkovich & Kjos, 1992a)]. A small proportion of polymicrogyria, probably less than 5 per cent, will be calcified. Anomalous venous drainage is common in areas of polymicrogyria (Barkovich, 1998) especially superficial to large infoldings of thickened cortex. This appearance should not be mistaken for vascular malformations; angiography is not indicated.

A number of articles have indicated that PET scanning or SPECT scanning (Henkes *et al.*, 1991) may be useful in detecting small areas of dysplastic cortex that may be cryptic to standard imaging (Chugani *et al.*, 1990; Newton *et al.*, 1993; Lee *et al.*, 1994; Swartz *et al.*, 1995; Chiron *et al.*, 1996; Richardson *et al.*, 1996). Generally this is more of a problem with focal cortical dysplasias than with polymicrogyria. The problem with PET and SPECT, with either FCD or polymicrogyria, is that they are non-specific: correlative MR imaging is always needed. Our approach is to use PET scanning in those patients who have some localization to their seizure disorder and a normal initial MR scan. If the PET study shows an area of hypometabolism, a high resolution MR scan with phased array surface coils is performed to generate images in multiple planes, preferably with partition size of less than 1 mm through the region of abnormality. The cortex in that area is then closely scrutinized for any irregularity of the cortical surface or gray–white junction.

References

Barkovich, A.J. (1988): Abnormal vascular drainage in anomalies of neuronal migration. *Am. J. Neuroradiol.* **9**, 939–942.

Barkovich, A.J. & Chuang, S.H. (1990): Unilateral megalencephaly: Correlation of MR imaging and pathologic characteristics. *Am. J. Neuroradiol.* **11**, 523–531.

Barkovich, A.J. & Kjos, B.O. (1992): Non-lissencephalic cortical dysplasia: correlation of imaging findings with clinical deficits. *Am. J. Neuroradiol.* **13**, 95–103.

Barkovich, A.J. & Kjos, B.O. (1992): Schizencephaly: correlation of clinical findings with MR characteristics. *Am. J. Neuroradiol.* **13**, 85–94.

Barkovich, A.J. & Kuzniecky, R.I. (1996) Neuroimaging of focal malformations of cortical development. *J. Clin. Neurophysiol.* **13**, 481–494.

Barkovich, A.J. & Linden, C.L. (1994): Congenital cytomegalovirus infection of the brain: imaging analysis and embryologic considerations. *Am. J. Neuroradiol.* **15**, 703–715.

Barkovich, A.J., Chuang, S.H. & Norman, D. (1987): MR of neuronal migration anomalies. *Am. J. Neuroradiol.* **8**, 1009–1017.

Barkovich, A.J., Jackson Jr, D.E. & Boyer, R.S., (1989): Band heterotopias: A newly recognized neuronal migration anomaly. *Radiology* **171**, 455–458.

Barkovich, A.J., Gressens, P. & Evrard, P. (1992): Formation, maturation, and disorders of brain neocortex. *Am. J. Neuroradiol.* **13**, 423–446.

Barkovich, A.J., Guerrini, R. & Battaglia, G, *et al.* (1994): Band heterotopia: correlation of outcome with MR imaging parameters. *Ann. Neurol.* **36**, 609–617.

Barkovich, A.J., Rowley, H.A. & Bollen, A. (1995): Correlation of prenatal events with the development of polymicrogyria. *Am. J. Neuroradiol.* **16**, 822–827.

Barkovich, A.J. , Kuzniecky, R.I., Dobyns, W.B., Jackson, G.D., Becker, L. E. & Evrard, P. (1996): A classification scheme for malformations of cortical development. *Neuropediatrics* **27 (2)**, 59–63.

Becker, P.S., Dixon, A.M. & Troncoso, J.C. (1989): Bilateral opercular polymicrogyria. *Ann. Neurol.* **25**, 90–92.

Bosman, C., Boldrini, R., Dimitri , L., Di Rocco, C. & Corsi, A. (1996): Hemimegalencephaly. Histological, immunohistochemical, ultrastructural and cytofluorimetric study of six patients. *Child. Nerv. Syst.* **12**, 765–775.

Chiron, C., Dulac, O., Nuttin, C. & Depas, G. (1996): *Functional imaging in cortical dysplasia: SPECT*, pp. 175–179. Philadelphia: Lippincott-Raven.

Chugani, H.T., Shields, W.D., Shewmon, D.A., Olson, D.M., Phelps, M.E. & Peacock, W.J. (1990): Infantile spasms: I. PET identifies focal cortical dysgenesis in cryptogenic csases for surgical treatment. *Ann. Neurol.* **27**, 406–413.

Cusmai, R., Curatolo, P., Mangano, S., Cheminal, R. & Echenne, B. (1990): Hemimegalencephaly and neurofibromatosis. *Neuropediatrics* **21**, 179–182.

De Volder, A.G., Gadisseux, J.-F., Michel, C.J. et al. (1994): Brain glucose utilization in band heterotopia: synaptic activity of 'double cortex'. Pediatr. Neurol. **11**, 290–294

Falconer, J., Wada, J., Martin, & W., Li, D. (1990): PET, CT, and MRI imaging of neuronal migration anomalies in epileptic patients. Can. J. Neurol. Sci. **17**, 35–39.

Fitz, C.R., Harwood-Nash, D.C. & Boldt, D.W. (1978): The radiographic features of unilateral megalencephaly. Neuroradiology **15**, 145–148.

Franzoni, E., Bernardi, B., Marchiani, V., Crisanti, A.F., Marchi, R. & Fonda, C. (1995): Band brain heterotopia. Case report and literature review. Neuropediatrics **26**, 37–40.

Griffiths, P.D., Welch, R., Gardner-Medwin, D., Gholkar, A. & McAllister, V. (1994): The radiological features of hemimegalencephaly including three cases associated with proteus syndrome. Neuropediatrics **25**, 140–144.

Gropman, A.L., Barkovich, A.J., Vezina, L.G., Conry, J.A., Dubovsky, E.C. & Packer, R.J. (1997): Pediatric congenital bilateral perisylvian syndrome: clinical and MRI features in 12 patients. Neuropediatrics **28**, 198–203.

Guerrini, R., Dravet, C., Raybaud, C. et al. (1992): Epilepsy and focal gyral anomalies detected by MRI: electroclinico-morphological correlations and follow-up. Dev. Med. Child Neurol. **34 (8)**, 706.

Guerrini, R., Dravet, C., Raybaud, C. et al. (1992b): Neurological findings and seizure outcome in children with bilateral opercular macrogyric-like changes detected by MRI. Dev. Med. Child Neurol. **34 (8)**, 694.

Guerrini, R., Dulac, O., Canapicchi, R. et al. (1994): Epilepsie révélatrice d'une dysplasie corticale occipito-pariétale parasagittale bilatérale. Epilepsies **6**, 131–139.

Guerrini, R., Dubeau, F., Dulac, O. et al. (1997): Bilateral parasagittal parietooccipital polymicrogyria and epilepsy. Ann. Neurol. **41**, 65–73.

Hager, B.C., Dyme, I.Z., Guertin, S.R., Tyler, R.J., Tryciecky, E.W. & Fratkin, J.D. (1991): Linear nevus sebaceous syndrome: megalencephaly and heterotopic gray matter. Pediatr. Neurol. **7**, 45–49.

Hallervorden, J. (1994): Ueber eine Kohlenoxydvergiftung im Fetalleben mit Entwicklunsstörung der Hirnrinde. Allg. Z. Psychiatr. **124**, 289–298.

Happle, R. (1991): How many epidermal nevus syndromes exist? A clinicogenetic classification. J. Am. Acad. Dermatol. **25**, 550–556.

Henkes, K., Hosten, N., Cordes, M., Neumann, K. & Hansen, M.-L. (1991): Increased rCBF in gray matter heterotopias detected by SPECT using 99mTc hexamethylpropylenamine oxime. Neuroradiology **33**, 310–312.

Kalifa, C.L., Chiron, C., Sellier, N. et al. (1987): Hemimegalencephaly: MR imaging in five children. Radiology **165**, 29–33.

Kuzniecky, R. (1994): Familial diffuse cortical dysplasia. Arch. Neurol. **51**, 307–310.

Kuzniecky, R., Andermann, F., Tampieri, D., Melanson, D., Olivier, A. & Leppik I. (1989): Bilateral central macrogyria: epilepsy, pseudobulbar palsy, and mental retardation – a recognizable neuronal migration disorder. Ann. Neurol. **25**, 547–554.

Kuzniecky, R., Andermann, F., & Guerrini, R. (1993): Congenital bilateral perisylvian syndrome: study of 31 patients. The congenital bilateral perisylvian syndrome multicenter collaborative study. Lancet **341**, 608–612.

Lee, N., Radtke, R., Gray, L. et al. (1994): Neuronal migration disorders: positron emission tomography correlations. Ann. Neurol **35**, 290–297.

Livingston, J.H. & Aicardi, J. (1990): Unusual MRI appearance of diffuse subcortical heterotopia or 'double cortex' in two children. J. Neurol. Neurosurg. Psychiatry **53**, 617–620.

Manz, H.J., Phillips, T.M., Rowden, G., & McCullough, D.C. (1979) Unilateral megalencephaly, cerebral cortical dysplasia, neuronal hypertrophy, and heterotopia: cytomorphometric, fluorometric, cytochemical, and biochemical analyses. Acta Neuropath. (Ber.) **45** 97–103.

Miura, K., Watanabe, K., Maeda, N. et al. (1993): MR imaging and positron emission tomography of band heterotopia. Brain Dev. **15**, 288–290.

Morell, F., Whisler, W., Hoeppner, T. et al. Electrophysiology of heterotopic gray matter in the 'double cortex' syndrome. Epilepsia (1992): **33 (Suppl. 3)**, 76.

Newton, M.R., Austin, M.C., Chan, J.G. et al. (1993): Ictal SPECT using 99m-Tc-HMPAO: methods for rapid preparation and optimal deployment of tracer during spontaneous seizures. *J. Nucl. Med.* **34,** 666–670.

Ono, J., Mano, T., Andermann, E. et al. (1997): Band heterotopia or double cortex in a male: bridging structures suggest abnormality of the radial glial guide system. *Neurology* **48,** 1701–1703.

Palmini, A., Andermann, F., Aicardi, J. et al. (1991a): Diffuse cortical dysplasia, or the 'double cortex' syndrome: the clinical and epileptic spectrum in 10 patients. *Neurology* **41,** 1656–1662.

Palmini, A., Andermann, F., Olivier, A., Tampieri, D. & Robitaille, Y. (1991b): Focal neuronal migration disorders and intractable partial epilepsy: results of surgical treatment. *Ann. Neurol.* **30,** 750–757.

Palmini, A., Andermann, F., Olivier, A. et al. (1991c): Focal neuronal migration disorders and intractable partial epilepsy: a study of 30 patients. *Ann. Neurol.* **30,** 741–749.

Pavone, L., Curatolo, P., Rizzo, R. et al. (1991): Epidermal nevus syndrome: a neurologic variant with hemimegalencephaly, gyral malformation, mental retardation, seizures, and facial hemihypertrophy. *Neurology* **41,** 266–271.

Peserico, A., Battistella, P.A., Bertoli, P. & Drigo, P. (1998): Unilateral hypomelanosis of Ito with hemimegalencephaly. *Acta Paediatr. Scand.* **77,** 446–447.

Pinard, J.M., Motte, J., Chiron, C., Brian, R., Andermann, E. & Dulac, O. (1994): Subcortical laminar heteropia and lissencephaly in 2 families: a single X-linked dominant gene. *J. Neurol. Neurosurg. Psychiatry* **57,** 914–920.

Raybaud, C., Girard, N., Canto-Moreira, N. & Poncet, M. (1996): High-definition magnetic resonance imaging identification of cortical dysplasias: micropolygyria versus lissencephaly. In: *Dysplasias of cerebral cortex and epilepsy,* ed. R. Guerrini, pp. 131–143. Philadelphia: Lippincott-Raven.

Renowden, S.A. & Squier, M. (1994): Unusual magnetic resonance and neuropathological findings in hemimegalencephaly: report of a case following hemispherectomy. *Dev. Med. Child Neurol.* **36,** 357–369.

Richardson, M.P., Koepp, M.J., Brooks, D.J., Fish, D.R. & Duncan, J.S. (1996): Benzodiazepine receptors in focal epilepsy with cortical dysgenesis: an 11C-Flumazenil PET study. *Ann. Neurol.* **40,** 188–198.

Rolland, Y., Adamsbaum, C., Sellier, N., Robain, O., Ponsot, G. & Kalifa, G. (1995): Opercular malformations: clinical and MRI features in 11 children. *Pediatr. Radiol.* **25,** S2–S8.

Ross, M.E., Allen, K.M., Srivastava, A.K. et al. (1997): Linkage and physical mapping of X-linked lissencephaly/SBH (XLIS): a gene causing neuronal migration defects in human brain. *Hum. Mol. Genet.* **6,** 555–562.

Sims J.M. (1835): On hypertrophy and atrophy of the brain. *Trans. Med. Chirurg. Soc. (Lond.)* **19,** 346–348.

Sarwar, M. & Schafer, M. (1988): Brain malformations in linear nevus sebaceous syndrome: an MR study. *J. Comput. Assist. Tomogr.* **12,** 338–340.

Swartz, B.E., Khonsari, A., Brown, C., Mandelkern, M., Simkins, F. & Krisdakumtorn, T. (1995): Improved sensitivity of 18FDG-positron emission tomography scans in frontal and 'frontal plus' epilepsy. *Epilepsia* **36,** 388–395.

Tagawa, T., Otani, K., Futagi, Y., Wakayama, A., Morimoto, K. & Morita, Y. (1994): Serial IMP-SPECT and EEG studies in an infant with hemimegalencephaly. *Brain Dev.* **16,** 475–479.

Townsend, J.J., Nielsen, S.L., & Malamud, N. (1975): Unilateral megalencephaly: hamartoma or neoplasm? *Neurology* **25,** 448–453.

Wolpert, S.M., Cohen, A. & Libenson, M. (1994): Hemimegalencephaly: a longitudinal MR study. *Am. J. Neuroradiol.* **15,** 1479–1482.

Chapter 13

Neuroradiology of malformations of cortical development: schizencephaly, periventricular heterotopia

Ludovico D'Incerti, Laura Farina,
Tiziana Granata* and Mario Savoiardo

*Divisione di Neuroradiologia Diagnostica, *Divisione di Neuropsichiatria Infantile,
Istituto Nazionale Neurologico 'C. Besta', Via Celoria 11, 20133 Milan, Italy*

Summary

Schizencephaly is a brain malformation characterized by clefts extending from the surface of the brain to the walls of the lateral ventricles. The clefts are lined by dysplastic cortex; in closed lip schizencephaly their margins are in opposition, in open lip schizencephaly they are separated. Schizencephaly may be uni- or bilateral, and may be isolated, or part of a more complex malformative picture. Closed lip schizencephalies have to be differentiated from infoldings of polymicrogyria, from nodules of cortical heterotopia reaching the brain surface and from focal transmantle cortical dysplasia. Large open lip schizencephalies have to be differentiated from destructive lesion of the developing brain resulting in porencephaly. Clinical presentation always consists of epilepsy and mental delay, associated with focal neurological signs of variable severity, related to the position of the malformation and to the amount of the affected brain. The association with dysplastic cortex suggests that schizencephaly and polymicrogyria are different expressions of the same pathogenetic mechanism. The identification of a gene mutation in schizencephaly patients confirms that genetic factors are involved in the pathogenesis. Cortical heterotopia consists of collections of neurones in abnormal positions. It is caused by an arrest of the radial migration of neurones. On the basis of the location, band heterotopia, focal subcortical, periventricular and subependymal heterotopias are recognized. Nodules of cortical heterotopia may have different size and location; they can be associated with deformities of the cerebral hemispheres and with distortion of the ventricles. On MRI they are always isointense with normal grey matter; this allows differentiation from tumours and, in the cases of subependymal nodules, from hamartomas of the tuberous sclerosis. The affected patients may have seizures and variable motor and intellectual disturbances.

Schizencephaly

Schizencephaly is a congenital brain malformation first described by Yakovlev in 1946, characterized by clefts extending through the hemispheres from the pial surface to the walls of the lateral ventricles. Two different forms of schizencephaly are recognized: closed lip schizencephaly, in which the margins of the clefts are opposed to one another, and open lip schizencephaly, in which the lips are separated and the CSF fills the space between the walls of the cleft (Yakovlev & Wadsworth, 1946a, b). The clefts may be unilateral or bilateral. Their more frequent location is in the fronto-parietal area. The clefts are lined by dysplastic cortex with morphologic features of polymicrogyria.

The malformation may be isolated, or associated with more extended areas of dysplastic cortex (Barkovich & Norman, 1988; Truwit & Barkovich, 1996). Epilepsy is the most frequent symptom; mental delay and focal neurological signs are always present, related to the position of the malformation and the amount of the affected brain.

Magnetic resonance imaging (MRI) has allowed description *in vivo* of an increasing number of cases and correlation of the morphologic features with the clinical findings and outcome (Barkovich & Norman, 1988; Granata *et al.*, 1997).

Closed lip schizencephaly

In closed lip schizencephaly, the walls of the cleft are in opposition and CSF space is obliterated: in small closed lip schizencephalies, the continuity between the ventricle and the brain surface may be difficult to recognize. On conventional MRI studies, the small fused lip clefts may be overlooked when they are included in sections parallel to the cleft itself. MRI studies for epilepsy or mental delay should always include at least two planes of acquisition or reformatted multiplanar images.

Even small schizencephalies are easily recognized by a dimple observed on the wall of the lateral ventricle where it communicates with the cleft (Fig. 1). The dimple may be the clue suggesting the malformation and is always useful to differentiate it from polymicrogyria and heterotopic gray matter. As the malformation is frequently associated with areas of dysplastic cortex with variable extension, closed lip schizencephaly must be differentiated from infoldings of polymicrogyria and from nodules of heterotopic gray matter reaching the brain surface. The differentiation is recognized by a band of normal white matter separating the abnormal cortex from the wall of the ventricle. In these cases the dimple of the lateral ventricle is always absent (Barkovich & Norman, 1988; Truwit & Barkovich, 1996).

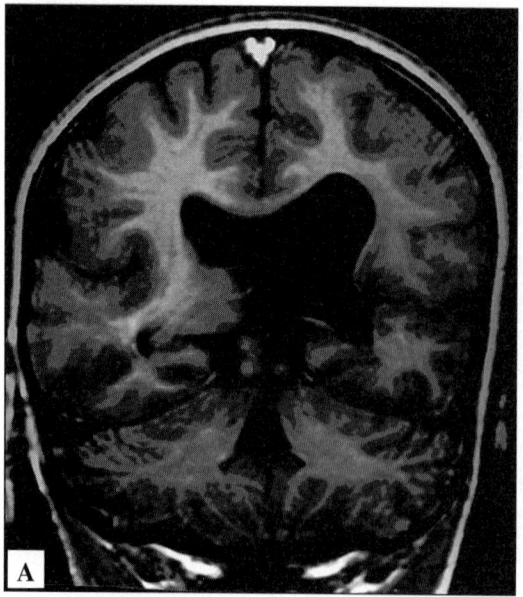
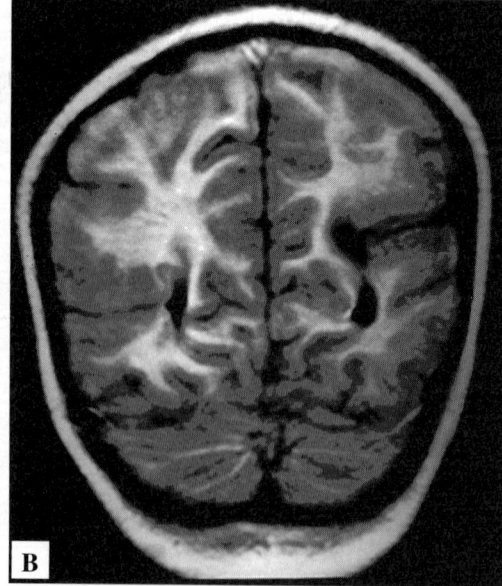

Fig. 1. Bilateral closed lip schizencephaly. On the left side the dimple of the lateral ventricle points to the malformation (A). A small dimple allows to recognize a small cleft on the opposite side, in more posterior location (B).

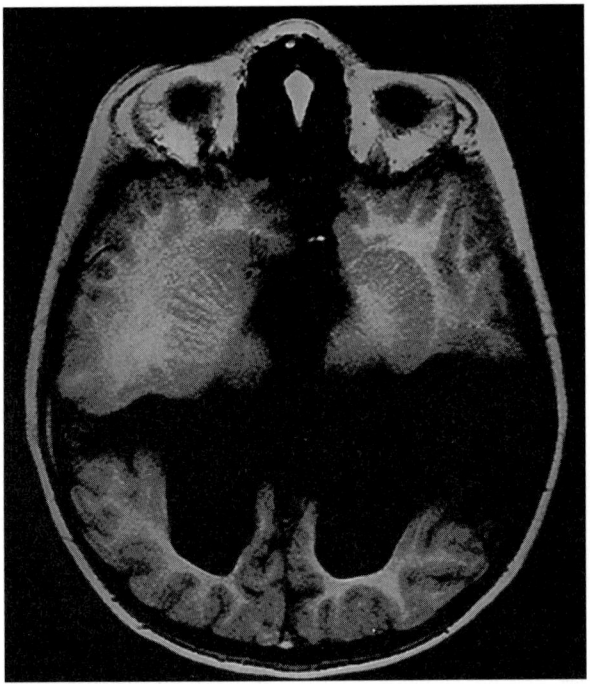

Fig. 2. Severe bilateral open lip schizencephaly.

The isointensity of the polymicrogiric cortex on the margins of the clefts with the normal gray matter allows differentiation of focal transmantle cortical dysplasia, a recently described malformation of cortical development. Focal transmantle cortical dysplasia is characterized by bands of heterotopic neurones mixed with 'balloon cells' of uncertain differentiation extended radially from the walls of the ventricles to the brain surface; these radial bands usually show dishomogeneous, mild hyperintensity in T2-weighted images and are associated with an abnormal gyral pattern of variable extension (Barkovich et al., 1997).

As schizencephaly is frequently a part of a complex malformative picture involving the whole brain, cortical dysplasia has always to be searched for also in the contralateral hemisphere in cases of unilateral cleft.

Open lip schizencephaly

The morphologic features of open lip schizencephalies are easily recognized on MRI studies. The malformative picture in these cases is usually severe and MRI frequently shows the association of schizencephaly with different malformative features (Fig. 2-3). (Barkovich & Norman, 1988; Granata et al., 1996; Truwit & Barkovich, 1996).

Partial or complete agenesis of the corpus callosum is frequently observed. The communication between the interhemispheric fissure and the third ventricle, sometimes associated with arachnoid cysts and with abnormal giration of the interhemispheric cortex, has not to be mistaken for open lip schizencephaly.

Callosal agenesis may also be associated with septo-optic dysplasia, consisting of optic nerve hypoplasia and deficiency of septum pellucidum, which is present in 20–45 per cent of patients with schizencephaly. The septum pellucidum is absent in 70–90 per cent of the affected patients. Of those with absence of the septum pellucidum, 30 per cent to 50 per cent have optic nerve hypoplasia. Therefore the chiasm and the optic nerves should always be scrutinized in these patients, especially when visual symptoms and hypothalamic–pituitary dysfunction are present (Truwit & Barkovich, 1996).

Large open lip schizencephalies should be differentiated from porencephalic cysts. Porencephaly is usually the result of an ischemic or haemorrhagic injury which may result in cysts communicating with the venticles or with the subarachnoid spaces or both, and in changes of the adjacent cortex including gyral abnormalities and sometimes polymicrogyria (Kuzniecky & Jackson, 1995). When these injuries occur in the early phase of brain development, reactive gliosis is minimal or absent and abnormal gyration or polymicrogyria on the margins of the cavity can be present. In these cases the morphologic features of porencephalic cysts may overlap with those of open lip schizencephaly.

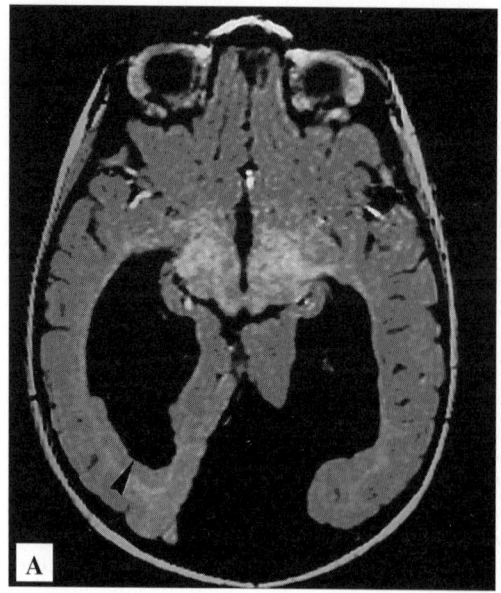
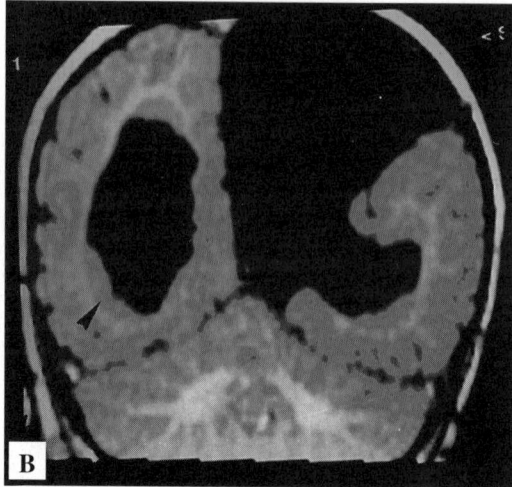

Fig. 3 A,B. Left occipital open lip schizencephaly, associated and with right subependymal nodular heterotopia (arrows).

When encephaloclastic lesions occur in the late phase of brain development, cortical dysplasia is not found; in full-term newborn, post-anoxic injuries to the cortex can result in ulegyria. MRI allows to differentiate the morphologic features of the 'mushroom gyri', this is typical of ulegyria, from the microgyri of cortical dysplasia. White matter post-anoxic changes, i.e. atrophy and reactive gliosis, are always associated with the mushroom gyri and are recognized as hyperintensity in T2-weighted images (Kuzniecky & Jackson, 1995; D' Incerti et al., 1997).

Different pathogenetic mechanisms have been proposed for schizencephaly. The irregular inner and outer surface of the cortex along the cleft suggested that schizencephaly is an extreme variant of polymicrogyria, in which the infolding of dysplastic cortex extends from the surface of the brain to the lateral ventricles (Barkovich et al., 1988).

The description of several familial cases of schizencephaly, however, has raised the possibility that genetic factors may be involved in its pathogenesis. A mutation in homeobox gene EMX2, recently described in schizencephaly patients, confirms this hypothesis and has been also demonstrated in our familial cases (Brunelli et al., 1996; Granata et al., 1997).

Periventricular heterotopia

Periventricular heterotopia is one of the forms in which grey matter heterotopia is classified. This entity is caused by an arrest of the radial migration of the neurones, resulting in the formation of collections of neurones in abnormal location. The nodules of heterotopic grey matter may have different size and distribution, and may be isolated or multiple, unilateral or bilateral. On the basis of the location of the nodules, the following forms are recognized: periventricular, focal subcortical and diffuse heterotopia, the last also known as band heterotopia or double cortex (Barkovich & Kjos, 1992; Truwit & Barkovich, 1996).

Patients with periventricular heterotopia almost always present with seizures, frequently of late onset. Patients with subependymal nodules tend to have mild clinical symptoms and normal development. Patients with more extended areas of heterotopic nodules, periventricular or subcortical, may have variable motor and intellectual disturbances; their severity is generally related to the extent of brain malformation cortex (Barkovich & Kjos, 1992; Truwit & Barkovich, 1996; Battaglia et al.,1997).

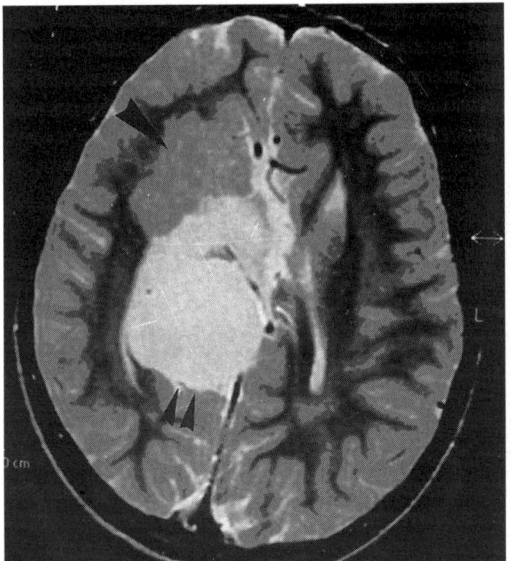
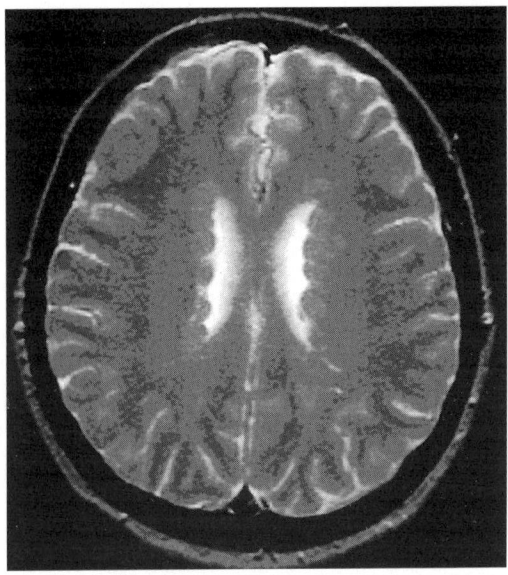

Fig. 4. Periventricular nodular heterotopia (arrow). Complete agenesys of the corpus callosum and an arachnoid cyst in the interhemispheric fissure (double arrow) are associated.

Fig. 5. Subependymal nodular heterotopia. Small nodules of heterotopic grey matter lines the walls of the lateral ventricles.

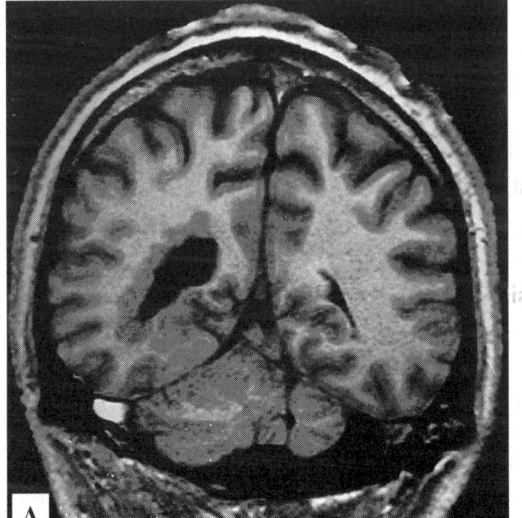
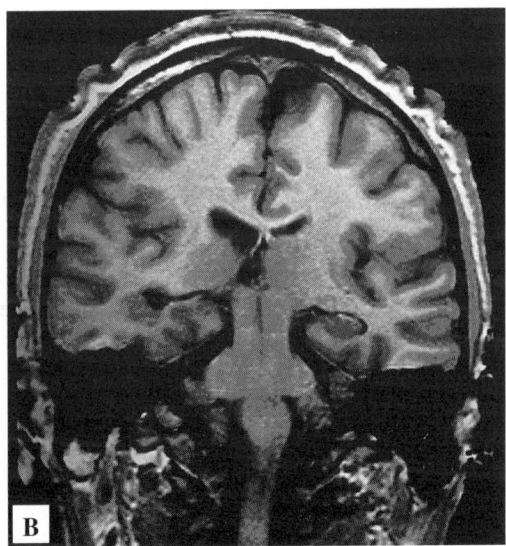

Fig. 6. Unilateral subependymal nodular heterotopia. Subependymal nodules are recognizable on the wall of the trigone (A) and of the temporal horn of the right lateral ventricle (B). The anatomy of the right hippocampus is not recognizable: compare with the normal hippocampus on the left side (B).

In MRI studies, cortical heterotopias appear as nodular areas of grey matter in the periventricular or subcortical regions, greatly variable in size and often associated with asymmetries of the brain hemispheres. When nodules are large, they may cause distortion of the ventricles. The clue for differentiation of heterotopic nodules from tumours is the signal isointensity to the normal grey matter on all imaging sequences (Fig. 4). In subependymal periventricular heterotopia, the nodules of heterotopic grey matter are usually of small size and bulge into the ventricular cavities, causing a characteristic indentation in the profile of the ventricles (Fig. 5).

Subependymal nodules may be single or multiple, unilateral or bilateral. The subependymal nodules of heterotopic grey matter are differentiated from the subependymal nodules of tuberous sclerosis by shape and extension, their signal isointensity to the normal cortex and by lack of calcifications cortex (Barkovich & Kjos, 1992; Truwit & Barkovich, 1996; Battaglia et al., 1997).

The overlaying cortex of the cerebral hemispheres is often normal. In other, although rare cases, subependymal nodules may be part of a more complex malformative picture, with association of neuronal migration disorders (Figs. 3-6).

References

Barkovich, A.J. & Kjos, B.O. (1992): Grey matter heterotopias: MR characteristics and correlation with developmental and neurologic manifestations. *Radiology* **182,** 493–499.

Barkovich, A.J., Kuzniecky, R.I., Bollen, A.W. & Ellen Grant, P. (1997): Focal transmantle dysplasia: a specific malformation of cortical development. *Neurology* **49,** 1148–1152.

Barkovich, A.J. & Norman, D. (1988): MR of schizencephaly. *AJNR* **9,** 297–302.

Battaglia, G., Granata, T., Farina, L., D' Incerti, L., Franceschetti, S. & Avanzini, G. (1997): Periventricular nodular heterotopia: epileptogenic findings. *Epilepsia* **38 (11),** 1173–1182.

Brunelli, S., Faiella, A. & Capra, V. (1996): Germline mutations in the homeobox gene EMX2 in patients with severe schizencephaly. *Nature genet.* **12,** 94–96.

D' Incerti, L., Chiapparini, L., Farina, L., Binelli, S., Villani, F., Spreafico, R. & Savoiardo, M. (1997): Ulegyria: MRI findings in three cases (abstract). *Neuroradiology* **39 (Suppl. 1),** 116.

Friede, R.L. (1989): *Developmental neuropathology*. Second edition, pp.28–44. Berlin: Springer-Verlag.

Granata, T., Battaglia, G., D'Incerti, L., Franceschetti S., Spreafico R., Savoiardo M. & Avanzini, G. (1996): Schizencephaly: neuroradiologic and epileptogenic findings. *Epilepsia* **37,** 1185–1193.

Granata, T., Farina, L., Faiella, A., Cardini, R., D'Incerti, L., Boncinelli, E. & Battaglia, G. (1997): Familial schizencephaly associated with EMX2 mutation. *Neurology* **48,** 1403–1406.

Kuzniecky, R.I. & Jackson, G.D. (1995): *Magnetic resonance in epilepsy*. pp. 213–234. New York: Raven Press.

Truwit, C.L. & Barkovich, A.J. (1996) : Disorders of brain development. In: *Magnetic resonance imaging of the brain and spine*, Second edition. ed. S.W. Atlas, pp.179–264. Philadelphia: Lippincott-Raven.

Yakovlev, P.I. & Wadsworth, R.C. (1946): Schizencephalies. A study of the congenital clefts in the cerebral mantle 1. Clefts with fused lips. *J. Neuropathol. Exp. Neurol.* **5,** 116–130.

Yakovlev, P.I. & Wadsworth, R.C. (1946): Schizencephalies. A study of the congenital clefts in the cerebral mantle. 2. Clefts with hydrocephalus and lips separated. *J. Neuropathol. Exp. Neurol.* **5,** 169–206.

Chapter 14

Neuronal migration disorders and epilepsy in infancy

Federico Vigevano

*Divisione di Neurofisiologia, Ospedale Bambino Gesù,
Piazza Sant'Onofrio 4, 00165 Rome, Italy*

Summary

Cortical development abnormalities cause cognitive delay, motor deficits and epilepsy. Epilepsy is very frequent and can worsen the prognosis. Although epilepsy pictures are not uniform, they do share general characteristics: seizures onset occurs early; characteristics of seizures and epilepsy depend on the type of malformation and the patient's age; resistance to drug treatment is frequent. Among the different types of malformation, focal cortical dysplasia seems to be the cause of most severe epilepsies. Neurophysiological study demonstrated the intrinsic epileptogenicity of dysplastic cortex.

Brain malformations cause cognitive delay, motor deficits and epilepsy. From a clinical and social point of view, epilepsy is very significant because it can worsen a prognosis that is often already very unfavourable.

The term 'neuronal migration' has been used frequently in a broad sense, almost as synonym of cortical development disorder. However, in the most recent classifications (Barkovich *et al.*, 1996), cortical development abnormalities are divided according to the type of embryological event mainly involved: neuronal and glial proliferation; neuronal migration; and cortical organization (dealt with in other chapters in this book). According to this classification, some disorders, such as focal dysplasia or polymicrogyria, are no longer considered true disorders of neuronal migration, but of neuronal proliferation and cortical organization respectively.

This chapter covers epilepsy associated with various forms of cortical development disorder. There are no systematic studies on the incidence of epilepsy in brain malformations. The data in the literature are not very reliable from an epidemiological standpoint, because cases with minimum symptoms may escape observation and also because epilepsy is often the main reason for the scientific study. However, data can be found referring to selected series of patients with particular malformations: epilepsy was found by Barkovich & Kjos (1992) in 74 per cent of focal cortical dysplasia cases, and by Kuzniecky *et al.* (1996) in 87 per cent of bilateral perisylvian syndrome cases, while Vigevano *et al.* (1996) observed it in 93 per cent of cases with hemimegalencephaly.

Brain malformations represent an etiological factor of 3–4 per cent in all epilepsies, but this percentage increases to 18–20 per cent in drug-resistant epilepsies, which is probably due to the fact that malformed brain tissue is highly epileptogenic. Brain malformations can be diffuse, multifocal or focal. When focal brain malformations are the cause of drug-resistant epilepsies, a good outcome can be obtained with neurosurgery.

General characteristics of epilepsy due to NMDs

Considering the large variation in cortical development abnormalities, epilepsy pictures are not uniform, but some general characteristics can be identified:

(1) seizure onset occurs early, very often during the first year of life;

(2) seizures and epilepsy show varying aspects, but share rather constant characteristics depending on the type of malformation and the patient's age;

(3) resistance to drug therapy is frequent.

In a series of 71 children with cortical development abnormalities, Dalla Bernardina *et al.* (1996) reported seizure onset in the first year of life in 55 cases, of which twenty were in the first month of life.

On average, epilepsy onset occurs earlier in generalized or multifocal forms than in focal disorders. On the other hand, Vigevano *et al.* (1996) demonstrated that in hemimegalencephaly, the cases with most severe epilepsy have an earlier onset, generally in the first month of life.

Various types of seizures have been described in the literature: partial motor, spasm, tonic, tonic–clonic, atonic, absence, positive and negative myoclonus. Various forms of epilepsy have also been described: neonatal epileptic encephalopathy with suppression-bursts; partial epilepsy, infantile spasms; epilepsy with continuous partial seizures; Lennox-Gastaut syndrome, epilepsia partialis continua.

These different forms of seizures and epilepsy can appear alone, but occur more commonly in the same patient at different ages. A single patient may have early epileptic encephalopathy with suppression-bursts in the neonatal period, then infantile spasms at about 3–4 months, followed by predominant partial seizures or by Lennox–Gastaut syndrome.

Certain forms of epilepsy are found more constantly in specific malformations: for example, infantile spasms in lissencephaly (Aicardi, 1991) or Lennox–Gastaut syndrome in subcortical band heterotopia (Ricci *et al.*, 1992).

Epilepsia partialis continua has been described exclusively in association with focal dysplasias or hemimegalencephaly (Fusco *et al.*, 1992b; Desbiens *et al.*, 1993). It also seems to have a higher incidence in cases where dysplasia involves the rolandic region. A similar point can be made for negative myoclonus, which is usually associated with localized cortical dysplasia.

In malformative disorders, partial seizures and spasms are often observed in the first months of life and can be isolated or closely correlated. Partial seizures are sometimes followed by spasms or, on the contrary, can have onset immediately after a spasm (Vigevano *et al.*, 1994).

In the first months of life, the semiology of partial seizures is often very subtle, being limited to eye deviation, mouth movements, grimaces and variations in breathing, and for this reason it is sometimes difficult to distinguish normal movements from ictal manifestations. Considering the surgical prospective, such as cortical resection and hemispherectomy, as well as the varying severity of epilepsy in the different types of malformation, it is crucial to know the characteristics of cases resistant to drug therapy. Wyllie (1996) used the term 'catastrophic epilepsy' to define intractable epilepsy in cases with focal cortical dysplasia. These cases presented a very early onset of partial seizures and spasms. In a series of 14 patients with hemimegalencephaly, Vigevano *et al.*

(1996) showed that the cases with most severe epilepsy, and therefore potential surgical candidates, had partial seizures and spasms, with onset in the first three months of life, more frequently in the first days of life, as well as EEG characterized by unilateral hypsarrhythmia and severe cortical pachygyria. Resistance to treatment was determined within the first year of age.

In the past, EEG aspects were considered very relevant, but with progress in neuroimaging, their role has now been re-evaluated. Nevertheless, it is worth remembering how descriptions were made of particular interictal EEG patterns, characteristic of malformations such as rhythmic delta waves and fast activity in holoprosencephaly and unusual fast activity in lissencephaly (Dalla Bernardina et al., 1996), hemispheric suppression-bursts or hypsarrhythmia in hemimegalencephaly (Paladin et al., 1989) and focal rhytmic discharges in focal cortical dysplasia (Gambardella et al., 1996).

General considerations

Cortical development abnormalities cause cognitive delay, motor deficits and epilepsy. The severity of these symptoms can vary considerably from one type of malformation to another, but also within selected groups with the same type of malformation. For example, a sporadic case of hemimegalencephaly (Fusco et al., 1992a) with normal cognitive development has been reported. This means that the degree of neuropathological alteration can vary markedly from case to case, even with the same type of brain malformation. Yet it is certain that cortical development abnormalities very frequently provoke epileptiform EEG abnormalities and epilepsy.

Kuzniecky & Barkovich (1996) analyzed the hypotheses regarding the pathogenesis of epilepsy. Without going into detail on a topic covered in another part of this book, we mention briefly that epilepsy can derive from an abnormality in inhibiting mechanisms, such as a decrease in GABA-ergic interneuronic or R2 glutamate receptors, or else from aberrant excitatory pathways at the axonal and synaptic level. What is significant is that the ability to provoke epilepsy, and especially resistant epilepsy, is not the same for all malformations.

Paglioli-Neto et al. (1996) compared a series of 18 patients with polymicrogyria with a series of 62 patients with focal dysplasia: seizure control was achieved in 50 per cent of patients in the first group and in only nine per cent of the second group. Status epilepticus was observed in one-third of the patients with focal dysplasia and in none of those with polymicrogyria.

The patient series of Palmini et al. (1996) also confirmed that focal cortical dysplasias with balloon cells are frequently the cause of resistant, severe epilepsies, and epilepsia partialis continua is found almost exclusively in this type of malformation.

Some studies (Mattia et al., 1995) have shown that the administration of the convulsant drug 4-aminopyridine induced spontaneous seizure-like discharges in slices of human dysplastic neocortex obtained from patients during neurosurgical procedures. By contrast, neocortical slices obtained from patients suffering from temporal lobe epilepsy with Ammon's horn sclerosis did not generate any epileptiform activity during administration of 4-aminopyridine. This study demonstrated the intrinsic epileptogenicity that characterizes the dysplastic cortex.

The extreme epileptogenicity of dysplastic lesions has been confirmed by neurophysiological studies. Gambardella et al. (1996) studied the scalp EEGs of 74 patients with intractable partial epilepsy. Rhythmic epileptiform discharges (REDs) were present in 15 (44 per cent) of the 34 patients with focal cortical dysplastic lesions and in none of the 40 patients with non-dysplastic structural lesions. An ECOG study evidenced the presence of continuous epileptiform discharges (CEDs) in a high percentage of patients with focal cortical dysplasia, with a strong relationship (80 per cent) between REDs and CEDs.

These studies provide several reasons for the exceptional epileptogenicity of these lesions and especially for the high frequency of intractability.

References

Aicardi, J. (1991): The agyria–pachygyria complex: a spectrum of cortical malformation. *Brain. Dev.* **13**, 1–8.

Barkovich, A.J. & Kjos, B.O. (1992): Nonlissencephalic cortical dysplasias: correlations of imaging findings with clinical deficits. *AJNR* **113**, 95–103.

Barkovich, A.J., Kuzniecky, R.I., Dobyns, W.B., Jackson, G.D., Becker, L.E. & Evrard, P. (1996): A classification scheme for malformations of cortical development. *Neuropediatrics* **27**, 59–63.

Dalla Bernardina, B., Pérez-Jiménez, A., Fontana, E., Colamaria, V., Piardi, F., Avesani, E., Santorum, E., Grimau-Merino, R. & Tassinari, C.A. (1996): Electroencephalographic findings associated with cortical dysplasias. In: *Dysplasias of cerebral cortex and epilepsy*. eds. R. Guerrini, F. Andermann, R. Canapicchi, J. Roger, B.G. Zifkin & P. Pfanner, pp. 235–245. Philadelphia: Lippincott-Raven Publishers.

Desbiens, R., Berkovic, S.F., Dubeau, F., Andermann, F., Laxer, K.D., Harvey, S., Leproux, F., Melanson, D., Robitaille, Y., Kalnins, R., Olivier, A., Fabinyi, G. & Barbaro, N.M. (1993): Life-threatening focal status epilepticus due to occult cortical dysplasia. *Arch. Neurol.* **50**, 695–700.

Fusco, L., Ferracuti, S., Fariello, G., Manfredi, M. & Vigevano, F. (1992): Hemimegalencephaly and normal intellectual development. *J. Neurol. Neurosurg. Psychiatry* **55**, 720–722.

Fusco, L., Bertini, E. & Vigevano, F. (1992): Epilepsia partialis continua and neuronal migration anomalies. *Brain Dev.* **14**, 323–328.

Gambardella, A., Palmini, A., Andermann, F., Dubeau, F., Da Costa, J.C., Quesney, L.F., Andermann, E. & Olivier, A. (1996): Usefulness of focal rhythmic discharges on scalp EEG of patients with focal cortical dysplasia and intractable epilepsy. *Electroenceph. Clin. Neurophysiol.* **98**, 243–249.

Kuzniecky, R., Andermann, F., Guerrini, R. & CBPS Multicenter Collaborative Study (1996): The congenital bilateral perisylvian syndrome. In: *Dysplasias of cerebral cortex and epilepsy*. eds. R. Guerrini, F. Andermann, R. Canapicchi, J. Roger, B. G. Zifkin, & P. Pfanner, pp. 271–277. Philadelphia: Lippincott-Raven Publishers.

Kuzniecky, R.I. & Barkovich, A.J. (1996): Pathogenesis and pathology of focal malformations of cortical development and epilepsy. *J. Clin. Neurophysiol.* **13**, 468–480.

Mattia, D., Olivier, A. & Avoli, M. (1995): Seizure-like discharges recorded in human dysplastic neocortex maintained in vitro. *Neurology* **45**, 1391–1395.

Paglioli-Neto, E., Palmini, A., Costa da Costa, J., Andermann, F., Dubeau, F., Gambardella, A., Paglioli, E., Olivier, A., Kim, H.I. & Chung, C.O. (1996): Histopathological pattern and putative pathogenetic mechanisms determine the degree of epileptogenicity in localized cortical dysplastic lesions. *Epilepsia* **37 (5)**, S142.

Paladin, F., Chiron, C., Dulac, O., Plouin, P. & Ponsot, G. (1989): Electroencephalographic aspects of hemimegalencephaly. *Dev. Med. Child Neurol.* **31**, 377–383.

Palmini, A., Costa da Costa, J., Andermann, F., Neto, P.R., Portuguez, M., Garcias-da Silva, L.F., Paglioli, E., Paglioli-Neto, E., Aesse, F. & Raupp, S. (1992): Focal electrographic ictal activity during acute cortical recording over dysplastic lesions in humans. *Epilepsia* **33 (3)**, S75.

Palmini, A., Gambardella, A., Andermann, F., Dubeau, F., Costa da Costa, J., Olivier, A., Tampieri, D., Gloor, P., Quesney, F., Andermann, E., Paglioli, E., Paglioli-Neto, E., Portuguez, M., Coutinho, L., Raupp, S., Leblanc, R. & Kim, H.I. (1996): The human dysplastic cortex is intrinsically epileptogenic. In: *Dysplasias of cerebral cortex and Epilepsy*. eds. R. Guerrini, F. Andermann, R. Canapicchi, J. Roger, B. G. Zifkin, & P. Pfanner, pp. 43–52. Philadelphia: Lippincott-Raven Publishers.

Ricci, S., Cusmai, R., Fariello, G., Fusco, L. & Vigevano, F. (1992): Double cortex a neuronal migration anomaly as a possible cause of Lennox-Gastaut syndrome. *Arch. Neurol.* **49**, 61–64.

Vigevano, F., Fusco, L., Ricci, S., Granata, T. & Viani, F. (1994): Dysplasias. In: *Infantile spasms and West syndrome*. eds. O. Dulac, H.T. Chugani, & B. Dalla Bernardina, pp. 178–191. London: WB Saunders Company Ltd.

Vigevano, F., Fusco, L., Granata, T., Fariello, G., Di Rocco, C. & Cusmai, R. (1996): Hemimegalencephaly: clinical and EEG characteristics. In: *Dysplasias of cerebral cortex and epilepsy*. eds. R. Guerrini, F. Andermann, R. Canapicchi, J. Roger, B. G. Zifkin, & P. Pfanner, pp. 285–294. Philadelphia: Lippincott-Raven Publishers.

Wyllie, E. (1996): Surgery for catastrophic localization-related epilepsy in infants. *Epilepsia* **37 (1)**, S22–S25.

Chapter 15

Schizencephaly: clinical and genetic findings in a case series

Tiziana Granata[1], Ludovico D'Incerti[2], Elena Freri[1], Silvana Franceschetti[3], Giuliano Avanzini[3], Antonio Faiella[4], Carlo Lenti[5] and Giorgio Battaglia[3]

[1] *Divisione di Neuropsichiatria Infantile*, [2] *Divisione di Neuroradiologia*,
[3] *Divisione di Neurofisiologia Sperimentale ed Epilettologia*,
Istituto Nazionale Neurologico,'C. Besta', Via Celoria 11, 20133 Milan, Italy,
[4] *DIBIT, Istituto Scientifico Ospedale S. Raffaele, Milan, Italy*,
[5] *Istituto di Neuropsichiatria Infantile, Università di Milano, Ospedale San Paolo, Milan, Italy*

Summary

We report neuroradiological, clinical and genetic findings in a series of 14 patients with schizencephaly. The extent of the anatomic malformation correlated closely with the severity of motor and mental impairment but not with the presence or severity of epilepsy. Patients with a unilateral closed or small open cleft had mild motor deficits, contralateral to the cleft, normal mental abilities, and focal epilepsy often resistant to the antiepileptic treatment. The epilepsy features were homogeneous in terms of age of onset, seizure characteristics and lack of secondary generalization. In contrast, patients with bilateral schizencephalies, which were always associated with extended brain malformations, had severe neurological deficits, but only rarely epilepsy, which when present was completely controlled by medication. The presence of heterozygous sequence abnormalities of the homeobox gene EMX2 in half the patients analysed, including two siblings, supports the relevance of this gene in the etiopathogenesis of at least some schizencephaly patients.

Introduction

Schizencephalies are congenital brain abnormalities characterized by the presence of a gray matter-lined cleft, spanning the cerebral hemisphere from the pial surface to the lateral ventricle. Following the original description by Yakovlev & Wadsworth (1946a, b), two types of schizencephaly are recognized: closed lip (type I) in which the walls of the cleft are in contact with each other, and open lip (type II) in which the lips are separated and the cleft is filled with cerebrospinal fluid.

Once thought to be an extremely rare disorder, schizencephaly has been increasingly recognized as a cause of neurological deficits and epilepsy since the advent of CT and MRI. More than a hundred cases have accumulated in recent literature, thus allowing delineation of anatomical features in relation to clinical characteristics (Miller *et al.*, 1984; Barkovich & Kjos, 1992; Granata *et al.*, 1996a; Packard *et al.*, 1997). Schizencephaly may be unilateral or bilateral, isolated, associated with other brain abnormalities, or part of more complex malformations also involving extracerebral structures. The main clinical manifestations are various degrees of motor deficit and mental retardation, as well as epileptic seizures (Granata *et al.*, 1996b).

The etiopathogenesis of schizencephaly is not fully understood. The most widely held theory is that schizencephaly results from an ischemic injury to the developing cortex during early postmigrational stages (Barth, 1987; Barkovich & Kjos, 1992). On the other hand, reports of some familial cases (Hosley *et al.*, 1992; Hilburger *et al.*, 1993; Haverkamp *et al.*, 1995; Muntaner *et al.*, 1997) and the recent finding of germ line mutations of the homeobox gene EMX2 in schizencephalic patients (Brunelli *et al.*, 1996; Faiella *et al.*, 1997; Granata *et al.*, 1997) raise the possibility that genetic factors are involved in the pathogenesis of this brain malformation.

In the present study we describe a series of 14 paediatric and adult patients with schizencephaly. Our aims were to clarify: (1) the relationship between morphological aspects of the malformation and clinical outcome; (2) the features and outcome of the associated epilepsy; and (3) the role of genetic vs. acquired factors in determining this brain malformation.

Patients and methods

The series consisted of six females and eight males, aged nine months to 68 years, referred to our Institute for the management of seizures, as well as motor and mental deficits, in whom schizencephaly was identified and assessed by MRI. The histories were reviewed with particular attention to family history, the presence of risk factors for brain malformations and epilepsy, and motor, mental and speech development. In the epileptic patients, epileptic histories and age and modality of seizure onset were carefully reviewed. The electroclinical features, clinical course and response to the antiepileptic treatment were followed prospectively. All patients underwent neurological evaluation, standardized psychometric tests (Wechsler Intelligence Scale or Griffith's Developmental Scale, according to age) and EEG recordings when awake and during slow sleep.

MR images were obtained with a 0.5 or 1.5 Tesla machine. Axial and coronal proton density and T2-weighted images (w.i.), and sagittal and coronal T1-w.i. were obtained in all cases. The patients were classified as having closed lip schizencephaly when an area of heterotopic gray-matter extended from the cerebral surface to the lateral ventricle, with a more or less evident infolding of the cortical surface and dimpling of the ventricular wall. Open lip schizencephaly was diagnosed when cerebrospinal fluid could be seen between the gray matter-lined walls throughout the entire length of the cleft (Byrd *et al.*, 1989; Barkovich & Kjos, 1992). Open lip clefts were small, medium, or large, according to the extent of lobar involvement as proposed by Barkovich & Kjos (1992). In each patient, we sought to relate clinical findings and epilepsy characteristics to side, location, extent and type of schizencephaly, as well as to any associated brain malformations.

Mutations in the EMX2 homeobox gene were investigated in 12 patients by single strand conformation polymorphism (SSCP) analysis of polymerase chain reaction products obtained by amplification of genomic DNA. Sequencing of the amplified fragments with altered migration was subsequently performed (Faiella *et al.*, 1997).

Results

Patients 1–9 had unilateral schizencephaly, and patients 10–14 had bilateral schizencephaly. Clinical, neuroradiological and genetic data for these two groups are reported in Table 1.

Table 1. Neuroradiological, clinical and genetic findings in patients with schizencephaly.

Case No.	Sex	Age (yrs)	Location and type of schizencephaly	Associated abnormalities	Neurological examination	Mental retardation	Epilepsy age at onset	EMX2 mutation
Unilateral schizencephaly								
1	M	30	L Parietal, closed lip	—	Mild right hemiparesis	—	Yes (21 years)	N.P.
2	F	27	L Temporo-occipital, closed lip	—	Mild right hemiparesis	—	Yes (17 yrs)	None
3	M	68	R Fronto-parietal, closed lip	Small right periventricular heterotopic nodules	Mild left hemiparesis	—	Yes (11 yrs)	i2, Single base deletion
4	M	17	L Parietal, closed lip	Arachnoid cyst in right middle cranial fossa	Mild right hemiparesis	—	Yes (11 yrs)	i2, Single base substitution
5	F	5	L Temporal, closed lip	L Parieto-occipital gray matter heterotopia	Right hemiparesis	—	Yes (18 mths)	e2, Synonymous substitution in the homeobox
6	F	22	L Frontal, small, open lip	—	Mild right hemiparesis	—	Yes (12 mths)	None
7	F	42	L Frontal, small, open lip	—	Right hemiparesis	±	No (I.Q.=89)	N.P.
8	F	32	L Rolandic, small, open lip	Small right rolandic polymicrogyria	Mild right hemiparesis	—	Yes (12 yrs)	None
9	F	9 m	L Parieto-occipital, large, open lip	ACC, ASP, Bilateral PNH, cerebellar dysplasia	Hypotonic syndrome Motor delay	++ (m.a. 6 m)	No	None
Bilateral schizencephaly								
10	M	5	Bilateral parietal, closed lip	Bilateral fronto-parietal dysplasia, ventricular enlargement	Right hemiparesis orofacial dyspraxia	+ (m.a. 3y 6m)	No	None
11	M	22	Bilateral fronto and parietal, closed lip	Large right parietal dysplasia, partial ACC	Left hemiparesis	++ (IQ = 58)	Yes (10 yrs)	None
12	M	8	L Fronto medium open lip R Frontal, closed lip	Bilateral frontal pachygyria, ASP	Spastic diplegia	+ (m.a. 6y 6m)	No (F.C. 22 mths)	e2, synonymous substitution in the homeobox
13*	M	8	Bilateral fronto-parietal, large closed lip	Partial ACC, ASP	Spastic tetraparesis	—	No	e2, deleterious point mutation 3' splice site
14*	M	10	Bilateral fronto-parietal, large open lip	Frontal lobe agenesis	Spastic tetraparesis	+++ (no test administrable)	No	e2, deleterious point mutation 3' splice site

* Patients 13 and 14 were siblings.
L = left; R = right; N.P = not performed; I.Q. = intelligence quotient; m.a. = mental age; ACC = agenesis of corpus callosum; ASP = agenesis of septum pellucidum; PNH = periventricular nodular heterotopia; F.C. = febrile convulsion

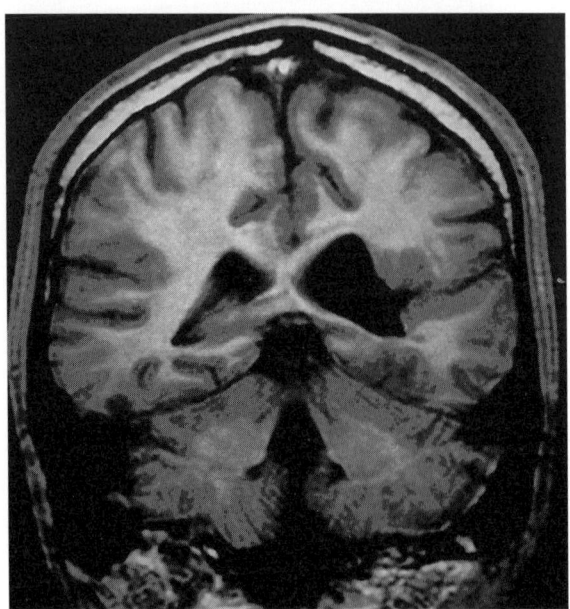

Fig. 1. Patient 1. Closed lip schizencephaly is present in the left posterior temporal region. Dimpling of the lateral ventricle and cortical dysplasia are evident along the margins of the cleft.

Unilateral schizencephaly

(Patients 1–9, Table 1.)

A family history of epilepsy was uncovered in patient 4, whose father suffered idiopathic partial epilepsy during childhood, and in patient 9 whose maternal grandfather had convulsive seizures as an adult. Patient 8 was an adopted child. For patients 3 and 4 modest vaginal bleeding was reported during the first trimester of each mother's pregnancy. In no case was maternal exposition to drugs, environmental toxins or viruses reported. The clefts were closed in five patients, small open in three, and large open in one. In four patients schizencephaly was the only brain abnormality (Fig. 1). In four other cases the cleft was associated with small circumscribed brain malformations that did not alter the general architecture of the brain; these associated malformations were in close anatomical association with the cleft in two cases, and contralateral to the cleft in two others. In patient 8 a small area of cortical dysplasia was located in the contralateral hemisphere at the same level as cleft. In the remaining case (patient 9), a large open lip schizencephaly was part of a complex malformation characterized by nodular bilateral periventricular heterotopia, agenesis of the corpus callosum and septum pellucidum, and dysplasia of the cerebellar cortex.

In the eight patients with closed lip or small open lip cleft, there were varying degrees of motor deficit on the side contralateral to the cleft but mental abilities were always within the normal range. Patient 9 with the large open lip cleft was more severely compromised, showing hypotonic–hyperreflexic syndrome and psychomotor delay. Her general developmental quotient as evaluated by Griffith's Scale was 67, indicative of a mental age of six months (at nine months).

Epilepsy was present in seven of the nine patients, with first decade onset in two cases and second decade onset in five (mean age 10.5 ± 6.9 years). In patients 3 and 4 convulsions during hyperthermia preceded epilepsy onset. Seizures were focal (elementary motor or complex) and not followed by secondary generalization – except in patient 1 who had only sporadic convulsive seizures during sleep, and patient 4 who had two convulsions during sleep before the initiation of treatment. Elementary motor fits had a postural onset followed by eye and head version; the side of these symptoms was consistent with the side of the schizencephaly. The focal complex seizures were characterized by loss of contact and simple motor automatisms.

In most patients the seizure rate was one per month or less, but patient 6 had a much higher seizure rate. In no case did the seizure rate worsen during the course of the disease. Epilepsy was completely controlled by drugs in three cases (patients 1, 4 and 5), in one of whom treatment is currently being withdrawn. In the other four cases seizures are refractory to AED treatment.

Interictal EEG recordings in the patients with partial seizures showed normal background activity and normal organization of sleep pattern, with the presence of focal epileptic abnormalities

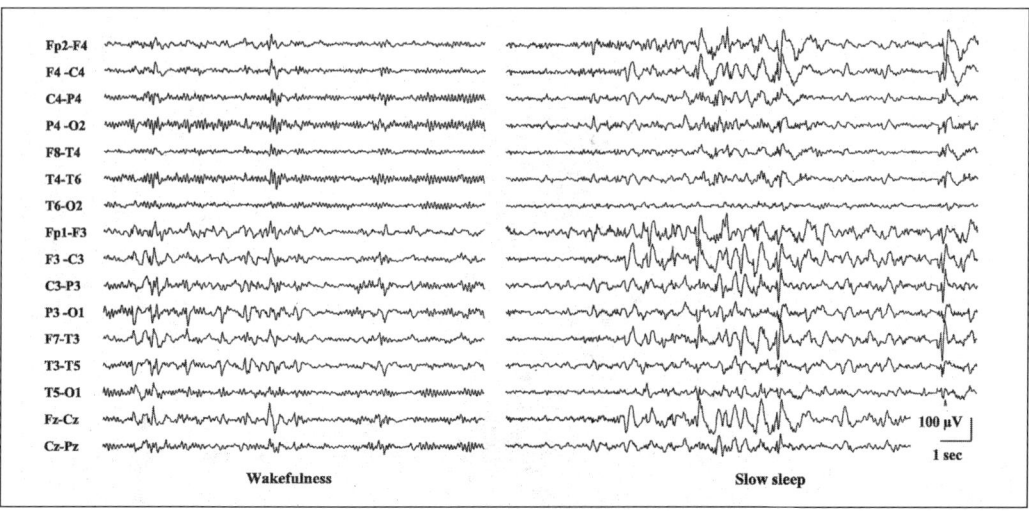

Fig. 2. Patient 8. This EEG recording shows interictal discharges of irregular sharp waves in the left hemisphere, more evident in the left fronto-central and temporal leads. This activity increases and diffuses during slow sleep.

consistent with the clinical ictal symptoms and cleft location (Fig. 2). No interictal epileptic abnormalities were recorded in patients without epilepsy. However in patient 9 bilateral fast activity, more evident and extensive during slow sleep, was consistently recorded.

Mutations in EMX2 gene were found in three of the seven patients analysed. Two carried a point mutation on the second intron (in patient 3 a single base pair was deleted; in patient 4 adenine substituted cytosine). In patient 5 there was a cytosine to adenine substitution in the homeobox which left the amino acid unaffected (arginine residue at position 3 of the homeodomain).

Bilateral schizencephaly

(Patients 10–14, Table 1).

Patients 13 and 14 were siblings, born to non-consanguineous parents. Patient 12 was an adopted child. All patients were born at term. Pregnancy was complicated by modest vaginal bleeding in the first trimester in patient 14, and by threatened miscarriage at the 26th week in patient 10. In no case was maternal exposure to drugs, environmental toxins or viruses reported.

The clefts always involved frontal or parietal lobes and in all cases large and complex brain malformations were also present resulting in severe alteration of general brain structure (Fig. 3). In patient 10 white matter abnormalities, suggesting periventricular leukomalacia, were also present.

Motor and mental deficits were present in all cases. The clinical picture ranged from spastic hemiparesis and mental retardation of medium degree in patients with close lip clefts, to spastic tetraparesis, severe mental retardation and absence of language in the patients with large open clefts.

One patient only (patient 11), now aged 22, had epilepsy. Three tonic/clonic seizures during sleep occurred at age 10; these were readily controlled by carbamazepine which was successfully withdrawn two years before. EEG recordings were always characterized by mildly impaired background activity but no evidence of epileptic abnormalities. Patient 12, now aged eight, had an isolated convulsion during hyperthermia at age 22 months; serial EEGs recorded between age two and eight were characterized by bilateral frontal discharges of sharp and slow-wave complexes, which

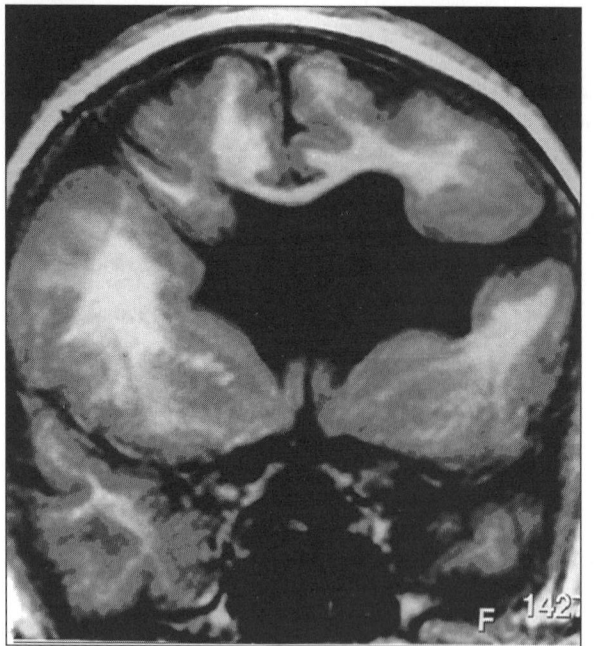

Fig. 3. Patient 12. Bilateral schizencephaly. Coronal T1 w.i. demonstrates left open lip and right closed lip schizencephaly. Agenesis of the septum pellucidum is also evident.

increased markedly during slow sleep. Right temporo-parieto-occipital spike and wave complexes, enhanced during slow sleep, were also consistently recorded in patient 10 (Fig. 4). In the two siblings (patients 13 and 14) with large bilateral schizencephaly, EEGs were characterized by severe bilateral impairment of background activity with no evidence of epileptic discharges.

Mutations in EMX2 were found in three of the five patients analysed, always affecting the second exon of the gene. Patient 12 carried an adenine to guanine substitution in the homeobox, but this was a synonymous mutation that left the arginine at position five of the homeodomain unchanged. The two siblings with large bilateral schizencephaly (patients 13 and 14) carried an identical mutation of the EMX2 gene, a guanine to thymidine substitution in the first position of the second exon, changing the amino acid from glycine to valine (Granata et al., 1997).

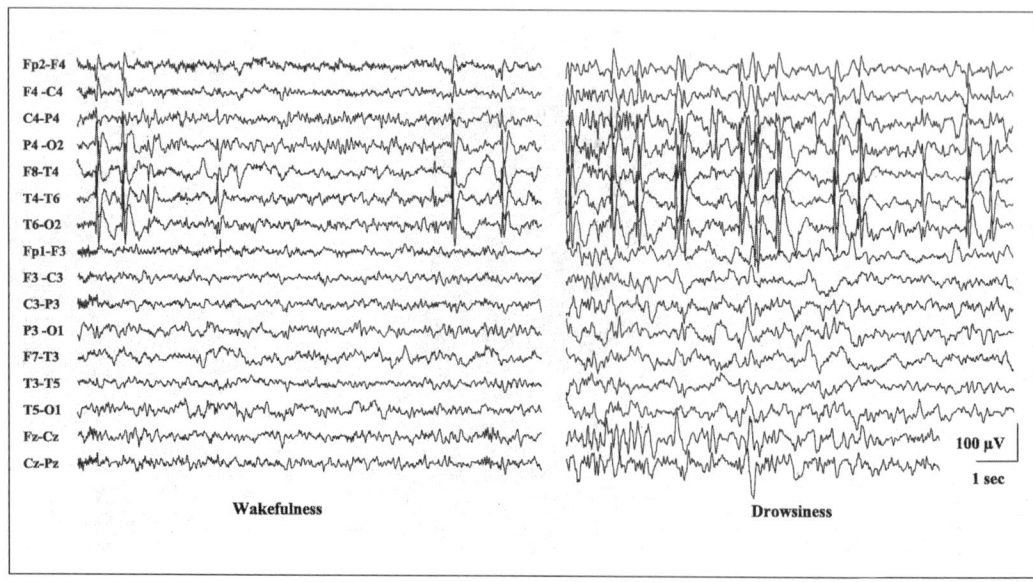

Fig. 4. Patient 10. This EEG recording shows interictal discharges of spikes and slow waves in the right parieto-occipital and temporal leads; slow activity is also evident, particularly on the temporal region. During drowsiness, the epileptic activity increases and diffuses, and is followed by signal attenuation mainly in the temporal region.

Discussion

Relation between neuroradiological findings and clinical outcome

Our findings confirm the broad spectrum of anatomical presentation of schizencephaly, as revealed by MRI, and also indicate that the severity of the malformations relates to the severity of neurological deficits (Barkovich & Kjos, 1992; Packard *et al.*, 1997). Thus, worse clinical compromise was observed in patients with large bilateral open lip cleft, and milder compromise was present in patients with unilateral closed or small open cleft. Our findings also suggest that the extent and complexity of the associated brain malformations are important in determining the overall clinical picture. This is exemplified by the favourable clinical outcome in patient 8, who had a small area of cortical dysplasia symmetrical and contralateral to a small open lip cleft, in contrast to the poor outcome in patient 9 in whom unilateral open lip schizencephaly was associated with widespread disorder of cortical development and involvement of the cerebellar cortex.

Epilepsy in schizencephaly

Epilepsy was present in 57 per cent of our patients and was well-controlled by treatment in half. Both these findings are consistent with more recent literature data (Barkovich & Kjos, 1992; Packard *et al.*, 1997). The relatively low incidence of drug-resistant epilepsy in schizencephaly is surprising in comparison to that associated with other structural brain abnormalities such as focal cortical dysplasia, which are usually associated with intractable and malignant focal seizures, often requiring surgery. This may be due to the absence, in schizencephalies, of the major cytological neuronal abnormalities observed in other types of cortical dysgenesis (Taylor *et al.*, 1971; Battaglia *et al.*, 1996; Spreafico *et al.*, 1998).

Our findings differ from those of other published results with regard to presence and severity of epilepsy in unilaterally versus bilaterally affected patients. Both Barkovich & Kjos (1992) and Packard *et al.* (1997) reported a higher incidence of epilepsy, with earlier onset and poorer prognosis in patients with bilateral schizencephaly than in those with unilateral clefts. In our series only one patient with bilateral schizencephaly had seizures, and these were sporadic and completely controlled by AEDs. Although some of our patients are young and may yet develop epilepsy, this discrepancy is not easy to explain. It may be speculated that the wide extent of brain damage in our bilaterally affected patients, coupled with agenesis of the corpus callosum, could have prevented the onset or diffusion of the hyperexcitability phenomena that eventually lead to the clinical appearance of seizures. In fact, the high incidence of interictal abnormalities in some of our bilaterally affected patients probably indicates the presence of neuronal hyperexcitability, which would not be sufficient for a clinical expression.

The electroclinical pictures of our epileptic patients shared some common features: usually late childhood or adolescent onset; postural and versive symptomatology, or loss of contact followed by simple motor automatisms; and lack of secondary generalization. The lack of generalization might be the consequence of anatomical rearrangement, provoked by presence of the cleft, of the cortico-cortical or cortico-subcortical pathways linking the two hemispheres, which could prevent the bilateral diffusion of epileptic discharges.

Genetic versus acquired factors in determining schizencephaly

The etiopathogenesis of schizencephaly and the precise timing of its occurrence are still unclear. Yakovlev & Wadsworth's original conjecture (1946a, b), that schizencephaly is a true malformation resulting from a primary disturbance in embryonic development, has been challenged by data suggesting a secondary compromise of development owing to the clastic effect of endogenous or exogenous factors acting prenatally (Barth, 1987; Barkovich & Kjos, 1992).

Our findings of EMX2 gene mutations in 6 out of 12 analysed patients support the first hypothesis. Like other genes coding for transcription factors, EMX2 is a regulatory gene. Its mouse analog, emx2, is specifically expressed in the proliferating cells of the ventricular zone during early ontogenesis and plays an important role in the structural patterning of the developing forebrain (Gulisano *et al.*, 1996). The point mutation in the second exon of the gene in the two siblings with large bilateral schizencephaly produces a splicing defect in the transcript, probably resulting in loss of function of the protein (Faiella *et al.*, 1997). In the remaining four sporadic cases with *de novo* EMX2 mutations, the sequence alterations could not be clearly associated with either loss of function or gain of abnormal function. However, it is worth noting that similar mutations have been detected in other schizencephaly patients (Brunelli *et al.*, 1996), but were absent in more than 1500 control individuals (Faiella *et al.*, 1997). Taken together, these data strongly indicate that the EMX2 gene plays a role in the pathogenesis of at least some schizencephaly cases.

However, the genetic hypothesis does not rule out the possibility of alternative etiopathogenetic mechanisms. *In utero* exposure to toxic agents including cocaine and other drugs (Dominguez *et al.*, 1991; Pati & Helmbrecht, 1994), prenatal CMV infections (Iannetti *et al.*, 1998), and vascular accidents (Kuijpers *et al.*, 1994; Landrieu & Lacroix, 1994; Suchet *et al.*, 1994) have been convincingly reported as causally related to schizencephaly, the common pathogenetic mechanism being an ischemic damage in the early postmigrational period. The vaginal bleeding reported for three of our patients, and the presence of MRI signs of periventricular leukomalacia in another case may be circumstantial evidence in support of this hypothesis. It is likely therefore that schizencephaly is caused by a variety of etiologic factors that impair mechanisms governing neuronal migration and cortical organization. The type, extent, and severity of the malformation and the resulting clinical pictures, may be related to complex pathogenetic processes involving genetic determinants, gene-environment interactions, and the timing of a causative pathologic event.

Acknowledgement

Supported by grant ICS 030.3/RF95/223 from the Italian Ministry of Health and by the Mariani Foundation for Paediatric Neurology, Milan.

References

Barkovich, A.J. & Kjos, B.O. (1992): Schizencephaly: correlation of clinical findings with MR characteristics. *Am. J. Neuroradiol.* **13**, 85–94.

Barth, P.G. (1987): Disorders of neuronal migration. *Can. J. Neurol. Sci.* **14**, 1–16.

Battaglia, G., Arcelli, P., Granata, T., Tampieri, D., Olivier, A., Avoli, M., Avanzini, G. & Spreafico, R. (1996): Neuronal migration disorders (NMDs) and epilepsy: a morphological analysis of three surgically treated patients. *Epilepsy Res.* **26**, 49–58.

Brunelli, S., Faiella, A., Capra, V., Nigro, V., Simeone, A., Cama, A. & Boncinelli, E. (1996): Germline mutations in the homeobox gene EMX2 in patients with severe schizencephaly. *Nature Genet.* **12**, 94–96.

Byrd, S.E., Osborn, R.E., Bohan, T.P. & Naidich, T.P. (1989): The CT and MR evaluation of migrational disorders of the brain. Part II. Schizencephaly, heterotopia and polymicrogyria. *Pediatr. Radiol.* **19**, 219–222.

Dominguez, R., Aguirre Vila-Coro, A., Slopis, J.M. & Bohan, T.P. (1991): Brain and ocular abnormalities in infants with in utero exposure to cocaine and other street drugs. *Am. J. Dis. Child.* **145**, 688–695.

Faiella, A., Brunelli, S., Granata, T., D'Incerti, L., Cardini, R., Lenti, C., Battaglia, G. & Boncinelli, E. (1997): A number of schizencephaly patients including two brothers are heterozygous for germline mutations in the homeobox gene EMX2. *Eur. J. Hum. Genet.* **5**, 186–190.

Granata, T., Battaglia, G., D'Incerti, L., Franceschetti, S., Spreafico, R., Battino, D., Savoiardo, M. & Avanzini, G. (1996a): Schizencephaly: neuroradiologic and epileptologic findings. *Epilepsia* **37**, 1185–1193.

Granata, T., Battaglia, G., D'Incerti, L., Franceschetti, S., Spreafico, R., Savoiardo, M. & Avanzini, G. (1996b): Schizencephaly: clinical findings. In: *Dysplasias of cerebral cortex and epilepsy*, eds. R. Guerrini, F. Andermann, R. Canapicchi, J. Roger & P. Pfanner, pp. 407–415, Philadelphia: Lippincott-Raven Publishers.

Granata, T., Farina, L., Faiella, A., Cardini, R., D'Incerti, L., Boncinelli, E. & Battaglia, G. (1997): Familial schizencephaly associated with EMX2 mutation. *Neurology* **48**, 1403–1406.

Gulisano, M., Broccoli, V., Pardini, C. & Boncinelli, E. (1996): Emx1 and Emx2 show different patterns of expression during proliferation and differentiation of the developing cerebral cortex in the mouse. *Eur. J. Neurosci.* **8**, 1037–1050.

Haverkamp, F., Zerres, K., Ostertun, B., Emons, D. & Lentze, M.J. (1995): Familial schizencephaly: further delineation of a rare disorder. *J. Med. Genet.* **32**, 242–244.

Hilburger, A.C., Willis, J.K., Bouldin, E. & Henderson-Tilton, A. (1993): Familial schizencephaly. *Brain. Dev.* **15**, 234–236.

Hosley, M.A., Abrams, I.F. & Ragland, R.L. (1992): Schizencephaly: case report of familial incidence. *Pediatr. Neurol.* **8**, 148–150.

Iannetti, P., Nigro, G., Spalice, A., Faiella, A. & Boncinelli, E. (1998): Cytomegalovirus infection and schizencephaly: case reports. *Ann. Neurol.* **43**, 123–127.

Kuijpers, R.W., Van den Ankers, J.N., Baerts, W. & von dem Borne, A.E. (1994): A case of severe neonatal thrombocytopenia with schizencephaly associated with anti-HPA-1b and anti-HPA-2a. *Br. J. Haematol.* **87**, 576–579.

Landrieu, P.& La Croix, C. (1994): Schizencephaly, consequence of a developmental vasculopathy? *Clin. Neuropathol.* **13**, 192–196.

Miller, G., Stears, J.C., Guggenheim, M.A. & Wilkening, G.N. (1984): Schizencephaly: a clinical and CT study. *Neurology* **34**, 997–1001.

Muntaner, L., Pérez-Ferròn, J.J., Herrera, M., Rosell, J., Taboada, D. & Climent, S. (1997): MRI of a family with focal abnormalities of gyration. *Neuroradiology* **39**, 605–608.

Packard, A.M., Miller, V.S. & Delgado, M.R.(1997): Schizencephaly: correlations of clinical and radiologic features. *Neurology* **48**, 1427–1434.

Pati, A. & Helmbrecht, G.D. (1994): Congenital schizencephaly associated with in utero warfarin exposure. *Reprod. Toxicol.* **8**, 115–120.

Spreafico, R., Battaglia, G., Arcelli, P., Andermann, F., Dubeau, F., Palmini, A., Olivier, A., Villemure, J.G., Tampieri, D., Avanzini, G. & Avoli, M. (1998): Cortical dysplasia. An immunocytochemical study of three patients. *Neurology* **50**, 27–36.

Suchet, I.B. (1994): Schizencephaly: antenatal and postnatal assessment with colour-flow Doppler imaging. *Can. Assoc. Radiol. J.* **45**, 193–200.

Taylor, D.C., Falconer, M.A., Bruton, C.J. & Corsellis, J.A.N. (1971): Focal dysplasia of the cerebral cortex in epilepsy. *J. Neurol. Neurosurg. Psychiatry* **34**, 369–387.

Yakovlev, P. & Wadsworth, R.C. (1946a): Schizencephalies. A study of the congenital clefts in the cerebral mantle. I. Clefts with fused lips. *J. Neuropath. Exp. Neurol.* **5**, 116–130.

Yakovlev, P. & Wadsworth, R.C.(1946b): Schizencephalies. A study of the congenital clefts in the cerebral mantle. II. Clefts with hydrocephalus and lips separated. *J. Neuropath. Exp. Neurol.* **5**, 169–206.

Chapter 16

Polymicrogyria and epilepsy

Renzo Guerrini

Divisione di Neuropsichiatria Infantile, IRCCS Fondazione Stella Maris, Università di Pisa,
Via dei Giacinti 2, 56018 Calambrone, Pisa, Italy

Introduction

The term polymicrogyria indicates an excessive number of small and prominent convolutions spaced out by shallow and enlarged sulci, giving the cortical surface a lumpy aspect. Both on direct brain inspection and MRI, it may be impossible to recognize polymicrogyria or to distinguish it from pachygyria, since the microconvolutions are packed and merged (Friede, 1989). However, when the malformation is conspicuous, it usually determines alterations of the gyral pattern that are macroscopically recognizable (Barkovich, 1996; Raybaud et al., 1996).

According to microscopic findings, two types of polymicrogyria are recognized. In *unlayered* polymicrogyria, the external molecular layer is continuous and does not follow the profile of the convolutions, and the underlying neurones have radial (or vertical) distribution but no laminar organization (Ferrer, 1984; Ferrer et al., 1986). Unlayered polymicrogyria is found in the border of schizencephalic clefts or in the cortex of Aicardi syndrome. It may be focal (Galaburda et al., 1985; Becker et al., 1989), multilobar, or diffuse (Billette de Villemeur et al., 1992) and is thought either to result from early exogenous insults (13 to 18th week of gestation) (Ferrer & Català, 1991) or to be genetically determined (Billette de Villemeur et al., 1992). In *four-layered* polymicrogyria, there are two neuronal layers under the molecular layer, separated by an intermediate layer with many fibres and few cells (Harding, 1992). Four-layered polymicrogyria is often responsible for localized cortical abnormalities. Its extent is extremely variable and the abnormal cortex may border abruptly on the normal cortex. Four-layered polymicrogyria is believed to result from a perfusion failure limited to one or more arterial vascular beds, occurring between the 20th and 24th weeks of gestation. This would lead to intracortical laminar necrosis with delayed damage of the distal section of glial radial fibres, with consequent late migration disorder and post-migratory overturning of cortical organization (Evrard et al., 1989). Damage to intermediate cortical layers would then produce a difference in growth rate between outer and inner cortical layers, with consequent excessive folding of the cortical surface (Richman et al., 1974). In this disorder, horizontal neuronal lamination is usually spared (Robain, 1996).

The spectrum of clinical manifestations that have been associated with polymicrogyria is very broad, and includes children presenting severe encephalopathies with spastic quadriparesis, profound mental retardation and intractable epilepsy, or normal individuals with selective impairment of higher-order neurological functions (Galaburda *et al.*, 1985; Cohen *et al.*, 1989). Here we will examine the main anatomoclinical syndromes resulting from polymicrogyria.

Aicardi syndrome

Aicardi syndrome (Aicardi *et al.*, 1965, 1969) is exclusively observed in females, and is therefore thought to be caused by an X-linked gene with lethality in the hemizygous male. However, the syndrome has also been observed in two males with two X chromosomes (Aicardi, 1996). Evidence for familial recurrence is limited to two affected sisters (Molina *et al.*, 1989). A possible locus for Aicardi syndrome is on the short arm of the X chromosome, according to numerous reports of the association of eye abnormalities and agenesis of the corpus callosum with translocations involving Xp22.3. In one study, the estimated survival rate was 75 per cent at six years and 40 per cent at 15 years (MacGregor *et al.*, 1993).

Clinical and neuroimaging features may involve severe mental retardation, infantile spasms, chorioretinal lacunae, agenesis of the corpus callosum and gray matter heterotopia. Neuropathological findings indicate early impairment of neuronal migration with: (1) a thin unlayered cortex, (2) diffuse unlayered polymicrogyria with fused molecular layers and (3) heterotopic nodules in the periventricular region and in the hemispheric white matter (Ferrer *et al.*, 1986; Billette de Villemeur *et al.*, 1992). The cortical pattern is irregular, with many small cauliflower-like convolutions. No laminar organization is recognizable in the cortex. Neurones have a radial arrangement, but the thickness of the cortex is irregular and difficult to measure because the neurones are scattered. As a result of the fusion of the molecular layers the microgyri are packed. Additional, less frequent, malformations such as agenesis of the anterior commissure, the fornix, or both, choroid plexus cysts, colobomata, and vertebral and costal abnormalities have also been described.

Specific electroclinical features of Aicardi syndrome include early onset of infantile spasms often associated with partial seizures. According to an overview by Chevrie & Aicardi (1986), spasms have been reported to be the only seizure type in 47 per cent of 184 patients recognizable in the literature. In 35 per cent of patients, spasms were associated with partial seizures. Often partial seizures begin in the first days of life preceding the onset of spasms. Aicardi syndrome has been suggested as one possible cause of "early infantile epileptic encephalopathy" (Ohtahara *et al.*, 1987). Hypsarrhythmia is observed in a minority of patients (about 18 per cent) (Aicardi, 1996). Interictal EEG abnormalities are typically asymmetric and asynchronous (split brain EEG), with or without suppression bursts during wakefulness and sleep. Seizure and EEG patterns change little, if at all, over time and seizures are almost always drug-resistant. Aicardi syndrome is a highly epileptogenic malformation in which there is evidence that seizure activity may originate from multiple cortical areas. There is a low tendency to develop epileptic syndromes typical of the older child.

Syndromes resulting from regional polymicrogyria

Based on site and extent of the polymicrogyric cortex, various polymicrogyria syndromes have been identified. Unlike the most severe malformations of cortical development, which can lead to premature death, most syndromes resulting from regional polymicrogyria are not accompanied by reduced lifespan. Therefore they are detected above all on MRI, and histopathological documentation remains scanty. Recent development of epilepsy surgery has contributed little to anatomic knowledge, probably because polymicrogyria patients are rarely operated by focal resection, on account of the type of epilepsy and extent of the lesions, often multilobar or bilateral.

Bilateral perisylvian polymicrogyria

This malformation involves bilaterally the gray matter bordering the lateral fissure which, in typical cases, is almost vertical and in continuity with the central or postcentral sulcus (Figs. 1 and 2). The

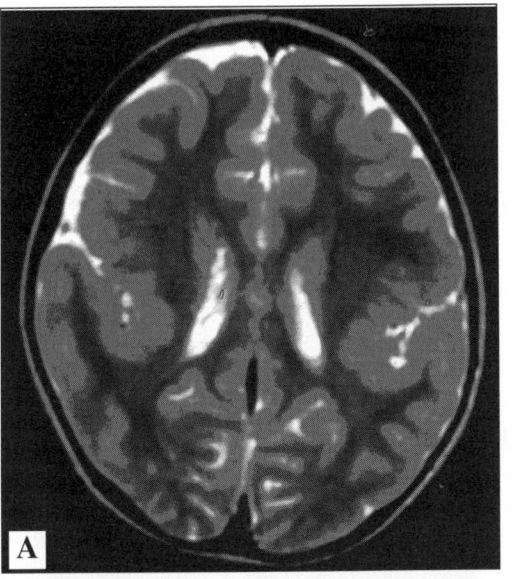
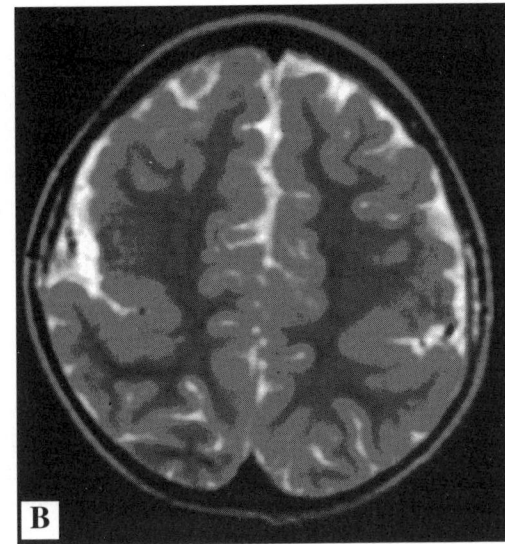
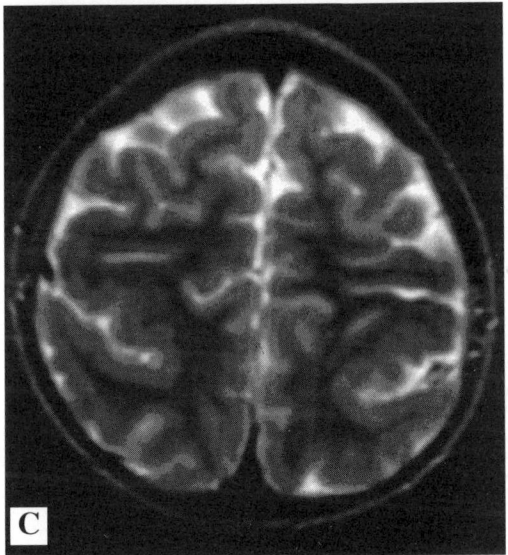

Fig. 1. A, B, C. Six-year-old girl with bilateral perisylvian syndrome. T2W images; 1.5T. The malformed cortex is thickened and smooth, and the gyral pattern is abnormal with a vertical sulcus replacing the sylvian and rolandic fissures.

cortical abnormality is usually symmetric but varies in extent among patients (Guerrini et al., 1992a; Kuzniecky et al., 1993). Neuropathologic studies have shown four-layered polymicrogyria in three cases (Kuzniecky et al., 1993; Ruton et al., 1994) and unlayered polymicrogyria in one (Becker et al., 1989). It is unclear whether these pathologically documented cases represent a single malformative spectrum with the same etiology or different malformations with the same topography. Although most cases are sporadic, two families have been reported, each with a pair of affected sibs (Andermann & Andermann, 1996), indicating possible autosomal recessive inheritance. A large pedigree has recently been reported which might indicate X-linked dominant transmission (Borgatti et al., 1997). However, no clear-cut sex predominance has been identified. Bilateral perisylvian polymicrogyria has also been reported in children born from monochorionic biamniotic twin pregnancies which were complicated by twin-twin transfusion syndrome with death of the co-twin between the 10th and 18th week of gestation (Baker et al., 1996; Van

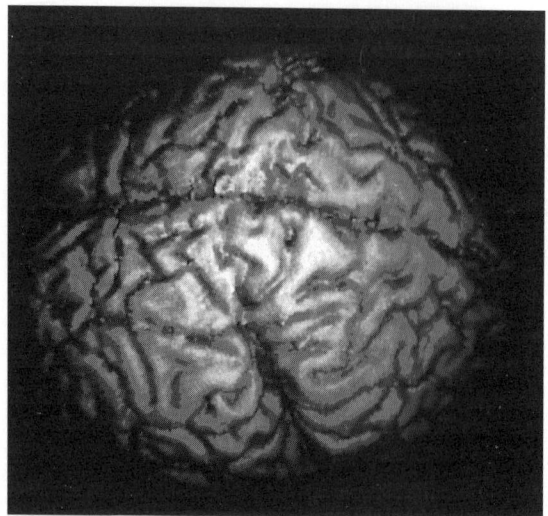

Fig. 2. 18-year-old woman with bilateral perisylvian syndrome. MRI. Three-dimensional surface reconstruction of the brain in a laterosuperior view. The frontal lobes are on the reader's hand right-hand side. Not the abnormally vertical sylvian sulcus surrounded by an abnormal gyral pattern.

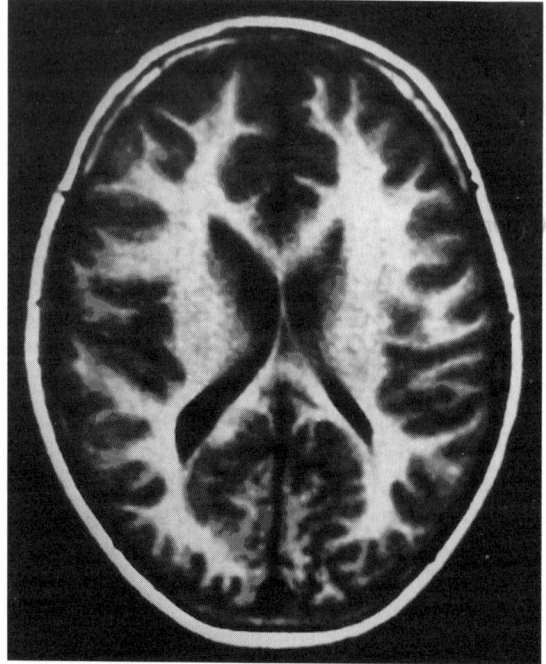

Fig. 3. Patient with bilateral parasagittal parieto-occipital polymicrogyria. IR axial image through the central portion of lateral ventricles. Bilateral thickening of mesial parieto-occipital cortex. Small interdigitations between gray and white matter.

Bogaert et al., 1996). In such cases the malformation could result from ischaemic injury secondary to hemodynamic changes induced by death of the co-twin. Parabiotic twin syndrome has also been associated with focal polymicrogyria involving the parieto-occipital cortex (Barth & van der Harten et al., 1985; Larroche et al., 1994; Sugama & Kusano, 1994).

Several studies have clarified the clinical spectrum of the bilateral perisylvian polymicrogyria syndrome (Kuzniecky et al., 1989, 1993, 1994; Guerrini et al., 1992a). Patients have facio-pharingo-glosso-masticatory diplegia, with dissociation of automatic (preserved) and voluntary (impaired) facial motility. Language impairment ranges from mild dysarthria in patients with mild or asymmetric cortical abnormality to complete absence of speech. Almost all patients have mental retardation and most have epilepsy. Seizures usually begin between age four and 12 years and are poorly controlled in about 65 per cent of patients. Atypical absences, tonic or atonic drop attacks and tonic–clonic seizures are the most frequent types, often occurring as Lennox–Gastaut-like syndromes. A minority of patients (26 per cent) have partial seizures, predominantly somatomotor, involving the lip, perioral or facial muscles, or complex partial seizures. Drug resistance is much less frequent in patients with partial seizures. Kuzniecky et al. (1994), reported on seven patients with disabling drop attack seizures who were treated by anterior callosotomy, with good results in five of these. Drop attack seizures due to bilateral synchronous involvement of the motor cortex are however replaced by lateralized seizures (Guerrini et al., in press).

Bilateral parasagittal parieto-occipital polymicrogyria

This malformation (Figs. 3 and 4) was recently observed on MRI in nine patients with partial epilepsy (Guerrini et al., 1997), most of whom had apparently normal 10 mm thick section CT scans.

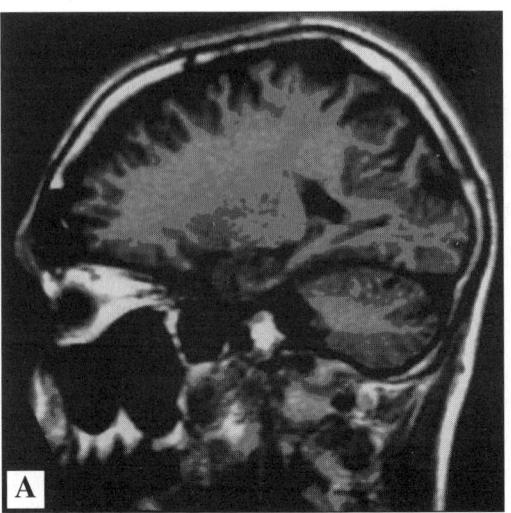 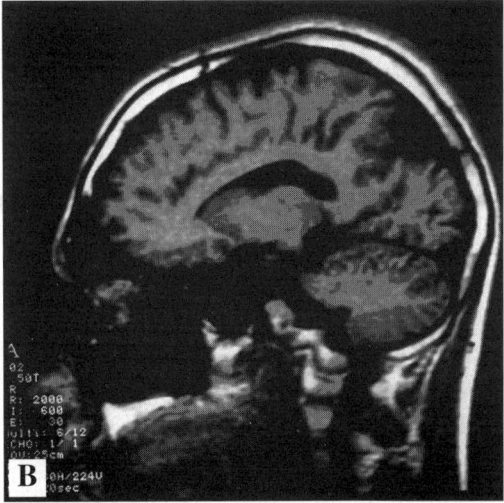

Fig. 4. 18-year-old man with bilateral parasagittal parieto-occipital polymicrogyria. MRI. IRW sagittal images through the right trigonus (A) and the parieto-occipital sulcus (B). Thickening and infolding of posterior parietal and superior occipital cortex. Small interdigitations between gray and white matter and widening of intervening sulci. The sylvian fissure was normal (not shown).

The abnormal cortex extended posteriorly to involve the occipital lobe just below the parieto-occipital sulcus (upper margin of the cuneus) and anteriorly to immediately behind the precuneus and superior parietal lobule. No familial distribution or etiologic factors were identified. Although location in a posterior watershed area between anterior, posterior and middle cerebral arteries could indicate perfusion failure as the underlying cause (Lyon & Robain, 1967), a mutation of regionally expressed developmental gene(s) (Dobyns & Truwit, 1995) cannot be excluded. IQs ranged from average to mild retardation. Several patients presented deficits in neuropsychological tasks requiring performance under time constraints, suggesting that this malformation may result in cognitive slowing. Seizures had started between ages 20 months and 15 years (mean nine years) and were intractable in seven patients. Most patients had complex partial seizures, which were preceded in some by sensory symptoms. Automatisms were not a prominent feature of seizure semiology. Clinical seizure symptomatology remained constant during follow-up in all patients.

Bilateral perisylvian and parieto-occipital polymicrogyria

Some patients have bilateral perisylvian polymicrogyria extending posteriorly, with the sylvian fissure prolonged across the entire hemispheric convexity up to the mesial surface (Fig. 5). The posterior portion of this malformation therefore bears strong similarity to parasagittal parieto-occipital polymicrogyria (see Figs. 4A and 5C) and the anterior portion to perisylvian polymicrogyria. This suggests the existence of a malformative pattern bordering a line passing through the sylvian fissure and directed posteriorly and upward to the mesial aspect of the hemispheric convexity. Polymicrogyria may involve only the anterior portion of this line (perisylvian), only the posterior portion (parieto-occipital), or both (perisylvian and parieto-occipital polymicrogyria). The rearrangement of the surrounding gyral pattern and the orientation of the abnormal sylvian fissure (usually more vertical than normal), are variable. Rarely, the malformation is asymmetric, with parieto-occipital extension on one side only. Patients with the most extensive form of the malformation often have severe epilepsies (Pupillo *et al.*, 1996) whose characteristics are similar to the bilateral perisylvian syndrome, with electroclinical patterns resembling the Lennox–Gastaut

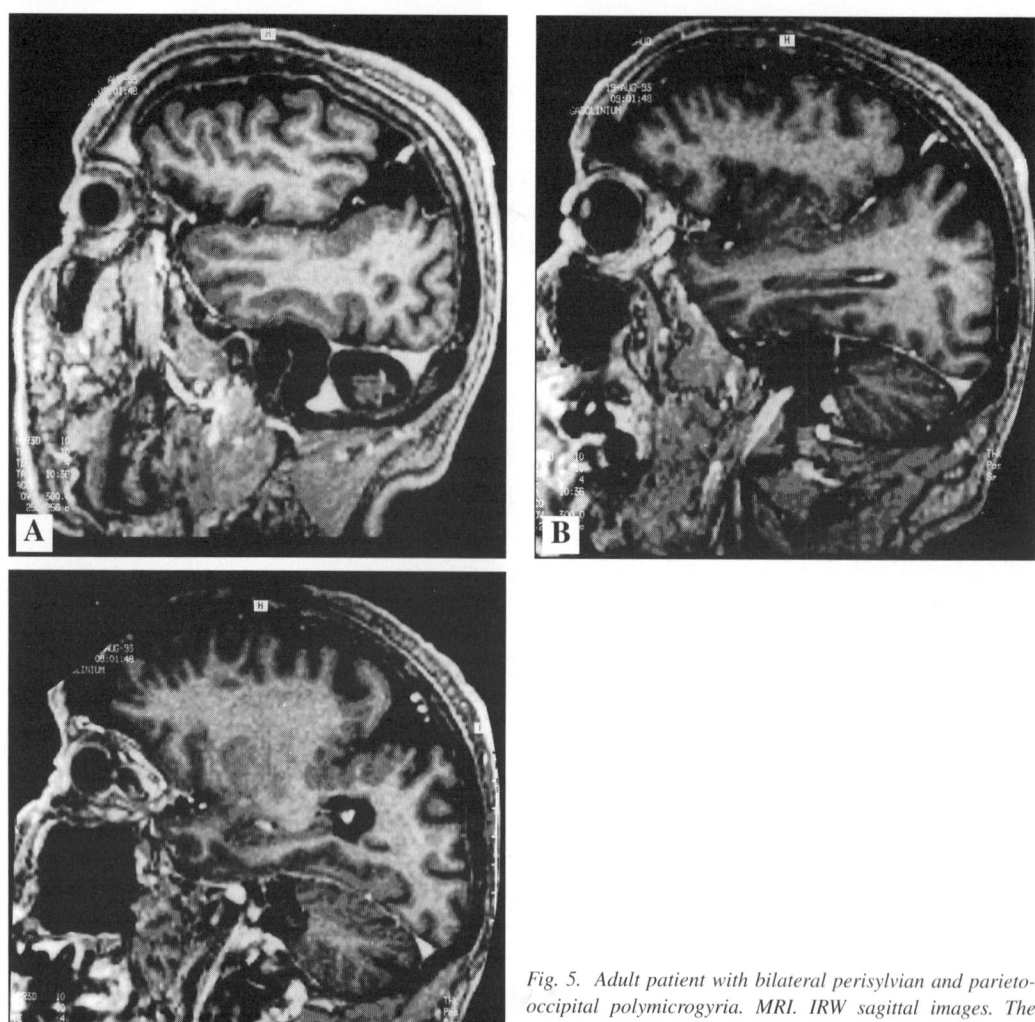

Fig. 5. Adult patient with bilateral perisylvian and parieto-occipital polymicrogyria. MRI. IRW sagittal images. The sylvian fissure is prolonged posteriorly and upward (A and B). Thickening of the insular cortex B. Infolding of the parasagittal parietal cortex (C).

syndrome. However, such patients may also have partial epilepsies with early ictal symptoms indicating onset in the occipital or parietal lobes. The only instance of familial occurrence was described in twin sisters (Avanzini *et al.*, 1997), but it is not known whether they were monozygotic or dizygotic.

Unilateral polymicrogyrias

Lateralized polymicrogyria may affect the whole hemisphere or part of it. Large malformations are associated with hypoplasia of the affected hemisphere (Fig. 6) and enlargement of the corresponding lateral ventricle. Subhemispheric forms are most frequently located in the perisylvian cortex. Polymicrogyria apparently shown to be lateralized on MRI (Fig. 7) may turn out to be bilateral and extensive on microscopic examination of the brain (Fig. 8) (Guerrini *et al.*, 1992b).

Clinical characteristics of lateralized polymicrogyria have been studied in a series of 20 patients (Guerrini *et al.*, 1996a): 75 per cent had seizures and mild to moderate hemiparesis, 70 per cent had

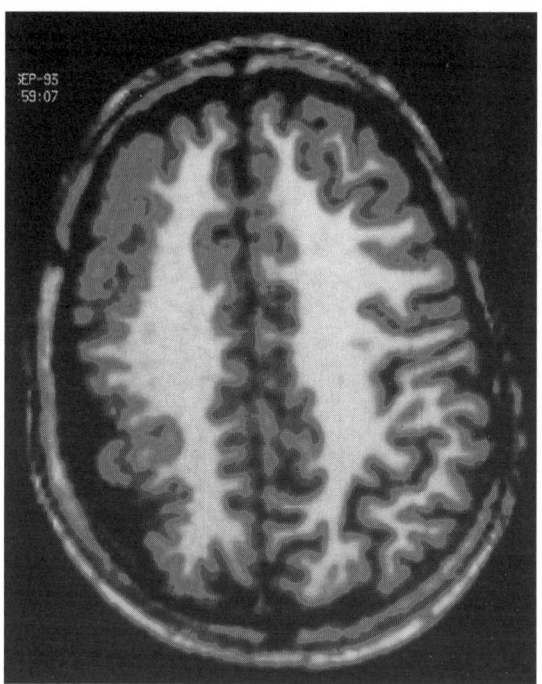

Fig. 6. Unilateral polymicrogyria. T1W axial section. The right hemisphere is hypoplastic, with an abnormal gyral pattern and irregular junction between gray and white matter.

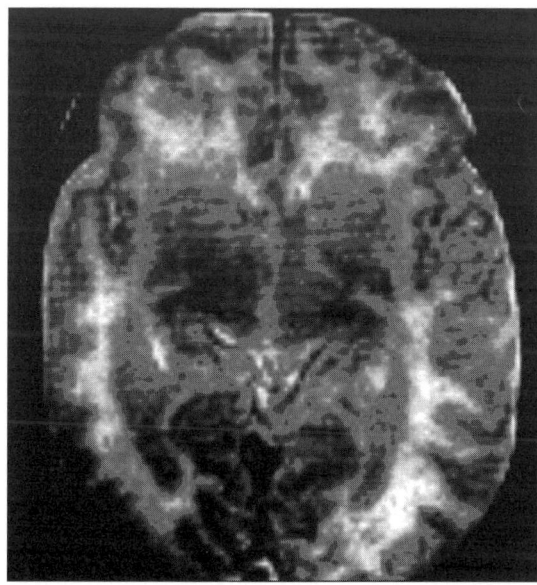

Fig. 7. Newborn. MRI. T2W image. Hypoplasia of the right temporal lobe which has smooth gyri and mild cortical thickening.

mild to moderate mental retardation. Hemiparesis was typically associated with prominent mirror movements of the affected limb. This feature has been attributed to ipsilateral cortical representation of the sensorimotor hand area (Maegaki *et al.*, 1995). In patients with interictal EEG abnormalities and seizures involving the motor cortex, hemiparesis worsened or became apparent with worsening of interictal epileptiform abnormalities or of seizures. Age at seizure onset ranged from one month to 19 years. At the last clinical evaluation epilepsy was severe in one-third of the 15 epilepsy patients still in follow-up, but had been considered intractable at some time in three other patients. The most common seizure types were partial motor seizures (73 per cent), atypical absences (47 per cent), generalized tonic–clonic seizures (27 per cent) and complex partial seizures (20 per cent). Epilepsy could be classified as partial in 80 per cent of patients and generalized in 20 per cent. Interictal EEG findings in most patients suggested greater cortical involvement than expected from MRI. Interictal EEG findings, coexistence of multiple seizure types, inclusion of the motor cortex in the epileptogenic zone, poor delimitation of the abnormal cortex and potential for more widespread cortical abnormality than recognized by MRI, make most patients with intractable epilepsy and lateralized polymicrogyria unlikely candidates for surgery.

Multilobar polymicrogyria is one possible cause of epilepsy with electrical status epilepticus during sleep (ESES) (Guerrini *et al.*, 1996b). Patients with this epilepsy syndrome have both partial motor and atypical absence seizures and both focal and generalized interictal discharges. Sleep recordings show continuous generalized SW complexes during slow-wave phases. The condition is usually detected between ages two and 10 years and may last for months to years. Age-related secondary bilateral synchrony is responsible for the generalized spike and wave EEG pattern in ESES (Dalla Bernardina *et al.*, 1989; Kobayashi *et al.*, 1994).

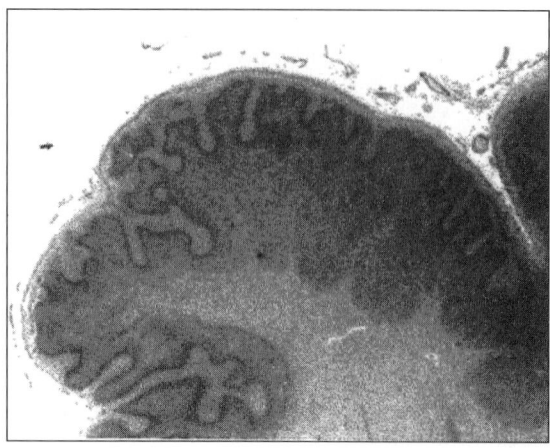

Fig. 8. Specimen of the right frontal lobe obtained from neuropathologic brain examination of the same patient as in Fig. 7. Typical four-layered polymicrogyria with areas of infolding of mycrogyri borders and zones of cortical thickening with loss of layering (Cresyl violet). This cortical pattern was recognizable throughout the cortical ribbon in both hemispheres.

Reported cases are almost equally divided between lesional and cryptogenic origin (Tassinari et al., 1992). The seizures can usually be controlled and tend to remit completely before adolescence. However, neuropsychological impairment, often emerging during the period of ESES, may persist indefinitely (Bureau et al., 1990; Tassinari et al., 1992). It is likely that the extent of eventual neuropsychological impairment is a function both of the underlying structural abnormality and duration of the ESES period. Although epilepsy with ESES is infrequent, its occurrence in patients with localized polymicrogyria does not appear to be extremely rare (Guerrini et al., 1998). This epileptic syndrome has never been reported to date in patients with other forms of cortical malformations. In a series of nine patients whose follow-up periods extended beyond cessation of ESES, seizure outcome was consistently good (Guerrini et al., 1998). In no patient was cognitive deterioration demonstrable after ESES compared with pre-ESES evaluation. However, assessment was carried out with different methods and in different centres, which may have influenced the ascertainment procedures.

The fact that ESES can be found among patients with polymicrogyria but not in those with other cortical malformations could be correlated with an anatomofunctional pattern unique to the polymicrogyric cortex. Selective damage to cortical layer V (Richman et al., 1974) could result in an imbalance between the excitatory activity of intrinsically bursting pyramidal neurones, situated in layers IV and V (Chagnac-Amitai & Connors, 1989) and consequently reduced in number, and the inhibitory activity of GABAergic interneurones, the latter being spared to some extent since they are distributed throughout the cortex. Enhanced excitation arising from the malformed cortex would thus lead to overwhelming hypersynchronous inhibitory neuronal discharges (Engel, 1995). Spared horizontal neuronal lamination (Robain, 1996) might then facilitate spread of SW activity leading to bilateral synchronous discharges (Blume & Pillay, 1985; Morrell, 1995). Age-related secondary bilateral synchrony underlying ESES in children without detectable brain lesions (Dalla Bernardina et al., 1989; Kobayashi et al., 1994) is likewise observed when ESES complicates polymicrogyria (Guerrini et al., 1998a). In other malformations, accompanied by severe disruption of cortical laminar organization, for example focal cortical dysplasia, only focal electroclinical manifestations occur (Guerrini et al., 1992b, 1996; Palmini et al., 1991a, 1991b, 1995) despite the high epileptogenicity (Mattia et al., 1995).

The role of resective surgery in epilepsy with ESES has not been specifically addressed, although it has been hypothesized that surgery may be effective when a focal abnormality is identified (Park et al., 1994). However, the good prognosis of epilepsy and the doubtful association with an acquired neuropsychological deficit should discourage early surgical procedures in patients with ESES and polymicrogyria. Multiple subpial transections (Morrell et al., 1989, 1995) with selective interruption of intracortical horizontal fibres could represent a rational option in patients with early onset ESES and evidence of incipient cognitive deterioration. Sleep EEG should be systematically performed in patients with polymicrogyria.

References

Aicardi, J., Chevrie, J.J. & Rousselle, F. (1969): Le syndrome agénésie calleuse, spasmes en flexion, lacunes chorio-rétiniennes. *Arch. Franc. Pédiatr.* **26,** 1103–1120.

Aicardi, J. (1996): Aicardi syndrome. In: *Dysplasias of cerebral cortex and epilepsy*, eds. R. Guerrini, F. Andermann, R. Canapicchi, J. Roger, B.G. Zifkin & P. Pfanner, pp. 211–216. Philadelphia: Lippincott-Raven.

Aicardi, J., Lefebvre, J. & Lerique-Koechlin, A. (1965): A new syndrome: spasms in flexion, callosal agenesis, ocular abnormalities. *Electroencephalogr. Clin. Neurophysiol.* **19,** 609–610.

Andermann, E. & Andermann, F. (1996). Genetic aspects of neuronal migration disorders. In: *Dysplasias of cerebral cortex and epilepsy,* eds. R. Guerrini, F. Andermann, R. Canapicchi, J. Roger, B. Zifkin, P. Pfanner, pp. 11–15. Philadelphia: Lippincott-Raven.

Avanzini, G., Granata, T., Farina, L., Girotti, F., Chiapparini, L., D'Incerti, L. & Battaglia, G. (1997): Bilateral parieto-occipital polymicrogyria: clinical and epileptological findings. *Epilepsia* **38 (Suppl. 3),** 230.

Baker, E.M., Khorasgani, M.G., Gardner-Medwin, D., Gholkar, A. & Griffiths, P.D. (1996): Arthrogryposis multiplex congenita and bilateral parietal polymicrogyria in association with the intrauterine death of a twin. *Neuropediatrics* **27,** 54–56.

Barkovich, A.J. (1996): Magnetic resonance imaging of lissencephaly, polymicrogyria, schizencephaly, hemimegalencephaly, and band heterotopia. In: *Dysplasias of cerebral cortex and epilepsy*, eds. R. Guerrini, F. Andermann, R. Canapicchi, J. Roger, B. Zifkin & P. Pfanner, pp. 115–129. Philadelphia: Lippincott-Raven.

Barth, P.G. & van der Harten, J.J. (1985): Parabiotic twin syndrome with topical isocortical disruption and gastroschisis. *Acta. Neuropathol.* **67,** 345–349.

Becker, P.S., Dixon, A.M. & Troncoso, J.C. (1989): Bilateral opercular polymicrogyria. *Ann. Neurol.* **25,** 90–92.

Billette de Villemeur, T., Chiron, C. & Robain, O. (1992): Unlayered polymicrogyria and agenesis of the corpus callosum: a relevant association? *Acta Neuropathol.* **83,** 265–270.

Blume, W.T. & Pillay, N. (1985). Electrographic and clinical correlates of secondary bilateral synchrony. *Epilepsia* **26,** 634–641.

Borgatti, R., Zucca, C., Triulzi, F., Piccinelli, P. & Giorda, R. (1997): Bilateral perisylvian polymicrogyria: description of two families suggestive of X-linked transmission. In: *Abnormal cortical development and epilepsy. Fourth international colloquium on childhood epilepsy. Venice, October 2–4, 1997. Mariani Foundation Book of abstracts.*

Bureau, M., Cordova, S., Dravet, Ch., Roger, J. & Tassinari, C.A. (1990): Epilepsie avec pointe-ondes continues pendant le sommeil lent (POCS). Evolution à moyen et long terme (à propos de 15 cas). *Epilepsies* **2,** 86–94.

Chagnac-Amitai, Y. & Connors B.W. (1989): Synchronized excitation and inhibition driven by intrinsically bursting neurones in neocortex. *J. Neurophysiol* **62,** 1149–1162.

Chevrie, J.J. & Aicardi J. (1986): The Aicardi syndrome. In: *Recent advances in epilepsy. Vol. 3*, eds. T.A. Pedley & B.S Meldrum, pp. 189–210. Edinburgh: Churchill Livingston.

Cohen, M., Campbell, R. & Yaghmai, F. (1989): Neuropathological abnormalities in developmental dysphasia. *Ann. Neurol.* **25,** 567–570.

Dalla Bernardina, B., Fontana, E., Michelizza, B., Colamaria, V., Capovilla, G. & Tassinari, C.A. (1989): Partial epilepsies of childhood, bilateral synchronization, continuous spike-waves during slow sleep. In: *Advances in epileptology: XVIIth Epilepsy International Symposium*, eds. J.Manelis, E. Bental, J.N Loeber & F.E. Dreifuss, pp. 295–302, New York: Raven Press.

Dobyns, W.B. & Truwit, C.L. (1995): Lissencephaly and other malformations of cortical development: 1995 update. *Neuropediatrics* **26,** 132–147.

Engel Jr., J. (1995): Inhibitory mechanisms of epileptic seizure generation. In: *Negative motor phenomena. Advances in Neurology, Vol. 67,* eds. S. Fahn, M. Hallett, O. Luders & C.D. Marsden, pp. 157–170. Philadelphia: Lippincott-Raven.

Evrard, P., De Saint-Georges, P., Kadhim, H. & Gadisseux, J.F. (1989): Pathology of prenatal encephalopathies. In: *Child neurology and developmental disabilities,* ed. J. French, pp. 153–176. Baltimore: Brookes.

Ferrer, I. (1984): A Golgi analysis ofunlayered polymicrogyria. *Acta Neuropathol.* **65,** 69–76.

Ferrer, I. & Català, I. (1991): Unlayered polymicrogyria: structural and developmental aspects. *Anat. Embryol.* **184,** 517–528.

Ferrer, I., Cusi, M.V., Liarte, A. & Campistol, J. (1986): A Golgi study of the polymicrogyric cortex in Aicardi syndrome. *Brain Dev.* **8,** 518–525.

Friede, R. L. (1989): *Developmental neuropathology,* 2nd edition, p. 577. New York: Springer-Verlag.

Galaburda, A.M., Sherman, G.F., Rosen, G.D., Aboitiz, F. & Geschwind, N. (1985): Developmental dyslexia: four consecutive patients with cortical anomalies. *Ann. Neurol.* **18,** 222–233.

Guerrini, R. (1997): Clinical epilepsy syndromes in focal cortical dysplasias. In: *Pediatric epilepsy surgery,* eds. H. Holthausen & I. Tuxhorn I, pp. 70–184. London: John Libbey.

Guerrini, R., Dravet, C., Raybaud, C., Roger, J., Bureau, M., Battaglia, A., Livet, M.O., Colicchio, G. & Robain, O., (1992a). Neurological findings and seizure outcome in children with bilateral opercular macrogyric-like changes detected by magnetic resonance imaging. *Dev. Med. Child. Neurol.* **34,** 694–705.

Guerrini, R., Dravet, Ch., Raybaud, Ch., Roger, J., Bureau, M., Battaglia, A., Livet, M.O., Gambarelli, D. & Robain, O. (1992b): Epilepsy and focal gyral anomalies detected by magnetic resonance imaging: electroclinico-morphological correlations and follow-up. *Dev. Med. Child. Neurol.* **34,** 706–718.

Guerrini, R., Dravet, C., Bureau, M., Mancini, J., Canapicchi, R., Livet, M.O. & Belmonte, A. (1996a): Diffuse and localized dysplasias of cerebral cortex: clinical presentation, outcome, and proposal for a morphologic MRI classification based on a study of 90 patients. In: *Dysplasias of cerebral cortex and epilepsy,* eds. R. Guerrini, F. Andermann, R. Canapicchi, J. Roger, B. Zifkin & P. Pfanner, pp. 255–269. Philadelphia: Lippincott-Raven.

Guerrini, R., Parmeggiani, A., Bureau, M., Dravet, C., Genton, P., Salas-Puig, X., Santucci, M., Bonanni, P. & Ambrosetto, G. (1996b): Localized cortical dysplasia: good seizure outcome after sleep-related electrical status epilepticus. In: *Dysplasias of cerebral cortex and epilepsy,* eds. R. Guerrini, F. Andermann, R. Canapicchi, J. Roger, B. Zifkin & P. Pfanner, pp. 329–335. Philadelphia: Lippincott-Raven.

Guerrini, R., Dubeau, F., Dulac, O., Barkovich, A.J., Kuzniecky, R., Fett, C., Jones-Gotman, M., Canapicchi, R., Cross, H., Fish, D., Bonanni, P., Jambaqué, I. & Andermann, F. (1997). Bilateral parasagittal parieto-occipital polymicrogyria and epilepsy. *Ann. Neurol.* **41,** 65–73.

Guerrini, R., Genton, P., Bureau, M., Parmeggiani, A., Salas-Puig, J., Santucci, M., Bonanni, P., Ambrosetto, G. & Dravet, C. (1998): Multilobar polymicrogyria, intractable drop attack seizures and sleep-related electrical status epilepticus *Neurology* **51,** 504–512.

Guerrini, R., Andermann, E., Avoli, M. & Dobyns, W.B. Cortical dysplasias, genetics and epileptogenesis. *Adv. Neurol.* [in press].

Harding, B.N. (1992): Malformations of the nervous system. In: *Greenfield's neuropathology,* eds. J.H. Adams & L.W. pp. 521–638. Duchen, London: Edward Arnold.

Kobayashi, K., Nishibayashi, N., Ohtsuka, Y., Oka. E. & Ohtahara, S. (1994): Epilepsy with electrical status epilepticus during slow sleep and secondary bilateral synchrony. *Epilepsia* **35,** 1097–1103.

Kuzniecky, R., Andermann, F., Tampieri, D., Melanson, D., Olivier, A. & Leppik, I. (1989): Bilateral central macrogyria: epilepsy, pseudobulbar palsy, and mental retardation – a recognizable neuronal migration disorder. *Ann. Neurol.* **25,** 547–554.

Kuzniecky, R., Andermann, F., Guerrini, R., & CBPS Multicentre Collaborative Study (1993) Congenital bilateral perisylvian syndrome: study of 31 patients. *Lancet* **341,** 608–612.

Kuzniecky, R., Andermann, F., Guerrini, R., & CBPS Multicentre Collaborative Study (1994) . The epileptic spectrum in the congenital bilateral perysilvian syndrome. *Neurology* **44,** 379–385.

Larroche, J. Cl., Girard, N., Narcy, F. & Fallet, C. (1994): Abnormal cortical plate (polymicrogyria), heterotopias, and brain damage in monozygous twins. *Biol. Neonate* **65,** 343–352.

Lyon G. & Robain O. (1967): Etude comparative des encéphalopathies circulatoires prénatales et para-natales. *Acta Neuropathol.* **9,** 79–98.

MacGregor, D.L, Menezes, A. & Buncic, J.R. (1993): Aicardi syndrome (AS): natural history and predictors of severity. *Can. J. Neurol.Sci.* **20 (Suppl. 2),** S36.

Maegaki, Y., Yamamoto, T. & Takeshita, K. (1995): Plasticity of central motor and sensory pathways in a case of unilateral extensive cortical dysplasia: investigation of magnetic resonance imaging, transcranial magnetic stimulation, and short-latency somatosensory evoked potentials. *Neurology* **45,** 2255–2261.

Mattia, D., Olivier, A. & Avoli, M. (1995): Seizure-like discharges recorded in the human dysplastic neocortex maintained *in vitro. Neurology* **45,** 1391–1395.

Molina, J.A., Mateos, F., Merino, M., Epifanio, J.L. & Gorrono, M. (1989): Aicardi syndrome in two sisters. *J. Pediatr.* **115,** 282–283.

Morrell, F., Whisler, W.W. & Bleck, T.P. (1989): Multiple subpial transection: a new approach to the surgical treatment of focal epilepsy. *J. Neurosurg.* **70,** 231–239.

Morrell, F. (1995): Electrophysiology of CSWS in Landau–Kleffner syndrome. In: *Continuous spikes and waves during slow sleep,* Mariani Foundation Paediatric Neurology Series, Vol. 3, eds. A. Beaumanoir, M. Bureau, T. Deonna, L. Mira & C.A. Tassinari. pp. 77–90. London: John Libbey.

Ohtahara, S., Ohtsuka, Y., Yamatogi, Y. & Oka, E. (1987). The early infantile epileptic encephalopathy with suppression burst: developmental aspects. *Brain Dev.* **9,** 371-376.

Palmini, A., Andermann, F., Olivier, A., Tampieri, D. & Robitaille, Y. (1991a): Focal neuronal migration disorders and intractable partial epilepsy: a study of 30 patients. *Ann. Neurol.* **30,** 741–749.

Palmini, A., Andermann, F., Olivier, A., Tampieri, D. & Robitaille, Y. (1991b): Focal neuronal migration disorders and intractable partial epilepsy: results of surgical treatment. *Ann. Neurol.* **30,** 750–757.

Palmini, A., Gambardella, A., Andermann, F., Dubeau, F., da Costa, J.C., Olivier, A., Tampieri, D., Gloor, P., Quesney, F., Andermann, E., Paglioli, E., Paglioli-Neto, E., Coutinho, L., Leblanc, R. & Kim, H.I. (1995): Intrinsic epileptogenicity of human dysplastic cortex as suggested by corticography and surgical results. *Ann. Neurol.* **37,** 476–487.

Park, Y.D., Hoffman, J.M., Radtke, R.A. & DeLong, G.R. (1994): Focal cerebral metabolic abnormality in a patient with continuous spike-waves during slow-wave sleep. *J. Child. Neurol.* **9,** 139–143.

Pupillo, G.T., Andermann, F., Dubeau, F., Tampieri. D., Guerrini, R., Dulac, O. & Lombroso, C. (1996): Bilateral sylvian parieto-occipital polymicrogyria. *Neurology* **46 (Suppl. 2),** A303.

Raybaud, Ch., Girard, N., Canto-Moreira, N. & Poncet, M. (1996): High definition magnetic resonance imaging identification of cortical dysplasias: micropolygyria versus lissencephaly. In: *Dysplasias of cerebral cortex and epilepsy,* eds. R. Guerrini, F. Andermann, R. Canapicchi, J. Roger, B. Zifkin & P. Pfanner, pp. 131–143. Philadelphia: Lippincott-Raven.

Richman, D.P., Stewart, R.M. & Caviness Jr, V.S. (1974): Cerebral microgyria in a 27-weeks foetus: an architectonic and topographic analysis. *J. Neuropathol. Exp. Neurol.* **33,** 374–384.

Robain, O. (1996): Introduction to the pathology of cerebral cortical dysplasia. In: *Dysplasias of cerebral cortex and epilepsy,* eds. R. Guerrini, F. Andermann, R. Canapicchi, J. Roger, B. Zifkin & P. Pfanner, pp. 1–9. Philadelphia: Lippincott-Raven.

Ruton, M.C., Expert-Besançon, M.C., Bursztyn, J., Mselati, J.C. & Robain, O. (1944). Polymicrogyrie biopericulaire associée à une ophtalmoplégie congénitale par atteinte du noyau du nerf moteur oculaire commun. *Rev. Neurol.* **150,** 363–369.

Sugama, S. & Kusano, K. (1994): Monozygous twin with polymicrogyria and normal co-twin. *Pediatr. Neurol.* **11,** 62–63.

Tassinari, CA., Bureau, M., Dravet, Ch., Dalla Bernardina, B. & Roger, J. (1992): Epilepsy with continuous spikes and waves during slow sleep - otherwise described as ESES (epilepsy with electrical status epilepticus during slow sleep). In: *Epileptic syndromes in infancy, childhood and adolescence,* 2nd edition, eds. J. Roger, M. Bureau, Ch. Dravet, F. Dreifuss, A. Perret & P. Wolf, pp. 245–256. London: John Libbey.

Van Bogaert, P., Donner, C., David, Phil., Rodesch, F., Avni, E.F. & Szliwowski, H.B. (1996): Congenital bilateral perisylvian syndrome in a monozygotic twin with intra-uterine death of the co-twin. *Dev. Med. Child. Neurol.* **38,** 166–171.

Chapter 17

Periventricular nodular heterotopia: further delineation of the clinical syndromes

François Dubeau, Li Min Li, Alexandre Bastos,
Eva Andermann and Frederick Andermann

*Department of Neurology and Neurosurgery, Montreal Neurological Institute and Hospital,
3801 University Street, Montreal, QC H3A 2B4, Canada*

Summary

High resolution imaging techniques, particularly MRI, demonstrated that gray matter heterotopias, like other neuronal migration disorders, have a broad spectrum of severity, including individuals with epilepsy, mild intellectual dysfunction and a normal life span. An increasing number of asymptomatic individuals has also been described.

Certain features of periventricular nodular heterotopias (PNH) have now become apparent and these are sufficient to recognize them as a distinct neuronal migration disorder. Periventricular heterotopias appear to be heterogeneous based on differences in sex ratio, location of the heterotopia and severity of symptoms. Periventricular heterotopia may be sporadic or familial. Onset of epilepsy in the second decade of life, normal intelligence or mild intellectual dysfunction, and the finding of female preponderance in both sporadic and familial cases, differentiate PNH from other cortical dysgenesis. An expanding number of other syndromes associated with PNH are also described.

Introduction

Cortical dysgeneses (CD), or malformations of cortical development, comprise a heterogenous group of disorders of cortical development often associated with epilepsy. Anatomical–radiological classifications divide cortical malformations into generalized, lateralized or focal types depending on gross lesion distribution seen at autopsy (Sarnat, 1991) or *in vivo*, based on MR imaging findings (Barkovich *et al.*, 1996). The classification system proposed by the latter categorizes the major malformations of cortical development on the basis of the three main steps in cortical development: malformations due to abnormal stem cell proliferation and differentiation; malformations due to abnormal neuronal migration; and those due to abnormal cortical organization. Included among these abnormalities are aberrations of gyration and sulcation (e.g. agyria, pachygyria, polymicrogyria), megalencephaly and hemimegalencephaly, focal cortical dysplasia, microdysgenesis, CD associated with neoplasia (e.g. dysembryoplastic neuroepithelial tumour, ganglioglioma), phacomatosis-associated dysplasia (e.g. neurofibromatosis type I, tuberous sclerosis) and cerebral heterotopia. Anatomical classifications are a useful first step in helping clarify the etiology and possible treatment approaches to the epilepsies associated with CD.

Heterotopic gray matter aggregates are clusters of neurones in abnormal locations. They presuppose an insult occurring during the period of active neuroblast migration, with these cellular elements thought to be arrested during the 10th to 17th weeks of gestation. These disorganized masses of neurones in the white matter usually occur in a periventricular position with a nodular morphology. They may also be found anywhere along the migration pathway resulting in nodules, laminae or bands of subcortical gray matter. Heterotopic neuronal masses are now classified into three groups: nodular, laminar and band heterotopia (Jakob, 1936; Barkovich *et al.*, 1989; Friede, 1989; Barkovich & Kjos, 1992).

The periventricular (or subependymal) nodular heterotopias (PNH) are abnormal islands of neurones that may be related to abnormalities of cell proliferation or non-radial migration in the developing ventricular and subventricular zones (Barkovich & Kjos, 1992; Sarnat, 1992). Heterotopia in the white matter, centrum semiovale or close to the cortex may be secondary to radial glial fibre migration disorders. The classification of dysplastic disorders may be further refined in some cases according to specific clinical syndromes, associated developmental malformations, neurological deficits, genetic profile, seizure patterns and electroencephalographic abnormalities (Guerrini *et al.*, 1996). In the classification system of Barkovich *et al.* (1996), gray matter heterotopia may be classified as generalized, including X-linked subcortical band heterotopia or double cortex syndrome (Dobyns *et al.*, 1996; Ross *et al.*, 1997) and X-linked bilateral periventricular nodular heterotopia (Eksioglu *et al.*, 1996); or as focal or multifocal, such as periventricular and subcortical nodular heterotopia. Both generalized and focal heterotopia may be found in association with organizational abnormality of the overlying cortex.

Before modern imaging, heterotopic gray matter was usually found at autopsy. The first report is attributed to Tüngel (1857), but Layton (1962) was the first to draw attention to the fact that heterotopia constitutes an anomaly which is not necessarily part of a gross defect but which may result in clinical symptoms. High resolution imaging techniques, particularly MRI, demonstrated that gray matter heterotopias have a broad spectrum of severity. Certain features of PNH have now become apparent and are sufficient to allow its recognition as a distinct neuronal migration disorder. However, patients with PNH represent a heterogeneous group, and several subgroups can be recognized based on location of the heterotopia, presence or absence of other brain and systemic malformations, sex distribution, and type and severity of symptoms (Dobyns *et al.*, 1996, 1997). They give rise to a broad spectrum of clinical pictures and various pathogenic mechanisms appear to be involved to explain their formation.

We reviewed the clinical, demographic and structural findings of 138 patients with PNH described in the literature, including 26 studied at our institution. Five underwent a pneumoencephalogram (Bergeron, 1967; Mueller, 1970), seven only a computerized-tomographic scan (Zimmerman *et al.*, 1983; Kamuro & Tenokuchi, 1993; Raymond *et al.*, 1994; Dubeau *et al.*, 1995), 105 a magnetic resonance imaging (Deeb *et al.*, 1985; Osborn *et al.*, 1987; Smith *et al.*, 1988, 1989; Martin Araguz *et al.*, 1989; Canapicchi *et al.*, 1990; Falconer *et al.*, 1990; Huttenlocher *et al.*, 1991; Zisch & Artmann, 1991; Barkovich & Kjos, 1992; Kamuro & Tenokuchi, 1993; DiMario *et al.*, 1993; Oda *et al.*, 1993; Huttenlocher *et al.*, 1994; Raymond *et al.*, 1994; Dubeau *et al.*, 1995; Jardine *et al.*, 1996; Thomas *et al.*, 1996; Battaglia *et al.*, 1997; Dobyns *et al.*, 1997; Li *et al.*, 1997) and 21 an autopsy (Tüngel, 1857; Meschede, 1866; Otto, 1887; Kernohan, 1930; Nezeloff *et al.*, 1976; Cupo *et al.*, 1981; Palm *et al.*, 1986; Eksioglu *et al.*, 1996; Joseph, 1997).

Description of malformations

Barkovich & Kjos (1992) were the first who attempted to classify PNH based on MRI criteria. They divided them according to the location, size and number of nodules. Periventricular nodular heterotopias are located along the walls of the lateral ventricles, along the trigones and the lateral

Table 1. Clinical data in patients with PNH.

	Literature	MNH/MNI series	Total
Number of patients	112	26	138
Unilateral focal PNH	24 (21%)	8 (31%)	32 (23%)
Bilateral focal PNH	22 (20%)	7 (27%)	29 (21%)
Bilateral diffuse PNH	66 (59%)	11 (42%)	77 (56%)
Female	72%	50%	68%
Seizures	76%	85%	78%
Developmental delay	22%	19%	21%
Associated CNS abnormalities	36%	23%	31%
Associated systemic malformations	10%	19%	16%

walls of the temporal and occipital horns. They are never described in the walls of the third or fourth ventricles. The nodules may be distributed diffusely, and are usually bilateral and contiguous (Fig. 1A, B). This pattern is now defined in the literature as bilateral periventricular nodular heterotopia or BPNH (Dobyns et al., 1996). Bilateral, diffuse and symmetrical PNH have been observed in multiple first degree relatives from several unrelated families. All these patients are female, and the gene for BPNH has been mapped to chromosome Xq28 (Eksioglu et al., 1996). The heterotopia may also be focal, clustered or even isolated, and these are often located along the posterior aspects of the lateral ventricles, the trigones and the temporal and occipital horns (Fig. 2A). They may be unilateral or bilateral. More rarely, a single nodule or scattered nodules may indent the lumen of one frontal, temporal or occipital horn (Fig. 2B, C). Hence, in addition to BPNH, we may classify PNH into two other groups: unilateral focal PNH and bilateral focal PNH.

The 138 cases were separated into three groups, depending on their periventricular distribution (Table 1): unilateral focal, bilateral focal and bilateral diffuse PNH (BPNH). These constituted approximately one-fourth, one-fourth and one-half of all cases, respectively. Eighty-one per cent of patients with bilateral focal PNH and 73 per cent of those with unilateral focal PNH present with a preponderance of PNH in the trigones and temporal and occipital horns. In addition, in patients with unilateral nodules only, a predilection of PNH for the right hemisphere was observed and 23 patients (72 per cent) of this group had a single or several nodules along the right lateral ventricle. Raymond et al. (1994) were the first to report this intriguing observation, and suggested that right-sided neuroblasts may complete migration slightly later than those on the left. The majority of the patients have no associated major brain developmental abnormalities and are therefore considered to have 'pure' PNH. Forty-three patients, however, had concomitant brain abnormalities including hypoplasia of the cerebellum ($n = 7$), mega cisterna magna (10), hypogenesis or agenesis of the corpus callosum (13) and hydrocephaly with or without stenosis of the aqueduct of Sylvius (15). Twenty-two patients had various systemic malformations including nine cardiac, five gastrointestinal and three urinary tract maldevelopment. Interestingly, an association with the Ehlers–Danlos syndrome was found in two patients (Cupo et al., 1981; Thomas et al., 1996).

On MRI, heterotopic nodules usually appear ovoid and smooth, are not calcified, and are isointense with normal gray matter on all imaging sequences. They cause little distortion of the rest of the brain. The surrounding white matter is usually normal, the deep gray matter nuclei have normal configuration, and the cerebral cortex has a normal gyral pattern. They are easy to differentiate from the classic, often calcified, subependymal lesions found in tuberous sclerosis. The latter are often elongated and irregular in shape, isointense or hypodense to white matter, and do enhance after gadolinium injection. In addition, patients with PNH do not have a family history or physical

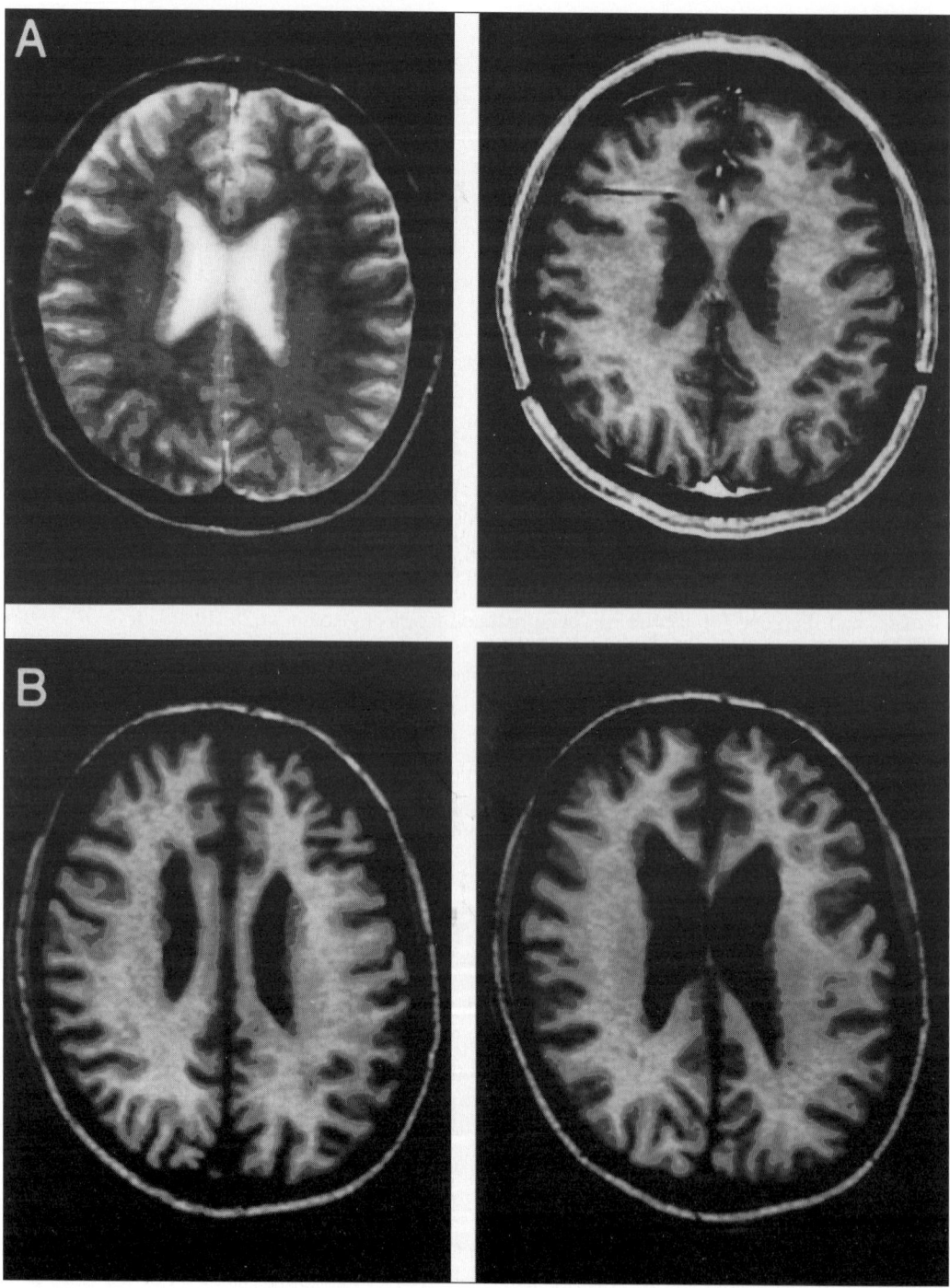

Fig. 1. Bilateral, diffuse periventricular nodular heterotopia. (A) A 36-year-old woman with epilepsy since age 13 and sporadic BPNH. Axial T2 (left) and T1-weighted (right) images show multiple periventricular nodules of gray matter symmetrically lining the lateral walls of the lateral ventricles. (B) A 28-year-old man with refractory seizures and sporadic BPNH. Axial T1-weighted (left and right) images. Note again multiple small ovoid nodules protruding into the lumina of the lateral ventricles.

Chapter 17 Periventricular nodular heterotopia

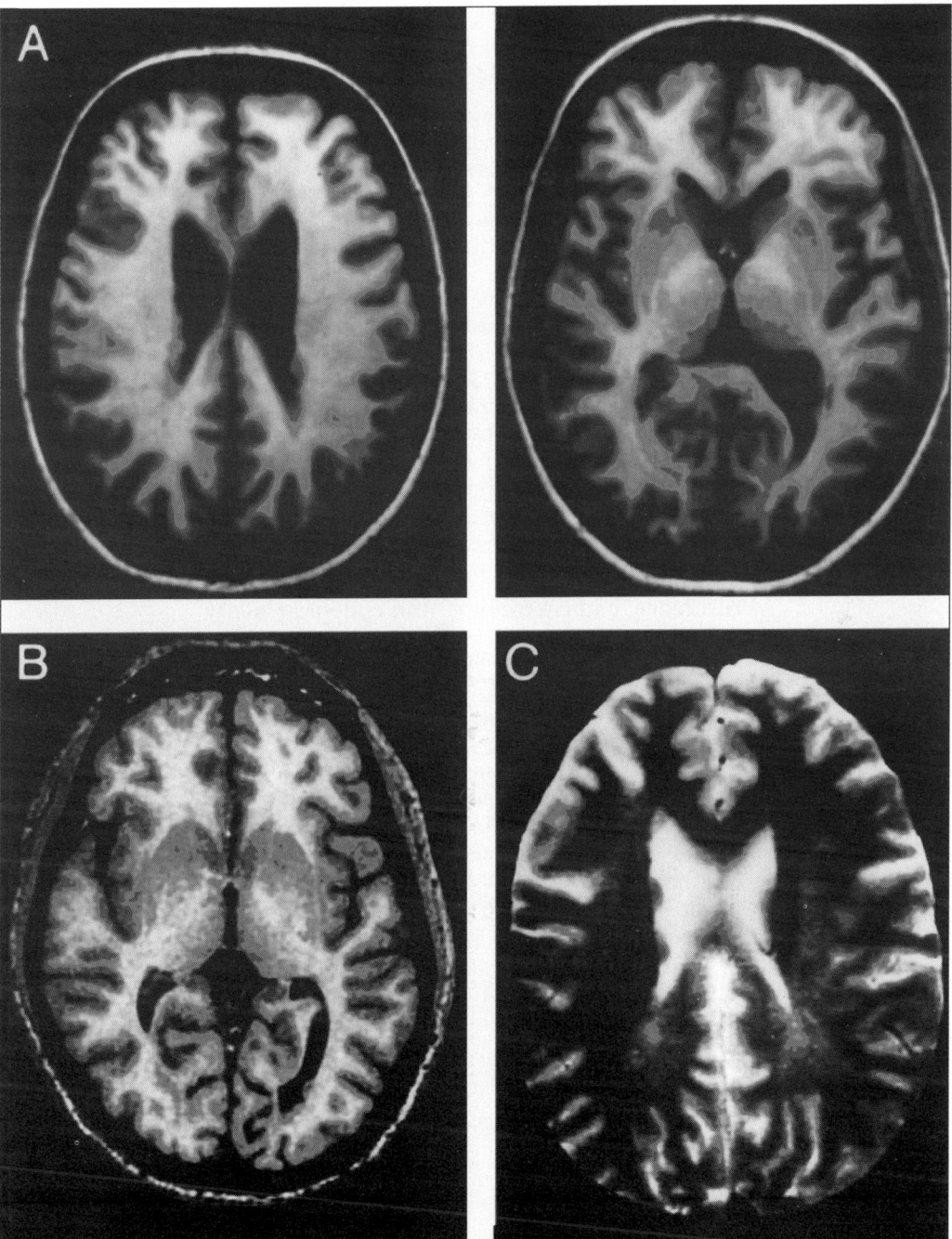

Fig. 2. Focal periventricular nodular heterotopia. (A) Bilateral focal PNH. A 40-year-old woman with normal development and intelligence but with a seizure disorder that began at age 20. Axial T1-weighted images (left and right) show that nodules clustered along the posterior aspect of both lateral ventricles including the trigones. (B) Unilateral focal PNH. A 38-year-old man with normal intelligence but intractable left temporo-occipital seizures. Axial T1-weighted image shows two small ovoid nodules along the lateral wall of the left occipital horn. (C) Unilateral focal PNH. A 23-old-man with normal intelligence and sensory seizures arising from the right hemisphere which started at age 17. Axial T2-weighted image shows two distinct nodules of gray matter protruding into the body of the right lateral ventricle.

stigmata of tuberous sclerosis (Barkovich & Kjos, 1992). It is also worth noting that positron emission tomography showed in a few cases that the gray matter heterotopia had a glucose utilization identical to that of the overlying cortex (Falconer et al., 1990; Lee et al., 1994; Dubeau et al., 1995).

Proton MR spectroscopy can measure N-acetyl-aspartate (NAA) localized exclusively in neurones and neuronal processes in the mature brain (Simmons et al., 1991). In heterotopia, because of the clustering of an abnormally high number of neurones, one would expect a relative increase of the NAA signal. However, Kuzniecky et al. (1997) and Li et al. (1998) found NAA to be variably normal or diminished in PNH suggesting that at least some of these apparently normal neurones are, in fact, dysfunctional.

Histopathological analysis of the few available surgical and autopsy specimens reveals that periventricular gray matter nodules are composed of normal appearing, mature, large and small pyramidal and non-pyramidal neurones with mild gliosis and no calcifications (Barkovich & Kjos, 1992; Dubeau et al., 1995; Eksioglu et al., 1996; Joseph, 1997). These neurones, however, are oriented in multiple directions and do not respect the habitual layering found in the normal cerebral cortex. In addition, a recent autopsy report on two elderly demented women with PNH (Joseph, 1997) showed that the morphologic features of the heterotopia recapitulated those of surrounding neocortex and displayed neurodegenerative changes similar to the ones found in the cortex. These findings again indicate that heterotopic neurones in PNH arise from cortical progenitor cells and that heterotopic tissue may degenerate like cerebral cortex.

Prevalence, clinical findings and epileptogenicity

The prevalence of PNH in patients with epilepsy is unknown. A large MRI series of 341 adults with epilepsy showed PNH in two per cent (Li et al., 1995). In our own series, PNH accounts for approximately 16 per cent (26 cases) of cortical dysgenesis (Table 2), of which 85 per cent had medically refractory seizures (Table 1). While most patients reported in the literature have also had refractory seizures, this may represent a referral bias, and some individuals (~ 22 per cent) have no seizures. Hence, these figures may represent underestimates, and reports of PNH may increase as the clinical relevance of these lesions is increasingly recognized. Patients usually demonstrated normal intelligence (Table 3). A higher proportion of male patients with low IQ (< 85) was found in all three groups (Table 3), particularly in the BPNH group. A larger proportion of males had associated brain malformations as compared to females, and this was also most marked in the BPNH group. These findings may be related to specific BPNH syndromes with mental retardation, which will be

Table 2. Types of cortical dysgenesis - an MNH/MNI series of 164 patients

	N (%)
Abnormalities of gyration	**48**
• Agyria/pachygyria	5 (3)
• Focal macrogyria	19 (11)
• Polymicrogyria	24 (15)
Hemimegalencephaly	**8 (5)**
Heterotopia	**55**
• Periventricular nodular	26 (16)
• Subcortical nodular	16 (10)
• Subcortical band	13 (8)
Focal cortical dysplasia	**53 (32)**

Table 3. Clinical findings according to PNH type.

	Ufocal (n=32)		Bfocal (n=29)		BPNH (n=77)	
Sex	♀	♂	♀	♂	♀	♂
	48%	52%	61%	39%	78%	22%
Seizures	93%	75%	92%	82%	68%	80%
Age at onset, years						
mean	16.3	12.5	13.4	10.6	14.1	11.2
median	17.0	14.5	14.0	9.0	15.0	14.0
range	0–30	2–17	0–28	0–25	0–24	0–25
Low IQ	0	19%	23%	33%	16%	53%
Associated brain malformations	20%	19%	29%	36%	30%	62%
Associated systemic malformations	13%	6%	12%	18%	15%	38%

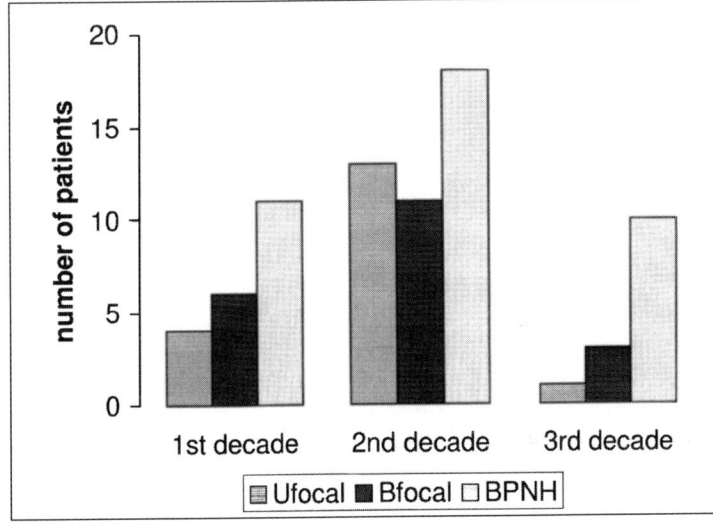

Fig. 3. Age of first seizure in patients with focal and diffuse PNH.

discussed later. The occurrence of strokes early in life in three members of a family with BPNH raises the question of whether stroke is part of the syndrome of periventricular heterotopia or due to a separate genetic defect (Huttenlocher et al., 1994). We did not find this association in other reports on either BPNH or focal periventricular heterotopia, as in our data.

The associated epilepsy syndrome is variable and may resemble generalized (Raymond et al., 1994) or localization-related epilepsy, often suggesting mesial or neocortical temporal and parieto-occipital onset (Raymond et al., 1994; Dubeau et al., 1995; Battaglia et al., 1997). Seizures usually begin during the second decade (Fig. 3 and Table 3) and relatively later than in other types of cortical dysgenesis, suggesting that PNH may be less epileptogenic. In our series, for instance, mean age of first seizure for patients with hemimegalencephaly was three years; with focal cortical dysplasia, five; with band heterotopia, six; with congenital bilateral perisylvian syndrome, eight; and with subcortical nodular heterotopia, ten. It is also our impression that the proportion of patients with PNH and epilepsy, and certainly with intractable epilepsy, is relatively lower when compared to patients with other types of CD (excluding patients with polymicrogyria).

Electroencephalographic data were available in 76 patients: in 37 (48 per cent) of those with BPNH, 16 (or 55 per cent) with bilateral focal PNH, and 23 (74 per cent) with unilateral focal PNH. The anatomic extent of the epileptogenic area was usually congruent with the detected periventricular structural anomaly. Patients with bilateral heterotopia tend to have bilateral or widespread interictal epileptiform activity, whereas those with unilateral and focal lesions tend to have an epileptogenic area restricted to that region. For instance, in the bilateral focal group, bilateral focal or generalized epileptiform abnormalities were described in 50 per cent of the patients, and unilateral abnormalities in 38 per cent. In the unilateral focal group, focal abnormalities were found in 61 per cent (usually but not necessarily ipsilateral to the lesion), and bilateral or generalized discharges in only 26 per cent. Patients with BPNH may have normal EEG (35 per cent), bilateral or widespread epileptiform activity (35 per cent), or unilateral spiking (30 per cent). Overall, the most consistent abnormalities are unilateral or bilateral temporal discharges described in 35 per cent of the patients with PNH, both in the unilateral and bilateral groups. On the other hand, generalized epileptiform activity appears to be relatively rare, and was described in only a small proportion of patients including those with BPNH (bilateral focal 12 per cent, unilateral focal five per cent and BPNH, nine per cent). Battaglia *et al.* (1997) made the interesting observation that all their patients with PNH showed photic driving of background activity, characterized by harmonic alpha rhythm frequencies which were often more evident after low-frequency stimulation. The photic driving was bilateral in those with bilateral lesions and unilateral in the majority with unilateral PNH. They suggested that this may be an indication of some neuronal hyperexcitability in posterior cortical regions close to or overlying the PNH, and due to possible structural cortical abnormalities or anatomic reverberating connections involving the PNH and adjacent cortical areas not identified by MRI studies. The authors reported the same EEG findings in a small subset of patients with unilateral or bilateral PNH and additional cortical abnormalities. These patients had unilateral or bilateral, predominantly trigonal, PNH with unilateral cortical hypoplasia or unilateral cerebral hypoplasia and parieto-occipital cortical dysplasia.

Our group (Li *et al.*, 1997) recently described 10 patients from several centres who had PNH and electroclinical features suggestive of temporal lobe epilepsy (TLE) and who were surgically treated for medically refractory seizures. Seven had bilateral PNH and six were studied with intracranial depth EEG recordings (including one with the radiological features of BPNH, Fig. 1A). None of the patients with a follow-up of more than 18 months remained seizure-free after temporal resection. Two, however, had only rare seizures after surgery including one who underwent an anterior temporal resection with a subtotal removal of the PNH. The other, with BPNH, had a right selective amygdalo-hippocampectomy. In this series, none of the six patients with intracranial depth electrode studies had an electrode contact placed in a periventricular nodule. Since this report, five more patients with partial intractable seizures and periventricular gray matter nodules were studied with invasive depth electrode recordings and, this time, at least one electrode contact placed in a periventricular nodule (Kothare *et al*, 1998; Dubeau *et al.*, unpublished data). In the three patients of Kothare *et al.* (1998), some or all seizures recorded originated in the PNH, and spread to the ipsilateral hippocampus before the amygdala. PNH were left occipital in one, left posterior in another and bilateral temporal in the third. The surgical outcome of these three patients was, however, not reported. In contrast, none of the seizures recorded in our two patients originated in the nodule and no interictal spiking could be seen from the nodules. In the first patient, PNH was in the right trigone and the epileptic discharge was left mesial temporal. In the second patient, two adjacent left occipital nodules (Fig. 2B) were found, and both interictal and ictal discharges were recorded from the overlying occipital cortex and ipsilateral amygdala and hippocampus. The first patient underwent a left selective amygdalo-hippocampectomy and had only one seizure eight days postoperatively with a follow-up of nine months. The second had three neighbourhood seizures postoperatively and one generalized attack 10 months later with a total follow-up of 13 months after the removal of the two nodules and overlying occipital cortex.

Functional and histological evidence has shown that neurones in PNH behave like normal neurones (Falconer *et al.*, 1990; Lee *et al.*, 1994; Dubeau *et al.*, 1995; Eksioglu *et al.*, 1996; Joseph, 1997;

Kuzniecky *et al.*, 1997; Li *et al.*, 1998). Their role in the genesis of seizures is, however, uncertain. A significant number of patients with PNH do not have seizures or epilepsy, and thus PNH may occur in individuals who are otherwise normal. As mentioned, the epilepsy syndrome described in patients with PNH is quite variable. Electroencephalographic data are conflicting, with normal or apparently contradictory EEG findings observed in many patients with either unilateral, bilateral or diffuse PNH. Finally, the clinical and electrographic features of PNH pointing to mesial temporal lobe origin are clearly misleading, and further recording from nodules and cortex as well as pathological studies should provide clarification. Periventricular nodular heterotopia may be part of a more widespread epileptogenic source, most apparent and manifested by temporal or by temporo-parieto-occipital epileptogenic discharges and clinical features. It is still unresolved whether PNH is to be regarded only as an index of a significant genetic or acquired insult (possibly ischemic) sustained by the developing brain, or whether it may represent an epileptogenic lesion and be directly responsible for the epilepsy. Interestingly, in one autopsy report of a patient with BPNH, fibre staining and immunohistochemical analysis demonstrated that the heterotopic neurones were richly innervated (Eksioglu *et al.*, 1996). It was not possible, however, to determine if the synaptic input was from within the nodules or from the cortex. This is certainly an important point: clarification may help determine the role of the nodules in the genesis of seizures describe in the majority of patients with PNH. It is also possible that in some patients there may be dual pathology with epileptogenic abnormalities arising in the temporal lobe, particularly the hippocampus (Raymond *et al.*, 1994; Cendes *et al.*, 1995; Li *et al.*, 1997; Battaglia *et al.*, 1997).

Dual pathology is defined as the presence of hippocampal atrophy in addition to an extrahippocampal lesion (Cendes *et al.*, 1995). The coexistence of hippocampal abnormalities, including hippocampal atrophy, is known to occur in some patients with CD. This was well demonstrated in particular in patients with intractable partial seizures and PNH (Raymond *et al.*, 1994), where ectopic gray matter was, at times, present in close anatomic contiguity with an atrophic or hypoplastic hippocampus. Our experience with surgical treatment of patients with dual pathology suggests that the best results are achieved when both the lesions and the atrophic hippocampus are resected (Li *et al.*, 1997). In our surgical series of 12 patients with PNH who had a temporal lobe resection, eight had histological or radiological hippocampal atrophy. Although they seemed to do better compared to patients with PNH only, none of them became seizure-free. All except one had focal unilateral or bilateral PNH.

Genetics and biology of PNH

The different types of periventricular nodular heterotopia appear to be heterogeneous, based on differences in the sex ratios (Table 3). However, the high incidence of females overall is striking (94 out of 138 are female). Bilateral and symmetric PNH (BPNH) have been observed in multiple individuals from several unrelated families. This was first described by Huttenlocher *et al.* (1991, 1994) who presented a family with six affected female members in four generations. After this initial description, seven other pedigrees were described with a total of 24 affected individuals (DiMario *et al.*, 1993; Oda *et al.*, 1993; Kamuro & Tenokuchi, 1993; Dubeau *et al.*, 1995; Eksioglu *et al.*, 1996; Jardine *et al.*, 1996). All these patients are female, and sex-linked dominant inheritance was suggested. The gene for BPNH has recently been mapped to chromosome Xq28 (Eksioglu *et al.*, 1996). Bilateral, symmetric and diffuse PNH is closely linked to markers on distal Xq28, and affected females represent obligate mosaics for the mutation. Male offspring of females with BPNH are normal, and have not been found to transmit the disorder. In addition, affected females exceeded normal females (11:6 in four pedigrees described by Eksioglu *et al.*, 1996), and there was a shortage of male offspring (the pedigrees included 17 females and only six males) and an excess of spontaneous abortions (approximately twice the expected rate of 20–25 per cent in normal pregnancies). The aborted fetus was always male in the few cases where the sex could be identified. The absence of affected males, the shortage of male offspring and the high miscarriage rate in the familial cases suggest that the defect may be lethal for males in this subgroup.

Recently, however, Dobyns *et al.* (1997) reported three unrelated boys with multiple congenital anomalies and mental retardation. They had BPNH, cerebellar hypoplasia, severe retardation, epilepsy, and syndactyly. Although clearly distinct from the classic BPNH syndrome found in females, they suggested that this disorder involves the same Xq28 locus and designated it as the BPNH/MR syndrome. The authors emphasized that BPNH may be observed in association with several other malformation syndromes including females with Ehlers–Danlos disease, and sporadic males with BPNH, mental retardation and other congenital abnormalities. They also included the BPNH–short gut syndrome described by Nezeloff *et al.* (1976) in two brothers; the BPNH–congenital nephrosis syndrome described in brothers by Palm *et al.* (1986); and the BPNH–frontonasal dysplasia syndrome recently observed by Guerrini (unpublished data) in two unrelated boys. These patients have heterotopia similar to those with 'classic BPNH' but they differ from it because of the male sex, the severe intellectual handicap, and the various congenital anomalies. Dobyns *et al.* (1997) hypothesized that all BPNH syndromes associated with significant mental retardation are or may be X-linked, as they have been only observed in males.

The same BPNH gene may be involved in both 'classic' BPNH and BPNH with mental retardation, where the latter represents either more severe expression in males with the same mutation, or a different mutations in the same gene. In the former case, since it is known that sex steroids play a role in brain development and maturation, males with the same mutation may be more severely affected. With respect to the genotype–phenotype correlations for different mutations, gross or submicroscopic deletions, as in the Miller–Dieker syndrome or other structural rearrangements, may produce a more severe phenotype than point mutations. Furthermore, mutations resulting in protein truncation, such as point mutations representing stop codons and base pair insertions and deletions resulting in a shift of the reading frame, are usually associated with a more severe phenotype than point mutations resulting in single amino acid substitutions. The location of the mutation along the gene is also important, since mutations in certain areas affect critical regions of the protein structure.

The female preponderance found in 'classic' BPNH also exists in sporadic BPNH. Analysis of 45 sporadic cases from the literature and our own series indicated that 76 per cent were female and the

Table 4. Types of periventricular nodular heterotopia

Type of PNH	Sex	Inheritance
1. *BPNH*		
• Classic or familial BPNH	Female	X-linked
• BPNH with Ehlers–Danlos syndrome	Female	?
• Sporadic BPNH	Female < male	? X-linked
• Associated with mental retardation and congenital anomalies		
BPNH/MR syndrome	Male	? X-linked
BPNH/short gut syndrome	Male	? X-linked
BPNH/nephrosis syndrome	Male	? X-linked
BPNH/frontonasal syndrome	Male	?
2. *Bilateral focal PNH*	Female and male with sex ratio skew	?
3. *Unilateral focal PNH*	Female and male with no sex ratio skew	?

Adapted from Dobyns *et al.* (1997).

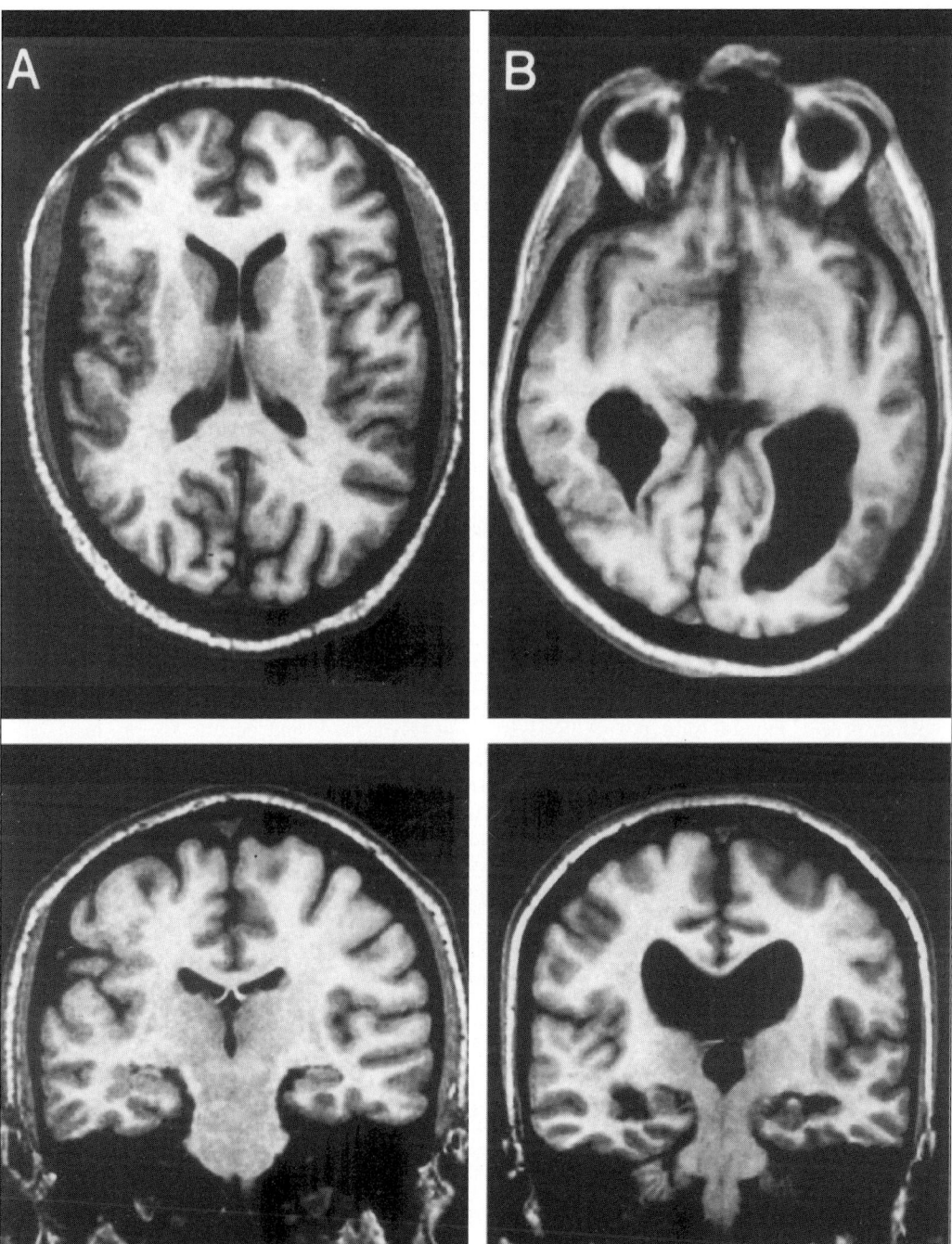

Fig. 4. Focal periventricular nodular heterotopia and associated polymicrogyria. (A) A 28-year-old man with normal development except for seizures that began at age 23. Axial and coronal T1-weighted images show nodules isointense to cortical gray matter, lining the lateral aspect of right temporal horn, with right perisylvian polymicrogyria. (B) A 25-year-old man with intellectual retardation and refractory seizures. Axial and coronal T1-weighted images show gray matter nodules lining both temporal and occipital horns, and bilateral temporo-occipital polymicrogyria. Note associated hippocampi hypoplasia, white matter hypoplasia and ventriculomegaly.

majority had a clinical picture which fits the classical description, i.e. average intelligence with seizures but without other neurological symptoms. However, some of the so-called sporadic cases in the literature may indeed have asymptomatic relatives with BPNH. Perhaps sporadic BPNH patients who otherwise resemble those with familial BPNH may also have abnormalities related to the same gene locus (Eksioglu *et al.*, 1996), but with different mutations resulting in decreased fertility.

Unilateral and bilateral focal PNH patients present with a somewhat different picture. Almost all the patients are sporadic, and the preponderance of females is not as striking, particularly in the unilateral focal group where both sexes are evenly represented. We have however seen a patient with focal periventricular nodules who responded poorly to temporal resection and whose mother also had poor outcome after temporal resection. Whether the mother also had periventricular nodules could not be demonstrated. In patients with focal PNH, seizures may occur more frequently, compared to patients with both 'classic' and sporadic BPNH (Table 3). These focal nodules show preferential location in the posterior temporal and trigonal-occipital regions, and this is difficult to explain on a genetic basis. However, the association of PNH with polymicrogyria found in a small number of patients (Fig. 4A, B., and Battaglia *et al.*, 1997), the vulnerable vascular watershed area of the trigonal and temporo-occipital regions (Guerrini *et al.*, 1997), and the possibility of increased prenatal risk factors which may lead to in utero impairment of perfusion in the developing brain, are arguments supporting an acquired basis for this type of PNH. Interestingly, however, Dobyns recently reported (unpublished data) two members of the same family with unilateral focal PNH.

Concluding remarks

The syndrome/s of periventricular nodular heterotopia is/are distinct from other types of migrational disorders. Several subtypes of PNH are now recognized, and genetic factors have been clearly defined in at least one: the 'classic' BPNH (Table 4). The identification of familial neuronal migration disorders is important not only for the insight these disorders may give into the mechanisms of cortical development, but also the genes involved may contribute to the etiology of epilepsy. Periventricular heterotopia represents a potentially important epilepsy susceptibility locus, since many affected individuals show only epilepsy with normal intelligence (Eksioglu *et al.*, 1996). It is unclear whether the heterotopic gray matter nodules are the epileptogenic source, or if the epilepsy is due to abnormalities in cortical wiring and neuronal function both during development and maturation. Pedigree analyses, biochemical and pathological studies, and direct recording of electrical activity from the nodules should provide further clarification. More definitive information will be available following the cloning of the gene(s) involved, and identification of the abnormal protein(s).

References

Barkovich, A.J. & Kjos, B.O. (1992): Gray matter heterotopias: MR characteristics and correlation with developmental and neurologic manifestations. *Radiology* **182**, 493–499.

Barkovich, A.J., Jackson Jr, D.E. & Boyer, R.S. (1989): Band heterotopia: a newly recognized neuronal migration anomaly. *Radiology* **171**, 455–458.

Barkovich, A.J., Kuzniecki, R., Dobyns, W., Jackson, G., Becker, L. & Evrard, L. (1996): A classification scheme for malformations of cortical development. *Neuropediatrics* **27 (2)**, 59–63.

Battaglia, G., Granata, T., Farina, L., D'Incerti, L., Franceschetti, S. & Avanzini, G. (1997): Periventricular nodular heterotopia: epileptogenic findings. *Epilepsia* **38 (11)**, 1173–1182.

Bergeron, R.T. (1967): Pneumoencephalographic demonstration of subependymal heterotopic cortical gray matter in children. *Am. J. Roentgenol. Radium Ther. Nucl. Med.* **101**, 168–177.

Canapicchi, R., Padolecchia, R., Puglioli, M., Collavoli, P., Marcella, F. & Valleriani, A.M. (1990): Eterotopie di sostanza grigia. *J. Neuroradiol.* **17,** 277–287.

Cendes, F., Cook, M.J., Watson, C., *et al.* (1995): Frequency and characteristics of dual pathology in patients with lesional epilepsy. *Neurology* **45,** 2058–2064.

Cupo, L.N., Pyeritz, R.E., Olson, J.L., McPhee, S.J., Hutchins, G.M. & McKusick, V.A. (1981): Ehlers–Danlos syndrome with abnormal collagen fibrils, sinus of Valsalva aneurysms, myocardial infarction, panacinar emphysema and cerebral heterotopias. *Am. J. Med.* **71,** 1051–1058.

Deeb, Z.L., Rothfus, W.E. & Maroon, J.C. (1985): MR imaging of heterotopic gray matter. *J. Comput. Assist. Tomogr.* **9 (6),** 1140–1141.

DiMario, F.J., Cobb, R.J., Ramsby, G.R. & Leicher, C. (1993): Familial band heterotopias simulating tuberous sclerosis. *Neurology* **43,** 1424–1426.

Dobyns, W.B., Andermann, E., Andermann, F., Czapansky-Beilman, D., Dubeau, F., Dulac, O., Guerrini, R., Hirsch, B., Ledbetter, D.H., Lee, N.S., Motte, J., Pinard, J.M., Radtke, R.A., Ross, M.E., Tampieri, D., Walsh, C.A. & Truwit, C.L. (1996): X-linked malformations of neuronal migration. *Neurology* **47,** 331–339.

Dobyns, W.B., Guerrini, R., Czapansky-Beilman, D.K., Pierpont, M.E.M., Breningstall, G., Yocks, D.H., Bonanni, P. & Truwit, C.L. (1997): Bilateral periventricular nodular heterotopia with mental retardation and syndactyly in boys: a new X-linked mental retardation syndrome. *Neurology* **49,** 1042–1047.

Dubeau, F., Tampieri, D., Lee, N., Andermann, E., Carpenter, S., Leblanc, R., Olivier, A., Radtke, R., Villemure, J.G. & Andermann F. (1995): Periventricular and subcortical nodular heterotopia: a study of 33 patients. *Brain* **118,** 1273–1287.

Eksioglu, Y.Z., Scheffer, I.E., Cardenas, P., Knoll, J., DiMario, F., Ramsby, G., Berg, M., Kamuro, K., Berkovic, S.F., Duyk, G.M., Parisi, J., Huttenlocher, P.R. & Walsh, C.A. (1996): Periventricular heterotopia: an X-linked dominant aberrant cerebral cortical development. *Neuron* **16,** 77–87.

Falconer, J., Wada, J.A., Martin, W. & Li, D. (1990): PET, CT, and MRI imaging of neuronal migration anomalies in epileptic patients. *Can. J. Neurol. Sci.* **17,** 35–39.

Friede, R.L. (1989): *Developmental neuropathology.* 2nd edition. Berlin: Springer-Verlag.

Guerrini, R., Dravet, C., Bureau, M., Mancini, J., Canapicchi, R., Livet, M.O. & Belmonte, A. (1996): Diffuse and localized dysplasias of cerebral cortex: clinical presentation, outcome, and proposal for a morphologic MRI classification based on a study of 90 patients. In: *Dysplasias of cerebral cortex and epilepsy,* eds. R. Guerrini, F. Andermann, R. Canapicchi, J. Roger, B. Zifkin & P. Pfanner, pp. 255–270. Philadelphia: Lippincott-Raven.

Guerrini, R., Dubeau, F., Dulac, O., Barkovich, A.J., Kuzniecky, R., Jones-Gotman, M., Canapicchi, R., Cross, H., Fish, D., Bonanni, P., Jambaqué, I. & Andermann, F. (1997): Bilateral parasagittal parietooccipital polymicrogyria and epilepsy. *Ann. Neurol.* **41,** 65–73.

Huttenlocher, P.R., Taravath, S. & Mojtahedi, S. (1991): Familial periventricular heterotopias and seizures in four generations (abstract). *Ann. Neurol.* **30,** 461.

Huttenlocher, P.R., Taravath, S. & Mojtahedi, S. (1994): Periventricular heterotopia and epilepsy. *Neurology* **44,** 51–55.

Jakob, H. (1936): Faktoren bei der Enstehung der normalen und der entwicklungsgestörten Hirnrinde. *Z. Ges. Neurol. Psychiat.* **155,** 1–39.

Jardine, P.E., Clarke, M.A. & Super, M. (1996): Familial bilateral periventricular nodular heterotopia mimics tuberous sclerosis. *Arch. Dis. Chil.* **74,** 244–246.

Joseph, J.T. (1997): Periventricular heterotopias display cortical degenerative neuropathology. *Neurology* **49,** 884–887.

Kamuro, K. & Tenokuchi, Y. (1993): Familial periventricular nodular heterotopia. *Brain Dev.* **15,** 237–241.

Kernohan, J.W. (1930): Cortical anomalies, ventricular heterotopias and occlusion of the acqueduct of Sylvius. *Arch. Neurol. Psychiat.* **23,** 460–480.

Kothare, S. V., Van Landingham, K., Armon, C., Friedman, A. & Radtke, R. (1998): Ictal EEG patterns from intracerebral depth electrodes placed within periventricular nodular heterotopias in 3 patients with gray matter heterotopias and refractory complex partial seizures (abstract). *Neurology* **50 (Suppl. 4),** A25.

Kuzniecky, R., Hetherington, H., Pan, J., Hugg, J., Palmer, C., Gilliam, F., Faught, E. & Morawetz, R. (1997): Proton spectroscopic imaging at 4.1 tesla in patients with malformations of cortical development and epilepsy. *Neurology* **48,** 1018–1024.

Layton, D.D. (1962): Heterotopic cerebral gray matter as an epileptogenic focus. *J. Neuropathol. Exp. Neurol.* **21,** 244–249.

Lee, N., Radtke, R.A., Gray, L., Burger, P.C., Montine, T.J., DeLong, G.R., Lewis, D.V., Oakes, W.J., Friedman, A.H. & Hoffman, J.M. (1994): Neuronal migration disorders: positron emission tomography correlations. *Ann. Neurol.* **35,** 290–297.

Li, L.M., Fish, D.R., Sisodiya, S.M. *et al.* (1995): High resolution magnetic resonance imaging in adults with partial or secondary generalised epilepsy attending a tertiary referral unit. *J. Neurol. Neurosurg. Psychiatry* **59,** 384–387.

Li, L.M., Dubeau, F., Andermann, F., Fish, D.R., Watson, C., Cascino, G.D., Berkovic, S.F., Moran, N., Duncan, J.S., Olivier, A., Leblanc, R., Olivier, A. & Harkness, W. (1997): Periventricular nodular heterotopia and intractable temporal lobe epilepsy: poor outcome after temporal lobe resection. *Ann. Neurol.* **41,** 662–668.

Li, L.M., Cendes, F., Bastos, A.C., Andermann, F., Dubeau, F. & Arnold, D.L. (1998): Neuronal metabolic dysfunction in patients with cortical developmental malformations – proton magnetic resonance spectroscopic imaging study. *Neurology* **50,** 755–759.

Martin Araguz, A., Moreno Martinez, J.M., Garrido Carrion, A. & Esteban Alonso, F. (1989): Heterotopias de sustancia gris: una causa infrecuente de epilepsia. *Arch. de Neurobiol.* **52 (3),** 140–143.

Meschede, F. (1866): Ein Fall von Heterotopie der grauen Substanz in den beiden Hemisphären des Grosshirns. *Arch. Path. Anat.* **37,** 567–570.

Mueller, C.F. (1970): Heterotopic gray matter. *Radiology* **94,** 357–358.

Nezeloff, C., Jaybert, F. & Lyon, G. (1976): Syndrome familial associant grêle court, malrotation intestinale, hypertrophie du pylore et malformation cérébrale: étude anatomo-clinique de trois observations. *Annales d'anatomie pathologique* **21,** 401–412.

Oda, T., Nagai, Y., Fujimoto, S., Sobajima, H., Kobayashi, M., Togari, H. & Wada, Y. (1993): Hereditary nodular heterotopia accompanied by mega cisterna magna. *Am. J. Med. Genet.* **47,** 268–271.

Osborn, R.E., Byrd, S.E., Naidich, T.P., Bohan, T.P. & Friedman, H. (1987): MR imaging of neuronal migrational disorders. *AJNR* **9,** 1101–1106.

Otto, R. (1887): Zur Hirnpathologie. *Virchows Arch. Path. Anat.* **110,** 81.

Palm, L., Hägerstrand, I., Kristoffersson, U., Blennow, G., Brun, A. & Jörgensen, C. (1986): Nephrosis and disturbances of neuronal migration in male siblings – a new hereditary disorder? *Arch. Dis. Child.* **61,** 545–548.

Raymond, A.A., Fish, D.R., Stevens, J.M., Sisodiya, S.M., Alsanjari, N. & Shorvon, S.D. (1994): Subependymal heterotopia: a distinct neuronal migration disorder associated with epilepsy. *J. Neurol. Neurosurg. Psychiatry* **57,** 1195–1202.

Ross, M.E., Allen, K.M., Srivastava, A.K., Featherstone, T., Gleeson, J.G., Hirsch, B., Harding, B.N., Andermann, E., Abdullah, R., Berg, M., Czapansky-Bielman, D., Flanders, D.J., Guerrini, R., Motte, J., Mira, A.P., Scheffer, I., Berkovic, S., Scaravilli, F., King, R.A., Ledbetter, D.H., Schlessinger, D., Dobyns, W.B. & Walsh, C.A. (1997): Linkage and physical mapping of X-linked lissencephaly/SBH (XLIS): a gene causing neuronal migration defects in human brain. *Hum. Mol. Genet.* **6 (4),** 555–562.

Sarnat, H.B. (1991): Cerebral dysplasias as expressions of altered maturational processes. *Can. J. Neurol. Sci.* **18,** 196–204.

Sarnat, H.B. (1992): Disorders of neuroblast migration. In: *Cerebral dysgenesis: embriology and clinical expression,* ed. H.B. Sarnat, pp. 245–274. New York: Oxford University Press.

Simmons, M.L., Frondoza, C.G. & Coyle, J.T. (1991): Immunocytochemical localization of N-acetyl-aspartate with monoclonal antibodies. *Neuroscience* **45,** 37–45.

Smith, A.S., Weinstein, M.A., Quencer, R.M., Muroff, L.R., Stonesifer, K.J., Li, F.C., Wener, L., Soloman, M.A., Cruse, R.P., Rosenberg, L.H. & Berke, J.P. (1988): Association of heterotopic gray matter with seizures: MR imaging. *Radiology* **168,** 195–198.

Smith, A.S., Ross, J.S., Blaser, S.I. & Weinstein, M.A. (1989): Magnetic resonance imaging of disturbances in neuronal migration: illustration of an embryologic process. *Radiographics* **9 (3),** 509–522.

Thomas, P., Bossan, A., Lacour, J.P., Chanalet, S., Ortonne, J.P. & Chatel, M. (1996): Ehlers–Danlos syndrome with subependymal periventricular heterotopias. *Neurology* **46,** 1165–1167.

Tüngel, C. (1857): Ein Fall von Neubildung grauer Hirnsubstanz. *Virchows Arch. Path. Anat.* **16,** 166–168.

Zimmerman, R.A., Bilaniuk, L.T. & Grossman, R.I. (1983): Computed tomography in migratory disorders of human brain development. *Neuroradiology* **25,** 257–263.

Zisch, R. & Artmann W. (1991): MRI in the diagnostic of heterotopic gray matter: report of three cases first discovered in adulthood. *Neuroradiology* **33,** 527–528.

Chapter 18

The clinical and pathophysiological relevance of evoked potentials study in neuronal migration disorders

Vidmer Scaioli[1], Tiziana Granata[2], Giorgio Battaglia[1], Ludovico D'Incerti[3], Roberto Spreafico[1], Ferruccio Panzica[1], Giuliano Avanzini[1] and Lucia Angelini[2]

[1]Divisione di Neurofisiopatologia; [2]Divisione di Neuropsichiatria Infantile; [3]Divisione di Neuroradiologia Diagnostica, Istituto Nazionale Neurologico 'C. Besta', Via Celoria 11, 20133 Milan, Italy.

Summary

We studied pattern and flash visual (VEP) and somatosensory evoked potentials (SEP) in 23 patients with various forms of neuronal migration disorder (NMD). The *in vivo* diagnosis was in all cases confirmed by magnetic resonance imaging (MRI). The neurophysiological findings were generally in agreement with the distribution of alterations revealed by MRI, although in some patients EP abnormalities were greater and in others less than expected from the MRI findings. Several kinds of changes were found on EP, including global abolition or severe deterioration of components, selective loss of SEP components, VEP changes depending on spatial orientation of stimulation, asymmetric distribution of EPs, and EPs arising in non-typical areas (VEPs from centro-parietal regions, SEP N20 component with unusual anterior frontal or parieto-occipital distribution) associated with asymmetry between the two sides. The latter finding, in patients with cortical polymicrogyria and unilateral paratrigonal heterotopia, indicates extensive reorganization of the cortical representation of certain sensory modalities. In the five patients with parietal bilateral polymicrogyria there was a close correlation between clinical symptoms and signs, MRI findings and neurophysiological changes. These findings indicate that EP studies are a useful and reliable means for exploring pathophysiological changes in NMDs and for revealing CNS plasticity. EP can be useful to identify functional cortical areas that must be preserved in NMD patients undergoing surgery.

Introduction

Developmental brain dysgeneses, commonly known as neuronal migration disorders (NMDs), are a heterogeneous group of central nervous system (CNS) disorders that include the severe form lyssencephaly, which often leads to early death, and more benign forms such as focal heterotopia. Clinical symptoms may be evident soon after birth or may appear later as seizures (often drug refractory), neurological syndromes, mental retardation and mood disorders (Barkovich, 1995).

Latest generation MRI can usually provide a definitive clinical diagnosis, and is sensitive enough to define the gross anatomical extent of the morphological abnormalities (Barkovich, 1995). However, subtle anatomo-functional changes can also occur, affecting intracortical neuronal connections and the organization of thalamo-cortical pathways.

In order to further explore functional changes in NMDs, we performed visual evoked potential (VEP) and median nerve somatosensory evoked potential (SEP) studies in a series of 23 patients with various forms of these disorders.

Material and methods

Patients

The 23 patients were grouped according to the *in vivo* MRI diagnosis. There were 12 patients with polymicrogyria, seven with heterotopia, two with diffuse pachygyria, one with lyssencephaly and one with complex cortical dysplasia (CD). In the patients with polymicrogyria (Table 1) the locations of morphological changes evidenced by MRI were: bilateral parietal parasagittal (five patients); bilateral parieto-occipital (two patients); frontal bilateral (one patient); diffuse and associated with encephalocele (one patient); right hemispheric (one patient); left hemispheric (one patient); and right temporal-insular (one patient).

The patients with heterotopia (Table 2) had bilateral and symmetrical periventricular nodular heterotopia (two patients); unilateral periventricular nodular heterotopia (on left and one right sided) (two patients); and band heterotopia (three patients). The third group of patients (Table 3) included those with pachygyria (two patients), lyssencephaly (one patient) and CD (one patient).

Table 1. Polymicrogyria

	Parietal SEP	Frontal SEP	Visual EP	Comments
Parietal parasagittal				
1 C.D./36/M	N20 changes	N30 preserved	Normal	SEP asymmetry
2 C.S./36/M	N20 changes	N30 preserved	Normal	SEP asymmetry
3 DE N.A./68/M	N20 changes	N30 deteriorated	Abnormal	SEP asymmetry
4 R.A./24/M	N20 deteriorated	N30 preserved	Mild changes	
5 G.R./54/M	N20 deteriorated	N30 preserved	Normal	
Parietal, bilateral				
6 B.D./13/M	Left N20 deteriorated	N30 deteriorated	Right/left asymmetry	SEP/VEP asymmetry
7 M.V./7/M	N20 deteriorated	N30 deteriorated	Abnormal	SEP asymmetry
Frontal, bilateral				
8 C.N./12/F	Right/left asymmetry	Right/left asymmetry	Right/left asymmetry	Global clockwise rotation
Diffuse				
9 S.S./13/M	Mild changes	Normal	Mild changes	
Right hemisphere				
10 M.F./12/M	Unilateral changes	Unilateral changes	Asymmetry	SEP/VEP asymmetry
Right temporo-insular				
11 P.M.G./51/F	Normal	Unilateral changes	Not performed	
Left hemisphere				
12 C.G.L./12/F	Unilateral changes	Unilateral changes	Asymmetry	SEP/VEP asymmetry

Visual evoked potentials

Pattern and flash VEP studies were performed. Pattern VEP employed monocular full-field pattern reversal stimulation by means of checkerboard and vertical and horizontal bars (60 minutes spatial frequency). In flash VEP binocular stimulation was performed with a Ganzfield stimulator producing white flashes of one joule intensity administered at the rate of 0.9 Hz. The average of two series of 100 individual responses were analysed.

Sensory evoked potentials

The right and left median nerve at the wrist were stimulated at the rate of 1.0 Hz. Stimulation intensity was set at the threshold of thumb muscle contraction. Two averaged series of 200–500 individual responses were obtained. Two additional series were obtained to study the brachial plexus N9, the spinal N11 and N13, and the P14–N18 subcortical components.

Recording

On the scalp the evoked signal was recorded by 16 electrodes, distributed according to the 10–20 system. Latencies and amplitudes of waveforms and components were evaluated and compared with control. In addition, spatial mappings of the evoked potentials were constructed by software manipulation of the neurophysiological signals.

Results

The main electrophysiological alterations found are summarized in Tables 1–3.

Table 2. Heterotopia

	Parietal SEP	Frontal SEP	Visual EP	Comments
Nodular periventricular, bilateral				
13 C.I./18/F	Normal	Normal	Normal	
14 R.A./36/F	Normal	Normal	Normal	
Nodular periventricular, right				
15 S.P.F./13/M	Left N20 changes	Left N30 changes	Right/left asymmetry	SEP/VEP global changes
Nodular periventricular, left				
16 F.G./43/F	Right N20 changes	Right N30 changes	Right/left asymmetry	Clockwise rotation
Band heterotopia				
17 D.E./2/F	Left N20 changes	Left N30 changes	Normal	SEP asymmetry
18 G.K./18/F	N20 changes	N30 deteriorated	Normal	
19 P.I./42/F	N20 changes	N30 deteriorated	Normal	

Table 3.

	Parietal SEP	Frontal SEP	Visual EP	Comments
Lissencephaly				
20 P.L./1F	N20 deteriorated	N3 deteriorated	Normal	Selective SEP changes
Pachygyria				
21 C.V./8/F	N20 mild changes	N30 deteriorated	Abnormal P-VEP	F-VEP P1 pronounced
22 C.A./12/F	Normal	N30 deteriorated	Deteriorated	
Complex CD				
23 R.M./22/M	N20 deteriorated	N30 deteriorated	Deteriorated	Global EPs changes

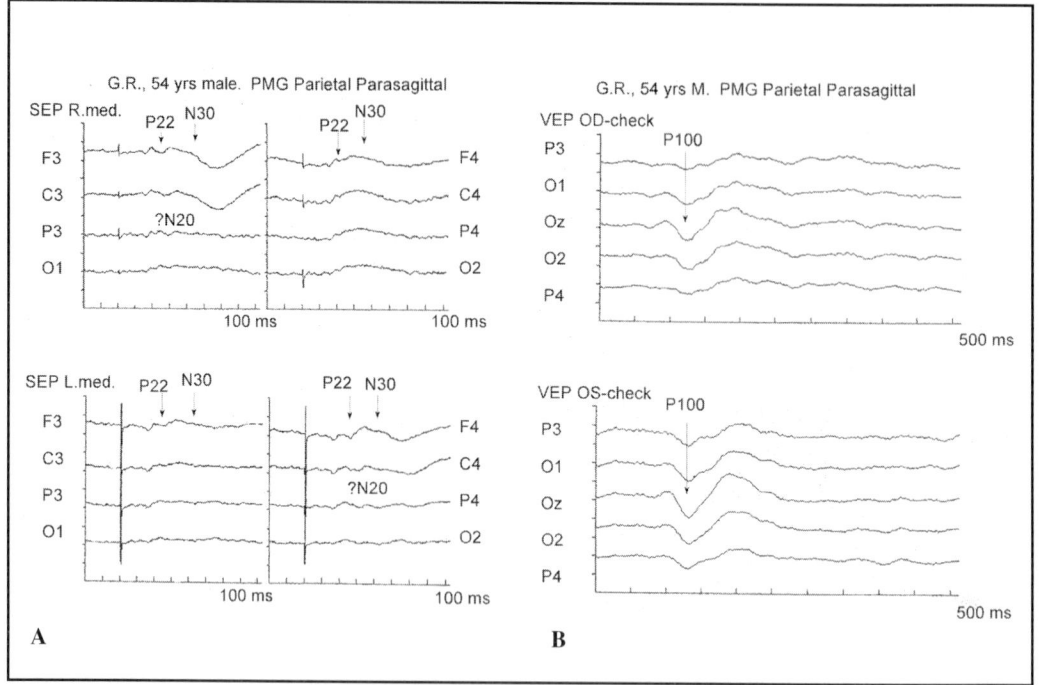

Fig. 1. (A) SEP recordings from patient 5. The patient has parietal and parasagittal polymicrogyria. In parieto-occipital leads no contralateral N20 cortical response was recognized; in frontal leads the P22 and N30 components were normal in shape and distribution. The patient had clinical symptoms of a defect in stereognosis, with preservation of elementary sensory functions. (B) Pattern VEP recordings from patient 5. The visual responses are normal in shape, wave form and distribution. P100 latency and amplitude are normal.

Polymicrogyria (PMG)

In this sub-group of patients, SEPs were characterized by deterioration or loss in components of cortical origin and VEPs were characterized by changes in waveform and distribution, and SEPs were more compromised than VEPs. Asymmetry of EP changes was another prominent feature present in most patients. In patient 8, asymmetry was marked and took the form of a global clockwise rotation of VEP and SEP locations.

Although in general the correlation between the MRI distribution of the anatomical alterations and EP results was satisfactory, in patients 4, 6 and 7 alterations were much more severe than would be expected from the MRI findings. By contrast, in patient 11 with temporo-insular involvement, in patient 8 with frontal and in patient 9 with diffuse involvement, cortical functionality was preserved in spite of gross abnormalities on MRI.

There was good correlation between MR and EP findings in the those (patients 1-5) with parietal parasagittal involvement; thus a defect in stereognosis was the only sensory impairment detected on clinical examination.

Figs. 1A and B show the SEP and VEP recordings of patient 5 which illustrate these findings.

Heterotopia

The two patients (12 and 13) with symmetrically distributed bilateral nodular periventricular heterotopia had normal evoked responses. By contrast, marked changes both in wave forms and in

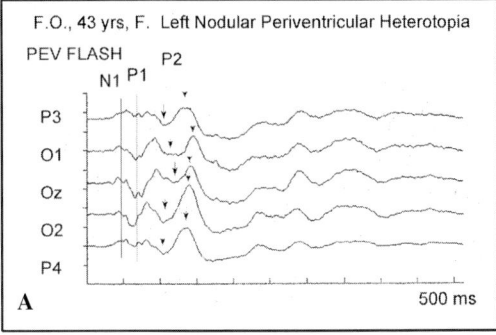

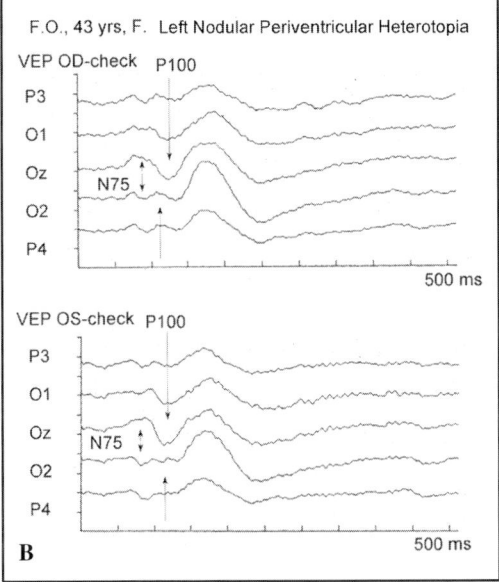

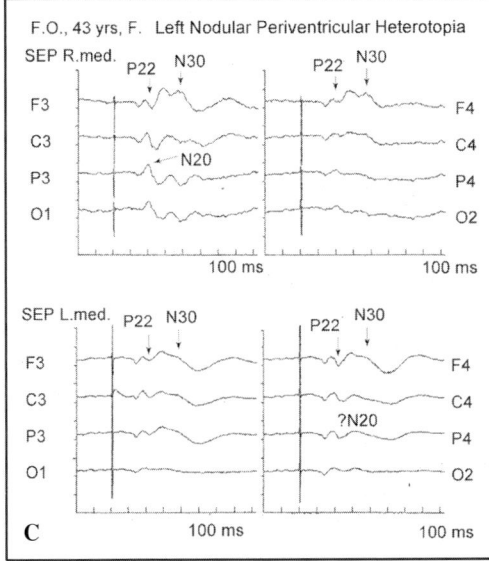

the cortical distribution of VEPs and SEPs were found in the two patients (14 and 15) with unilateral periventricular heterotopia, correlated with the side of the abnormality. P-VEPs and F-VEPs were markedly asymmetric between left and right hemispheres. Figs. 2A-C illustrate these findings in patient 15.

The three patients (patients 16–18) with band heterotopia had normal or mildly altered VEPs, while SEPs revealed clear evidence of centroparietal or frontal origin alteration. These findings are illustrated in Figs. 3A and B which show recordings from patient 18.

Pachygyria

The two non-twin sisters with pachygyria (patients 20 and 21) showed severely deteriorated VEPs and SEPs; however the centroparietal SEP components were quite well preserved. Recordings from patient 21 are shown in Figs. 4A-C.

The patient with lyssencephaly had normal VEPs in spite of severe bilateral SEP alterations. The patient with CD complex had global EP deterioration, and in particular no waveforms of cortical origin could be identified.

Fig. 2. (A) Flash VEP in patient 16. The patient has left periventricular nodular heterotopia. While the early negative component is symmetrically distributed across the midline, subsequent waves, labelled P1 and P2, are clearly asymmetric in distribution. P1 has greater amplitude than P2. (B) Pattern VEP obtained in patient 16. In the mid-occipital lead the P100 component is normal in shape and latency. However, N75 and P100 are asymmetrically distributed across the mid-occipital region, and show an uncrossed-asymmetry pattern. No definite visual clinical signs were present. (C) SEP recordings in patient 16. In frontal leads P22 and N30 components are normal. A mild asymmetry of N20 amplitude is evident in centroparietal leads. Sub-cortical P14 and N18 components are clearly recognizable. No clinical symptoms or signs were found on clinical examination.

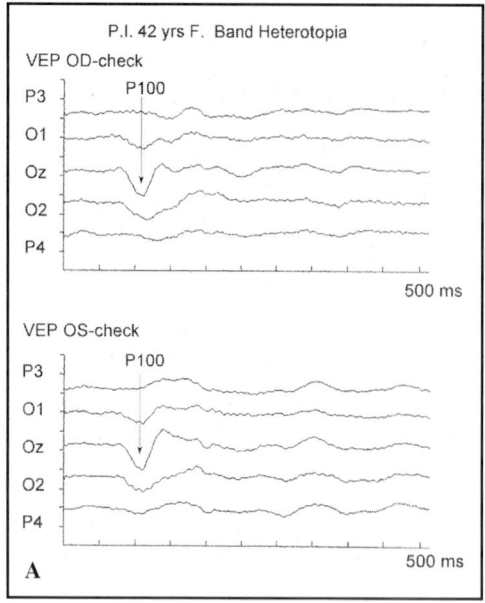

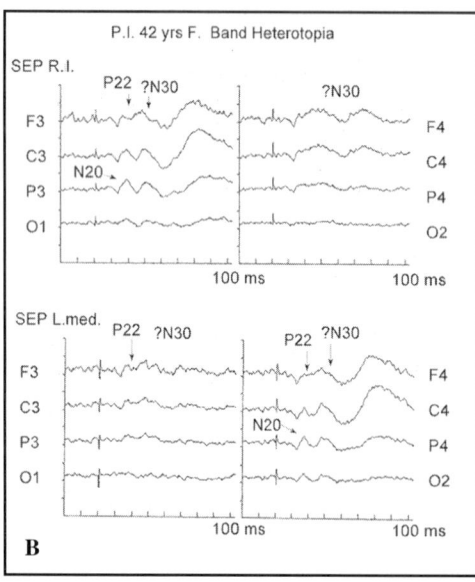

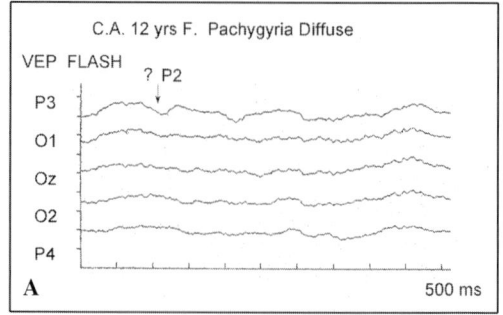

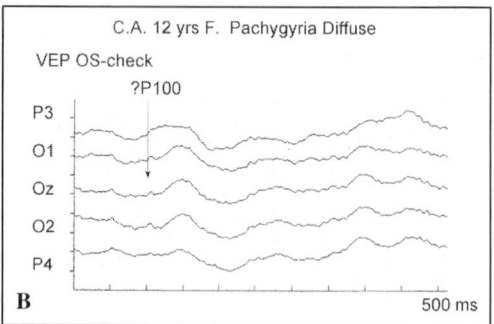

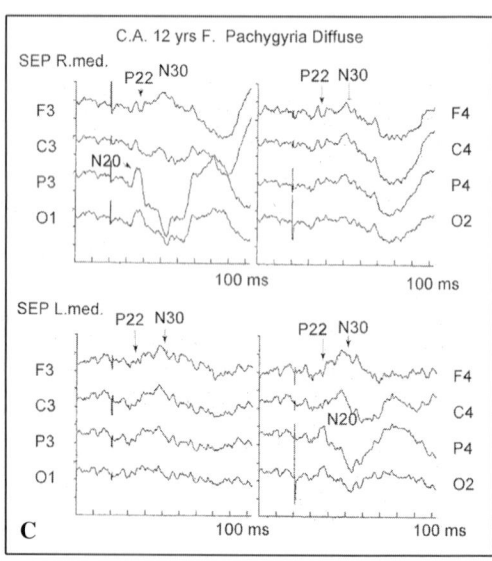

Fig. 3. (A) Pattern VEPs in patient 19 with band heterotopia. The P100 component is normal in shape, latency, amplitude and distribution. (B) SEPs in patient 19. The centro-parietal N20 component is normal; in frontal leads P22 is normal but it is difficult to distinguish the following N30.

Fig. 4. (A) Flash VEPs in patient 22. The patient has diffuse pachygyria. Occipital responses totally absent; only in the parietal region is a questionable positive component present. (B) Pattern VEPs in patient 22. The waveform appear totally absent and no definite P100 component is present. (C) SEP recording in patient 22. The N20 and frontal P22 and N30 are normal or show minimal desynchronization.

Discussion

This study of NMD patients revealed various neurophysiological changes in NMDs attributable to different pathophysiological mechanisms (de Rijk-van Andel et al., 1993; Nishimura & Nishimura, 1995). In all but one of the polymicrogyria cases, the EP abnormalities were consistent with cortical involvent in somatosensory-specific areas. The clockwise rotation of the cortical distribution of EPs could be explained, in the patient with frontal PMG, by a global reorganization of subcortical/cortical sensory connections, rather than intracortical re-arrangement.

In the five patients with parietal bilateral polymicrogyria, the relations between clinical clinical symptoms and signs, MRI findings and neurophysiological changes were impressive; thus, while elementary sensory functions were preserved, there was a selective disturbance in stereognosis which correlated with disorganization of parietal SEP components. A similar finding was reported by Mauguière et al. (1983) and Raymond et al. (1997) .

In patients with unilateral nodular heterotopia, cortical functions in the areas close to the nodular dysplastic tissue (located subcortically) were deteriorated and were associated with a displacement of the cortical representation of the VEPs, SEPs or both. By contrast the alterations observed in patients with band heterotopia were confined to the central SEP components, and no evidence of dysfunction in occipital and frontal areas was found.

In the lyssencephaly patient, SEPs findings were similar to those reported by Di Capua et al. (1993); however in our patient, occipital cortical functionality, as revealed by VEP findings, was well preserved. This could be due to the better anatomical preservation of the occipital lobes as shown by MRI. This would agree with the results of Barkovich's (1995) MRI study on a larger series of lyssencephaly patients.

In accordance with the results of Coupland & Sarnat et al., (1990) and de Rijk-van Andel et al. (1993), who reported abnormal VEP findings in 3/3 CD patients (including lyssencephaly and pachygyria), we observed marked VEP changes in the patients with pachygyria.

By comparing MRI abnormal findings with EPs results, we were able to identify normal functional areas and their cortical distribution in several cases where the *in vivo* MRI findings indicated gross abnormality suggesting the utility of EP studies in planning surgery in NMD patients; such studies can identify cortical areas specifically concerned with a given sensory modality, and which therefore have to be preserved during the operation. Finally, in the same patients, neurophysiological investigation of NMDs patients can reveal unexpected plasticity in the supplementary areas (Maegaki et al., 1995; Valeriani et al., 1997) and contribute to our understanding of cortical sensory functionality and organization (Pruel et al., 1997; Spreafico et al., 1998).

In conclusion, the present study shows that different pathophysiological mechanisms are involved in NMDs. Functional changes in NMDs can be the result of reorganization of thalamo-cortical projection systems or intracortical functional changes.

Acknowledgement

Supported by the Mariani Foundation for Paediatric Neurology, Milan and by grant ICS 030.3/RFBS/223 from the Italian Ministry of Health.

References

Barkovich, J.A. (1995): Disorders of neuronal migration and organization. In: *Magnetic resonance in epilepsy*, eds. R.I. Kuzniecky & G.D. Jackson. New York: Raven Press.

Coupland, S.G. & Sarnat, H.B. (1990): Visual and auditory evoked potentials correlates of cerebral malformations. *Brain and Development* **12**, 466–472.

de Rijk-van Andel, J.F. Arts, W.F. & de Weerd, A.W. (1993): EEG and evoked potentials in a series of 21 patients with lissencephaly type I. *Neuropediatrics* **23 (1),** 4–9.

Di Capua, M., Vigevano, F. & Wisniewski, K. (1993): Somatosensory evoked potentials in hemimegalencephaly and lyssencephaly: anatomo-functional correlations. *Brain Dev.* **15,** 253–257.

Maegaki, Y., Yamamoto, T. & Takeshita, K. (1995): Plasticity of central motor and sensory pathways in a case of unilateral extensive cortical dysplasia: investigation of magnetic resonance imaging, trancranial magnetic stimulation and short-latency somatosensory evoked potentials. *Neurology* **45(12),** 2255–2261

Mauguière, F., Desmedt, J.E. & Courjon, J. (1983): Astereognosis and dissociated loss of frontal or parietal components of somatosensory evoked potentials in hemispheric lesions: detailed correlations with clinical signs and computerized tomographic scanning. *Brain* **106,** 271–311.

Nishimura, S. & Nishimura, M. (1995): Somatosensory evoked potentials in severely handicapped patients. *No to Hattatsu (Brain and Development)* **27 (3),** 197–292.

Preul, M.C., Leblanc, R., Cendes. F., Dubeau, F., Reutens, D., Spreafico, R., Battaglia, G., Avoli, M., Langevin, P., Arnold, D. & Villemure, J.G. (1997): Functional and organization in dysgenetic cortex. *J. Neurosurgery* **87,** 113-121.

Raymond, A.A., Joned, S.J., Fish, D.R., Stewart, J., Stevens, J.M. (1997): Somatosensory evoked potentials in adults with cortical dysgenesis and epilepsy. *Electroenceph. Clin. Neurophysiol.* **104,** 132–142.

Spreafico, R., Battaglia, G., Arcelli, P., Anderman, F., Dubeau, F., Palmini, A., Olivier, A., Villemure, J.G., Tampieri, D., Avanzini, G. & Avoli, M. (1998): Cortical dysplasia. An immunocytochemical study of three patients. *Neurology* **50,** 27–36.

Valeriani, M., Restuccia, D., Di Lazzaro, V., Le Pera, D., Scerrati, M., Tonali, P. & Mauguière, F. (1997): Giant central N20–P22 with normal area 3b N20–P20: an argument in favour of an area 3a generator of early median nerve cortical SEPs? *Electroenceph. Clin. Neurophysiol.* **104,** 60–67.

Chapter 19

Surgical pathology of cortical dysplasia, tuberous sclerosis and dysembryoplastic neuroepithelial tumours: experience with 55 cases in a recent series of 230 patients with chronic epilepsy

Basile Pasquier[1], Michel Peoc'h[1], Raphaelle Barnoud[1], Dominique Pasquier[1], Philippe Kahane[2], Dominique Hoffmann[2], Alim Louis Benabid[2] and Claudio Munari[2]

[1]Service d'Anatomie Pathologique, Centre Hospitalier Régional et Universitaire CHU, B.P. 217X, 38043 Grenoble Cedex 9, France
[2]Dipartimento di Scienze Neurologiche, Centro Regionale per la Chirurgia dell'Epilessia, Ospedale Niguarda Ca' Granda, Piazza Ospedale Maggiore 3, 20162 Milan, Italy

Summary

In a recent series of 230 consecutive patients who underwent surgery in our institution for medically-intractable epilepsy, 15 were identified with cortical dysplasias (CD), five with tuberous sclerosis (TS) and 35 with dysembryoplastic neuroepithelial tumours (DNETs). Among the 15 cases of CD, 14 revealed changes consistent with focal cortical dysplasia (FCD): localized disruption of the normal cortical lamination by large bizarre neurons; close mixture of giant neurons and 'ballooned' cells in both deeper layers of cortex and subcortical white matter. In the one remaining case, CD was characterized by a hypercellular molecular layer with increased numbers of neurons and glia associated with clusters of neurons in the cortex. In five children, the characteristic lesions of TS were present consisting of multifocal cortical tubers (CTs) and subependymal giant cell astrocytomas (SEGAs). CTs appeared as firm nodular and often calcified lesions. Histologically, CTs exhibited abnormal cortical lamination, neuronal dysmorphism with giant neurons and variable numbers of large and eosinophilic cells looking like 'ballooned' cells of FCD. All SEGAs were localized near the anterior or medial part of the ventricular system. The tumoural population was made of large spindle to epithelioid cells and of giant ballon-like cells with a striking perivascular clustering. In 35 surgical specimens DNETs were identified. The main pathological characteristics consisted of intracortical location, multinodular pattern with mucoid substance accumulation, and a 'specific glioneuronal element'. An inconstant additional feature was an oligoglial, astrocytic or mixed oligoastrocytic nodularity. Various 'dysplastic' features mainly consisting of atypical multinucleated giant cells (15 cases) and CD (14 cases) were also observed in the cerebral tissue adjacent to DNETs. Herein we have focused on the main pathological features of CD, TS, and DNETs according to the most recent literature.

Introduction

Epilepsy, one of the most common neurological disorders, is a major problem of public health. In an increasing number of countries, surgery is now considered as an acceptable treatment for selected patients with partial drug-resistant seizures (Kahane et al., 1993; Wolf & Wiestler, 1993). Modern epilepsy surgery requires specialized centres with a multidisciplinary team of highly trained physicians among whom pathologists bring today a major contribution (Plate et al., 1993; Wolf & Wiestler, 1993; Vital et al., 1994 Pasquier et al., 1996). We report our experience with a recent series of patients who underwent surgery for medically-intractable epilepsy due to three pathological conditions: cortical dysplasia (CD), tuberous sclerosis (TS) and dysembryoplastic neuroepithelial tumours (DNETs). Hereafter, we will focus on the main pathological features encountered in the central nervous system (CNS) lesions of these three major epileptogenic disorders.

Patients, materials and methods*

Between March 1, 1990 and January 31, 1996, 230 consecutive patients underwent surgical treatment for partial drug-resistant epilepsy at the Department of Neurosciences, University of Grenoble. The presurgical procedures were conducted in order to plan a tailored cortical excision (corticectomy) of the epileptic zone and/or lesional excision (lesionectomy). A detailed description of the surgical techniques used in our centre has been published elsewhere (Munari et al., 1995). All tissue specimens of 26 lesionectomies, 93 corticectomies and 111 combined lesionectomies and corticectomies were fixed in 10% buffered formalin, embedded in paraffin. In each case, sections were cut at 2–3 µm thick and stained for each case with hematoxylin-erythrosin-saffron (HES). In selected cases, additional special stains (Bielschowsky silver method for axons; luxol-fast-blue stain combined with hematoxylin-erythrosin: LFB/HE) and immunohistochemical reactions (glial fibrillary acidic protein: GFAP; synaptophysin; neuron-specific enolase: NSE; neurofilament protein; and S-100 protein) were performed. Tumours were classified according to the revised World Health Organization (WHO) classification for tumours of the CNS (Kleihues et al., 1993).

Results

Table 1 gives the main clinicopathological results for each group of patients. In 15 cases the pathological findings were consistent with cortical dysplasia (CD). Among them, 14 revealed changes characteristic of focal or nodular cortical dysplasia (FCD). In 8 FCD, the pathological findings were localized in the frontal areas and in all 14 cases the focal disorder was unilateral. The cortical surface appeared normal to the naked eye in 6 FCD and in eight cases there was thickening of the cortical ribbon and blurring of the grey–white matter junction. Histologically, all 14 cases revealed the following features with some minor individual variations: localized disruption of the normal cortical lamination (Fig. 1) by large bizarre neurons (Fig. 2); abnormalities of shape and orientation of these giant neurons (Fig. 3), present in all but the first cortical layer; close mixture of giant neurons and 'ballooned' cells in both deeper layers of cortex (Figs. 4 and 5) and subcortical white matter (Fig. 6). In two cases of FCD, randomly distributed Rosenthal fibres in the white matter were also identified. In the remaining case, CD was characterized by a hypercellular molecular layer with increased numbers of neurons and glia associated with clusters of neurons in the cortex (without giant neurons and/or 'ballooned' cells). This latter case was classified among CD, in the broadest sense. In five children under the age of six years, brain lesions characteristic of tuberous sclerosis (TS) were present, consisting of multifocal cortical tubers (CTs) and subependymal giant cell astrocytomas (SEGAs; WHO grade I). CTs appeared as firm nodular (Fig. 7) and often calci-

---

* In order to present a more comprehensive illustration of the CNS lesions of TS we have added to the above mentioned surgical specimens an unpublished and demonstrative autopsy case of this condition. This typical case was from a 18-month-old girl referred to our hospital for uncontrollable seizures from birth to death in March, 1996.

Chapter 19 Surgical pathology of CD, TS and DNETs

Table 1. Main clinicopathological characteristics of cortical dysplasia, tuberous sclerosis and dysembryoplastic neuro-epithelial tumours in a series of 230 patients with chronic epilepsy.

Pathological diagnosis	Number of cases of lesions	Anatomical location (no. of cases)	Median age of patients (yrs)		Mean duration of seizures (yr)
			at onset of seizures	at surgery	
Cortical dysplasia	15	T (3), TF (1), TO (1), F (4), FP (3), P (2), PO (1)	3.7	21.2	17.5
Tuberous sclerosis*	5	TF (1), F (4)	1.3	3.9	2.6
Dysembryoplasic neuroepithelial tumours	35	T (22), TO (2), TP (1), TPO (1), C (2), F (3), O (2), P (2)	8.9	21.7	12.8

C, central; F, frontal; FP, frontoparietal; T, temporal; TF, temporofrontal; TP, temporoparietal; TPO, temporoparietooccipital O, occipital; P, parietal; PO, parietooccipital; yr = year.
*: topography of subependymal giant cell astrocytomas associated in each case with multifocal cortical tubers.

Table 2. Main pathological features in 35 dysembryoplastic neuroepithelial tumours.

Pathological features	Number of cases
Tumour location	
neocortical area*	26
mesial temporal structures	9
Tumour involvement	
cortex	35
white matter	28
pia	7
Specific glioneuronal element	35
Nodularity	
oligoglial	10
astrocytic	9
oligoglial and astrocytic	5
Calcification	14
Vascular proliferation	4
Mitosis	4
Necrosis	0

* See Table 1 for the cerebral lobar repartition.

fied lesions within the cerebral cortex. Histologically CTs exhibited abnormal cortical lamination (Fig. 8), neuronal dysmorphism (Figs. 9 and 10) with variable numbers of large and eosinophilic cells (Fig. 11) looking like 'ballooned' cells of FCD. These large and eosinophilic cells often expressed GFAP (Fig. 12) and some of them both glial and neuronal markers. All SEGAs were localized near the anterior or mesial part of the ventricular system. The tumoural population was made up of large spindle to epithelioid cells and of giant balloon-like cells (Fig. 13) with a striking perivascular clustering (Fig. 14). Large amounts of calcification (Fig. 15) were also present as well as scattered mastocytes within a fibrovascular stroma. Occasional neurone-like cells possessed vesicular nuclei with prominent nucleoli. Rare mitotic figures were also noted. All five SEGAs showed variable immunoreactivity for GFAP (Fig. 15), S-100 protein and neuronal markers (Fig. 16). In the autopsy case, coronal sections of the brain revealed bilateral CTs as well as multiple subependymal nodules and several foci of nodular cortical heterotopia (Figs. 17 and 18). In 35 surgical specimens and mainly from the temporal areas (26 cases) DNETs (WHO grade I) were

229

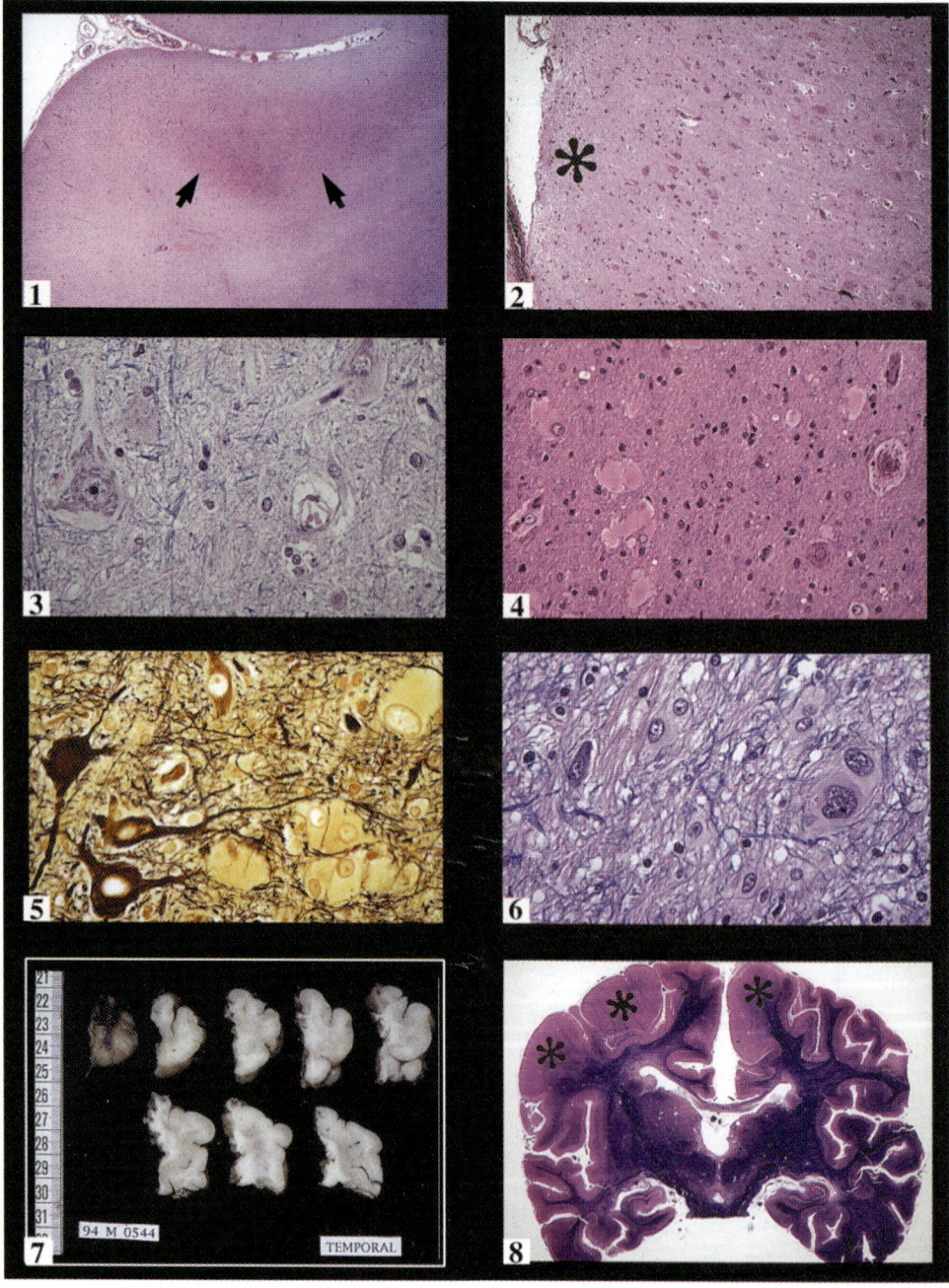

Fig. 1. Focal cortical dysplasia: focal widening (arrows) of a gyrus (HES ×25).
Fig. 2. Focal cortical dysplasia: giant neurons in all layers except the first one (asterisk) (LFB/HE ×100),
Fig. 3. Focal cortical dysplasia: giant neurons with coarse Nissl bodies and processes (LFB/HE×400)
Fig. 4. Focal cortical dysplasia: giant neurons and balloon cells in the deeper cortex (HES ×200).
Fig. 5. Focal cortical dysplasia: silver impregnation giant neurons (brown); balloon cells appear as round to polygonal with a yellow cytoplasm (Bielschowsky ×200)
Fig. 6. Focal cortical dysplasia: balloon cells with atypical nuclei in the subcortical white matter (LFB/HE ×200)
Fig. 7. Tuberous sclerosis: serial cut sections of a temporal gyrus showing a pale and nodular cortical tuber.
Fig. 8. Tuberous sclerosis: total coronal slice of the brain showing multifocal cortical tubers (asterisks) (LFB/HE ×0.6).

Chapter 19 Surgical pathology of CD, TS and DNETs

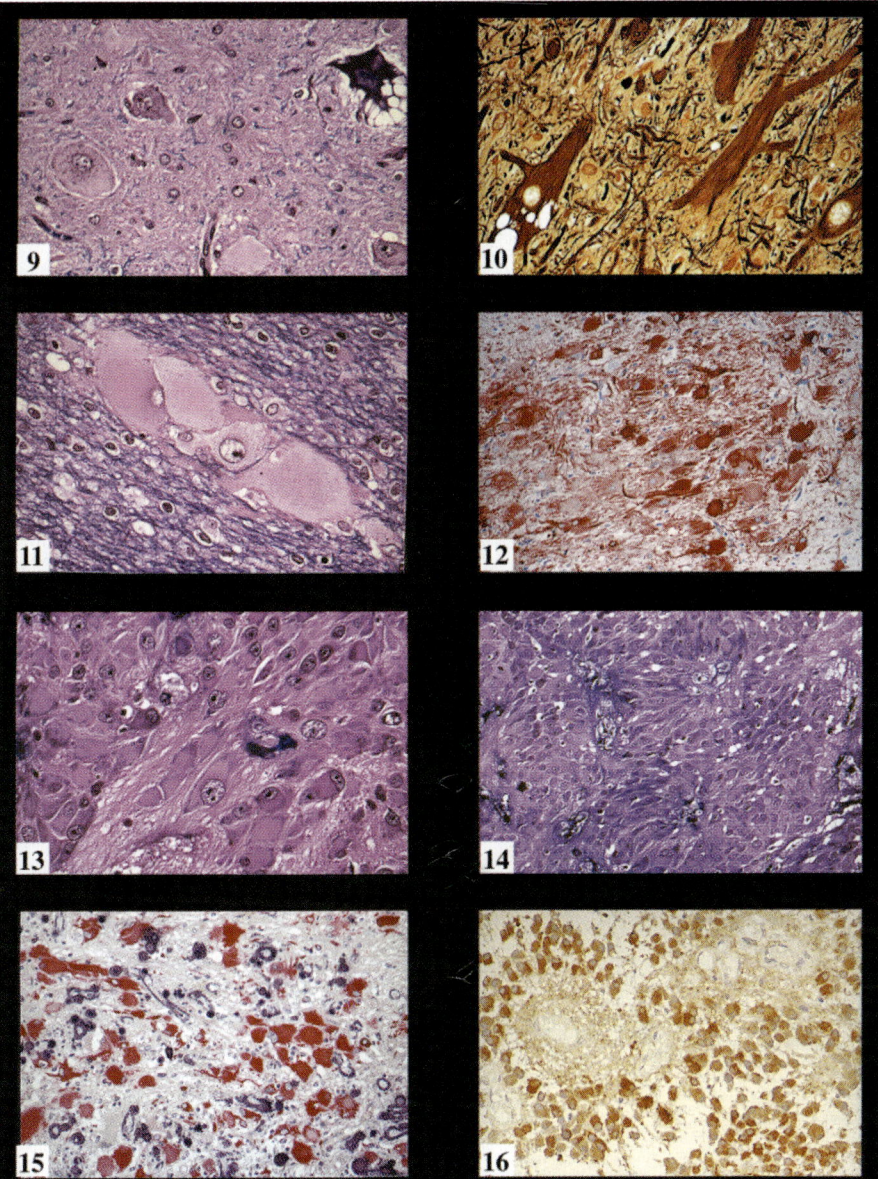

Fig. 9. Tuberous sclerosis: neuronal dysmorphism in a cortical tuber; a large eosinophilic cell is observed in the middle of the bottom (LFB/HE ×400).
Fig. 10. Tuberous sclerosis: silver impregnation of giant dysmorphic and sometimes multivacuolated neurons in cortical tuber (Bielschowsky ×400).
Fig. 11. Tuberous sclerosis: collection of large and eosinophilic cells in the subcortical white matter (LFB/HE ×400).
Fig. 12. Tuberous sclerosis: immunostaining of large eosinophilic cells for GFAP (Immunoperoxidase ×200).
Fig. 13. Tuberous sclerosis: large spindle to polygonal or ganglion-like cells in a subependymal giant cell astrocytoma (LFB/HE ×400).
Fig. 14. Tuberous sclerosis: perivascular distribution of elongated cells in a subependymal giant cell astrocytoma (LFB/HE ×200).
Fig. 15. Tuberous sclerosis: GFAP positive cells (red) and amounts of calcification (blue) in a subependymal giant cell astrocytoma (Immunoperoxidase ×200).
Fig. 16. Tuberous sclerosis: immunostaining of tumoural cells (brown) for NSE in a subependymal giant cell astrocytoma (Immunoperoxidase ×200).

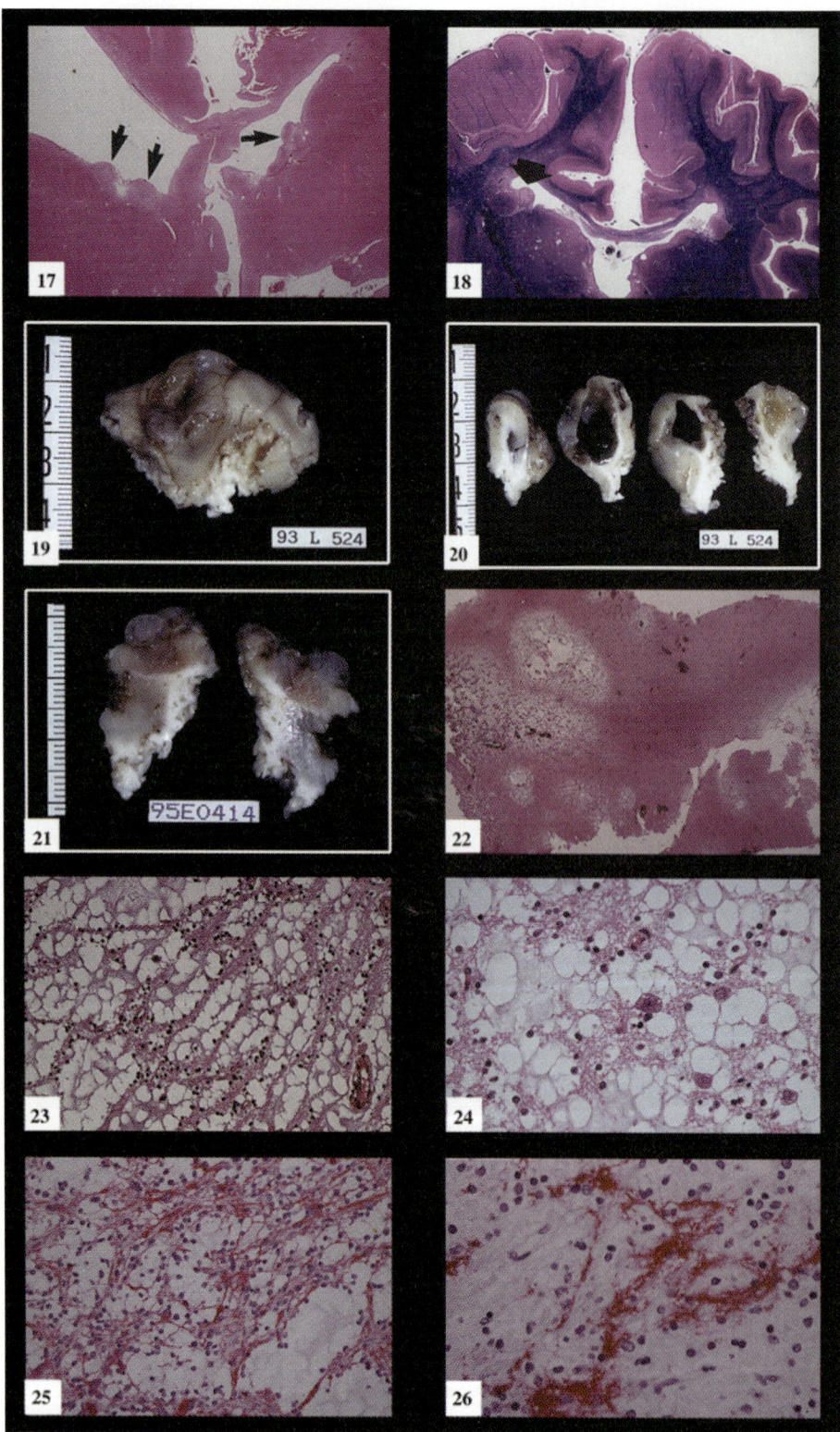

Fig. 16. Tuberous sclerosis: immunostaining of tumoural cells (brown) for NSE in a subependymal giant cell astrocytoma (Immunoperoxidase ×200);

Fig. 17. Tuberous sclerosis: coronal slice showing several subependymal nodules (arrows) in the anterior part of the cerebral ventricles (HES ×0.9)

Fig. 18. Tuberous sclerosis: coronal slice showing two cortical tubers, a single subependymal nodule (arrow) in the right caudate nucleus region and foci of cortical heterotopia in the left centrum semi-ovale (LFB/HE ×0.8)

Fig. 19. Dysembryoplastic neuroepithelial tumour: diffuse expansion of a cortical gyrus with a central blister-like nodule.

Fig. 20. Dysembryoplastic neuroepithelial tumour: cystic nodule with a gelatinous translucid material on the internal surface (cut section).

Fig. 21. Dysembryoplastic neuroepithelial tumour: cortical, exophytic, solid and mushroom-like tumoural nodule (cut section).

Fig. 22. Dysembryoplastic neuroepithelial tumour: intracortical and multinodular architecture (HES ×25).

Fig. 23. Dysembryoplastic neuroepithelial tumour: specific glioneuronal element with a columnar/alveolar appearance and fluid-filled spaces (HES ×100),

Fig. 24. Dysembryoplastic neuroepithelial tumour: specific glioneuron element made of a mixture of small oliodendrocyte-like cells and of neurons floating with mucin pools (HES ×250).

Fig. 25. Dysembryoplastic neuroepithelial tumour: some tumoural cells are immunoreactive for GFAP (red) (Immunoperoxidase ×100)

Fig. 26. Dysembryoplastic neuroepithelial tumour: synaptophysin staining (red) for some rare cell membranes as well as the fibrillary background (Immunoperoxidase ×200).

Table 3. Dysplastic features observed in the cerebral tissue neighbouring dysembryoplastic neuroepithelial tumours.

Dysplastic features	Number of cases
Atypical multinucleated giant cells (probably neuronal) in cortex	15
Cortical dysplasia (CD)	14
Binucleated neurons	9
Nests of neuroblasts or primitive neuroepithelial cells in temporal neocortex or mesial structures	2
Duplication of the fascia dentata	1
Nodular cortical heterotopia (NCH)	1
Hemimegalencephaly + CD + NCH	1

identified. The main pathological characteristics consisted of an intracortical location (Figs. 19, 20 and 21), a multinodular pattern (Fig. 22) with mucoid substance accumulation (Fig. 23) and a 'specific glioneuronal element' made of a mixture of glial-like cells and neurons 'floating' within mucous pools (Fig. 24). A small number of cells showed immunoreactivity for GFAP (Fig. 25) and focally for synaptophysin (Fig. 26). A more complete histological description is summarized in Table 2 and some 'dysplastic' features commonly observed in our series are mentioned in Table 3.

Discussion

It is well-known that a wide spectrum of abnormalities of development and organizational abnormalities of the cerebral cortex are commonly associated with long-standing epilepsy (Bruton, 1988; Andermann & Guerrini, 1996). This heterogeneous group of lesions includes various subtypes of cortical dysgenesis, sometimes coexisting with phacomatosis and/or tumours (Cavanagh, 1958; Daumas-Duport et al., 1988; Prayson et al., 1993; Vinters et al., 1993; Wolf & Wiestler, 1993; Wolf et al., 1993; Vital et al., 1994; Raymond et al., 1995; Pasquier et al., 1996). From a practical point of view CD, TS and DNETs represent three major developmental and/or tumoural conditions encountered in the field of chronic epilepsy and account for approximately 24% of all cases in our series of 230 patients.

Table 4. A non-exhaustive list of lesions (*) referred to as cortical dysplasia in the literature (the term most commonly used appears in capitals)

MICRODYSGENESIS
    mild cortical dysplasia; cortical dysplasia
    cortical-subcortical aberration
    heterotopia/ectopia; hamartia

FOCAL CORTICAL DYSPLASIA
    cortical dysplasia; focal dysplasia
    cortical dysplasia with neuronal cytomegaly
    hamartoma/hamartia

MACROGYRIA
    focal cortical dysplasia

POLYMICROGYRIA (unlayered and four-layered cortex)

PACHYGYRIA

AGYRIA (lissencephaly type 1)

WALKER–WARBURG SYNDROME (lissencephaly type 2)

HEMIMEGALENCEPHALY

* The main sources are the following: Honavar & Meldru, 1997 in *Greenfield's neuropathology*; Robain, 1996; Robain & Gelot; Prayson & Estes, 1995; Mischel *et al.*, 1995

Cortical dysplasia

Terms such as cortical dysplasia (CD) or dysplasia encompass a wide range of lesions affecting the cerebral cortex and/or white matter, making recognition and classification difficult. A classic textbook of neuropathology, e.g., *Greenfield's neuropathology* (Honavar & Meldrum, 1997) and numerous published data include various pathological disorders or defects of neuronal migration and/or differentiation under this heading (Table 4). Among them, microdysgenesis (focal absence of neurons or neuronal clustering in the temporal neocortex; neuronal ectopia in the leptomeninges or white matter; Meencke & Janz, 1985) is still a matter of debate. According to Hardiman *et al.*, (1988), severe ectopia, defined by more than 8 neurons/mm^2 white matter, is present in 43% of surgical specimens in chronic epilepsy, but not in controls. In contrast, Babb *et al.* (1984), quoted by Honavar & Meldrum (1997), did not find any significant difference between the temporal neocortex of epileptic patients and of normal controls, when comparing the volumetric neurone density. By extension, and incorrectly in our opinion, some other microscopic abnormalities have been included among CDs: small grey matter heterotopias; perivascular amounts of glia; duplication of fascia dentata or dispersion of its granule cell component (Armstrong, 1993); glioneuronal hamartia (Wolf *et al.*, 1993; 1995). In the same manner, some tuberous-like lesions (Wolf *et al.*, 1996) are better classified as focal cortical dysplasia (FCD). We feel that FCD, as described by Taylor *et al.* (1971), unquestionably remains the best defined entity among the accumulation of disorders (see Table 4) described under the inaccurate term of CD. We confirm, as previously mentioned by Janota (1996), a frontal predominance and a frequent normal external appearance of lesions. Occasionally, FCD appears as a focal widening of a gyrus with blurring, on cut section, of the grey–white matter junction (Taylor *et al.*, 1971; Pasquier *et al.*, 1996; Honavar & Meldrum, 1997). In some cases, a zone of partial lissencephaly may be associated with FCD (Janota, 1996). Histologically, the main characteristic corresponds to a focal disruption of the normal cortical ribbon by collections of large, bizarre neurons typically present in all cortical layers except the first one (Taylor *et al.*, 1971). These giant neurons with prominent coarse dendrites are haphazardly oriented and usually accompanied by a various number of large and also bizarre, ballooned cells. Giants neurons, measuring up to 80 µm, contain coarse, peripheral or perinuclear Nissl bodies and may be bipolar or binucleate (Robain, 1996). Ballooned cells show an abundant, eosinophilic, glassy cytoplasm and large often multiple and atypical nuclei. Both types of cells may be usually identified throughout the cortex (mainly in the deeper portions) and the subjacent white matter. Occasionally, giant neurons and/or ballooned cells may be found in the brain adjacent to the main focus or in association with hemimegalencephaly (Robain & Gelot, 1996). Various other (probably degenerative) abnormalities are rarely observed: Rosenthal fibres formation, astrocytic gliosis, dark mineral particles accumulation, loss of nerve fibres, and cavitation (Janota, 1996). Giant neurons are immunoreactive with antibodies against neurofilament epitopes, tau and ubiquitin (Farrell *et al.*, 1992; Duong *et al.*, 1994). Balloon cells contain intracytoplasmic filaments 20 nm thick and 400–600 nm in length (Farrell *et al.*, 1992) and express GFAP inconsistently (Honavar & Meldrum, 1997). Some balloon cells are also immunoreactive for both glial and neuronal markers (Farrell *et al.*, 1992; Vital *et al.*, 1994). Because of the morphological and immunohistochemical similarities between the cells of FCD and of cortical tubers (CTs), the relationship between a forme fruste of TS and FCD has been considered (Palmini *et al.*, 1991) but remains, up to now, not clearly established. Usually, FCD is a unifocal disorder with a mild tendency to cavitation and without calcification or tumoural association. Conversely, CTs are often multifocal, calcified and have a marked tendency to cavitation. In TS, furthermore, a frequent association of CTs with subependymal nodules and/or giant cell astrocytomas is well known. A practical approach of CD including FCD has been realized by Mischel *et al.* (1995) based upon specimens of 77 patients and with a proposal for a grading system (mild, moderate and severe CD). Histologically, nine specific and easily identifiable abnormalities have been defined, i.e. cortical laminar disorganization; single heterotopic white matter neurons; neurons in the cortical molecular layer; persistant remnants of the subpial granular cell layer; marginal glioneuronal heterotopia; polymicrogyria; white matter neuronal heterotopia; neuronal cytomegaly with associated cytoskeletal abnormalities; and balloon cell change. Interestingly, there is some correlation between the category of pathological features, the presumed approximate time of their development and the frequency of seizures. Therefore, FCD can be considered as an early developmental event corresponding clinically to severe CD. Conversely the lesions of 'cortical microdysgenesis' (cortical disorganization; heterotopic white matter neurons; neurons in molecular layer; persistent subpial granular layer) are classified among abnormalities of late development. An intermediate group is composed of marginal heterotopia and polymicrogyria.

Tuberous sclerosis

In Bourneville's disease or TS complex (Gomez, 1988), CNS is the most frequently affected system (Harding & Copp, 1997). The neuropathological hallmarks of TS are glioneuronal hamartomas named cortical tubers (CTs), subependymal nodules (SENs) and/or giant cell astrocytomas (SEGAs), and white matter heterotopias. Usually cerebral and multiple (up to 40), CTs are sometimes cerebellar. Firm, pale, nodular, potato-like and often calcified, they may be wide and flat or round and dimpled (Pellizzi, 1901, quoted by Gomez, 1995) measuring from millimetres to several centimetres. Histologically they are characterized by an effacement of cortical lamination due to collections of large bizarre cells looking like abnormal, maloriented and often vacuolated giant neurons and of atypical astrocytes. These latter cells often multinucleated eosinophilic and giant are reminiscent of balloon cells of FCD. A marked subpial gliosis, demyelination and cystic formation within the adjacent white matter may also occur, as well as diffuse calcification of CTs ('brainstones'). On immunohistochemical studies, dysmorphic neurons usually express neurofilament proteins and eosinophilic cells demonstrate a frequent coexpression of both glial and neuronal markers (Hirose *et al.*, 1995). These findings have been corroborated by ultrastructural data suggesting the presence of astrocytic, neuronal, or combined glial–neuronal differentiation in CTs (Hirose *et al.*, 1995; Harding & Copp, 1997). SENs may occur as a single nodule, usually measuring less than one centimetre in diameter or in rows ('candle gutterings'). Firm, calcified and stony hard, they arise mainly around the lateral ventricles, near the caudate nucleus and thalamic region, or in the third ventricle. SENs may protrude into the ventricular cavity, occasionally within the fourth ventricle, and even the aqueduct. Histologically, SENs are similar to SEGAs and by convention, nodules larger than one centimeter or clinically symptomatic are considered as SEGAs (Giannini & Scheithauer, 1997), the most common tumours of TS (6 per cent of affected patients: Shepherd et al., 1991). They typically arise in children and young patients (under 20 years of age) in the caudate nucleus region with a frequent obstruction of the foramen of Monro. Intraventricular, well circumscribed and often heavily calcified they are composed of a mixture of three major cell populations: small spindle-shaped or elongated cells; polygonal or 'gemistocytic-like' cells of intermediate size; globoid or ganglion-like cells (Lantos et al., 1997). In some areas elongated cells have a striking perivascular distribution reminiscent of ependymal pseudorosettes. In other regions, the tumoural cells look like astrocytes and/or neurons showing prominent nucleoli or eccentric and often multiple nuclei. Most often, nuclear atypia, mitoses, necrosis and vascular hyperplasia are rare. The immunophenotype of SEGAs is, up to now, poorly understood, showing a diffuse S-100 protein reactivity, a variable GFAP staining and a frequent expression of neuronal and neuroendocrine markers (Hirose et al., 1995; Lopes et al., 1996; Giannini & Scheithauer, 1997). In other words, SEGAs reveal a mixed glial–neuronal differentiation with a capacity of neuroendocrine differentiation but without apparent immunohistochemical co-localization (Lantos et al., 1997; Giannini & Scheithauer, 1997). From a practical point of view, the survival of patients with SEGAs reaches nearly 80 per cent at both five and 15 years (Shepherd et al., 1991). Other tumoural conditions are exceptional in TS (glioblastoma; astrocytoma; ganglioglioma; ependymoma; gliomatosis cerebri; spongioblastoma or hemangioma: Russell & Rubinstein, 1989; Giannini & Scheithauer, 1997). On the other hand, collections of abnormal neurons and/or eosinophilic giant cells in the white matter adjacent to CTs are frequent findings. Other non-tumoural conditions include hemimegalencephaly, agenesis of the corpus callosum and subcortical cystic degeneration.

Dysembryoplastic neuroepithelial tumours

DNETs are a new clinicopathological entity first identified among patients with chronic intractable epilepsy (Daumas-Duport et al., 1988). Nowadays more than 200 cases (Hasegawa et al., 1991; Nishio et al., 1992; Prayson & Estes, 1992; Daumas-Duport, 1993; Gottschalk et al., 1993; Hirose et al., 1994; Leung et al., 1994; Raymond et al., 1994; Kuchelmeister et al., 1995; Lellouch-Tubiana et al., 1995; Taratuto et al., 1995; Wolf et al., 1995; Daumas-Duport, 1996; Pasquier et al., 1996; Cervera-Pierot et al., 1997; Itoh et al., 1997) have been documented, but the actual incidence of these lesions is probably underestimated. In its initial description, DNET is considered as a supratentorial glioneuronal tumour found in young patients (usually children or young adults) without neurological deficit nor mental retardation or stigmata of phacomatosis. Typically, the clinical presentation is a long-standing partial and pharmacoresistant epilepsy with early onset (before the age of 20 years). The tumour preferentially involves the temporal lobe with a striking cortical location and a frequent focal cranial deformity. The tumoural size ranges from some millimetres to several centimetres. On gross examination, except in cases with exclusive involvement of the temporal mesial structures, DNET is often easily identified at the cortical surface. The most bulky and characteristic examples show a diffuse enlargement of the cortical gyrus with a central blister-like nodule mainly cystic on cut section. The internal surface of the cyst consists of a gelatinous, translucid and friable material. In other well preserved specimens, a more localized exophytic and solid tumoural nodule looking like a mushroom is jutting out over the cortical ribbon. Histologically, DNET exhibits specific features: predominant cortical topography; multinodular architecture; presence of a 'specific glioneuronal element'; frequent foci; dysplastic cortical disorganization. Multinodularity is made of several (up to 12 in our experience) cortical nodules sometimes resembling astrocytomas (often pilocytic), oligodendrogliomas or oligoastrocytomas. The 'specific glioneuronal element' consists of a diffuse proliferation of small, round oligodendrocyte-like cells (OLCs) often distributed in a columnar/alveolar pattern within an accumulation of mucin pools. OLCs exhibit a uniform round and hyperchromatic nuclei with occasional minute nucleoli, and a scanty cytoplasm with an inconstant perinuclear halo. A variable number of astrocytes, often of pilocytic type is associated with OLCs as well as neurons of varying size 'floating' within the fluid-filled spaces. A glomeruloid capillary proliferation realizing vascular arcades is often present in astrocytic components. The adjacent cerebral cortex shows frequent foci of dysplastic disorganization qualified as CD (Daumas-Duport *et al.*, 1988). This above described subtype of DNET corresponds to the 'complex form' according to Daumas-Duport, 1993 and is usually identified from large surgical specimens. Another subtype for which only a 'specific glioneuronal element' can be observed is classified as 'simple form', often from stereotactic biopsy material. Nuclear atypia, rare mitosis and occasional foci of necrosis can be present in DNET without any pejorative connotation. Immunohistochemical studies reveal that the majority of OLCs are immunoreactive for S-100 protein and inconsistently for GFAP. In approximately 40% of cases these same cells may express classe III-*B* tubulin considered as an early neuronal differentiation without immunoreactivity for neurofilament protein epitopes and synaptophysin (Hirose *et al.*, 1994; Lantos *et al.*, 1997). The MIB1/Ki 67 labelling index usually ranges from 0.1 to 1.0% (Wolf *et al.* 1995). OLCs sometimes reveal ultrastructural features of both neuronal and oligoglial lineages, in varying proportion from case to case (Daumas-Duport, 1993; Hirose *et al.*, 1994; Leung *et al.* 1994). Other rare OLCs appear to be astrocytic and a major part of this cell population has no characteristic ultrastructural features (Hirose *et al.*, 1994). Since the initial description of DNETs, extraneocortical tumoural locations have been observed in the caudate nucleus region (Cervera-Pierot *et al.*, 1997), the quadrigeminal plate (unpublished personal case), the cerebellum (Kuchelmeister *et al.*, 1995) as well as in multifocal CNS involvement (namely: left temporal lobe, third ventricle and basal ganglia in case one, and right temporal lobe, both thalami, pons and right cerebellar hemisphere in case two of Leung *et al.*, 1994; left frontal, parietal and temporal independent localizations in case one of Lellouch-Tubiana *et al.*, 1995). A unusual association with neurofibromatosis type one has also been reported in two cases (Lellouch-Tubiana *et al.*, 1995) and, more recently, a new subset of DNETs ('non-specific form': Daumas-Duport, 1996; Daumas-Duport *et al.*, 1996) has been introduced. The clinical presentation and post-operative follow-up of the three subtypes of DNETs are identical. Histologically, the 'non-specific' variety looks like a conventional glioma (astrocytoma; oligoglioma; oligoastrocytoma or unclassable glioma) without the 'specific glioneuronal element' but with frequent foci of CD. According to their putative histogenesis and dysembryoplastic origin, DNETs may derive from secondary germinal layers (subpial and subependymal granular layers; external granular layer of the cerebellum; fascia dentata: Daumas-Duport, 1988; Daumas-Duport, 1996; Cervera-Pierot *et al.*, 1997), as previously suggested by Cavanagh (1958). From a practical point of view DNETs remain stable and surgically curable lesions with an excellent prognosis. A high incidence of DNETs in young patients with partial drug-resistant epilepsy (Daumas-Duport *et al.*, 1996; Pasquier *et al.*, 1996) needs to be considered to prevent the application of useless radio- or chemotherapy.

References

Andermann, F. & Guerrini, R. (1996): The cortical dysplasias and epilepsy: an overview. In: *Dysplasias of cerebral cortex and epilepsy*, eds. R. Guerrini, F. Andermann, R. Canapicchi, J. Roger, B.G. Zifkin & P. Pfanner, pp. 151–162. Philadelphia: Lippincott-Raven.

Armstrong, D.D. (1993): The neuropathology of temporal lobe epilepsy. *J. Neuropath. Exp. Neurol.* **52**, 433–443.

Bruton, C.J. (1988): *The neuropathology of temporal lobe epilepsy*. Maudsley Monographs No. 31. Oxford: Oxford University Press.

Cavanagh, J.B. (1958): On certain small tumours encountered in the temporal lobe. *Brain* **81**, 389–405.

Cervera-Pierot, P., Varlet, P., Chodkiewicz, J.P., Daumas-Duport, C. (1997): Dysembryoplastic neuroepithelial tumours located in the caudate nucleus area: report of four cases. *Neurosurgery* **40**, 1065–1069.

Daumas-Duport, C. (1993): Dysembryoplastic neuroepithelial tumours. *Brain Pathol.* **3**, 283–295.

Daumas-Duport, C. (1996): Dysembryoplastic neuroepithelial tumours in epilepsy surgery. In: *Dysplasias of cerebral cortex and epilepsy*, eds. R. Guerrini, F. Andermann, R. Canapicchi, J. Roger, B.G. Zifkin & P. Pfanner, pp. 71–80. Philadelphia: Lippincott-Raven.

Daumas-Duport, C., Scheithauer, B.W., Chodkiewicz, J.P., Laws Jr, E.R. & Vedrenne, C. (1988): Dysembryoplastic neuroepithelial tumour: a surgically curable tumour of young patients with intractable partial seizures. Report of thirty-nine cases. *Neurosurgery* **23**, 545–556.

Daumas-Duport, C, Varlet, P., Cervera, P. & Chodkiewicz, J.P. (1996): Non-specific histological forms of dysembryoplastic neuroepithelial tumours (DNTs): a study of 40 cases. *Neuropathol. Appl. Neurobiol.* **22 (Suppl. 1)**, 1–18.

Duong, T., De Rosa, M.J., Poukens, V., Vinters, H.V. & Fisher, R.S. (1994): Neuronal cytoskeletal abnormalities in human cerebral cortical dysplasia. *Acta Neuropathol.* **87**, 493–503.

Farrell, M.A., De Rosa, M.J., Curran, J.G., Lenard Secor, D., Cornford, M.E., Comair, Y.G., Peacock, W.J., Shields, W.D. & Vinters, H.V. (1992): Neuropathologic findings in cortical resections (including hemispherectomies) performed for the treatment of intractable childhood epilepsy. *Acta Neuropathol.* **83**, 246–259.

Giannini, C. & Scheithauer, B.W. (1997): Classification and grading of low-grade astrocytic tumours in children. *Brain Pathol.* **7**, 785–798.

Gomez, M.R. (1988): Criteria for diagnosis. In: *Tuberous sclerosis*, ed. M.R. Gomez, pp. 9–19. New-York: Raven Press.

Gomez, M.R. (1995): History of the tuberous sclerosis complex. *Brain Dev.* **17 (Suppl)**, 55–57.

Gottschalk, J., Korves, M., Skotzek-Konrad, B., Goebel, S. & Cervos-Navarro, J. (1993): Dysembryoplastic neuroepithelial micro-tumour in a 75-year-old patient with long-standing epilepsy. *Clin. Neuropathol.* **12**, 175–178.

Hardiman, O., Burke, T., Phillipps, J., Murphy, S., O' Moore, B., Staunton, H. & Farrell, M.A. (1988): Microdysgenesis in resected temporal neocortex: incidence and clinical significance in focal epilepsy. *Neurology* **38**, 1041–1047.

Harding, B. & Copp, A.J. (1997): Tuberous sclerosis (Bourneville's disease). In: *Greenfield's neuropathology, Volume 1*, eds. D.I. Graham & P.L. Lantos, pp. 497–502. London: Edward Arnold.

Hasegawa, H., Bitoh, S., Koshino, K., Obashi, J. & Kobayashi, Y. (1991): Dysembryoplastic neuroepithelial tumour: a case report. *No Shinkei Geka* **19**, 553–557.

Hirose, T., Scheithauer, B.W., Lopes, B.S. & Vandenberg, S.R. (1994): Dysembryoplastic neuroepithelial tumour (DNT): an immunohistochemical and ultrastructural study. *J. Neuropath. Exp. Neurol.* **53**, 184–195.

Hirose, T., Scheithauer, B.W., Lopes, M.B.S., Gerber, H.A., Altermatt, H.J., Hukee, M.J., Vandenberg, S.R. & Charlesworth, J.C. (1995): Tuber and subependymal giant cell astrocytoma associated with tuberous sclerosis: an immunohistochemical, ultrastructural, and immunoelectron microscopic study. *Acta Neuropathol.* **90**, 387–399.

Honavar, M. & Meldrum, B.S. (1997): Defects of neuronal migration. In: *Greenfield's neuropathology, Volume 1*, eds. D.I. Graham & P.L. Lantos, pp. 936–938. London: Edward Arnold.

Itoh, M., Morita, T., Houdou, S., Kato, S., Ohama, E., Mizushima, M. & Hori, T. (1997): Two cases of dysembryoplastic neuroepithelial tumours with intractable complex partial seizures. *J. Child. Neurol.* **12**, 67–70.

Janota, I. (1996): Cortical dysplasia in surgical specimens. In: *Dysplasias of cerebral cortex and epilepsy*, eds. R. Guerrini, F. Andermann, R. Canapicchi, J. Roger, B.G. Zifkin & P. Pfanner, pp. 53–55. Philadelphia: Lippincott-Raven.

Kahane, P., Francione, S., Tassi, L., Hoffmann, D., Lo Russo, G., Garrel, S., Feuerstein, C., Perret, J., Benabid, A.L. & Munari, C. (1993): Traitement chirurgical des épilepsies partielles graves pharmaco-résistantes: approches diagnostiques et thérapeutiques (rapport préliminaire sur trois années d'activité a Grenoble). *Epilepsies* **5**, 179–204.

Kleihues, P., Burger, P.C. & Scheithauer, B.W. (1993): International histological classification of tumours. *Histological typing of tumours of the central nervous system*, 2nd edition. Berlin: Springer-Verlag.

Kuchelmeister, K., Demirel, T., Schlorer, E., Bergmann, M. & Gullotta, F. (1995): Dysembryoplastic neuroepithelial tumour of the cerebellum. *Acta Neuropathol.* **89**, 385–390.

Lantos, P.L., Vandenberg, S.R. & Kleihues, P. (1997): Subependymal giant cell tumours. In: *Greenfield's neuropathology, Volume 2*, eds. D.I. Graham & P.L. Lantos, pp. 625–627. London: Edward Arnold.

Lellouch-Tubiana, A., Bourgeois, M., Vekemans, M. & Robain, O. (1995): Dysembryoplastic neuroepithelial tumours in two children with neurofibromatosis type 1. *Acta Neuropathol.* **90**, 319–322.

Leung, S.Y., Gwi, E., Ng, H.K., Fung, C.F. & Yam, K.Y. (1994): Dysembryoplastic neuroepithelial tumour. A tumour with small neuronal cells resembling oligodendroglioma. *Am. J. Surg. Pathol.* **18**, 604–614.

Lopes, M.B.S., Altermatt, H.J., Scheithauer, B.W., Shepherd, C.W. & Vandenberg, S.R. (1996): Immunohistochemical characterization of subependymal giant cell astrocytomas. *Acta Neuropathol.* **91**, 368–375.

Meencke, J.J. & Janz, D. (1985): The signifiance of microdysgenesia in primary generalized epilepsy : an answer to the considerations of Lyon and Gastaut. *Epilepsia* **26**, 368–371.

Mischel, P.S., Nguyen, L.P. & Vinters, H.V. (1995): Cerebral cortical dysplasia associated with pediatric epilepsy. Review of neuropathologic features and proposal for a grading system. *J. Neuropath. Exp. Neurol.* **54**, 137–153.

Munari, C., Francione, S., Kahane, P., Hoffmann, D., Tassi, L., Lo Russo, G. & Benabid A.L. (1995): Multilobar resections for the control of epilepsy. In: *Operative neurosurgical techniques. Indications, methods and results, Volume 2*, eds. H.H. Schmidek & W.H. Sweet, pp. 1323–1339. Philadelphia: W.B. Saunders.

Nishio, S., Takeshita, I., Kaneko, Y. & Furui, M. (1992): Cerebral neurocytoma. A new subset of benign neuronal tumours of the cerebrum. *Cancer* **70**, 531–537.

Palmini, A., Andermann, F., Olivier, A., Tampieri, D. & Robitaille, Y. (1991): Focal neuronal migration disorders and intractable partial epilepsy: a study of 30 patients. *Ann. Neurol.* **30**, 741–749.

Pasquier, B., Bost, F., Péoc'h, M., Barnoud, R. & Pasquier, D. (1996): Données neuropathologiques dans l'épilepsie partielle pharmacorésistante. Etude d'une série de 195 observations. *Ann. Pathol.* **16**, 174–181.

Plate, K.H., Wieser, H.G., Yasargil, M.G. & Wiestler, O.D. (1993): Neuropathological findings in 224 patients with temporal lobe epilepsy. *Acta Neuropathol.* **86**, 433–438.

Prayson, R.A. & Estes, M.L. (1992): Dysembryoplastic neuroepithelial tumour. *Am. J. Clin. Pathol.* **97**, 398–401.

Prayson, R.A. & Estes, M.L. (1995): Cortical dysplasia: a histopathological study of 52 cases with partial lobectomy in patients with epilepsy. *Hum. Pathol.* **26**, 493–500.

Prayson, R.A., Estes, M.L. & Morris, H.H. (1993): Coexistence of neoplasia and cortical dysplasia in patients presenting with seizures. *Epilepsia* **34**, 609–615.

Raymond, A.A., Halpin, S.F.S., Alsanjari, N., Cook, M.J., Kitchen, N.D., Fish, D.R., Stevens, J.M., Harding, B.N., Scaravilli, F., Kendall, B., Shorvon, S.D. & Neville, B.G.R. (1994): Dysembryoplastic neuroepithelial tumour. Features in 16 patients. *Brain* **117**, 461–475.

Raymond, A.A., Fish, D.R., Sisodiya, S.M., Alsanjari, N., Stevens, J.M. & Shorvon, S.D. (1995): Abnormalities of gyration, heterotopias, tuberous sclerosis, focal cortical dysplasia, microdysgenesis, dysembryoplastic neuroepithelial tumour and dysgenesis of the archicortex in epilepsy. Clinical, EEG and neuroimaging features in 100 adult patients. *Brain* **118**, 629–660.

Robain, O. (1996): Introduction to the pathology of cerebral cortical dysplasia. In: *Dysplasias of cerebral cortex and epilepsy*, eds. R. Guerrini, F. Andermann, R. Canapicchi, J. Roger, B.G. Zifkin & P. Pfanner, pp. 1–9. Philadelphia: Lippincott-Raven.

Robain, O. & Gelot, A. (1996): Neuropathology of hemimegalencephaly. In: *Dysplasias of cerebral cortex and epilepsy*, eds. R. Guerrini, F. Andermann, R. Canapicchi, J. Roger, B.G. Zifkin & P. Pfanner, pp. 89–92. Philadelphia: Lippincott-Raven.

Russell, D.S. & Rubinstein, L.J. (1989): *Pathology of tumours of the nervous system.* London: Edward Arnold.

Shepherd, C.W., Scheithauer, B.W., Gomez, M.R., Altermatt, H.J. & Kaltzmann, J.A. (1991): Subependymal giant cell astrocytoma: a clinical, pathological and flow cytometry. *Neurosurgery* **28**, 864–868.

Taratuto, A.L., Pomata, H., Sevlever, G., Gallo, G. & Monges, J. (1995): Dysembryoplastic neuroepithelial tumour: morphological, immunocytochemical, and desoxyribonucleic acid analyses in a pediatric series. *Neurosurgery* **36**, 474–481.

Taylor, D.C., Falconer, M.A., Bruton, C.J. & Corsellis, J.A.N. (1971): Focal dysplasia of the cerebral cortex in epilepsy. *J. Neurol. Neurosurg. Psychiat.* **34**, 369–387.

Vinters, H.V., Armstrong, D.L., Babb, T.L., Daumas-Duport, C., Robitaille, Y., Bruton, C.J. & Farrell, M.A. (1993): The neuropathology of human symptomatic epilepsy. In: *Surgical treatment of the epilepsies*, ed. J. Engel, Jr. New York: Raven Press.

Vital, A., Rivel, J., Loiseau, H., Marchal, C., Rougier, A. & Vital, C. (1994): Histopathologie de 110 cortectomies pour épilepsie pharmacorésistante. *Rev. Neurol.* **150**, 33–38.

Wolf, H.K. & Wiestler, O.D. (1993): Surgical pathology of chronic epileptic seizure disorders. *Brain Pathol.* **3**, 371–380.

Wolf, H.K., Campos, M.G., Zentner, J., Hufnagel, A., Schramm, J., Elger, C.E. & Wiestler, O.D. (1993): Surgical pathology of temporal lobe epilepsy. Experience with 216 cases. *J. Neuropath. Exp. Neurol.* **52,** 499–506.

Wolf, H.K., Wellmer, J., Muller, M.B., Wiestler, O.D., Hufnagel, A. & Pietsch, T. (1995): Glioneuronal malformative lesions and dysembryoplastic neuroepithelial tumours in patients with chronic pharmacoresistant epilepsies. *J. Neuropath. Exp. Neurol.* **54,** 245–254.

Wolf, H.K., Normann, S., Green, A.J., von Bakel, I., Blumcke, I., Pietsch, T., Wiestler, O.D. & von Deimling, A. (1996): Tuberous sclerosis-like lesions in epileptogenic human neocortex lack allelic loss at the TSC 1 and TSC2 regions. *Acta Neuropathol.* **93,** 93–36.

Chapter 20

Immunocytochemical studies in epileptogenic dysplastic tissue

Rita Garbelli[1], Basile Pasquier[2], Lorella Minotti[2], Laura Tassi[4], Silvia De Biasi[3], Alim L. Benabid[2], Giorgio Battaglia[1], Claudio Munari[4,5] and Roberto Spreafico[1]

[1]*Divisione di Neurofisiologia Sperimentale ed Epilettologia, Istituto Nazionale Neurologico 'C. Besta', Milan, Italy;*
[2]*Service d'Anatomie Pathologique, Centre Hospitalier Régional et Universitaire CHU, B.P. 217X, 38043, Grenoble Cedex 9, France;*
[3]*Dipartimento di Fisiologia Generale e Biochimica, Università di Milano, Italy;*
[4]*Dipartimento di Scienze Neurologiche, Centro Regionale per la Chirurgia dell'Epilessia, Ospedale Niguarda Ca' Granda, Piazza Ospedale Maggiore 3, 20162 Milan, Italy*
[5]*Dipartimento di Neurochirurgia, Università di Genova, Italy*

Abstract

Thanks to high resolution imaging techniques, cortical abnormalities are increasingly diagnosed *in vivo*, particularly in patients affected by intractable epilepsy and thus candidates for epilepsy surgery. This present paper reports an immunocytochemical analysis, by means of antisera recognizing specific neuronal and glial markers, of two patients with cortical dysplasia (as revealed by MRI), and operated on for intractable epilepsy. Surgical samples of the lesional area and of the epileptogenic surrounding zone, revealed by SEEG recording, were processed for routine histology and immunocytochemistry. The neuropathological examinations of the first case showed a cortical laminar disruption and the presence of aggregate of fusiform cells resembling neuroblasts, suggesting a disturbance of migratory events and subsequent impairment of neuronal differentiation. In the second case, the main characteristics of the specimens examined were: cortical laminar disruption; presence of giant hypertrophic neurones in gray matter and heterotopic neurones in white matter filled by neurofilaments; balloon cells, particularly abundant in the deep portion of the gray matter and in the white matter, labelled with glial and neuronal markers. In this case the presence of balloon cells suggests that precursor cells fail to mature sufficiently prior to migration and may not migrate normally. The present data demonstrate that morphological abnormalities can be different in different cortical dysplasia and suggest possible basic mechanisms leading to epilepsy in these patients.

Introduction

The cerebral cortex in adult mammals is a multilayered highly ordered structure resulting from very complex, multistep sequences of cellular migration that take place during the foetal period. The first structure recognized in the developing cortex is the primordial plexiform layer (Marín-Padilla, 1978). This layer, the primordium of the future layer I, formed by the earliest generated neurones and by the apical portion of the radial glial fibres, is thought to be the switcher for the subsequent migratory events of later generated neurones (Marín-Padilla, 1984). Subsequently the primordial plexiform layer is split into two different structures, the subpial marginal zone and the subplate, by the incoming postmitotic neurones which climb the radial glia fibres and eventually form the cortical plate (Luskin & Shatz, 1985; Bayer & Altman, 1991; Marín-Padilla, 1978). This newly generated structure, enriched by successive migratory waves of postmitotic neuroblast following an inside-out gradient, will generate the future cortical layers II–VI.

In humans, the marginal zone is recognized as early as the 5th gestational week and by the 5th lunar month the migratory events forming the cortical plate are supposed to be concluded. Although the human cerebral cortex is considered to have received the full complement of nerve cells by the middle of gestation, a considerable number of neuronal elements are found below the cortical layers residing in the subplate and intermediate zone during the last trimester and even after birth (see Sidman & Rakic, 1973 for details).

During the second semester the dissolution of some transient structures, such as the subplate, subventricular and ventricular zones, is paralleled by the enlargement of the cortical layers as a result of the progressive differentiation of neuronal and glia elements, arborization of dendrites and axons, incoming fibres and synaptogenesis (Kostovic & Rakic, 1990). However the ventricular zone, although dramatically reduced, persists and continues to function as a germinal area (Jammes et al., 1973; Sidman & Rakic, 1973). Although the intimate mechanisms controlling the proliferation, migration and differentiation are not fully understood, it is clear that both genetic and environmental factors are involved and their respective importance changes along the different steps of cortical maturation (McConnell, 1988).

Any factor, either genetic or environmental (i.e. traumatic, vascular, toxic, metabolic or infective), interfering in a step of the developmental processes may cause focal or generalized disruption of the cortical organization, leading to morphological and functional alteration of the cortex. In the past, cortical malformations were mainly detected during autopsy and sometimes in surgical specimens from patients affected by epilepsy associated with different degrees of neurological and mental deficits. In the last ten years however, the advent of high resolution imaging techniques, namely MRI, has allowed the recognition *in vivo* of most, although not all, of the cortical abnormalities (Barkovich et al., 1987; Kuzniecky et al., 1995).

Despite the higher resolution of the modern imaging techniques versus the previously used neuroradiological tools (CT scan), only the general features of the anomalies can be evaluated *in vivo*, while the intimate organization of the dysplastic area cannot be recognized yet. Nevertheless, thanks to MRI, an increasing number of drug-resistant epileptic patients can be surgically treated with satisfactory results (Fried & Cascino, 1993; Palmini et al., 1994). The ablated tissue can be analyzed by routine neuropathological techniques and by specific immunocytochemical procedures, thus allowing a better understanding of the origin of the malformation and of the relationship between dysplastic area and epilepsy (Farrell et al., 1992; Ferrer et al., 1992; De Felipe et al., 1993; Duong et al., 1994; Mischel et al., 1995). Furthermore a correlation between radiological and neuropathological findings could help the clinicians and radiologists towards a more accurate *in vivo* diagnosis.

In the present report we describe the immunocytochemical findings on two patients, operated on at the Hôpital de Grenoble (France), and affected by intractable epilepsy. One of these patients has been previously reported (Spreafico et al., 1998b).

Methods

The presented cases are part of a large series of drug-resistant epileptic patients operated on at the department of Neurosurgery, CHU in Grenoble. All the patients underwent, in addition to a careful clinical examination and scalp EEG, an MRI and stereo-EEG (SEEG) analysis. Cortical samples processed for immunocytochemical study were part of the tissue removed, after informed consent, for strictly therapeutic reasons and used for routine neuropathological exam. Surgical technique and stereotactic methodology were similar to those described by Talairach et al. (1974), partially modified by Munari & Bancaud (1985). Surgical strategy was aimed at ablating not only the lesion revealed by MRI but also the cortical regions, although not involved by the lesion, defined as 'epileptogenic zones' by the SEEG findings.

Surgical specimens were immediately fixed by immersion in 10 per cent neutral buffered formalin, subsequently dehydrated in graded alcohol, embedded in paraffin and cut in 4–10 µm thick sections. Some paraffin sections were stained with hematoxylin and eosin, thionin, Luxol fast blue, or Bielschowsky, while others were processed using immunocytochemistry. For immunocytochemical procedures, after an incubation with 10 per cent (v/v) normal horse serum to mask non-specific adsorption sites, the sections were incubated in primary antisera: (a) monoclonal antibody raised in mouse against microtubule associated protein-2 (MAP 2; Boehringer Mannheim; dilution 1:500); (b) monoclonal antibody raised in mouse against non-phosphorylated neurofilaments (SMI 311; Sternberger Monoclonals Incorporated; dilution 1:250); (c) monoclonal antibody raised in mouse against glial fibrillary acid protein (GFAP; Boehringer Mannheim; dilution 1:100); (d) monoclonal antibody raised in mouse against vimentin (VIM; Dako; dilution 1:20); (e) mouse monoclonal antibodies against calcium binding proteins (CaBPs) parvalbumin (PV; Swant; dilution 1:2000), calbindin (CB; Swant; dilution 1:1500); and (f) polyclonal antibody against calretinin (CR; Swant; dilution 1:1500). For details of the ICC procedures see Spreafico et al. (1998a).

Results

In the present report two patients are described, in which MRI was showing a localized signal alteration in the cortical mantle suggestive of localized cortical dysplasia. They were referred to the department of Neurosurgery, CHU in Grenoble. In both patients the MRI visible lesion was ablated and corticectomies of the epileptogenic zones (as defined on the basis of the SEEG recordings) were performed. In this paper only the neuropathological finding of the lesion will be reported, although cortical abnormalities, not detected by MRI, were observed also in some of the epileptogenic areas revealed by the SEEG.

Patient Z.R.

After a normal delivery and normal psychomotor development, this female patient started having partial complex seizures at the age of nine. Since that time, despite the tested antiepileptic drugs, the semiology of the seizures did not modify but their frequency increased to more than five daily. A CT scan demonstrated only a mild ventricular asymmetry while the MRI disclosed a cortical lesion, hyperintense in T2 weighted signal, in the right temporal area. The first operation was addressed to a complete lesionectomy revealed by neuroradiological images. One year later the seizures, although reduced, were still present and a second surgery was performed preceded by SEEG recordings showing epileptogenic zones not only in the areas closed to the previous lesionectomy but also in other regions of the temporal lobe, including the hippocampus, the temporal pole, T_2 and T_3. Ablation of these areas was performed. The patient is now seizure-free after almost two years of follow up.

Neuropathological examination of the ablated tissue showed, in the MRI visible lesion, a disorganized cytoarchitecture of the cortex. In sections processed for routine histology no cortical layers were recognized except layer I (Fig. 1A). Numerous neurones were found in the white matter, while the deep cortical layers contained aggregates of small round-shaped or fusiform cells with a large nucleus surrounded by a thin rim of cytoplasm. These cells had the morphological aspect of immature neuroblasts (Fig. 1D). Large vascular trunks perpendicular to the pial surface with only few collateral branches were present and particularly visible in the superficial layers. These

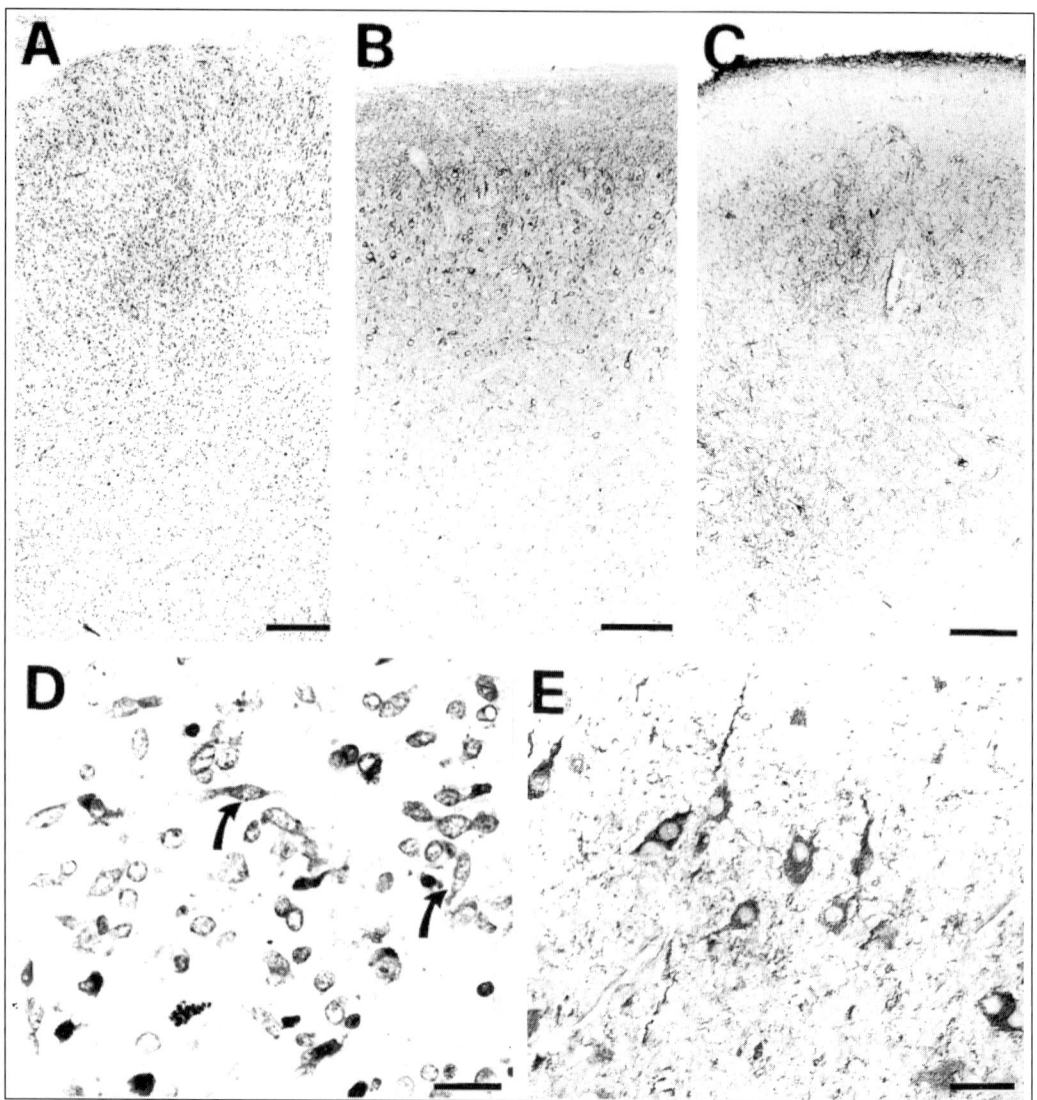

Fig. 1. (A) Low power photomicrograph of a thionin stained section showing the laminar disruption of the cortical mantle (scale bar: 200 μm). (B) The laminar disorganization is also visible in the MAP 2 stained section (scale bar: 110 μm). (C) Low power photomicrograph showing a cortical gliosis as revealed by GFAP immunostaining (scale bar : 110 μm). (D) High power photomicrograph showing an aggregation of poorly differentiated cells (neuroblasts, arrows) within the cortical gray matter (scale bar: 20 μm). (E) Misplaced and disoriented MAP 2 positive neurons in the cortical mantle (scale bar: 30 μm).

observations were confirmed by the immunocytochemistry. SMI 311 and MAP 2 immunoreactive (ir) neurones were dishomogeneously distributed through the cortex with no laminar organization (Fig. 1B). Neurones were weakly labelled by both the antisera; misplaced and disoriented neurones (particularly with pyramidal shape) were present throughout the cortex and in the white matter (Fig. 1E). Immunostaining performed with GFAP showed a moderate gliosis through all the thickness of the sample but particularly around blood vessels and in the white matter (Fig. 1C). Neither giant neurones nor balloon cells were found. A reduced number of CaBPs-positive neurones and terminals was observed as compared to those reported in normal human cortex (not shown).

Patient C.O.

This male patient, born after normal delivery, started having partial seizures at the age of seven. Initially he was treated with Carbamazepine with reduction of seizures but, at age 15, seizures increased and were incompletely controlled by other antiepileptic drugs. EEG recording showed interictal discharges of spikes and waves in the parietal region of the right hemisphere. CT scan was normal. MRI showed, in the T2 weighted signal, hyperintensity in the right cortical area of the parieto-occipital region, defined as focal cortical dysplasia. After SEEG recording, the patient was operated on and the dysplasia was removed along with the epileptogenic areas (corticectomy) revealed by the SEEG findings.

In the dysplastic region revealed by MRI a complete disorganization of cortical lamination was found so that any layer except layer I could have been recognized (Figs. 2 and 3A). In thionin (Fig. 3A, B) and Bielschowsky stained sections, numerous abnormal and heavily stained neurones were present. Large, round-shaped neurones were scattered throughout the cortex, but particularly at the border with the white matter, while giant pyramidal cells, some with inverted polarity, predominated in the superficial layers. The neurones showed an intense immunoreactivity for MAP 2 and particularly for SMI 311 (Fig. 3C). Numerous large SMI 311 in neurones were also present in the white matter. In this region, thionin (Fig. 4A) and Bielschowsky staining revealed the presence of many binucleated, large balloon cells. These cells also invaded the deep portion of the gray matter, and their morphology and location were identical to those of the balloon cells described by

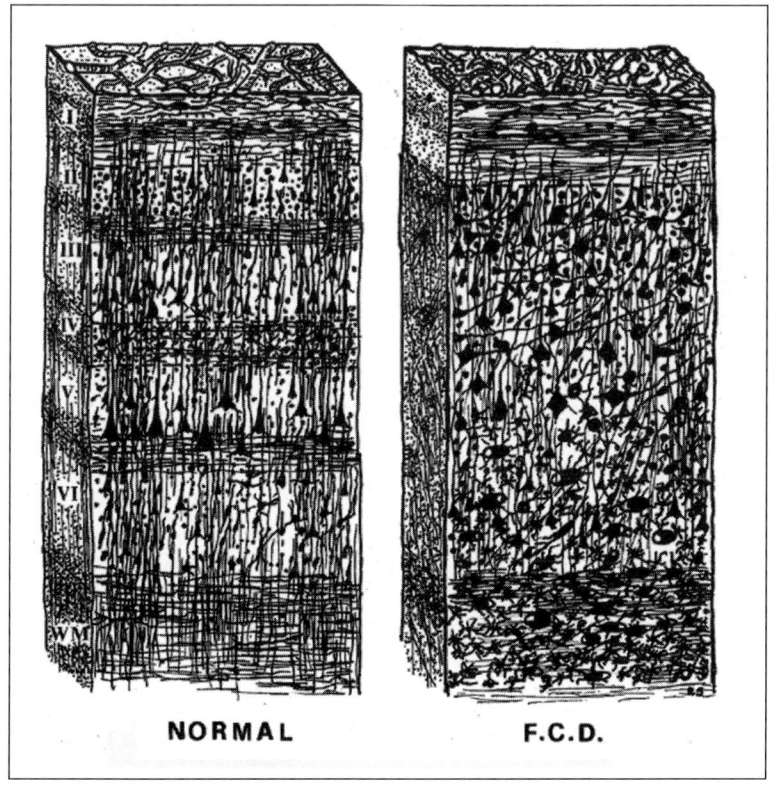

Fig. 2. Drawing showing the disorganization of cortical layers with presence of giant cells in Taylor's focal cortical dysplasia (F.C.D.) as compared to normal cortex.

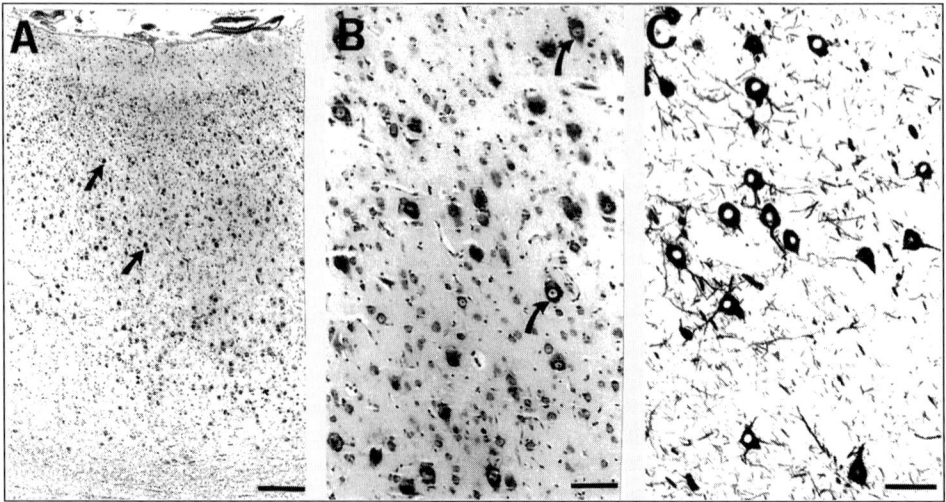

Fig. 3. Low (A) and high power (B) photomicrographs showing the disorganized cellular arrangement as visible in thionin stained sections. Note the heavily stained hypertrophic neurons (arrows) scattered throughout the gray matter (scale bars: 200 and 80 μm respectively). (C) Large and disoriented neurons stained by SMI 311 antibody (scale bar: 100 μm).

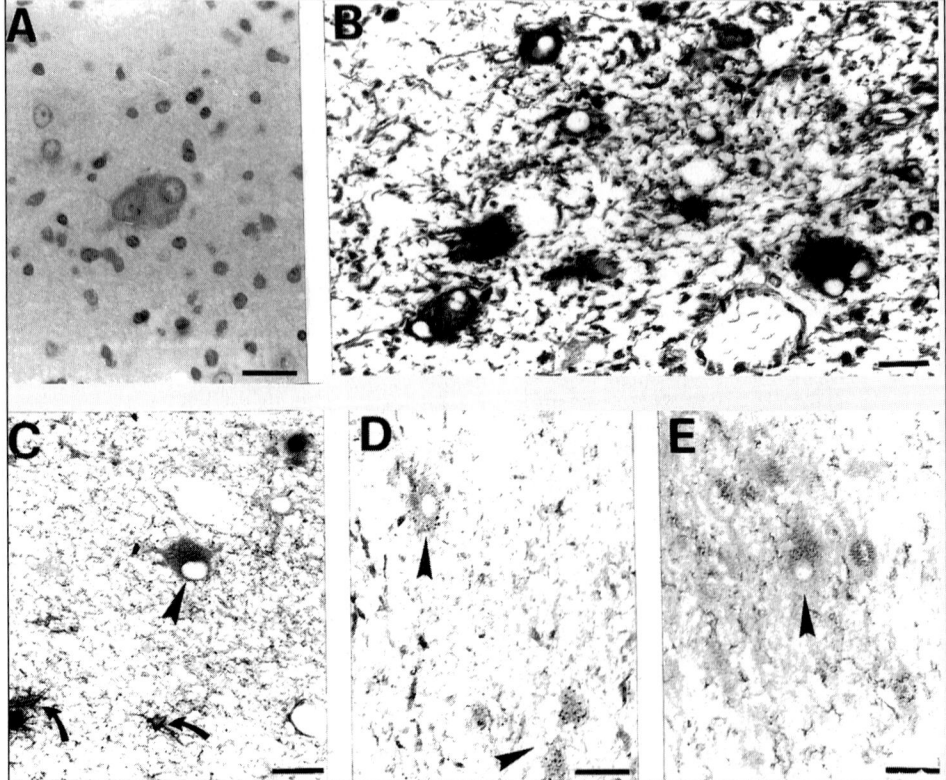

Fig. 4. Schematic drawing showing the distribution of parvalbumin immunoreactive neurons and terminals in the normal cortex and in Taylor's focal cortical dysplasia (F.C.D.). Note the reduction of immunopositive terminals in F.C.D. frequently clustered around large immunonegative neurons.

Taylor *et al.* (1971). Balloon cells were heavily labelled by anti-Vimentin and anti-GFAP antibodies (Fig. 4B and C) and a light immunoreactivity for SMI 311 and MAP 2 was also present in most, if not all, of these cells (Fig. 4D and E).

In sections processed for GFAP immunocytochemistry, numerous astrocytes were found in the white matter and in the subpial region, suggesting a moderate degree of gliosis. Balloon cells were however less intensely labelled as compared to the reactive astrocytes (Fig. 4C).

A particular reduction of immunoreactive neurones and neuropil was observed in sections processed with antibodies against CaBPs (not shown). Despite this fact, neurones labelled by PV, CR and CB had apparently normal morphology and were heavily labelled. However, the typical distribution of PV-ir terminals observed in normal human cortex was completely disrupted and immunoreactive puncta appeared particularly concentrated around PV-negative perikarya of giant, round-shaped and pyramidal neurones. This peculiar distribution and arrangement of PV-positive puncta was especially evident in the superficial layers and at the border between gray and white matter (Fig. 5). The abnormal distribution of CaBPs and particularly of PV immunoreactivity was identical to that reported by Spreafico *et al.* (1998a) in three other patients with similar neuropathological and radiological findings.

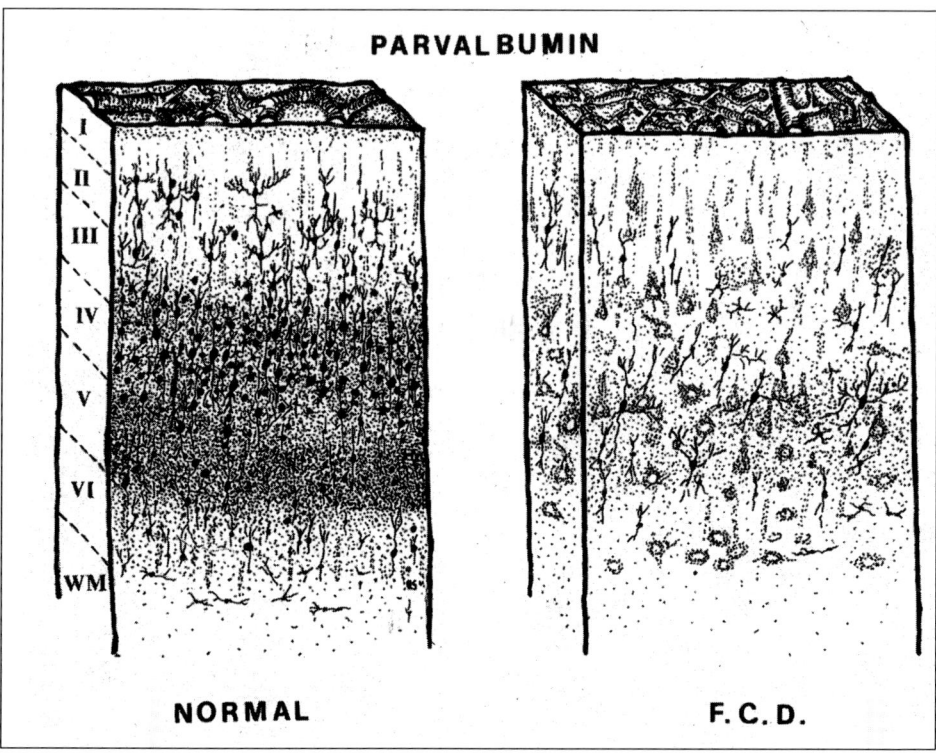

Fig. 5. (A) Binucleated large balloon cells in the white matter (scale bar: 20 μm). (B) Balloon cells are heavily stained by Vimentin antibody (scale bar: 20 μm). (C) GFAP immunoreactivity showing the presence of both reactive astrocytes (arrows) and balloon cells (arrowhead, scale bar: 20 μm). (D and E) Arrowheads point to some balloon cells lightly stained by SMI 311 and MAP 2 respectively (scale bars: 30 μm).

Discussion

The present data report the neuropathological differences observed in two epileptic patients presenting, localized cortical dysplastic lesions at the MRI investigation. Before discussing neuropathological peculiarities, some electroclinical and radiological considerations must be emphasised. In some areas, particularly those close to the visible lesion, a disrupted cortical organization similar to that found in the MRI detected lesion, although less intense was found. This finding suggests that, despite the high resolution of the MRI, some pathological cortical areas can escape neuroradiological investigation, leading to the risk of leaving epileptogenic tissue in place despite an apparently complete 'lesionectomy'. Although not described in detail in this report, it should be mentioned also that in both cases, epileptogenic areas as detected by SEEG included not only cortical areas within the visible lesion but also zones apparently normal in the neuropathological investigation. Consequently in our opinion SEEG recordings are mandatory at least in those patients in which the semiology of seizures is not evident.

Despite the fact that in both patients the dysplastic lesions were quite localized, and the term 'focal cortical dysplasia' could have been applied, a more accurate analysis of MRI selected sections revealed some differences. In the first case the lesion appeared more dishomogeneous than in the second case, while in the second patient a blurring between gray and white matter was present. These differences could be attributed to the different neuropathological process observed at the microscopical level. In fact in the first patient (Z.R.) a disruption of cortical layers was found with the presence of islands of immature neurones and diffused moderate gliosis. By contrast, in C.O. the alteration of layers was associated with the presence of giant hypertrophic neurones and balloon cells not visible in Z.R. The high content of neurofilament in giant neurones, and the presence of balloon cells in the deep layers and in the white matter, could explain the hyperintense signal and the blurring of the gray–white matter junction visible at MRI (Barkovich et al., 1997; Bronen et al., 1997).

These neuropathological findings were reported originally by Taylor et al. (1971) and subsequently described by other authors (Rorke, 1994, Duong et al., 1994; Mischel et al., 1995; Prayson & Estes, 1995; Crino et al., 1997; Spreafico et al., 1998a) thus defining a peculiar form of cortical dysplasia generally termed focal cortical dysplasia (or Taylor's focal cortical dysplasia). In agreement with these data we concur that this term should be applied only to this form of dysplasia, where neuropathological observations disclose hypertrophic neurones and balloon cells in association with dislamination of the cortex. In fact the dysplasia observed in the first patient was radiologically and neuropathologically different from that observed in the second case. In Z.R. the cortical disruption was associated with the presence of immature cells interspersed within the cortical mantle and of numerous neurones in the white matter, but neither giant neurones nor balloon cells were detected. These aspects suggest a disturbance of migratory events with presumably a subsequent impairment of neuronal differentiation. Thus, in our opinion, this lesion could be appropriately named as a neuronal migration disorder.

The second case, namely Taylor's focal cortical dysplasia, seems to be a more complex disorder than the previous one. The presence of giant hypertrophic neurones filled by a large amount of neurofilaments and the large distribution of balloon cells suggest that more complex mechanisms are involved in the generation of this dysplasia. In particular, the balloon cells immunoreactive for Vimentin antibody, recognizing early intermediate filaments of the glial lineage, and for SMI 311 and MAP 2 suggest that these cells could represent cellular elements that have not accomplished their final fate (Taylor et al., 1971; De Rosa et al., 1992; Doung et al., 1994; Crino et al., 1997). It should be noted that the present findings are very similar to those we reported on three other epileptic patients, thus confirming previous observations (Spreafico et al., 1998a).

In both the presented patients, a decrease of CaBPs immunoreactivity was observed and this finding is in agreement with other reports on the cortices of epileptic patients (Ferrer et al., 1992,

1994; Marco et al., 1996). However a peculiar distribution of the PV immunoreactivity, never observed in other forms of dysplasia, was detected only in patients affected by Taylor's type cortical dysplasia (Battaglia et al., 1996; Preul et al., 1997; Spreafico et al., 1998a) thus confirming the particular identity of this dysplastic lesion.

Acknowledgements

Supported by grant ICS 030.3/RF95/223 from the Italian Ministry of Health and by the Mariani Foundation for Paediatric Neurology, Milan. Thanks are due to M. Denegri for typing and editing support.

References

Barkovich, A.J., Chuang, S.H. & Norman, D. (1987): MR of neuronal migration anomalies. *Am. J. Neuroradiol.* **8**, 1009–1017.

Barkovich, A.J., Kuzniecky, R.I., Bollen, A.W. & Grant, P.E. (1997): Focal transmantle dysplasia: a specific malformation of cortical development. *Neurology* **49**, 1148–1152.

Battaglia, G., Arcelli, P., Granata, T., Selvaggio, M., Andermann, F., Dubeau, F., Olivier, A., Tampieri, D., Villemure, J.G., Avoli, M., Avanzini, G. & Spreafico, R. (1996): Neuronal migration disorders and epilepsy: a morphological analysis of three surgically treated patients. *Epilepsy Res.* **26**, 49–58.

Bayer, S.A. & Altman, J. (1991) *Neocortical development*. New York: Raven Press.

Bronen, R.A., Vives, K.P., Kim, J.H., Fulbright, R.K., Spencer, S.S. & Spencer, D.D. (1997): Focal cortical dysplasia of Taylor, balloon cell subtype: MR differentiation from low-grade tumors. *Am. J. Neuroradiol.* **18**, 1141–1151.

Crino, P.B., Trojanowski, J.Q. & Eberwine, J. (1997): Internexin, MAP1B, and nestin in cortical dysplasia as markers of developmental maturity. *Acta Neuropathol.* **93**, 619–627.

De Felipe, J., Sola, R.G., Marco, P., del Rio, M.R., Pulido, P. & Ramon y Cajal, S. (1993): Selective changes in the microorganization of the human epileptogenic neocortex revealed by parvalbumin immunoreactivity. *Cerebral Cortex* **3**, 39–48.

De Rosa, M.J., Secor, D.L., Barsom, M., Fisher, R.S. & Vinters, H.V. (1992): Neuropathologic findings in surgically treated hemimegalencephaly: immunohistochemical, morphometric, and ultrastructural study. *Acta Neuropathol.* **84**, 250–260.

Duong, T., De Rosa, M.J., Poukens, V., Vinters, H.V. & Fisher, R.S. (1994): Neuronal cytoskeletal abnormalities in human cerebral cortical dysplasia. *Acta Neuropathol.* **87**, 493–503.

Farrell, M.A., De Rosa, M.J., Curran, J.C., Lenard Secor, D., Cornford, M.E., Comair, Y.G., Peacock, W.J., Shields, W.D. & Vinters, H.V. (1992): Neuropathologic findings in cortical resections (including hemispherectomies) performed for the treatment of intractable childhood epilepsy. *Acta Neuropathol.* **83**, 246–259.

Ferrer, I., Tuñón, T., Soriano, E., del Rio, A., Iraizoz, I., Fonseca, M. & Guionnet, N. (1992): Calbindin immunoreactivity in normal human temporal neocortex. *Brain. Res.* **572**, 33–41.

Ferrer, I., Oliver, B., Russi, A., Casas, R. & Rivera, R. (1994): Parvalbumin and calbindin-D28K immunocytochemistry in human neocortical epileptic foci. *J. Neurol. Sci* **123**, 18–25.

Fried, I. & Cascino, G. (1993): Lesional surgery. In: *Surgical treatment of the epilepsies*, 2nd edition, ed. J. Engel Jr., pp. 501–509. New York: Raven Press.

Jammes, J.L., Gilles, F.H. & Yakovlev, P.I. (1973): Measures of development of matrix and of isocortex and allocortex in the human foetus (abstract). *Neurology* **23**, 401–402.

Kostovic, I. & Rakic, P. (1990): Developmental history of the transient subplate zone in the visual and somatosensory cortex of the macaque monkey and human brain. *J. Comp. Neurol.* **297**, 441–470.

Kuzniecky, R., Morawetz, R., Faught, E. & Black, L. (1995): Frontal and central lobe focal dysplasia: clinical, EEG and imaging features. *Dev. Med. Child Neurol.* **37**, 159–166.

Luskin, M.B. & Shatz, C.J. (1985): Studies of the earliest generated cells of the cat's visual cortex: cogeneration of subplate and marginal zones. *J. Neurosci.* **5**, 1062–1075.

Marco, P., Sola, R.G., Pulido, P., Alijarde, M.T., Sánchez, A., Cajal, R.S. & De Felipe, J. (1996): Inhibitory neurones in the human epileptogenic temporal neocortex. An immunocytochemical study. *Brain* **119**, 1327–1347.

Marín-Padilla, M. (1978): Dual origin of the mammalian neocortex and evolution of the cortical plate. *Anat. Embryol.* **152**, 109–126.

Marín-Padilla, M. (1984): Neurones of layer I: A developmental analysis. In: *Cerebral cortex, Vol. 1*, eds. A. Peters & E.G Jones, pp. 447–478. New York: Plenum Press.

McConnell, S.K. (1988): Development and decision-making in the mammalian cerebral cortex. *Brain Res. Rev.* **13**, 1–23.

Mischel, P.S., Nguyen, L.P. & Vinters, H.V. (1995): Cerebral cortical dysplasia associated with pediatric epilepsy. Review of neuropathologic features and proposal for a grading system. *J. Neuropathol. Exp. Neurol.* **54**, 137–153.

Munari, C. & Bancaud, J. (1985): The role of stereo-EEG in the evaluation of partial epileptic seizures. In: *The epilepsies*, eds. M.L. Morselli & R.J. Porter, pp. 267–306. London: Butterworths.

Palmini, A., Andermann, E. & Andermann, F. (1994): Prenatal events and genetic factors in epileptic patients with neuronal migration disorders. *Epilepsia* **35**, 965–973.

Prayson, R.A. & Estes, M.L. (1995): Cortical dysplasia: a histopathologic study of 52 cases of partial lobectomy in patients with epilepsy. *Hum. Pathol.* **26**, 493–500.

Preul, M.C., Leblanc, R., Cendes, F., Dubeau, F., Reutens, D., Spreafico, R., Battaglia, G., Avoli, M., Langevin, P., Arnold, D.L. & Villemure, J.-G. (1997): Function and organization in dysgenic cortex. Case report. *J. Neurosurg.* **87**, 113–121.

Rorke, L.B. (1994): A perspective: the role of disordered genetic control of neurogenesis in the pathogenesis of migration disorders. *J. Neuropathol. Exp. Neurol.* **53**, 105–117.

Sidman, R.L. & Rakic, P. (1973): Neuronal migration disorders, with special reference to developing human brain: a review. *Brain Res.* **62**, 1–35.

Spreafico, R., Battaglia, G., Arcelli, P., Andermann, F., Dubeau, F., Palmini, A., Olivier, A., Villemure, J.-G., Tampieri, D., Avanzini, G. & Avoli, M. (1998a): Cortical dysplasia. An immunocytochemical study of three patients. *Neurology* **50**, 27–36.

Spreafico, R., Pasquier, B., Minotti, L., Garbelli, R., Kahane, P., Grand, S., Benabid, A.L., Tassi, L., Avanzini, G., Battaglia, G. & Munari, C. (1998b): Immunocytochemical investigation on dysplastic human tissue from epileptic patients. *Epilepsy Res.* **32**, 34–48.

Talairach, J., Bancaud, J., Szikla, G., Bonis, A., Geier, S. & Vedrenne, C. (1974): Exploration fonctionnelle stéréotaxique (SEEEG). In: *Approche nouvelle de la neurochirurgie de l'épilepsie. Méthodologie stéréotaxique et résultats thérapeutiques*, eds. J. Talairach, J. Bancaud, G. Szikla, S. Geier, C. Vedrenne, pp. 99–130. Paris: *Neurochirurgie* **20** (Suppl. 1).

Taylor, D.C., Falconer, M.A., Bruton, C.J. & Corsellis, J.A.N. (1971): Focal dysplasia of the cerebral cortex in epilepsy. *J. Neurol. Neurosurg. Psychiatry* **34**, 369–387.

PART V

GENETIC STUDIES IN NEURONAL MIGRATION DISORDERS

v

Chapter 21

The role of homeobox genes in NMDs

Edoardo Boncinelli[1,2], Antonio Faiella[1], Michela Zortea[3], Francesca Albani[4]

[1]*DIBIT, Istituto Scientifico H San Raffaele, Via Olgettina 58, 20132 Milan, Italy;* [2]*Centro di Farmacologia Cellulare e Molecolare, CNR, Via Vanvitelli 32, 20129 Milan, Italy;* [3]*Divisione di Radiologia, Ospedale Bambino Gesù, Piazza Sant'Onofrio 4, 00165 Rome, Italy;* [4]*Istituto di Neuropsichiatria Infantile, Fondazione Stella Maris, Università di Pisa, Via dei Giacinti 2, 56018 Calambrone, Pisa, Italy*

Summary

Many genes playing a role in the control of the development of the central nervous system of vertebrates are homeobox genes. Among them there are the *Hox* (HOX in humans) genes which collectively control regionalization and cell identity in the developing hindbrain and spinal cord. Other homeobox gene families, including the *Otx* and *Emx* genes, control brain development. More specifically, *Otx2* appears to play a crucial role in the early establishment of the rostral brain; *Otx1* and *Otx2* cooperate to define the posterior boundary of midbrain; and *Emx1* and *Emx2* play a major role in the developing cerebral cortex. Understanding the role of these genes or of other developmental genes acting under their control may be relevant for deciphering the etiopathological basis of some congenital brain defects and multifactorial brain disorders.

In the past few years the cellular and molecular mechanisms by which specific types of neurones are generated and organized in the central nervous system (CNS) have been explored. A number of developmental pathways have been elucidated and many principles have been discovered, most of which are conserved in evolution. All events of differentiation and patterning at the level of single cells or groups of cells are preceded by developmental decisions that involve entire regions of the developing nervous system. Some of these events have received particular attention. Among them, the regionalization of the CNS along its anterior–posterior axis, the establishment and maintenance of a dorso-ventral polarity of the neural tube, the process of segregation of the presumptive cerebral cortex from basal ganglia and the lamination of the cerebral cortex. Most alterations in one of these processes are likely to cause major developmental defects or contribute to some multifactorial disorders of the nervous system.

A key role in the regionalization of the CNS and in the specification of the various anatomical and functional neural domains is played by regulatory genes. These genes act through the control of the expression of other genes lying hierarchically downstream from them and sometimes termed 'target genes'. Regulatory genes generally encode transcription factors, i.e. nuclear proteins able to recognize specific DNA sequences, bind to them and modulate the level of expression of the corresponding target genes. A relatively large proportion of regulatory genes are homeobox genes (Boncinelli *et al.*, 1998).

Homeobox genes are regulatory genes characterized by the presence of a specific DNA sequence termed homeobox, able to code for a protein domain of some 60 amino acid residues, termed homeodomain. It is through the action of their homeodomain that the protein products of the homeobox genes, the homeoproteins, bind to the regulatory regions of specific genes and control their expression. Among the vertebrate homeobox genes, those belonging to the *Hox* family (McGinnis & Krumlauf, 1992; Krumlauf, 1994 for reviews) stand out. The 39 homeobox genes belonging to the *Hox* family are structurally and functionally homologous to the *Drosophila* homeotic genes. In mice and humans, they are organized in four genomic clusters of about 100 kb in length, termed *Hox* loci (HOXA, HOXB, HOXC and HOXD in man), each containing several genes arranged in a homologous sequence. Corresponding genes in the four loci belong to any one of 13 homology groups. *Hox* genes collectively control the identity of the various regions along the body axis from the branchial area through the tail. This action occurs in a collinear way, with 3' *Hox* genes expressed early in development and controlling anterior regions; and progressively more 5' genes expressed later in development and controlling progressively more posterior regions. In particular, 3' *Hox* genes of the four loci belonging to groups 1-4 primarily control the development of the branchial area and of the rhombencephalon, the embryonic region corresponding to the future hindbrain, and its orderly regionalization into 7-8 neural segments termed rhombomeres. Central *Hox* genes of groups 5-8 control the thoracic portion of the body, whereas 5' *Hox* genes of groups 9-13 control the lumbo-sacral region, including analia and genitalia. Conversely, these genes do not seem to play any significant role in the head and in brain regions anterior to the hindbrain.

Actually, development of the anteriormost body domain corresponding to the anterior head has remained relatively obscure also in flies (Finkelstein & Boncinelli, 1994). Nevertheless, at least three genes have been identified that play a role in the development and regionalization of the *Drosophila* head: *empty spiracles (ems)*, *orthodenticle (otd)* and *buttonhead (btd)*. The first two are homeobox genes and four vertebrate homologues have been isolated and characterized. These four genes are *Emx1* and *Emx2* (Simeone et al., 1992a, b), related to *ems*, and *Otx1* and *Otx2* (Simeone et al., 1992a, 1993; Finkelstein & Boncinelli 1994), related to *otd*. The four vertebrate genes are expressed in extended regions of the developing rostral brain of mouse embryos, including the presumptive cerebral cortex and olfactory bulbs.

At day 10 of development (E10) the entire neural tube consists of neuroepithelial cells in active proliferation and most of the specific differentiative events have not yet occurred. All four genes are already expressed. Their expression domains (Simeone et al., 1992a) are continuous regions of the developing brain contained within each other in the sequence $Emx1 < Emx2 < Otx1 < Otx2$. The $<Emx1<$ expression domain includes the dorsal telencephalon with a posterior boundary slightly anterior to that between presumptive diencephalon and telencephalon. *Emx2* is expressed in dorsal and ventral neuroectoderm with an anterior boundary overlapping that of *Emx1* and a posterior boundary within the roof of presumptive diencephalon. The *Otx1* expression domain contains the *Emx2* domain. It covers a continuous region including part of the telencephalon, the diencephalon and the mesencephalon with an anterior boundary approximately coincident with that of *Emx2*. The posterior boundary of *Otx1* domain practically coincides with that of the mesencephalon. Finally, the *Otx2* expression domain contains the *Otx1* domain, both dorsally and ventrally, and covers the entire fore- and midbrain.

In summary, analysis of E10 brain shows a pattern of nested expression domains of the four genes in brain regions defining an embryonic rostral, or pre-isthmic, brain, including the fore- and midbrain, as opposed to hindbrain and spinal cord. The first appearance of transcripts of the four genes is also sequential: *Otx2* is already expressed in the implanted blastocyst at E5.5, followed by *Otx1* and *Emx2* in E8-8.5 and finally by *Emx1* in E9.5 mouse embryos (Simeone et al., 1992a). It seems reasonable to postulate a role of the four homeobox genes in establishing the identity of the various embryonic brain regions. In this respect, the specification of the regions of the early rostral brain seems to be a discrete process with its focal point in the dorsal telencephalon.

Otx1 and *Otx2* are also expressed in restricted regions of diencephalon: epithalamus, dorsal thalamus and mammillary region of posterior hypothalamus. Both *Otx* genes are also expressed in developing special sense organs, that is in the olfactory epithelium, as well as in the developing inner ear and in the developing eye, including the external sheaths of the optic nerve (Boncinelli *et al.*, 1993; Simeone *et al.*, 1993). It has to be emphasized that *Otx* and *Emx* genes are by no means the only genes expressed in the developing brain. Many other regulatory or structural genes are also expressed here, even if not exclusively (Rubenstein & Puelles, 1994; Rubenstein *et al.*, 1994; Shimamura *et al.*, 1995 and references therein). Partly on the basis of the expression domains of all of these genes, a model has been proposed for the subdivision of the developing rostral brain in neuromeres, namely the so-called prosomeric model (Rubenstein *et al.*, 1994). It entails a subdivision of the embryonic forebrain into six neuromeres, termed prosomeres, p1 to p6, from posterior to anterior. Three of these, p1 to p3, subdivide the diencephalon and three subdivide what these authors call secondary prosencephalon, that is telencephalon and hypothalamic regions.

All four genes are expressed between E9.5 and E10.5 in the presumptive cerebral cortex. Starting from E10.75, *Otx2* expression progressively disappears from this region, whereas *Emx1*, *Emx2* and *Otx1* remain expressed in the presumptive cerebral cortex in an extended developmental period corresponding to major events in cortical neurogenesis (Simeone *et al.*, 1992b). *Emx1* expression domain comprises cortical regions including primordia of neopallium, hippocampal and parahippocampal archipallium. *Emx1* expression seems characteristic of cortical regions, mainly but not exclusively hexalaminar in nature. In the same period, the *Emx2* expression domain comprises presumptive cortical regions including neopallium, hippocampal and parahippocampal archipallium and selected paleopallial localisations. (Simeone *et al.*, 1992b). *Otx1* expression domain in forebrain (Simeone *et al.*, 1993; Frantz *et al.*, 1994; Gulisano *et al.*, 1996) includes dorsal telencephalon but also extends to basal regions.

It is interesting to consider the temporal pattern of expression of the *Emx* genes in the various zones of the forming cerebral cortex (Gulisano *et al.*, 1996). Here, at least three major zones can be defined: the germinal neuroepithelium or ventricular zone, where cortical neurones proliferate, a transitional field, and finally the forming cortical plate from which the cortical gray matter will subsequently develop (Bayer & Altman, 1991). At the beginning and up to E12.5 the germinal neuroepithelium is practically the sole component of the prosencephalic wall. Then a transitional field appears. This includes the subventricular zone and the intermediate zone to which differentiating cortical cells translocate before migrating to outer regions. As development proceeds, the thickness of the cortical plate progressively increases. Both the transitional field and the cortical plate develop at the expense of the neuroepithelium according to specific spatial and temporal gradients within the forming cortex. Two major neurogenetic and morphogenetic gradients can be observed: one progressing anterior to posterior and a second progressing ventrolateral to dorsomedial. The various cortical layers are then formed in an inside-out pattern (Bayer & Altman, 1991). Cell tracing experiments have shown that neurones destined to occupy the depth of the cortex are generated first and that the subsequently generated waves of neurones bypass the earlier ones by active migration and settle above them.

In mouse embryos of all stages, *Emx2* expression coincides with cells of the germinal neuroepithelium (Gulisano *et al.*, 1996; Mallamaci *et al.*, 1998). In E12.5 embryos, the *Emx2* hybridization signal is uniformly distributed across the cortex without major differences, but starting from E13.5 it appears to be confined to the germinal neuroepithelium of the ventricular zone, excluding both the transitional field and the cortical plate. From day 14.5 on, *Emx2* cortical expression progressively declines in anterior and ventrolateral regions and by the end of gestation is solely confined to specific cell layers in the hippocampus. It is conceivable that *Emx2* plays a role in the control of proliferation of cortical neuroblasts, and thus the regulation of their subsequent migration process, since it is known that these cells reach their final destination in the mature cortex according to their birthdate.

Conversely, *Emx1* is expressed in most cortical neurones, whether proliferating, migrating, differentiating, or fully differentiated and organized in a mature cerebral cortex (Briata *et al.*, 1996; Gulisano *et al.*, 1996). On the other hand, no *Emx1* expression is detectable in ventral forebrain regions and in particular in the developing basal ganglia. These observations suggest that *Emx1* may be involved in the definition of a specific cellular identity in the cerebral cortex.

It is interesting to note that *Emx2* is expressed in the ventricular zone of midgestation mouse embryos according to an anterior–posterior gradient of intensity, higher in posterior cortical regions than in anterior ones (Gulisano *et al.*, 1996; Mallamaci *et al.*, 1998). This expression gradient of *Emx2* is suggestive of a contribution of *Emx2* to cortical polarization in the framework of an arealization process taking place in the ventricular zone (O'Leary *et al.*, 1994). As a regulatory gene encoding a transcription factor, *Emx2* is an ideal candidate for generating and/or maintaining a position-dependent signal within the cortex.

Transgenic mice lacking *Otx2* gene products are early embryonic lethal (Acampora *et al.*, 1995; Ang *et al.*, 1996; Matsuo *et al.*, 1995). Therefore, they do not provide useful information about the role of this gene in late brain development. Conversely, transgenic mice lacking the gene products of *Otx1*, *Emx1* and *Emx2* are born and their brain can be analyzed. All show major disturbances in the architecture of various brain regions, including the cerebral cortex. Particularly noticeable is the altered patterning of hippocampus and the total absence of dentate gyrus in *Emx2* null mice (Pellegrini *et al.*, 1996). A detailed anatomical and functional analysis of these mutants is underway.

In the meantime, mutations in the human *Emx2* gene, more correctly designated EMX2, have been reported (Brunelli *et al.*, 1996; Boncinelli, 1997; Faiella *et al.* 1997; Granata *et al.*, 1997) in sporadic cases of schizencephaly, a human congenital defect of the cerebral cortex. The schizencephalies are congenital brain malformations characterized by clefts of the cerebral mantle, extending from the pial surface to the lateral ventricles and lined by heterotopic polymicrogyric gray matter (Yakovlev & Wadsworth, 1946a, b). The schizencephaly patients are clinically characterized by motor and mental deficits of varying degree, according to the severity and extent of the brain malformation, and they are frequently affected by epilepsy. The malformation may be unilateral or bilateral, the latter being usually symmetric in location, but not in size (Guerrini *et al.*, 1996). Based on the space separating the walls of the fissure, an open-lip form and a closed-lip form can be distinguished. The cortex is covered with a membrane resulting from the fusion between the pia and the ventricular ependyma (pial–ependymal seam). The cleft can be detected in any encephalic site, but it is far more frequent in the perisylvian area (Barkovich & Kjos, 1992). In 80 per cent of cases the septum pellucidum is also absent (Chamberlain *et al.*, 1990). Septo-optic dysplasia (agenesis of the septum pellucidum and optic nerve hypoplasia) is observed in about one-third of cases (Barkovich & Norman, 1988; Hosley *et al.*, 1992).

Close examination of both mouse and human phenotypes associated with *Emx2* mutations suggests an implication of cell migration as well as cell proliferation in the cerebral cortex. With this in mind, we very recently analysed in detail the distribution of the EMX2 homeoprotein (Mallamaci *et al.*, 1998) and found it to be also present in the nuclei of Cajal–Retzius cells localized in the developing cortical layer I. These relatively large cells are thought to be instrumental in organizing the fibres of radial glia necessary for the appropriate migration of cortical neurones (Marín-Padilla, 1998). In this light, human cortical disorders arising from EMX2 mutations may be attributable to defects in both proliferation and migration processes of cortical neurones.

The finding of EMX2 mutations in two siblings, and not in their neurologically normal parents, provides further evidence that, at least in some cases, schizencephalies are determined by deleterious mutations of this homeobox gene (Granata *et al.*, 1997). The genetic hypothesis does not rule out the possibility of alternative pathogenetic mechanisms. A genetic analysis of a larger series of schizencephaly patients (Faiella *et al.*, 1997) demonstrated that only some schizencephaly patients carried EMX2 mutations. Therefore, some cases of schizencephaly may not be related to loss of

Table 1. Summary of cases analysed

Patient	Schizencephaly	Association	Nature/position of the mutation	Mechanism
BA	severe, bilateral	agenesis cc, sp	base insertion within the hb	nonsense
DZ	severe, bilateral	agenesis cc, sp	synonymous substitution within the hb	unknown
GM	severe, bilateral	agenesis cc, sp	deletion of two bases in the intron i2	unknown
ME	severe, bilateral	agenesis cc, sp	substitution at the 3' splice site of intron i1	splice site
MI	severe, bilateral	agenesis cc, fl	substitution at the first base of exon e2	splice site, missense
MM	severe, bilateral	hypoplasia cc	substitution at the first base of exon e2	splice site, missense
PN	severe, bilateral	hydr, dysgenesis cc	substitution at the 3' splice site of intron i1	splice site
FA	severe, bilateral	polymicrogyria	none	
BV	mild, unilateral	partial epilepsy	synonymous substitution within the hb	unknown
DCS	mild, unilateral	partial epilepsy	synonymous substitution within the hb	unknown
PC	mild, unilateral	partial epilepsy	synonymous substitution within the hb	unknown
VF	mild, unilateral	partial epilepsy, mMR	synonymous substitution within the hb	unknown
MB	mild, unilateral	partial epilepsy	deletion of one base within intron i2	unknown
PB	mild, unilateral	partial epilepsy	base substitution within intron i2	unknown
RB	mild, unilateral	partial epilepsy	none	
MC	mild, unilateral	partial epilepsy	none	
OD	mild, unilateral	partial epilepsy	none	
CG	mild, unilateral	partial epilepsy	none	

cc, corpus callosum; fl, frontal lobe; hb, homeobox; hydr, hydrocephalus; mMR, mild mental retardation; sp, septum pellucidum.

function of EMX2 gene, but may be acquired encephaloclastic lesions resulting, like porencephalies, from focal infarction in the territory of a major cerebral artery (Sarnat, 1992).

Patients with bilateral clefts usually have microcephaly, and severe developmental delay with spastic quadriparesis (Barkovich & Kjos, 1992; Granata et al., 1996). Open-lip clefts result in more severe impairment, with seizures being present in most patients, usually beginning before three-years of age. Unilateral clefts are accompanied by a much less severe clinical phenotype. Epilepsy is estimated to occur in equal proportion in patients with unilateral or bilateral cleft (about 80 per cent) (Granata et al., 1996). However, early seizure onset and seizure intractability are much more frequent when the malformation is bilateral (81 per cent vs 63 per cent and 50 per cent vs 27 per cent, respectively). Epilepsy is always partial, and there are no distinctive electroclinical patterns.

Classification and molecular analysis of the various *Emx2* mutations implicated in schizencephaly is likely to provide useful information for both clinical practice and understanding of the pathogenesis of these types of diseases (Table 1). Preliminary data (Capra et al., 1997; Faiella et al., 1997; Granata et al., 1997) point in the direction of a correlation between the nature of the molecular defect, the severity of the phenotype and the presence of particular clinical features. In fact, severe molecular defects, such as frameshift mutations or mutations affecting the splicing pattern, are invariably associated with severe, open-lip, bilateral schizencephaly, whereas subtle or leaky mutations are associated with mild, closed-lip, seemingly unilateral schizencephaly (Table 1). In view of the difficulties of the differential diagnosis of schizencephaly versus similar cortical dysplasias, it would be extremely valuable to be able to devise a molecular differential diagnosis to distinguish schizencephaly from other similar cortical dysplasias and to further discriminate between different clinical forms of schizencephaly. Results of this analysis are likely to be of primary relevance for our understanding of the genetic component of epilepsy and possibly of other multifactorial congenital defects of the brain.

Acknowledgements

We are indebted to G. Battaglia, A. Cama, T. Granata and R. Guerrini for a number of helpful comments and suggestions. This work was supported by grants from the EC BIOTECH and BIOMED Programmes, the Telethon-Italia Programme and the Italian Association for Cancer Research (AIRC).

References

Acampora, D., Mazan, S., Lallemand, Y., Avantaggiato, V., Maury, M., Simeone, A. & Brulet P. (1995): Forebrain and midbrain regions are deleted in *Otx2* mutants due to a defective anterior neuroectoderm specification during gastrulation. *Development* **121**, 3279–3290.

Ang, S.-L., Jin, O., Rhinn, M., Daigle, N., Stevenson, L. & Rossant, J. (1996): A targeted mouse *Otx2* mutation leads to severe defects in gastrulation and formation of axial mesoderm and to deletion of rostral brain. *Development* **122**, 243–252.

Barkovich, A.J. & Kjos, B.O. (1992): Schizencephaly: correlation of clinical findings with MR characteristics. *AJNR* **13**, 85–94

Barkovich, A.J. & Norman, D. (1988): MR of schizencephaly. *AJNR* **9**, 297–302.

Bayer, S.A. & Altman, J. (1991): *Neocortical development*. New York: Raven Press.

Boncinelli, E. (1997): Homeobox genes and disease. *Curr. Opin. Genet. Dev.* **7**, 331–337.

Boncinelli, E., Gulisano, M. & Broccoli, V. (1993): Emx and Otx genes in the developing mouse brain. *J. Neurobiol.* **24**, 1356–1366.

Boncinelli, E., Mallamaci, A. & Broccoli, V., (1998): Body plan genes and human malformation. *Adv. Genet.* **38**, 1–29.

Briata, P., Di Blas, E., Gulisano, M., Mallamaci, A., Iannone, R., Boncinelli, E. & Corte, G. (1996): EMX1 homeoprotein is expressed in cell nuclei of the developing cerebral cortex and in axons of the olfactory sensory neurones. *Mech. Dev.* **5**, 169–180.

Brunelli, S., Faiella, A., Capra, V., Nigro, V., Simeone, A., Cama, A. & Boncinelli, E. (1996): Germline mutations in the homeobox gene EMX2 in patients with severe schizencephaly. *Nature Genet.* **12**, 94–96.

Capra, V., De Marco, P., Moroni, A., Faiella, A., Brunelli, S., Tortori-Donati, P., Andreussi, I., Boncinelli, E. & Cama, A. (1997): Schizencephaly: surgical features and new molecular genetic results. *Eur. J. Ped. Surg.* **6 (Suppl.)** 27–29.

Chamberlain, M.C., Press, G.A. & Bejar, R.F. (1990): Neonatal schizencephaly: comparison of brain imaging. *Pediatr. Neurol.* **6**, 382–387.

Faiella, A., Brunelli, S., Granata, T., D'Incerti, L., Cardini, R., Lenti, C., Battaglia, G. & Boncinelli, E. (1997): A number of schizencephaly patients including two brothers are heterozygous for germline mutations in the homeobox gene EMX2. *Eur. J. Hum. Genet.* **5**, 186–190.

Finkelstein, R. & Boncinelli, E. (1994): From fly head to mammalian forebrain: the story of *Otd* and *Otx*. *Trends Genet.* **10**, 310–315.

Frantz, G.D., Weimann, J.M., Levine, M.E. & McConnell, S.K. (1994): *Otx1* and *Otx2* define layers and regions in developing cerebral cortex and cerebellum. *J. Neurosci.* **14**, 5725–5740.

Granata, T., Battaglia, G., D'Incerti, L., Franceschetti, S., Spreafico, R., Savoiardo, M. & Avanzini, G. (1996): Schizencephaly: clinical findings. In: *Dysplasias of cerebral cortex and epilepsy* eds. R.Guerrini, F. Andermann, R. Canapicchi, J. Roger, B. Zifkin & P. Pfanner, pp. 407–415. Philadelphia: Lippincott-Raven.

Granata, T., Farina, L., Faiella, A., Cardini, R., D'Incerti, L., Boncinelli, E. & Battaglia, G. (1997): Familial schizencephaly associated with EMX2 mutation. *Neurology* **48**, 1403–1406

Guerrini, R., Andermann, F., Canapicchi, R., Roger, J., Zifkin, B. & Pfanner, P. (eds.) (1996): *Dysplasias of cerebral cortex and epilepsy*. Philadelphia: Lippincott-Raven.

Gulisano, M., Broccoli, V., Pardini, C. & Boncinelli, E. (1996): *Emx1* and *Emx2* show different patterns of expression during proliferation and differentiation of the developing cerebral cortex. *Eur. J. Neurosci.* **8**, 1037–1050.

Hosley, M.A., Abroms, I.F. & Ragland, R.L. (1992): Schizencephaly: case report of familial incidence. *Pediatr. Neurol.* **8,** 148–150.

Krumlauf, R. (1994): *Hox* genes in vertebrate development. *Cell* **78,** 191–201.

Mallamaci, A., Iannone, R., Briata, P., Boncinelli, E. & Corte, G. (1999): EMX2 protein in the developing brain. *Mech. Dev.* [in press].

Marín-Padilla, M. (1998): Cajal–Retzius cells and the development of the neocortex. *Trends Neurosci.* **21,** 64–71.

Matsuo, I., Kuratani, S., Kimura, C., Takeda, N. & Aizawa, S. (1995): Mouse *Otx2* functions in the formation and patterning of rostral head. *Genes Dev.* **9,** 2646–2658.

McGinnis, W. & Krumlauf, R. (1992): Homeobox genes and axial patterning. *Cell* **68,** 283–302.

O'Leary, D.D.M., Schlaggar, B.L. & Tuttle, R. (1994): Specification of neocortical areas and thalamocortical connections. *Ann. Rev. Neurosci.* **17,** 419–39.

Pellegrini, M., Mansouri, A., Simeone, A., Boncinelli, E. & Gruss, P. (1996): Dentate gyrus formation requires *Emx2*. *Development* **122,** 3893–3898.

Rubenstein, J.L.R., Martinez, S., Shimamura, K. & Puelles, L. (1994): The embryonic vertebrate forebrain: the prosomeric model. *Science* **266,** 578–580.

Rubenstein, J.L.R. & Puelles, L. (1994): Homeobox gene expression during development of the vertebrate brain, *Curr. Top. Dev. Biol.* **29,** 1–63.

Sarnat, H.B. (1992): *Cerebral dysgenesis: embryology and clinical expression.* New York: Oxford University Press.

Shimamura, K., Hartigan, D.J., Martinez, S., Puelles, L. & Rubenstein, J.L.R. (1995): Longitudinal organization of the anterior neural plate and neural tube. *Development* **121,** 3923–3933.

Simeone, A., Acampora, D., Gulisano, M., Stornaiuolo, A. & Boncinelli, E. (1992a): Nested expression domains of four homeobox genes in developing rostral brain. *Nature* **358,** 687–690.

Simeone, A., Gulisano, M., Acampora, D., Stornaiuolo, A., Rambaldi, M. & Boncinelli, E. (1992b): Two vertebrate homeobox genes related to the *Drosophila empty spiracles* gene are expressed in the embryonic cerebral cortex. *EMBO J.* **11,** 2541–2550.

Simeone, A., Acampora, D., Mallamaci, A., Stornaiuolo, A., D'Apice, M.R., Nigro, V. & Boncinelli, E. (1993): A vertebrate gene related to *orthodenticle* contains a homeodomain of the bicoid class and demarcates anterior neuroectoderm in the gastrulating mouse embryo. *EMBO J.* **12,** 2735–2747.

Yakovlev, P. & Wadsworth, R.C. (1946a): Schizencephalies: a study of the congenital clefts in the cerebral mantle, I. Clefts with fused lips. *J. Neuropathol. Exp. Neurol.* **5,** 116–130.

Yakovlev, P.L. & Wadsworth, R.C. (1946b): Schizencephalies: a study of congenital clefts in the cerebral mantle, II. Clefts with hydrocephalus and lips separated. *J. Neuropathol. Exp. Neurol.* **5,** 169–206.

Chapter 22

The genetic basis of malformations of neuronal migration: molecular mechanisms and clinical correlation

William B. Dobyns

Institute of Human Genetics, The University of Chicago, Chicago, IL, USA

Introduction

Development of the cerebral cortex has been studied in some detail during the past several decades, but little is known about the molecular signals that control this complex process. Many different malformations of cortical development have been described. The inherited malformations in this group provide a unique opportunity to identify genes that control these processes. We have therefore attempted to isolate developmental genes associated with different human cortical malformations, and plan to use these as tools to study the molecular steps involved in neuronogenesis and gliogenesis, neuronal migration and subsequent cortical organization.

New classification and recent progress

The first step was to classify all known cortical malformations into three main groups based on the three fundamental embryologic events of cortical formation: (1) cellular proliferation in the germinal zones; (2) migration of cells to the cortical plate; and (3) vertical and horizontal organization of cells within the cortex (Barkovich *et al.*, 1996). We have chosen to classify malformations which demonstrate abnormalities in several steps of cortical development based upon the first identified abnormal step. Our current classification is shown in Table 1.

From among these disorders, progress has been made in delineation of several new or at least newly recognized malformations, including microcephaly with simplified gyral pattern and microlissencephaly, and lissencephaly with cerebellar hypoplasia. Several genes associated with human or mouse cortical malformations have been isolated or mapped to specific chromosomes. This paper will review three new cortical malformations and the status of gene studies in four established syndromes.

New malformations

Microcephaly with simplified gyral patterns and microlissencephaly

We recently reviewed clinical and brain imaging studies of 22 patients with severe congenital microcephaly defined as less than -3 standard deviations below the mean, and abnormal gyral

Table 1. Classification of malformations of cortical development

I. Malformations due to abnormal neuronal and glial proliferation

    A. Generalized

        1. Decreased proliferation

            (a) Microcephaly with simplified gyral pattern

            (b) Microlissencephaly - normal or thin cortex

            (c) Microlissencephaly - thick cortex

        2. Increased + dysplastic proliferation - NONE KNOWN

        3. Dysplastic proliferation (abnormal cell types) - NONE KNOWN

    B. Focal or Multifocal

        1. Decreased proliferation - NONE KNOWN

        2. Increased + dysplastic proliferation

            (a) Hemimegalencephaly

                (i) isolated

                (ii) epidermal nevus syndrome

                (iii) Hypomelanosis of Ito

                (iv) Neurofibromatosis Type 1

            (b) Focal transmantle dysplasia

        3. Dysplastic proliferation (abnormal cell types)

            (a) Tuberous sclerosis, types 1 and 2

            (b) Focal cortical dysplasia with balloon cells

        4. Dysplastic + neoplastic

            (a) DNET

            (b) Ganglioglioma

            (g) Gangliocytoma

II. Malformations due to abnormal neuronal migration

    A. Generalized

        1. Classical (Type 1) lissencephaly (agyria-pachygyria-band spectrum)

            (a) Chromosome 17-linked

                (i) Miller-Dieker Syndrome†

                (ii) Isolated Lissencephaly Sequence (ILS17)†

            (b) X-linked

                (i) X-linked Lissencephaly††

                (ii) Subcortical Band Heterotopia††

            (c) Other Loci

                (i) Isolated Lissencephaly Sequence

                (ii) Other Syndromes

        2. Cobblestone (Type 2) Lissencephalies

            (a) Fukuyama Congenital Muscular Dystrophy

            (b) Walker–Warburg Syndrome*

            (c) Muscle-Eye Brain Disease*

        3. Lissencephaly - not otherwise classified

            (a) Lissencephaly with ambiguous genitalia

            (b) Lissencephaly with cerebellar hypoplasia

Table 1. Continued

    4. Heterotopia
        (a) Subependymal
            (i) X-linked bilateral periventricular nodular heterotopia
            (ii) Sporadic
        (b) Cortical infolding (symmetric)
        (c) Neurones in molecular layer/Marginal glioneuronal heterotopia

  B. Focal or Multifocal Malformations of Neuronal Migration
    1. Focal Agyria/Pachygyria (partial lissencephaly)
        (a) Bilateral posterior pachygyria
        (b) Bilateral parietal pachygyria

    2. Focal or Multifocal Heterotopia
        (a) Focal subependymal nodular
        (b) Focal subcortical nodular
        (c) Focal mixed subcortical/subependymal
        (d) Cortical infoldings (unilateral)
        (e) Neurones in molecular layer/Marginal glioneuronal heterotopia
            (i) Fetal alcohol syndrome
            (ii) Other

    3. Focal or Multifocal Heterotopia with Organizational Abnormality of the Cortex
        (a) Focal subependymal nodular
        (b) Focal subcortical nodular
        (c) Focal mixed subcortical/subependymal
            (i) Aicardi syndrome
            (ii) Peroxisomal disorders
        (d) Cortical infolding (unilateral or asymmetric)
        (e) Neurones in molecular layer/Marginal glioneuronal heterotopia

    4. Excessive Single Ectopic White Matter Neurones

III. Malformations due to Abnormal Cortical Organization

  A. Generalized
    1. Polymicrogyria (PMG), diffuse

  B. Focal or Multifocal
    1. Polymicrogyria/Schizencephaly
        (a) Bilateral symmetric polymicrogyria
            (i) Bilateral frontal PMG
            (ii) Bilateral perisylvian PMG
            (iii) Bilateral posterior PMG
        (b) Asymmetric PMG
        (c) Schizencephaly and mixed schizencephaly/PMG
    2. Focal or Multifocal Cortical Dysplasia without Balloon cells
    3. Microdysgenesis

IV. Malformations of Cortical Development, Not Otherwise Classified

Modified from Barkovich (1996)

patterns in an attempt to differentiate them from children with better recognized malformations (Barkovich et al., 1998). All infants were found to have fewer and shallower sulci than normal neonates on MRI compared to age-matched normal infants, and all were severely microcephalic at birth, with head circumferences ranging from 22–31 cm. This group comprises a subset of those children who might previously have been diagnosed to have primary microcephaly or 'microcephaly vera'. However, our review of the literature found no consistent definition of microcephaly vera, and no classification that helped clinicians classify and establish prognoses for micrencephalic infants.

Our review clearly showed that these criteria identified a heterogeneous group of malformations. We divided them into six groups based on a combination of clinical and imaging criteria. Groups 1–4 had reduced numbers of gyri of normal width and shallow sulci, for which we introduced the term. These groups were separated based on clinical criteria and differences in myelination status and depth of sulci. Groups 5 and 6 had reduced numbers of abnormally broad gyri (clearly greater than 1.5 cm in at least some brain regions) with shallow sulci, for which we had previously introduced the term microlissencephaly (MLIS) (Barkovich et al., 1996). The cortex was normal or thin by imaging in group 5, but abnormally thick in group 6. The latter was sometimes associated with cerebellar hypoplasia, which thus overlaps with the malformation discussed in the next section. Several children previously reported to have 'lissencephaly with extreme neopallial hypoplasia' (Barth et al., 1982) or Norman–Roberts syndrome, patient 1 in Norman et al. (1976) probably fit in the MLIS spectrum. The six groups are summarized in Table 2.

Table 2. Microcephaly with simplified gyral pattern and microlissencephaly groups and characteristics

Group	Imaging findings	Exam/Course
1	Simplified gyral pattern Normal myelination Normal cortical thickness	Normal neonatal course Mild corticospinal tract signs in infancy No seizures
2	Simplified gyral pattern Shallow sulci Delayed myelin	Breech presentation Abnormal neonatal course Severe neonatal hypertonia Neonatal seizures
3	Simplified gyral pattern Normal myelin Shallow sulci Heterotopia	Abnormal neonatal course Severe neonatal hypertonia Neonatal myoclonic seizures
4	Simplified gyral pattern Shallow sulci Normal myelin	Multiple congenital anomalies Seizure onset at 2-3 weeks Severe neonatal hypertonia One neonatal death
5	Very simplified gyral pattern Large subarachnoid spaces Reduced white matter volume Delayed myelination Thin cerebral cortex	Abnormal neonatal course Neonatal hypotonia No neurologic development Neonatal seizures
6	Agyria or pachygyria Thick cortex Cerebellar hypoplasia in some Callosal hypogenesis/agenesis	Abnormal neonatal course Neonatal hypertonia Neonatal seizures

Note: Simplified gyral pattern means that too few sulci are present and that the sulci are abnormally shallow (1/3 to 1/2 of normal sulcal depth)

Lissencephaly with cerebellar hypoplasia

Lissencephaly with cerebellar hypoplasia (LCH) consists of lissencephaly which appears similar to classical lissencephaly except for the added presence of cerebellar hypoplasia (Dobyns & Truwit, 1995). We have reviewed records and scans on 16 patients with LCH. Among this group, birth head circumference was at or below the 2nd percentile in almost all, which is smaller than in most children with classical lissencephaly. It thus overlaps with group six microlissencephaly; we have not yet determined how best to separate these two groups, although several had head circumferences between -2 and -3 standard deviations below the mean. MRI scans usually showed widespread agyria with only restricted areas of pachygyria. The cortex was very thick, about 1–1.5 cm, which is comparable to classical lissencephaly. The entire cerebellum was hypoplastic in all but one of these children, frequently with upward rotation of the vermis. The remaining child had hypoplasia and upward rotation of the vermis only. None had other changes of cobblestone lissencephaly, so that Walker–Warburg and related syndromes could be excluded. FISH testing with the D17S379 probe has been performed in four of these children, always with negative results. None have had affected sibs, although I am aware of one anecdotal report of affected sibs. Thus, the pattern of inheritance is unknown, although it could be autosomal recessive. This malformation could also be causally heterogeneous.

Progress in genetic studies

To date, four genes (EMX2 and LIS1 in humans, and *reeler* and *scrambler* in mouse) associated with cortical malformations have been cloned, and three others (BPNH, FCMD and XLIS) have been mapped (Table 3). Molecular studies of the EMX2 gene in schizencephaly are reported elsewhere in this volume, while studies of FCMD, *reeler* and *scrambler* have been reported by other groups. The following sections will review the molecular genetics of classical lissencephaly and bilateral periventricular nodular heterotopia.

Table 3. Genes associated with cortical development, 1998

Chromosome	Gene	Protein	Syndrome	References
Xq22.2-q23	XLIS	Double cortin	X-linked lissencephaly and subcortical band heterotopia	Ross et al., 1997; Gleeson et al., 1998; Eksioglu et al., 1996
Xq28	BPNH	Filamin 1	Bilateral periventricular nodular heterotopia	
1q25	ASTN	Astrotactin	None known	
7q22	reeler	reelin	*reeler* mouse	
9q31	FCMD	Fukutin	Fukuyama congenital muscular dystrophy	
10q26.1	EMX2	empty spiracles homologue 2	schizencephaly	
17p13.3	LIS1	PAFA β subunit*	isolated lissencephaly sequence	
17p13.3	LIS1	PAFA β subunit*	Miller-Dieker syndrome	
????	mdab 1	Disabled – I	*scrambler* mouse	

*PAFA b subunit, brain isoform of platelet activating factor acetylhydrolase (PAFA) β subunit

Classical lissencephaly and subcortical band heterotopia

Classical lissencephaly (smooth brain) is a human brain malformation which consists of diffuse agyria and pachygyria, an abnormally thick 1–1.5 cm cortex, and associated changes such as hypogenesis of the corpus callosum and enlarged posterior portions of the lateral ventricles (Barkovich et al., 1991; Dobyns et al., 1992, 1996; Norman et al., 1995). The thick cortex consists of a marginal layer, a superficial cellular layer which is largely unlaminated but corresponds to the true cortical plate, a cell sparse layer, and a deep cellular layer containing large numbers of heterotopic neurones. At the milder end of this spectrum, it merges with a malformation known as subcortical band heterotopia (SBH). The latter consists of bilateral and symmetric ribbons of gray matter located in the central white matter just below the cortex and well above the ventricular walls (Barkovich et al., 1994; Dobyns et al., 1996). The bands are separated from both by distinct layers of white matter. This malformations has sometimes been called the 'double cortex syndrome', which is a misnomer as the heterotopic layer looks nothing like the true cortex.

The clinical manifestations of classical lissencephaly consist of severe or profound mental retardation, feeding problems and intractable epilepsy including frequent infantile spasms (Dobyns et al., 1992, 1996). It most often occurs as the only major anomaly in affected children, in which case it is known as isolated lissencephaly sequence (ILS). But it has also been observed in several multiple congenital anomaly syndromes, especially Miller–Dieker (MDS) and Baraitser–Winter (BWS) syndromes. The phenotype of SBH consists of variable mental retardation and epilepsy which may be intractable. A recent survey of the literature showed that mental retardation was observed in 85 per cent of cases (severe 20 per cent, moderate 24 per cent, mild 32 per cent, and borderline 9 per cent), while the remaining 15 per cent had normal intelligence (Dobyns et al., 1996). Lissencephaly and SBH have been observed in the same brain, indicating that they belong to a single 'agyria-pachygyria-band' spectrum of malformations (Dobyns & Truwit, 1995).

Malformation syndromes associated with classical lissencephaly

Most children with ILS have subtle bitemporal hollowing and a slightly small jaw with an otherwise normal facial appearance (Dobyns et al., 1992). However, this is clearly a heterogenous disorder which may be caused by mutations of more than one gene, with subtle clinical differences between them (Dobyns et al., 1996). We have therefore assigned numbers to the different forms as has been done for other multilocus disorders: ILS17 associated with chromosome 17 (LIS1) mutations, and ILSX associated with mutations of the *XLIS* gene. Some children with ILS17 who have deletions of chromosome 17p13 involving the LIS1 gene also have subtle facial changes reminiscent of MDS but not sufficient for diagnosis (Dobyns et al., 1992; 1995). They may also have minor hand anomalies such as clinodactyly or transverse palmar crease, and sacral dimples. Boys with ILSX may have subtle facial changes such as low nasal bridge and epicanthal folds, although this observation is based on limited experience to date. Other congenital anomalies are rare in all forms of ILS.

Children with MDS have characteristic facial abnormalities, especially prominent forehead, bitemporal hollowing, short nose with upturned nares, low nasal bridge with prominent lateral nasal folds, flat midface, thick upper lip with downturned vermillion border and small jaw, and sometimes other birth defects (Dobyns et al., 1991). Other common abnormalities include telecanthus, epicanthal folds, low-set and posteriorly rotated ears, malformed ears, high and narrow palate, mild congenital heart malformations, omphalocele, genital hypoplasia, undescended testes (in males), transverse palmar creases, clinodactyly and mild distal contractures. Almost all have a prominent sacral dimple.

Children with BWS have shallow orbits, ptosis, colobomas of the iris and choroid, trigonocephaly, and mental retardation (Ramer et al., 1996). Several affected children have had other congenital anomalies such as hearing loss, congenital heart malformations and hemivertebrae. However, only three of six BWS patients in whom scans were done had classical lissencephaly. This therefore might represent another microdeletion syndrome in which a second autosomal lissencephaly gene is variably deleted.

Genetic studies of XLIS and LIS1

X-linked lissencephaly and subcortical band heterotopia (XLIS) is a malformation syndrome which causes SBH in heterozygous carrier females and classical lissencephaly in hemizygous males. The existence of this syndrome was first suspected based on a striking skew of the sex ratio in SBH with more than 90 per cent being female (51 females and only three males), and several families in which mildly affected women with SBH had daughters with SBH, sons with lissencephaly, or both (Dobyns et al., 1996). The gene responsible for XLIS has recently been mapped between Xq21.3 and Xq24, flanked by markers DXS990 and DXS1001, with a maximum two point lod score of approximately 3.3 (Ross et al., 1997). This region was refined to a 1 Mb region in Xq22.3-q23 by physical mapping of an X-autosomal translocation in a girl with classical lissencephaly. Most recently, a physical map has been constructed across this region which should allow cloning of the *XLIS* gene within the relatively near future (see Table 3).

Miller–Dieker syndrome was first mapped to chromosome 17p13.3 by discovery of small deletions in two of three affected children in 1983 (Dobyns et al., 1983). We have subsequently found visible chromosomal deletions or other rearrangements in 29 of 45 (64.4 per cent) patients (unpublished data). Submicroscopic deletions were first identified using restriction fragment length polymorphisms, but have been detected by fluorescence *in situ* hybridization (FISH) with probes for locus D17S379 (ONCOR, Inc.) for several years. This probe is known to be located 100-150 kb telomeric to the LIS1 gene. Of a further 13 patients tested by FISH, 11 had a submicroscopic deletion at D17S379, resulting in a deletion detection rate of 95.2 per cent in these patients (W.B. Dobyns and D.H. Ledbetter, unpublished data). In all of these patients, the deletion involves the LIS1 gene and at least 150 kb telomeric to LIS1, suggesting that deletion of other genes besides LIS1 contribute to the phenotype.

ILS was first suspected to be mapped to the same region of chromosome 17 as MDS based on the close similarity of the phenotype to MDS. This was confirmed in 1992 when the first submicroscopic deletions were detected, defining a subset of children we now refer to as ILS17 (Ledbetter et al., 1992). Further studies eventually led to isolation of the gene in this region responsible for classical lissencephaly, which was assigned the name *LIS1* (Reiner et al., 1993). Cloning of the gene has led to development of better FISH probes for detecting deletions. Molecular diagnosis of ILS17 by FISH using probes for locus D17S379 (ONCOR, Inc.) detects deletions in about 20 per cent of children with ILS. More recent FISH studies using probes from the *LIS1* region detect deletions in about 40 per cent of children with ILS (Pilz et al., 1998a). In addition, small intragenic mutations of LIS1 have been detected in several children.

The *LIS1* gene extends over about 80 kb of genomic DNA and contains 11 exons (Lo Nigro et al., 1997). Intron one is about 50 kb in size which is unusually large, so many deletion breakpoints fall within this segment of the gene (Chong et al., 1997). *In situ* studies of RNA and more recently LIS1 protein have demonstrated expression in the brain and spinal cord at all ages, but especially in the developing cerebral and cerebellar cortical plates, with the highest expressin in Cajal–Retzius cells, some subplate neurones, thalamic neurones and the ventricular neuroepithelium (Mizuguchi et al., 1995; Reiner et al., 1995; Albrecht et al., 1996; Clark et al.,1997).

LIS1 encodes the 45kD brain isoform of the non-catalytic β subunit of platelet activating factor (PAF) acetylhydrolase, an enzyme which inactivates and thus regulates the intracellular levels of PAF (Hattori et al., 1994). The effects of high or low levels of intracellular PAF have not yet been studied in migrating neurones. However, excessively high levels of intracellular PAF are known to cause collapse of axonal growth cones by affecting the microtubular structure (Clark et al., 1995). If the same mechanism occurs in the leading processes of migrating neurones, abnormalties of migration might be expected to result.

The *LIS1* gene was isolated in part based on its homology to the WD repeat family of genes which contain 4–8 tandem WD repeats (Reiner et al., 1993). Each repeat contain an initial variable sequence followed by a core sequence of 27–45 amino acids which terminate with the dipeptide tryptophan-aspartate (WD). The LIS1 protein itself contains eight such repeats. This large family of genes is involved in a variety of regulatory functions such as regulation of cell division, transcription, transmembrane signalling and mRNA modification. A subset of this family function as G proteins, which are particularly involved in transmembrane signalling. G proteins typically exist as trimers with α, β and γ subunits coded by different genes. When activated by a cell surface receptor, the trimer will separate into Gα and G$\beta\gamma$ subunits, which serve as intracellular second messengers. Thus, the LIS1 protein may function by regulating intracellular levels of PAF, or by serving as the second messenger in an as yet unknown pathway.

Classical BPNH and the BPNH/MR syndrome

Bilateral periventricular nodular heterotopias (BPNH) are nodular masses of gray matter which line the ventricular walls and protrude into the lumen (Dobyns et al., 1996). They may be diffuse and contiguous, or regional and non-contiguous, and are separated from each other by layers of myelinated fibres. Patients with the classical form of BPNH have normal intelligence (78 per cent) or borderline retardation (22 per cent), and epilepsy with multiple seizure types which may or may not prove difficult to control. Several asymptomatic individuals have been found during family evaluations. The sex ratio is also skewed such that about 73 per cent of patients are female, and several families with multiple affected individuals have been reported in which all affected persons are females. Some of these families have a striking increase in the rate of miscarriages, most of which appear to be male foetuses.

X-linked inheritance of classical BPNH was first suggested by the skewed sex ratio, and has been confirmed by linkage studies in several multiplex families which mapped the BPNH gene to chromosome Xq28 with a maximal multipoint lod score of 5.37 with no recombinants (theta = 0) for polymorphic markers in distal Xq28 including DXS1108 and F8c (Factor VIII), and a suggested critical region of <7 Mb (Eksioglu et al., 1996). No liveborn males with BPNH or other neurodevelopmental problems were observed in any of these families, although one liveborn male died from overwhelming spontaneous bleeding (Huttenlocher et al., 1994).

We recently reported a new presumably X-linked BPNH syndrome in three boys which consists of BPNH and associated anomalies such as dysplasia of the corpus callosum and ventriculomegaly, focal or regional cortical dysplasia, cerebellar hypoplasia, severe mental retardation, epilepsy which may be intractable, clinodactyly, and partial syndactyly of the hands or feet (Dobyns et al., 1998). The hand and foot anomalies were subtle in one of the three boys, but were always present with a careful examination. We refer to this disorder as the BPNH/MR syndrome to distinguish it from the more common classical BPNH syndrome observed predominately in females, and from several other BPNH syndromes.

High resolution chromosome analysis revealed a subtle abnormality of Xq28 in one of the three boys with BPNH/MR syndrome (Fink et al., 1997). FISH studies in prometaphase and interphase cells using cosmids and yeast artificial chromosomes from Xq28 further characterized this abnormality as a 2.25–3.25 Mb inverted duplication. The proximal breakpoint was located between markers DXS15 and L1CAM, while the distal breakpoint was located very near the telomere. The two possible mechanisms of mutation include simple gene overdosage in which case the gene could be located anywhere within the duplicated segment, or disruption by one of the two breakpoints. Three boys with larger 5 Mb duplications involving the same region of Xq28 had mental retardation and other abnormalities without recognized BPNH (Lahn *et al.*, 1994), at least in the two boys who had CT or MRI scans of the head (Fink *et al.*, 1997). This observation favors disruption of the BPNH gene by one of the two duplication breakpoints (see Table 3).

References

Albrecht, U., Abu-Issa, R., Ratz, B., Hattori, M., Aoki, J., Arai, H., Inoue, K. & Eichele, G. (1996): Platelet-activating factor acetylhydrolase expression and activity suggest a link between neuronal migration and platelet-activating factor. *Dev. Biol.* **180**, 579–593.

Barkovich, A.J., Koch, T.K. & Carrol, C.L. (1991): The spectrum of lissencephaly: report of ten cases analyzed by magnetic resonance imaging. *Ann. Neurol.* **30**, 139–146.

Barkovich, A.J., Guerrini, R., Battaglia, G., Kalifa, G., N'Guyen, T., Parmeggiani, A., Santucci, M., Giovanardi-Rossi, P., Granata, T. & D'Incerti, L. (1994): Band heterotopia: correlation of outcome with magnetic resonance imaging parameters. *Ann. Neurol.* **36**, 609–617.

Barkovich, A.J., Kuzniecky, R.I., Dobyns, W.B., Jackson, G.D., Becker, L.E. & Evrard, P. (1996): A classification scheme for malformations of cortical development. *Neuropediatrics* **27**, 59–63.

Barkovich, A.J., Ferriero, D.M., Barr, R.M., Gressens, P., Dobyns, W.B., Truwit, C.L. & Evrard, P. Microlissencephaly and microgyrencephaly: heterogeneous malformations of cortical development. *Neuropediatrics* [submitted].

Barth, P.G., Mullaart, R., Stam, F.C. & Slooff, J.L. (1982): Lissencephaly with extreme neopallial hypoplasia. *Brain Dev.* **4**, 145–151.

Brunelli, S., Faiella, A., Capra, V., Nigro, V., Simeone, A., Cama, A. & Boncinelli E. (1996): Germline mutations in the homeobox gene EMX2 in patients with severe schizencephaly. *Nature Genet.* **12**, 94–96.

Chong, S.S., Pack, S.D., Roschke, A.V., Tanigami, A., Carrozzo, R., Smith, A.C.M., Dobyns, W.B. & Ledbetter, D.H. (1997): A revision of the lissencephaly and Miller–Dieker syndrome critical regions in chromosome 17p13.3. *Hum. Mol. Genet.* **6**, 147–155.

Clark, G.D., McNeil, R.S., Bix, G.J. & Swann, J.W. (1995): Platelet-activating factor produces neuronal growth cone collapse. *Dev. Neurosci.* **6**, 2569–2575.

Clark, G.D., Mizuguchi, M., Antalffy, B., Barnes, J. & Armstrong, D. (1997): Predominant localization of the LIS family of gene products to Cajal–Retzius cells and ventricular neuroepithelium in the developing human cortex. *J. Neuropath. Exp. Neurol.* **56**, 1044–1052.

Dobyns, W.B. & Truwit, C.L. (1995): Lissencephaly and other malformations of cortical development: 1995 update. *Neuropediatrics* **26**, 132–147.

Dobyns, W.B., Stratton, R.F., Parke, J.T., Greenberg, F., Nussbaum, R.L. & Ledbetter, D.H. (1983): Miller–Dieker syndrome and monosomy 17p. *J. Pediatrics* **102**, 552–558.

Dobyns, W.B., Curry, C.J.R., Hoyme, H.E., Turlington, L. & Ledbetter, D.H. (1991): Clinical and molecular diagnosis of Miller–Dieker syndrome. *Am. J. Hum. Genet.* **48**, 584–594.

Dobyns, W.B., Elias, E.R., Newlin, A.C., Pagon, R.A. & Ledbetter, D.H. (1992): Causal heterogeneity in isolated lissencephaly. *Neurology* **42**, 1375–1388.

Dobyns, W.B., Andermann, E., Andermann, F., Czapansky-Beilman, D., Dubeau, F., Dulac, O., Guerrini, R., Hirsch. B., Ledbetter, D.H., Lee, N.S., Motte, J., Pinard, J.-M., Radtke, R.A., Ross, M.E., Tampieri, D., Walsh, C.A. & Truwit, C.L. (1996): X-linked malformations of neuronal migration. *Neurology* **47**, 331–339.

Dobyns, W.B., Guerrini, R., Czapansky-Beilman, D.K., Pierpont, M.E.M., Breningstall, G., Yock, J. D.H., Bonanni, P. & Truwit, C.L. (1997): Bilateral periventricular nodular heterotopia (BPNH) with mental retardation and syndactyly in boys: a new X-linked mental retardation syndrome. *Neurology* **49**, 1042–1047.

Eksioglu, Y.Z., Scheffer, I.E., Cardenas, P., Knoll, J., DiMario, R., Ramsby, G., Berg, M., Kamuro, K., Berkovic, S.F., Duyk, G.M., Parisi, J., Huttenlocher, P.R. & Walsh, C.A. (1996): Periventricular heterotopia: an X-linked dominant epilepsy locus causing aberrant cerebral cortical development. *Neuron* **16**, 77–87.

Fink, J.M., Dobyns, W.B., Guerrini, R. & Hirsch, B.A. (1997): Identification of a duplication of Xq28 associated with bilateral periventricular nodular heterotopia (BPNH). *Am. J. Hum. Genet.* **61**, 379–387.

Fox, J.W., Lamperti, E.D., Eksioglu, Y.Z., Hong, S.E., Feng, Y., Graham, G.A., Scheffer, I.E., Dobyns, W.B., Hirsch, B.A., Radtke, R.A., Berkovich, S.F., Huttenlocher PR. & Walsh C.A. Mutations in *Filamin 1* prevent migration of cerebral neurones in human periventricular heterotopia. *Neuron* [in press].

Gleeson J.G., Allen, K.A., Fox, J.W., Lamperti, E.D., Berkovic, S., Scheffer, I., Cooper, E.c., Dobyns, W.b., Minnerath, S., Ross, M.E. & Walsh, C.A. (1998): Doublecortin, a brian-specific gene mutated in human X-linked lissencephaly and double cortex syndrome, encodes a putative signalling protein. *Cell* **92**, 63–72.

Hattori, M., Adachi, H., Tsujimoto, M., Arai, N. & Inoue, K. (1994): Miller–Dieker lissencephaly gene encodes a subunit of brain platelet-activating factor acetylhydrolase. *Nature* **370**, 216–218.

Hirotsune S., Takahara, T., Sasaki, N., Hirose, K., Yoshiki, A., Ohashi, T., Kusakabe, M., Murakami, Y., Watanabe, S., Nakao, K., Katsuki, M. & Hayashizaki, Y. (1995): The *reeler* gene encodes a protein with an EGF-like motif expressed by pioneer neurones. *Nature Genet.* **10**, 77–83.

Huttenlocher, P.R., Taravath, S. & Mojtahedi, S. (1994): Periventricular heterotopia and epilepsy. *Neurology* **44**, 51–55.

Kobayashi, K., Nakahori, Y., Miyake, M., Matsumura, K., Kondo-Iida, E., Nomura, Y., Segawa, M., Yoshioka, M., Saito, K., Osawa, M., Hamano, K., Sakakihara, Y., Nonaka, I., Nakagome, Y., Kanazawa, I., Nakamura, Y., Tokunaga, K. & Toda, T. (1998): An ancient retrotransposal insertion causes Fukuyama-type congenital muscular dystrophy. *Nature* **394**, 388–392

Lahn, B.T., Ma, N., Breg, W.R., Stratton, R., Surti, U. & Page, D.C. (1994): Xq-Yq interchange resulting in supernormal X-linked gene expression in severely retarded males with 46,XYq karyotype. *Nature Genet.* **8**, 243–250.

Ledbetter, S.A., Kuwano, A., Dobyns, W.B. & Ledbetter, D.H. (1992): Microdeletions of chromosome 17p13 as a cause of isolated lissencephaly. *Am. J. Hum. Genet.* **50**, 182–189.

Lo Nigro, C., Chong, S.S., Smith, A.C.M., Dobyns, W.B. & Ledbetter, D.H. (1997): Point mutations and an intragenic deletion in LIS1, the lissencephaly causative gene in isolated lissencephaly sequence and Miller–Dieker syndrome. *Hum. Mol. Genet.* **6**, 157–164.

Mizuguchi, M., Takashima, S., Kakita, A., Yamada, M. & Ikeda, K. (1995): Lissencephaly gene product: localization in the central nervous system and loss of immunoreactivity in Miller–Dieker syndrome. *Am. J. Pathol.* **147**, 1142–1151.

Norman, M.G., Roberts, M., Sirois, R.J. & Tremblay, L.J.M. (1976): Lissencephaly. *Can. J. Neurol. Sci.* **3**, 39–46.

Norman, M.G., McGillivray, B.C., Kalousek, D.K., Hill, A. & Poskitt, K.J. (1995): *Congenital malformations of the brain: pathological, embryological, clinical, radiological and genetic aspects.* New York: Oxford University Press.

Pilz, D.T., Macha, M.E., Precht, K.S., Smith, A.C.M., Dobyns, W.B. & Ledbetter, D.H. (1998a): FISH analysis on 110 patients with isolated lissencephaly sequence (ILS): significantly increased deletion detection rate with *LIS1* specific probes. *Genet. Medicine* **1**, 29–33.

Pilz, D.T., Matsumoto, N., Minnerath, S., Mills, P., Gleeson, J.G., Allen, K.A., Walsh, C.A., Barkovich, A.J., Dobyns, W.B., Ledbetter, D.H. & Ross M.E. (1998b): *LIS1* and *XLIS (DCX)* mutations cause most human classical lissencephaly, but different patterns of malformation. *Hum. Molec. Genet.* **7**, 2029–2037.

Ramer, J.C., Lin, A.E., Dobyns, W.B., Ayme, S., Pallotta, R. & Ladda, R. (1996) Shallow orbits, ptosis, coloboma, trigonocephaly, gyral abnormalities, mental and growth retardation: a possible new syndrome with features of the CHARGE association. *Am. J. Med. Genet.* **57**, 403–409.

Reiner, O., Carrozzo, R., Shen, Y., Wehnert, M., Faustinella, F., Dobyns, W.B., Caskey, C.T. & Ledbetter, D.H. (1993): Isolation of a Miller–Dieker lissencephaly gene containing G protein beta-subunit-like repeats. *Nature* **364**, 717–721.

Reiner, O., Albrecht, U., Gordon, M., Chianese, K.A., Wong, C., Gal-Gerber, O., Sapir, T., Siracusa, L.D., Buchberg, A.M., Caskey, C.T. & Eichele, G. (1995): Lissencephaly gene (LIS1) expression in the CNS suggests a role in neuronal migration. *J. Neurosci.* **15**, 3730–3738.

Ross, M.E., Allen, K.M., Srivistava, A.K., Featherstone, T., Gleeson, J.G., Hirsch, B., Harding, B.N., Abdullah, R., Andermann, E., Berg, M., Czapansky Beilman, D., Flanders, D.J., Guerrini, R., Motté, J., Puche Mira, A., Scheffer, I., Berkovic, S., King, R.A., Ledbetter, D.H., Schlessinger, D., Dobyns, W.B. & Walsh, C.A. (1997): Linkage and physical mapping of X-linked lissencephaly/SBH (XLIS): a gene causing neuronal migration defects in human brain. *Hum. Mol. Genet.* **6,** 555–562.

Ware, M., Fox, J., Gonzalez, J., Davis, N., Lambert de Rouvroit, C., Chua, S., Goffinet, A. & Walsh, C. (1997): Aberrant splicing of a mouse disabled homolog, mdab1, in the scrambler mouse. *Neuron* **19,** 1–20.

Zheng, C., Heintz, N. & Hatten M.E. (1996): CNS gene encoding astrotactin, which supports neuronal migration along glial fibres. *Science* **272,** 417–419.

PART VI

SURGICAL APPROACHES – HOW, WHY, WHEN?

Chapter 23

Surgical treatment of cortical dysplasias and migration disorders

André Olivier, Warren Boling, Frederick Andermann and François Dubeau

Montreal Neurological Institute and Hospital, McGill University,
3801 University Street, Montreal, QC H3A 2B4, Canada

Introduction

The advent of Magnetic Resonance Imaging (MRI) has virtually opened a new field in the surgery of epilepsy, namely that of intractable seizures due to cortical dysplasias. Although long recognized as a source of focal epilepsy, particularly in the temporal lobe (Hardiman *et al.*, 1988; Mathieson, 1975; Talairach *et al.*, 1974; Taylor *et al.*, 1971) cortical dysplasias were usually fortuitous discoveries at surgery or autopsy (Janota & Polkey, 1992; Norman, 1967; Staunton *et al.*, 1983). Falconer (Taylor *et al.*, 1971) was the first to recognize developmental lesions of the temporal lobe as a cause of surgically treatable epilepsies. This has been further documented by his coworkers (Avoli *et al.*, 1996; Bruton, 1988; Janota & Polkey, 1992; Norman, 1967). Perot, Weir and Rasmussen in 1966 presented the concept of the forme fruste of tuberous sclerosis, with isolated dysplastic lesions strongly resembling tubers, the classical lesions found in tuberous sclerosis (Perot *et al.*, 1966). Talairach and Bancaud, in their 1974 monograph (Talairach *et al.*, 1974) referred to 18 cases of cortical dysplasia. Andermann *et al.*, in 1987, presented the first report on the surgical treatment of diffuse cortical dysplasias. This chapter is an extension of a previous report dealing with a series of 85 cases of migration disorders (Olivier *et al.*, 1996).

While CT scanning on occasion revealed the more obvious lesions, most would remain undetected or would await surgical confirmation. With MRI it is now possible to recognize these cortical developmental defects, to localize them more accurately and to assess their gross extent with precision. Some of the more discrete lesions no doubt will continue to escape diagnosis because of their small size or because the more subtle forms can look so much like normal cortex.

There are several specific problems encountered in the surgery of cortical dysplasia. First there is an obvious ambiguity of terminology and nomenclature. This problem concerns all workers in the field and has been addressed elsewhere (Robain, 1996). There is a definite need for a clearer definition of entities such as dysplasia, hamartoma, heterotopia, microdysgenesis, and migration disorders. Another area which needs further analysis is the borderland between cortical dysplasias and 'dysplastic' tumours such as gangliogliomas and dysembryoplastic tumours (Daumas-Duport, 1993; Gueneau *et al.*, 1982; Haddad *et al.*, 1992; Khajavi *et al.*, 1994; Russell & Rubinstein, 1989). This diversity in terminology is a reflection of a large spectrum of anomalies ranging from gross lesions to undetectable ones.

Among the many characteristics of dysplasias, their location, size, extent and relationship to the ECoG findings are the most important factors from the surgical standpoint. The lesions may be superficial or deep. They can range from small to large size. They may be obvious on MR scanning or remain undetected by this modality. The differences or boundaries between normal and abnormal tissue may be very discrete on MRI and clearly undetectable at surgery.

From the purely technical standpoint, they present a considerable challenge. As already mentioned, at the time of surgery, with the cortex exposed, it may be difficult or impossible to localize small lesions or to identify the edges of the larger ones. Indeed, their appearance may be deceptive, as they may look strikingly like normal cortex. The symptomatic lesions frequently encroach on highly functional areas of the brain, and because of their location and extent, only a limited resection can be performed. The diffuse bilateral dysplasias, which are clearly non-resectable present a different problem, namely that of deciding which patients could benefit from a palliative procedure such as callosotomy (Kuzniecki *et al.*, 1990) or a partial resection of the most abnormal portion of the lesion.

Finally, one of the surgical challenges presented by cortical dysplasias is to correlate electrically, with the aid of electrocorticography or stereotactic intracranial recording the area of maximal firing within the area of dysplastic cortex (Munari *et al.*, 1996; Palmini *et al.*, 1996).

The purpose of this chapter is to review our experience with the resection of these lesions, to present the effect of surgical removal on the seizure tendency according to the different regions involved and to see if strategies can be developed to eventually improve the surgical outcome. Work from our Institution has already demonstrated that the more radical the resection of the dysplasia the better the surgical results (Andermann *et al.*, 1987; Olivier *et al.*, 1996; Palmini *et al.*, 1991; Palmini *et al.*, 1995; Perot *et al.*, 1966; Prayson *et al.*, 1993). It has been clearly shown that these lesions present an intrinsic epileptogenicity (Avoli *et al.*, 1996) which can be detected reliably by electrocorticography and also less frequently by EEG. In order to accomplish an adequate and more complete removal of these lesions we have applied the technique of MRI-guided frameless stereotaxy (Olivier *et al.*, 1996). This approach uses the capabilities of MRI technology to display the morphological characteristics of cortical dysplasia, and to use 3-D reconstructions of the brain for precise stereotaxic guidance during surgery (Olivier *et al.*, 1996; Olivier *et al.*, 1994).

Material, patients and methods

Distribution according to regions and pathology

Our surgical material which comprises a series of 129 patient has been divided according to the localization of the lesions as seen on MRI, the area of resection during surgery, and according to pathology.

A series of illustrative patients is presented according to location of the lesion. These characteristic cases will help illustrate the problems confronted by the neurosurgeon in dealing with cortical dysplasias in specific areas and present some possible solutions. All patients were operated by the same surgeon (A.O.).

Dysplasia of temporal area

Patient Z.J.
Z. J. was a 26 year old woman at the time of surgery with intractable epilepsy since nine months of age. Her development was normal until two years of age when she began exhibiting signs of mental retardation and autistic behaviour. Prior to her presentation for surgery her conduct was increas-

Chapter 23 Surgical treatment of cortical dysplasias and migration disorders

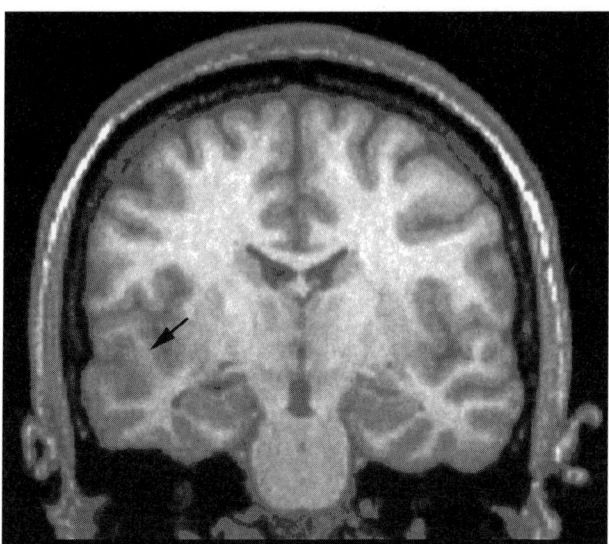

Fig. 1. Case Z.J. Preop. coronal MRI, showing macrogyria of the right temporal area.

ingly troublesome to manage with persistent agitation and impulsive behaviour requiring round the clock supervision and psychotropic medication. Her seizures occurred several times per week and were characterized by a moan or cry, followed by staring, myoclonic jerks of the left hand and face, and tonic extension of one or both of the arms. She was unable to describe an aura. The seizure frequency was several per week and they were intractable to medication. She had been hospitalized twice for status epilepticus. Her neurologic exam demonstrated a mild left hemiparesis. She was able to follow only simple commands, and her language abilities consisted of simple naming with a very limited vocabulary. Scalp EEG revealed poorly localized ictal onset and interictal activity predominating in the right temporal and centrotemporal areas. The MRI showed a hyperintense T2 signal lesion in the right anterior temporal neocortical structures in addition to enlarged lateral temporal gyri compared to the contralateral side (Fig. 1).

With the hypothesis that the lesion in the temporal lobe was the cause of the seizures, the patient underwent a right frontotemporal craniotomy. ECoG revealed no spiking on the surface but rhythmic spiking in the deepest contacts of electrodes inserted to the amygdala and hippocampus with frameless stereotactic guidance. A temporal resection including an amygdalohippocampectomy was performed encompassing the lesion demonstrated on the MRI (Fig.2A, B). The temporal resection measured 5 cm along the Sylvian fissure and 6 cm along the floor of the middle fossa and included most of the amygdala and 3 cm of the hippocampus. Pathology of the lateral temporal specimen revealed large balloon cells, heterotopic neurons within the white matter, large bizarre neurons in the cortex, and cortical dyslamination. Postoperatively she had one brief staring spell in the past nine months which was not clearly an epileptic event. The parents reported her behaviour was markedly improved. She was more relaxed with better concentration and more in contact with people in her environment. This allowed her to stop the psychotropic medication and made caring for her much easier.

This case illustrates the striking effect that complete removal of a visible lesion can have on the seizure tendency. Additionally we are increasingly recognizing the beneficial effect that seizure control can have on behaviour in patients like this one.

Dysplasia of Frontal Area

Patient S.G.

S.G. was a 13-year-old left handed girl in 1997 with intractable epilepsy since three years of age, of unknown aetiology. Her neurological exam was normal. Neuropsychological assessment revealed an average IQ but a significant decline in intellectual abilities, especially verbal, since her previous testing in 1990. Her seizure pattern initially consisted of spinning in circles with deviation of the eyes to the left. Later the predominant seizure pattern was a loss of contact, vocalization, left

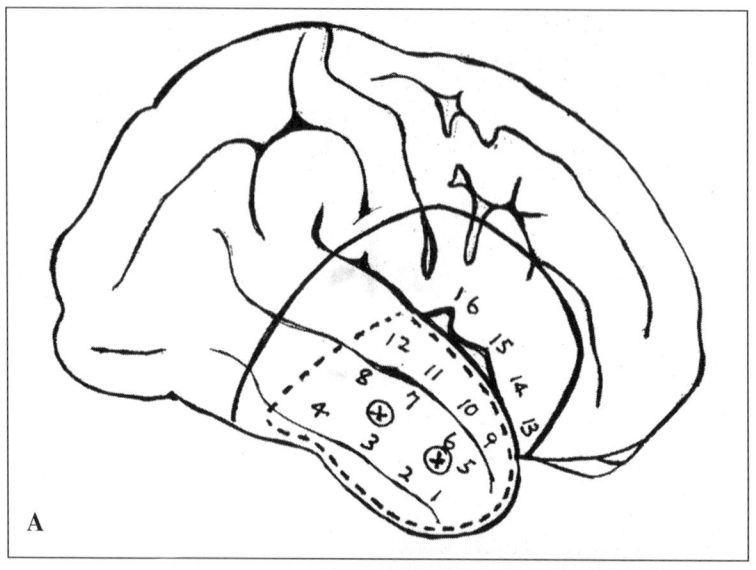
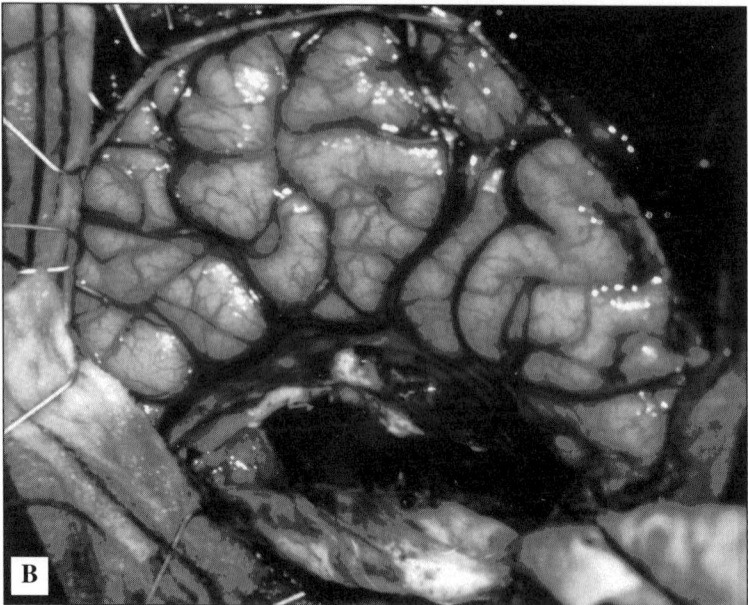

Fig. 2. (A) Case Z.J. Operative diagram showing position of surface and depth electrodes. Dotted line indicates the extent of the resection. (B) Case Z.J. Operative photograph showing temporal resection which included the grossly dysplastic cortex, the amygdala and anterior hippocampus.

side adversion, and tonic posturing with elevation of her upper extremities. She denied any warning. The seizures were frequent and intractable. They occurred from 50 times each day to primarily nocturnal seizures of one to four each night. The frequency followed a seasonal pattern with the greatest seizure tendency in the spring. Scalp EEG showed a diffuse ictal onset with predominant right frontocentral epileptiform activity. The interictal activity demonstrated a paroxysmal disturbance of cerebral activity from the right frontocentral convexity and parasagital locations. The MRI revealed a subtle abnormality in the right frontal lobe which was evaluated further with an

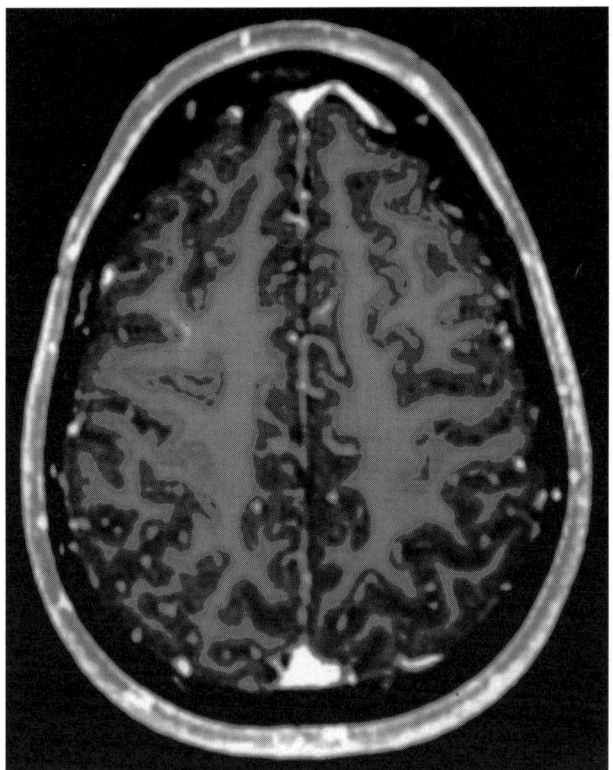

Fig. 3. Case S.G. MRI-transverse section showing lesion in bottom of superior frontal sulcus. Left side of the picture is left side of the brain.

MRI surface coil study. The lesion's appearance was of a thickened cortex and blurred gray/white junction in the depth of the superior frontal sulcus (Fig. 3). A PET study was performed to evaluate speech and sensorimotor localization. Language tasks activated the speech areas on the left and amytal testing confirmed left hemisphere speech dominance. Ictal SPECT was attempted but no useful results were obtained.

Since the scalp EEG only provided a gross localization to the right frontocentral region, she underwent a study with intracranial electrodes (stereo-electro-encephalography) to prove that the subtle lesion corresponded to the seizure focus and that the seizures were not arising in a zone outside the lesion such as the supplementary motor area (SMA). Stereoelectroencephalography was performed with multicontact electrodes targeting the cingulate gyrus, the SMA, the fronto-orbital region, and the frontal lesion on the right. Recordings confirmed the presence of an active epileptic focus in the contacts of the lesion electrode which was positioned in the middle frontal gyrus with secondary spread to the SMA. A right frontal craniotomy was performed revealing a normal appearance of the cortex on the surface (Fig. 4A, B). MRI-guided frameless stereotaxy was required to identify the location and extent of the lesion around the bottom of the superior frontal sulcus and it was selectively resected through a linear incision preserving a large bypassing ascending frontal vein (Figs. 5A, B; 6). Histological studies confirmed the diagnosis of cortical dysplasia with the presence of balloon cells in addition to subpial and white matter neuronal heterotopias. She has been seizure free for one year since surgery.

This case illustrates that a subtle but obvious dysplastic cortical lesion in a patient with intractable epilepsy can be the origin of severe seizures and that resection of such a lesion can bring total arrest of these seizures. Improved imaging studies have benefited patients like this one by discovering previously unrecognized subtle migrational abnormalities. In the past this patient would have been diagnosed with cryptogenic epilepsy and she may have undergone a right frontal lobectomy. A large resection may have had the same positive effect on her seizure tendency, but we believe the selective removal of a lesion is beneficial for the patient because it reduces the risk of neurologic complications and spares the surrounding normal cortex and white matter.

Patient T.O.
Patient T. O. was a right handed 15 year old boy at the time of surgery. The seizure onset was at five years with an unknown etiology. The boy had a warning of fear and tachycardia before each attack. They occurred predominantly at night and in clusters of many repetitive seizures separated

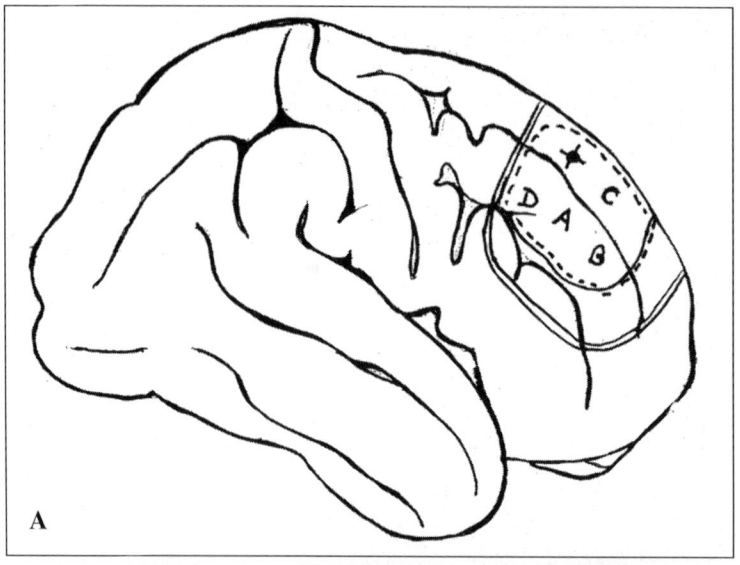

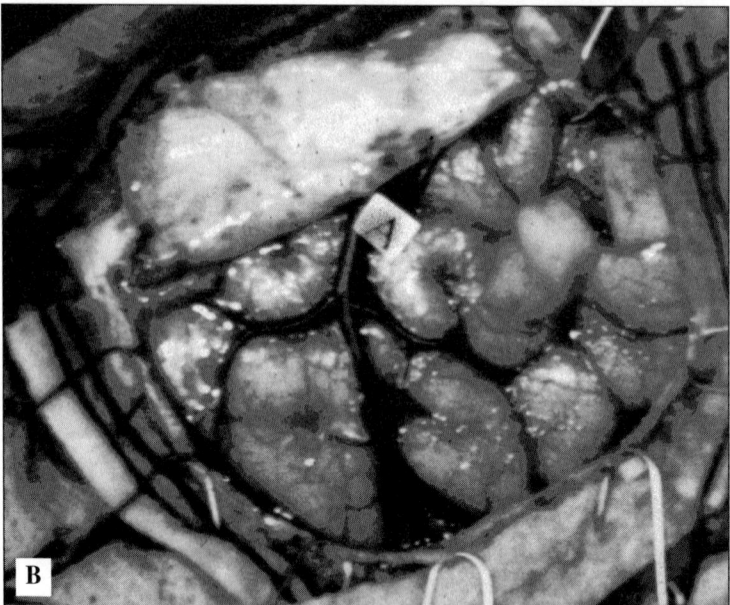

Fig. 4. (A) Case S.G. Brain map showing site of restricted craniotomy using computer image guidance. The epileptiform activity (A,B,C,D) overlies the cortical lesion as demarcated with the stereotactic pointer. (B) Case S.G. Corresponding photograph showing the exposed cortex. No lesion is seen. A large ascending vein traversing the field was left intact.

by seizure free intervals of one to two months. The seizures could come every five minutes and up to 50 to 60 per day. Each attack lasted from five to 15 seconds and was characterized by lying prone on the floor or in bed, moaning, rolling side to side, kicking his legs and banging his head. This was followed by postictal confusion. The seizures were refractory to multiple anticonvulsant medications. Scalp EEG demonstrated interictal abnormalities of high amplitude slow sharp activity over the fronto-central region with left side predominance. Ictal EEG events were consistently obscured

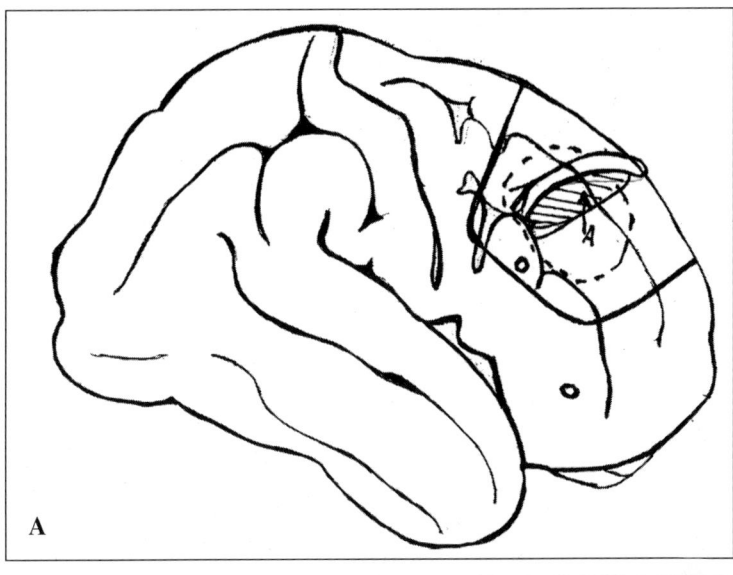

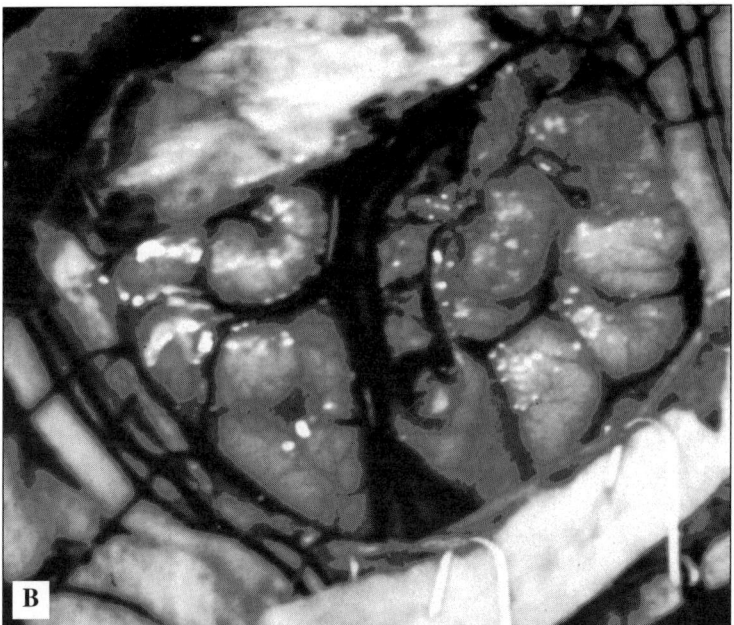

Fig. 5. (A) Case S.G. Orientation diagram for figure 5B. Dotted line shows extent of resection anterior and posterior to the ascending vein. (B) Case S.G. The area of cortical dysplasia around a deep superior frontal sulcus was resected through a linear incision anterior to the large vein.

by movement artifact. MRI showed a restricted zone of thickened cortex in the anterior left frontal cingulate gyrus (Figs. 7A; 8A).

Since the patient had an obvious lesion and congruent scalp EEG findings, removal of the lesion was expected to bring significant reduction in the seizure frequency. He underwent a left frontal craniotomy with MRI image guidance. Pre-excision ECoG was performed with recording electrodes placed over the surface of the frontal lobe and one depth electrode inserted through the superior

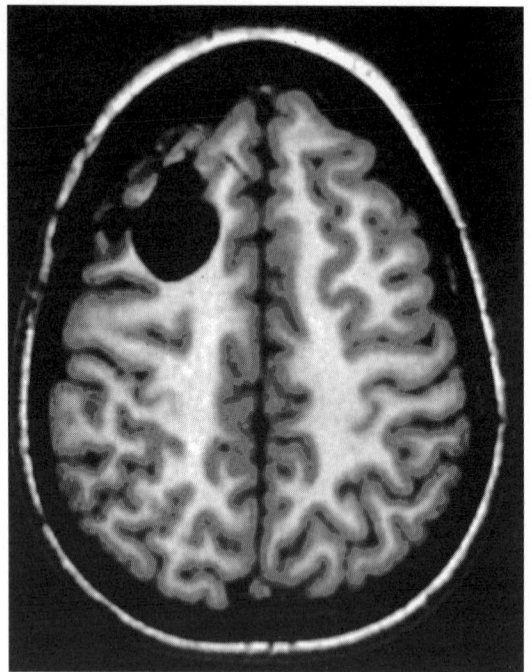

Fig. 6. Case S.G. Post-op MRI showing extent of resection in the right frontal lobe; compare with Figure 3.

frontal gyrus (F1) into the anterior cingulate lesion (Fig. 9A-C). Very rhythmic sharp waves were recorded from the deepest contacts of the depth electrode in addition to slow and sharp waves over the surface of F1. With MRI-guided frameless stereotaxy and using an interhemispheric approach a selective resection was performed of the anterior cingulate lesion measuring 3 cm in diameter (Figs. 7B; 8B). There was no postoperative deficit and the patient has remained seizure free for the last three years since surgery except for a single generalized convulsion. Pathological analysis confirmed the diagnosis of cortical dysplasia.

This case illustrates again the striking effect the selective removal of a cortical dysplastic lesion can have on seizure tendency. It also demonstrates the importance of MRI-guided frameless stereotaxy in the removal of dysplasia. Small areas of dysplasia visible on MRI usually can not be differentiated from the normal cortical surface at operation. In order to reliably identify the cortical dysplastic lesion and its borders, MRI-guided frameless stereotaxy is essential. The technique can also be used for selective intralesional recording.

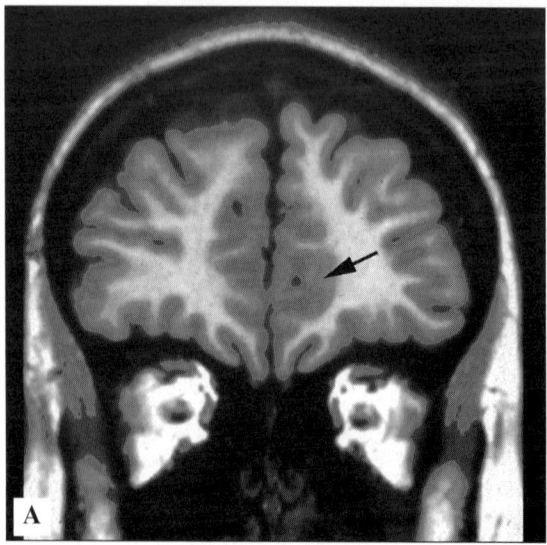
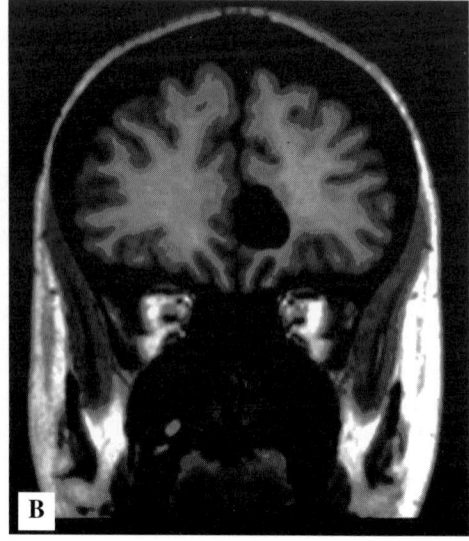

Fig. 7. (A) Case T.O. Coronal pre-op MRI showing area of dysplasia in anterior left cingulate area. (B) Case T.O. Coronal post-op MRI in the same plane showing selective resection of left cingulate lesion through an interhemispheric approach.

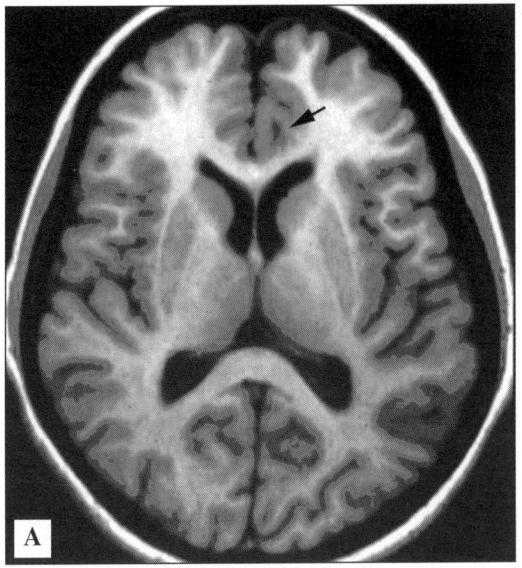 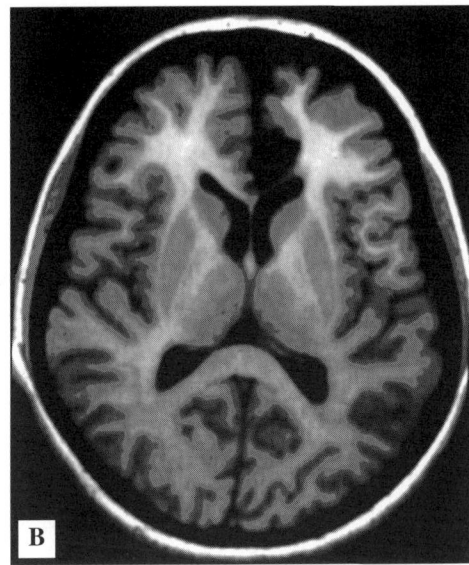

Fig. 8. (A) Case T.O. Transverse pre-op MRI showing area of dysplasia in the left anterior cingulate area. (B) Case T.O. Transverse post-op MRI showing resection.

Dysplasia of central area

Patient J.L.

At the time of surgery, J.L. was a 17 year old right handed male patient with a seven year history of intractable epilepsy of unknown etiology. Initially the seizures were heralded by a sensation that his left hand was becoming 'as big as the hospital'. The sensation of macropsia ended soon after seizure onset and at his presentation to the MNI, he was describing an aura of numbness in the whole left hand with a sharp demarcation of the paraesthesia at the wrist without a march. The seizures were predominantly nocturnal and the pattern consisted of abruptly sitting up, eye blinking, and tonic extension of the left arm. The frequency was almost daily. Surface EEG showed right centroparietal interictal spiking. The MRI revealed no lesion. Ictal SPECT demonstrated hyperperfusion in the right lower central area.

Because of the initial aura of macropsia and the curious somatosensory sensation involving the whole hand without a march of symptoms, it was postulated the seizure origin was either in the primary somatosensory cortex of the post central gyrus or in an area posterior to it. In an attempt to better define the seizure origin and spread, stereoelectroencephalography was performed (Fig. 10). Two multicontact depth electrodes were inserted within the frontal lobe targeted to the supplementary motor area (SMA) and the anterior cingulate area. One multicontact depth electrode was inserted through the inferior parietal lobule and targeted at the mesial parietal cortex. A series of epidural cortical electrodes were placed over the central and pericentral area (Fig. 10). To obtain greater precision in mapping the central area, the patient had a PET activation study of hand motor function and the data integrated with MRI for target selection. The seizure origin was localized to the right lower central area. At surgery under local anaesthesia a right frontotemporoparietal craniotomy was performed using MRI-guided frameless stereotaxy. The Sylvian fissure, central region, and parietal lobe were well exposed. ECoG recording from the cortical surface demonstrated a clear focus of spike activity at the lower postcentral and supramarginal gyrus (Fig.11A, B). Cortical stimulation was used to map the somatosensory areas of the tongue and hand. Stimulation of the supramarginal gyrus elicited a hand paresthesia similar to his usual aura. At stimulation of point S

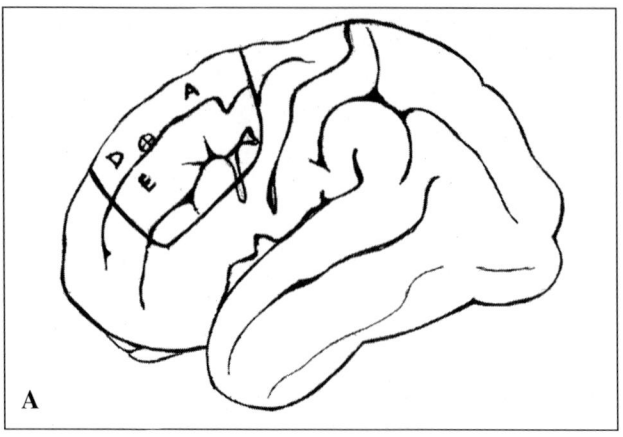

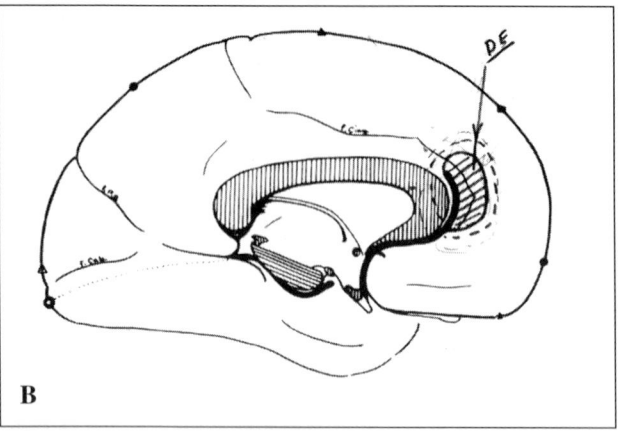

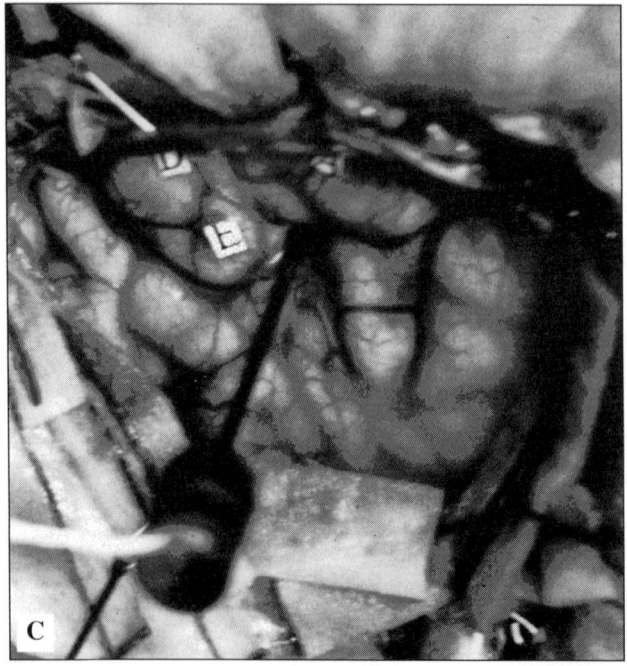

Fig. 9. (A) Case T.O. Operative diagram for orientation showing left frontal craniotomy and sites of epileptiform activity on the surface. The small circle with the cross corresponds to the entry site of a recording depth electrode inserted into the cingulate lesion. A, D and E represent the site of maximum paroxismal rhythmic activity recorded from the surface EcoG. (B) Case T.O. Operative diagram of the mesial surface showing site of the lesion and the trajectory of the depth electrode. The dotted line corresponds to the extent of the resection. (C) Case T.O. Operative photograph (See Fig. 9 A for orientation). A,D,E represent sites of epiletiform activity. The electrode was directed to the lesion with computer guidance.

Chapter 23 Surgical treatment of cortical dysplasias and migration disorders

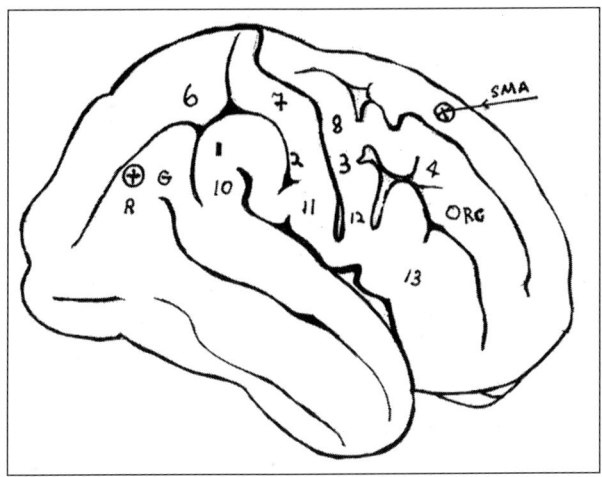

Fig. 10. Case J.L. Diagram showing the placement of intracranial electrode inserted over predetermined sites with the frameless stereotactic technique, SMA depth electrode directed at the supplementary motor area, depth electrode going through the parietal lobe. Interictal and ictal activity was recorded at electrodes 11 and 12.

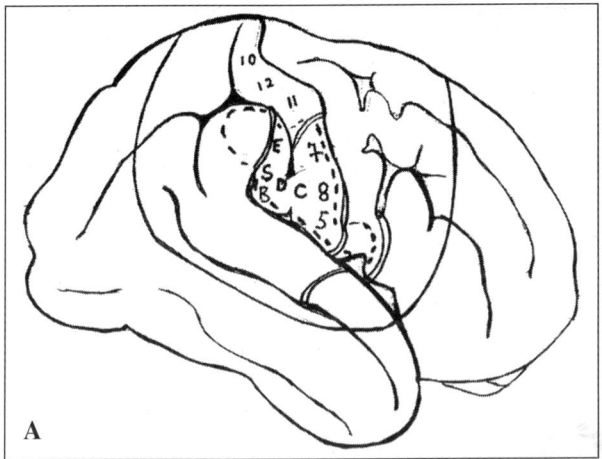

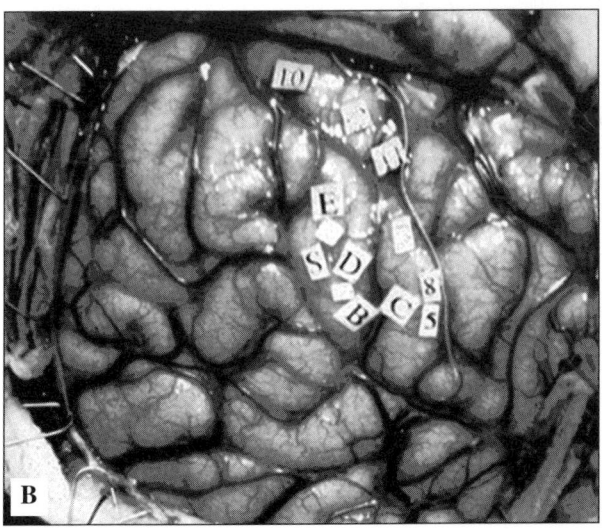

Fig. 11. (A) Case J.L. Operative diagram showing results of brain mapping, stimulation and EcoG. Stimulation at letter S produced a typical seizure. Dotted line shows extent of resection. (B) Case J.L. Operative photograph (See Fig. 11 A for orientation). The white thread corresponds to the central sulcus.

285

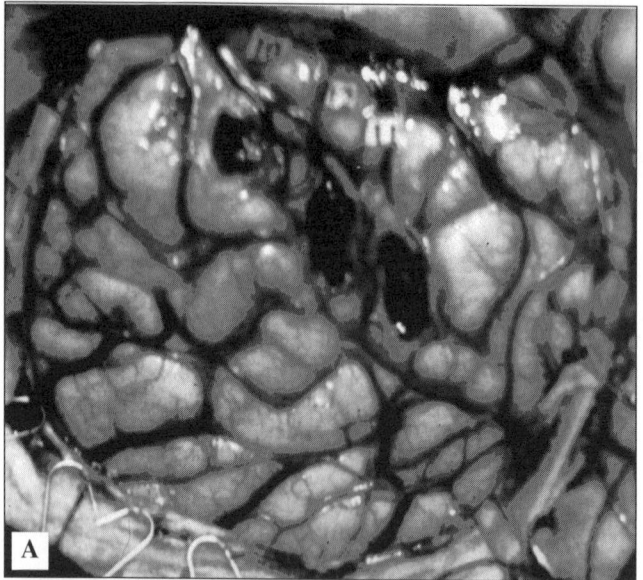

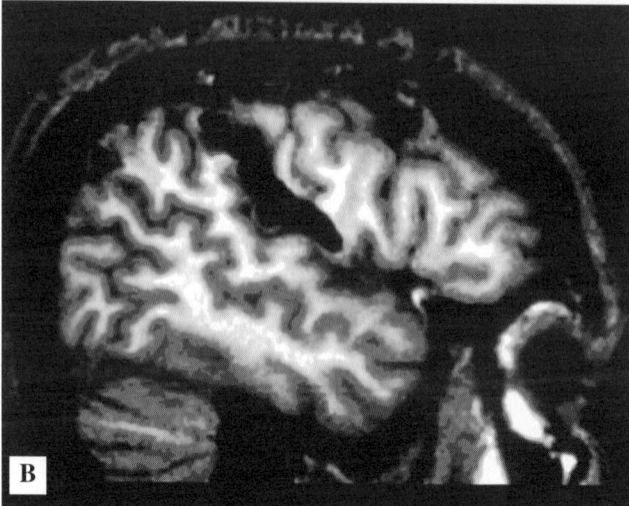

Fig. 12. (A) Case J.L. Operative photograph showing the actual resection. Note that the endopial resection was performed through separate compartments and that all the bypassing arteries and veins were left intact. (B) Case J.L. Post-op MRI showing extent of operative resection. Compare with operative photograph 12 A. The end result of the endopial emptying is shown.

over the lower post-central gyrus (Fig. 11A, B) the patient had a focal motor seizure involving the left upper limb which was aborted with I.V. Brietal.[1] He subsequently underwent a removal of the lower central area, up to the hand region, and resection of the supramarginal gyrus by the technique of subpial microdissection leaving intact all of the pial vessels passing through the central area (Fig. 12A, B). The histological specimen revealed neuronal heterotopia. There were no post-operative complications and the patient has remained seizure free with a follow-up now of nine months.

Dysplasia is inherently epileptogenic and this is often detected when recording from the brain surface. This case demonstrates the ability of ECoG to delineate a clear epileptic focus even though a lesion was not identified. The element of dysplasia present in this patient was too subtle to be resolved by the MRI but a resection of the epileptogenic area determined by ECoG brought an excellent result in seizure control.

Patient S.R.

S.R. was a nine year old right handed boy at the time of surgery with the onset of his intractable epilepsy at six years of age. Neurological examination revealed a decreased ability to perform rapid movements with the left hand and foot. His school performance showed a decline after the onset of his epilepsy. The seizure pattern was characterized by either generalized convulsions or a stare followed by left upper extremity tonic posturing and eye blinking. He described an aura of shock like sensations starting in the back of the tongue and zigzagging from side to side as the sensation traveled forward. He sometimes had a left side postictal paresis and the seizure frequency was three to five per day. Scalp EEG showed interictal

---

[1] Eli Lilly Canada Inc., Ontario, Canada

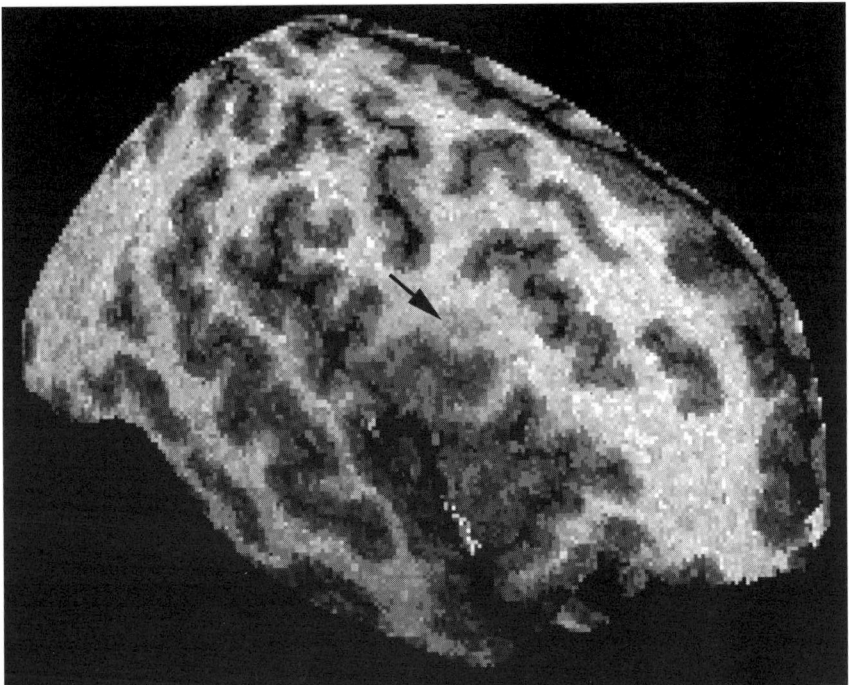

Fig. 13. Case S.R. Preoperative MRI. Curvilinear reconstruction showing area of dysplasia in lower central area.

abnormalities in the right frontocentrotemporal region and the ictal activity originating from the right frontocentral area. Dipole analysis was also consistent with a right central area seizure focus. The initial MRI revealed only asymmetry of the temporal horns but without hippocampal atrophy or other lesions. A fine cut MRI performed with curvilinear reconstruction demonstrated an area of thickened cortex and blurred gray/white junction consistent with dysplasia in the right inferior frontal gyrus and lower central area (Fig. 13). FDG-PET and ictal SPECT were congruent with seizure localization to this area. Amytal testing showed left hemisphere speech dominance.

A right frontocentral craniotomy was performed under general anaesthesia. ECoG recorded a continuous epileptic discharge, consistent with cortical dysplasia, from a depth electrode stereotactically placed in the lesion. Surface ECoG recorded bursts of polyspike activity over the posterior inferior frontal gyrus (F3) and the lower central area (Fig. 14A, B). MRI-guided frameless stereotaxy allowed the margins of the dysplasia as outlined on the MRI to be correlated to the brain surface to guide the resection. The lesion along with the surrounding region of active spike discharge was removed. The resection encompassed the lower central area, extending 2.5 cm above the Sylvian fissure, and the posterior portion of F3 (Fig. 15A-C). The patient had no deficit after surgery. Pathology revealed cortical dysplasia with dyslamination, large abnormal neurons, and gliosis. The patient has been seizure free for 10 months since surgery.

This case demonstrates the importance of ECoG in identifying active epileptogenic areas which may be found adjacent to visible dysplastic lesions. Presumably these active areas represent additional points of dysplasia too small for resolution by MRI. Because dysplasia is highly epileptogenic even these microscopic abnormalities must be removed to ensure the best outcome in reducing the seizure frequency.

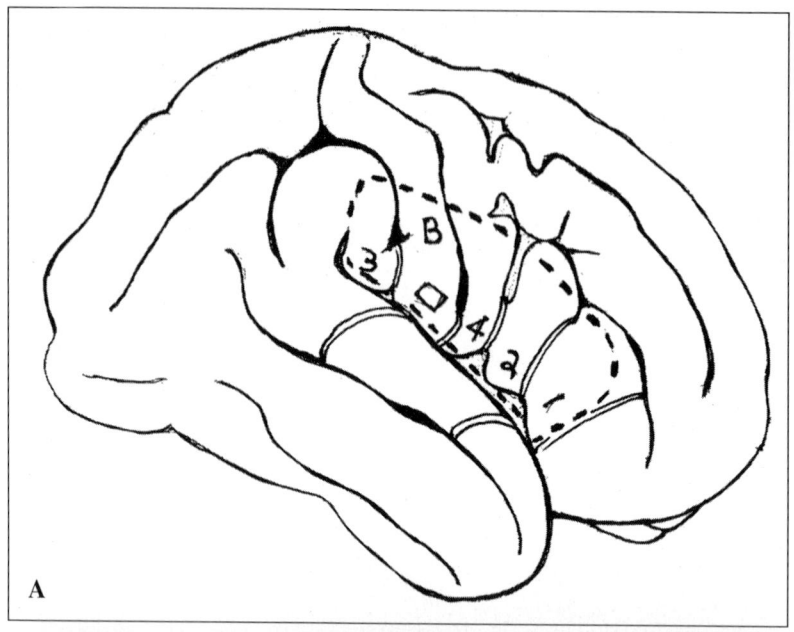
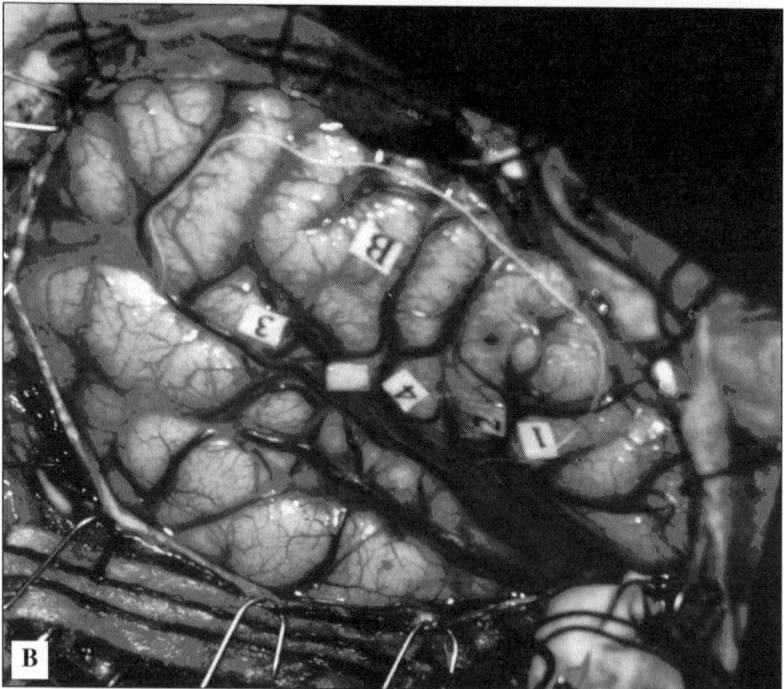

Fig. 14. (A) Case S.R. EcoG diagram: showing physiological response and EcoG data. 1,2,3 and 4 represent the location of maximum rhythmic slow wave activity recorded from the cortical surface. (B) Case S.R. Operative photograph showing EcoG data: See Fig. 14 A for orientation.

Chapter 23 Surgical treatment of cortical dysplasias and migration disorders

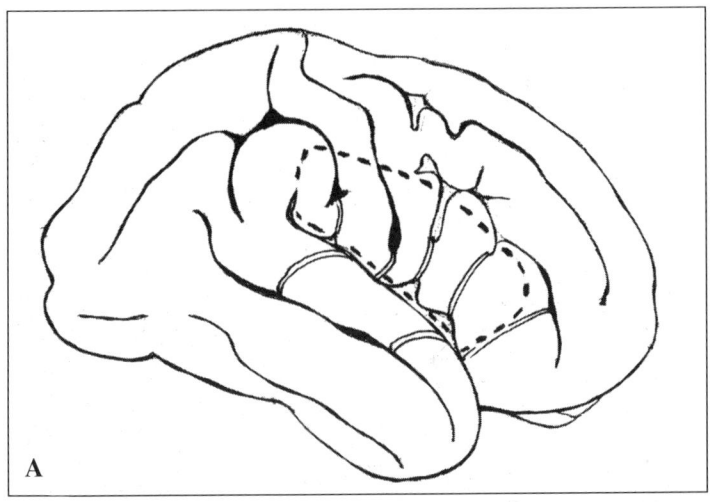

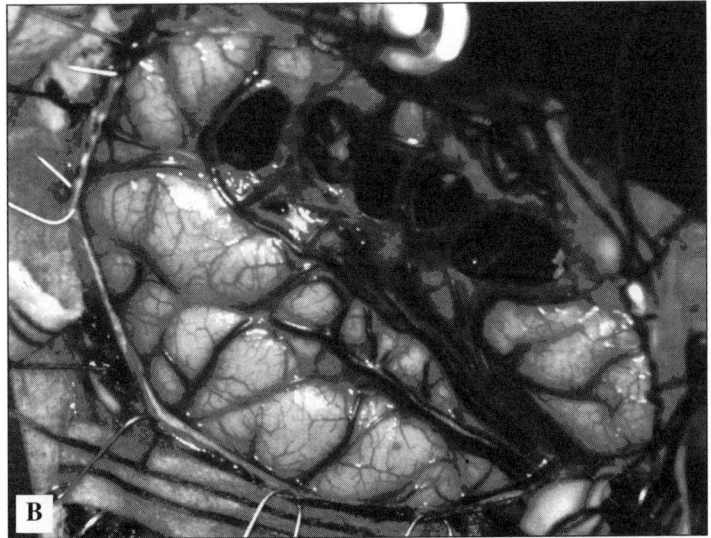

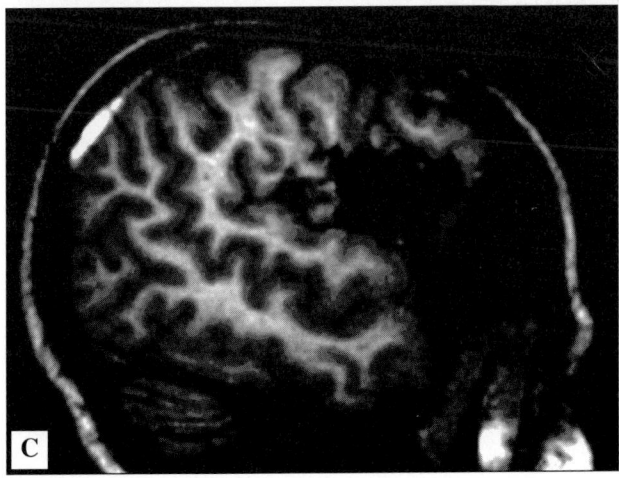

Fig. 15. (A) Case S.R. Diagram showing extent of resection. (B) Case S.R. Operative photograph showing resection (see 15 (A) for orientation). An other example of endopial resection performed through separate compartments. All ascending bypassing vessels have been left intact. (C) Case S.R. Post-op MRI (sagittal): compare with operative photograph showing resection (Fig. 15 B).

Dysplasia of occipital area

Patient J.G.

J. G. was a right handed 39 year old male at the time of surgery. His seizures began at the age of eight years with a pattern predominantly of a partial complex type. Most of the seizures began with an aura of a visual sensation described as a blurring in the right upper quadrant. In a minority of attacks the aura was a feeling of fear or an ascending epigastric sensation. The seizures then proceeded to a loss of contact, staring, and dystonic posturing of the right hand. During a seizure he may have grasped at objects with either hand or walked around the room. The partial complex seizures occurred twice a week and the generalized convulsions once a month. The seizures were uncontrolled with medication. Scalp EEG recorded many seizures showing onsets in the left inferomesial temporal, lateral temporal, posterior temporal, occipital, and parietooccipital areas. Neuropsychological testing was consistent with lateral cortical dysfunction in the left hemisphere as well as less severe dysfunction of the left mesial temporal structures. There was no visual field defect and the remainder of the neurological examination was normal. The initial MRI study demonstrated mild cortical atrophy of the left temporal pole without hippocampal atrophy. With additional fine cut MRI studies and curvilinear reconstruction a small subependymal nodule was discovered in the lateral wall of the left occipital horn consistent with dysplasia (Fig. 16A).

Although the occipital lesion was small, its location was consistent with the seizure generator on the scalp EEG. The resection of a deep seated occipital lesion would carry an almost certain risk of some visual deficit. Therefore, to confirm the lesion as the site of seizure onset and to rule out other potential sites of onset, stereoelectroencephalography was performed. Four multicontact depth electrodes were inserted in the left hemisphere, one directed at the amygdala, one at the posterior hippocampal area, and one at the mesial structures between the lesion and the posterior hippocampus. Another depth electrode was inserted within the subependymal nodule. Intracranial recording demonstrated the seizures arising from the region of the nodule. A left occipital craniotomy was performed. A transcortical microsurgical approach was used to the occipital horn using MRI-guided

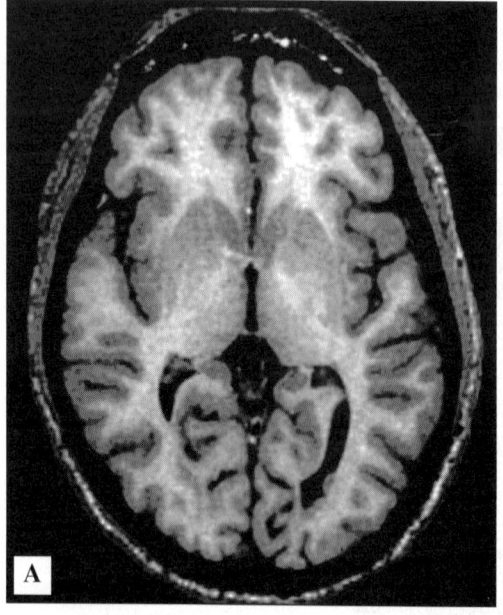 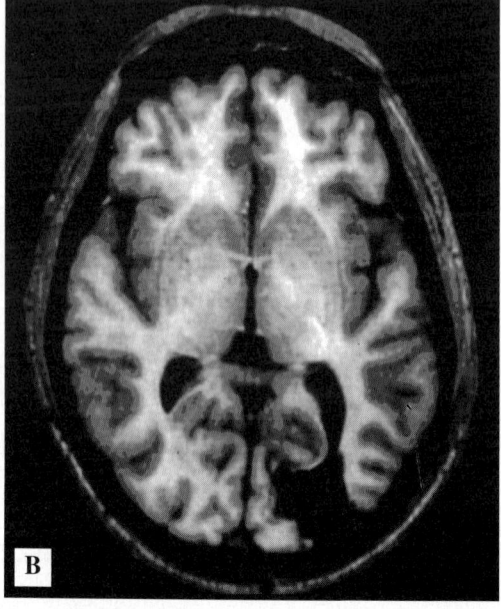

Fig. 16. (A) Case J.G. Pre-op MRI showing left paraventricular (subependymal) occipital heterotopia. (B) Case J.G. Post-op MRI showing removal of lesion. Compare with Fig. 16 (A).

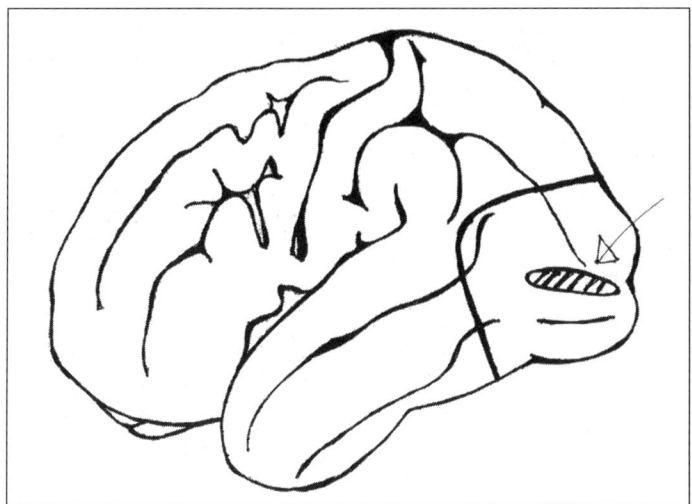

Fig. 17. Case J.G Operative diagram (for orientation see Fig. 18).

frameless stereotaxy (Fig. 17). The ependymal brownish lesion was well identified and a selective resection of the nodule was accomplished (Fig. 16B). After surgery visual field testing revealed an incomplete right lower homonymous field defect. At one year follow-up the patient has been seizure free except for a single nocturnal generalized convulsion.

This case illustrates again the effectiveness of selectively removing small areas of dysplasia proven to be the site of seizure origin. It also illustrates clearly the potential for subependymal lesions to be the cause and origin of seizures. It also demonstrates the not uncommon occurrence of an isolated convulsion after surgery in a patient who predominantly had partial complex seizures. The absence of his habitual partial complex type seizure is a positive indication of future excellent seizure control and the patient was reassured of this. However, patients with dysplasia must be very cautious in tapering of their antiepileptic medication. Epilepsy resulting from dysplasia is usually very severe and more prone to status than other common aetiologies (Palmini *et al.*, 1996).

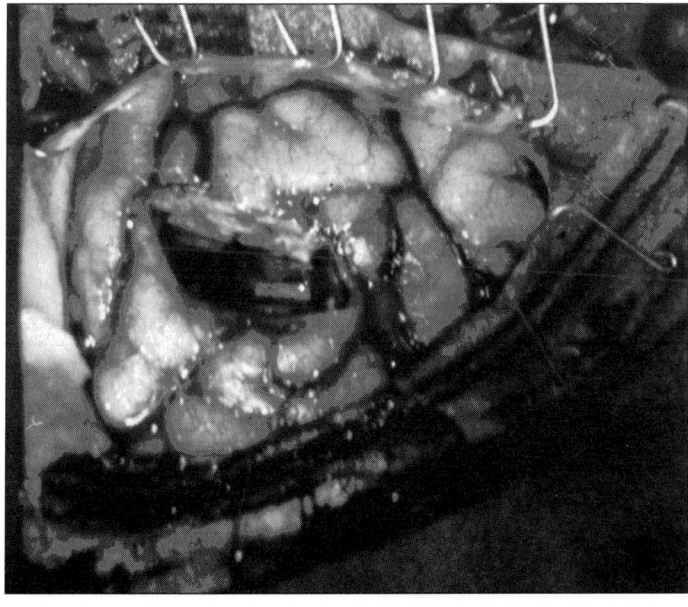

Fig. 18. Case J.G. Operative photograph showing cortical incision (See Fig. 17).

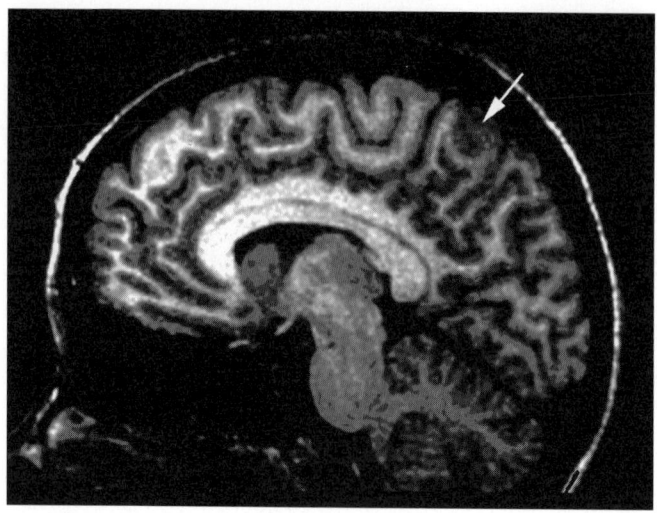

Fig. 19. Case A.H. Sagittal cut showing spherical lesion in parieto-central parasagittal area.

Dysplasia of parietal area

Patient A. H.

A. H. was a 19 year old woman at the time of surgery. She had febrile convulsions at 14 months of age but was well controlled with anticonvulsants for three years. Her medication was then tapered off and she remained asymptomatic for nine years. At 13 years old her seizures recurred with a generalized convulsion. However, her predominant seizure pattern became an elevation and tonic clonic contractions of the right upper limb with rotation of the head towards the right side. This was followed by a slow fall to the ground. She had no warning of these attacks. Despite multiple drug regimens her seizure frequency remained one per month. EEG telemetry revealed a frequent paroxysmal disturbance of cerebral activity recorded from the midcentral and parietal regions. Her neurologic examination was normal and the initial MRI scans did not reveal a focal abnormality. However, fine cut MRI with curvilinear reformatting performed at the MNI revealed a 1 cm spherical lesion in the left mesial precuneus with a close relationship to the paracentral lobule (Figs. 19, 21A). Actual involvement of the postcentral gyrus could not be excluded.

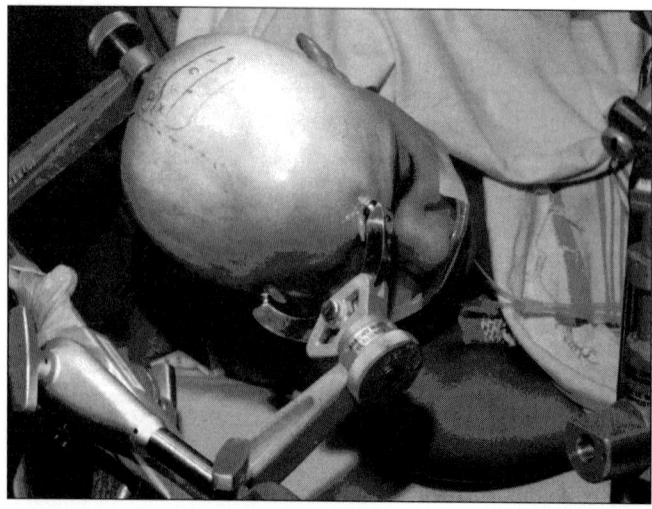

Fig. 20. Case A.H. Operative set-up under local anaesthesia, neuroloepanalgesia and neuronavigation.

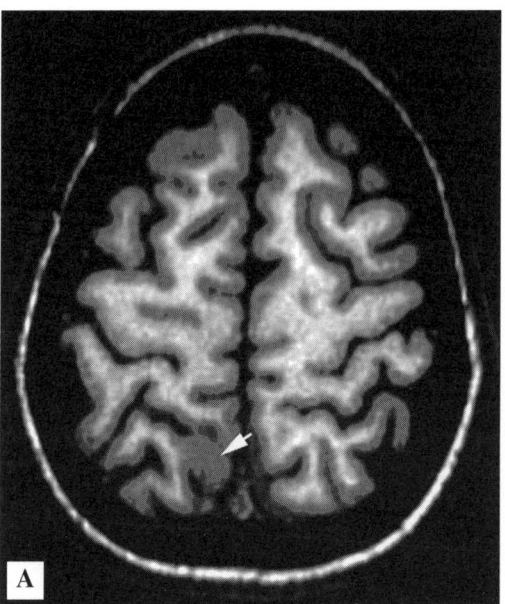 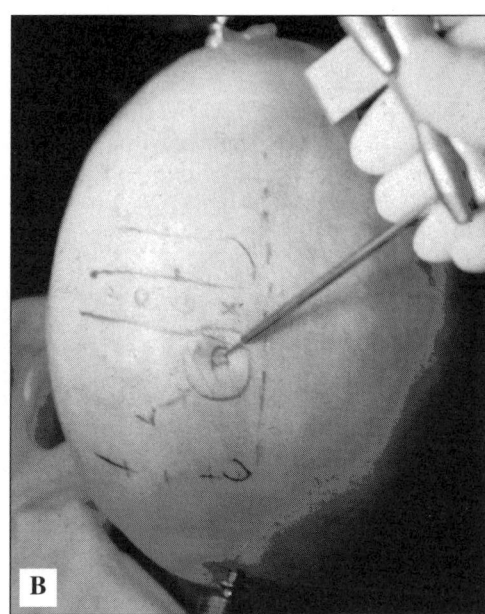

Fig. 21. (A) Case A.H. Transverse pre-op MRI showing lesion in sagittal parieto-central area (left side). (Compare with Fig. 21B). (B) Case A.H. Stereotactic wand pointing to the lesion over the scalp.

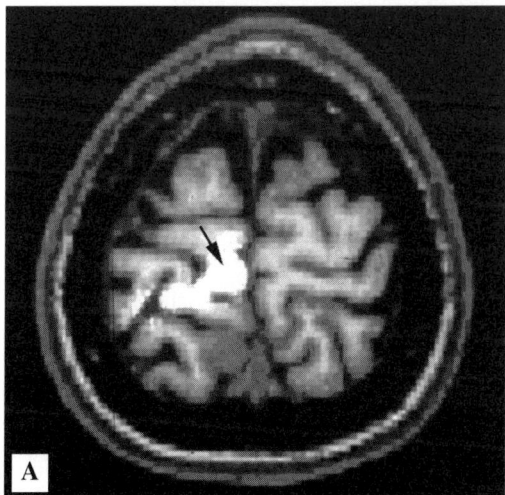 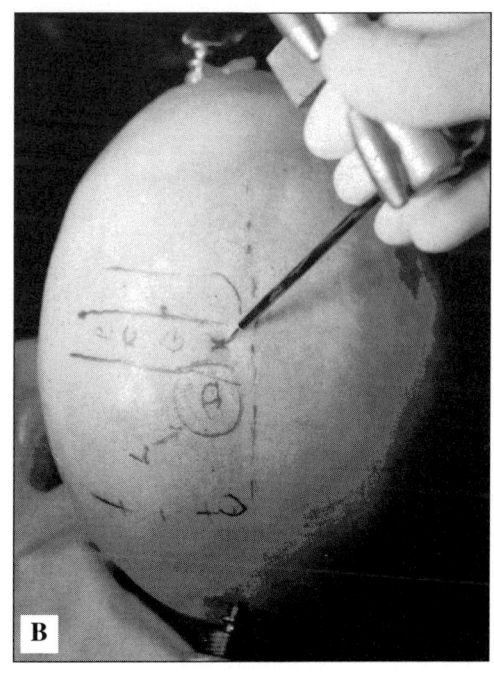

Fig. 22. (A) Case A. H. Transverse PET showing zone of foot sensory activation. (Compare with Fig. 22B). (B) Case A.H. Stereotactic wand pointing to the foot activation area over the scalp. Planning of scalp incision and craniotomy. Midline is indicated.

To determine the relationship of the lesion to foot function, a PET activation study was performed. This revealed foot sensory representation to be located in the gyrus immediately anterior to the lesion (Fig. 22A). A left parietocentral craniotomy was performed under local anaesthesia and with the frameless stereotactic neuronavigation system. The presumed position of the lesion and PET activation were displayed over the scalp to optimize the location and extent of the craniotomy

(Figs. 20; 21A, B; 22A, B). MRI-guided frameless stereotaxy was also used to locate the lesion and define its margins. Surface ECoG showed polymorphic slow wave activity over the lesion and a depth electrode inserted to the lesion revealed sharper activity. Following Brietal injection, low amplitude spikes were recorded from the same lesion. Stimulation of the post central gyrus at 1 and 1.5 volts was used to map thumb, finger, and foot areas (Fig. 23 A, B). A response of tingling in the foot obtained from postcentral gyrus stimulation corresponded to the site of PET activation (Fig. 23A, B). All of the apparent greyish/brownish lesion was selectively removed preserving the functioning cortex in the postcentral gyrus and adjacent draining veins (Fig. 24A). Pathology analysis

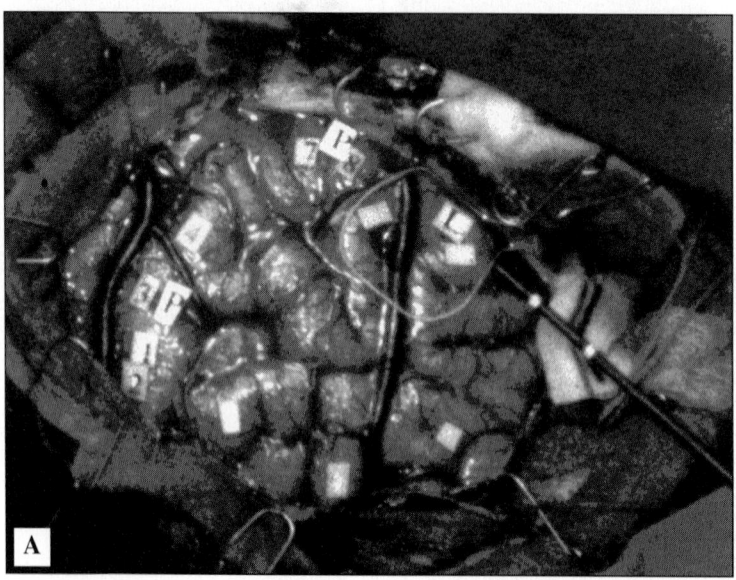

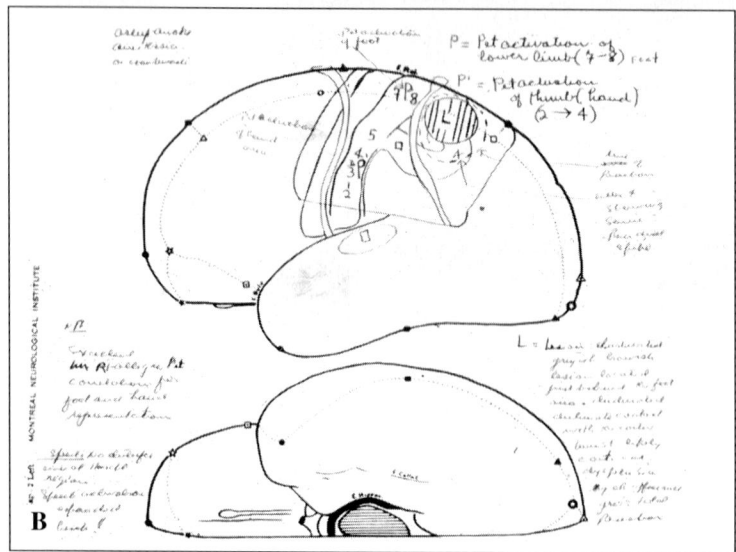

Fig. 23. (A) Case A.H. Exposed cortex at surgery. A recording electrode is inserted into the lesion. (See Fig. 23 B for orientation). (B) Case A.H. Brain map showing physiological responses to stimulation, correlation with PET scan and the location of lesions.

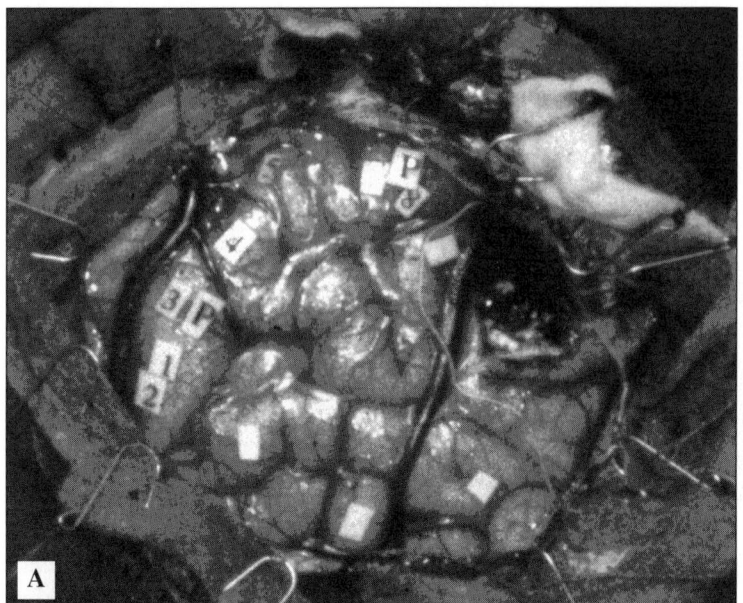

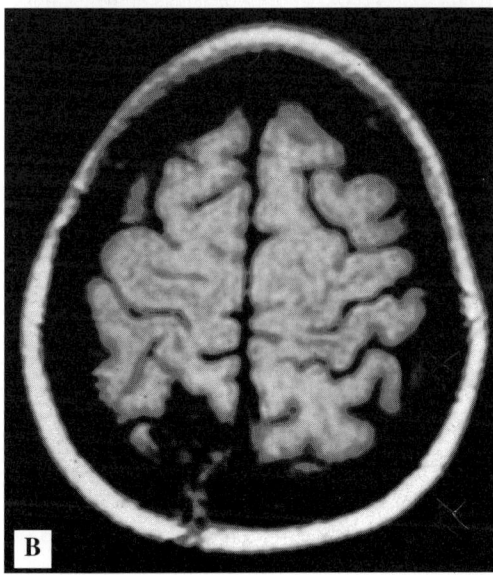

Fig. 24. (A) Case A.H. Operative photograph showing the resection. Note that a large central ascending vein has been left intact. (B) Case A.H. Transverse post-op MRI showing removal of the lesion.

revealed cortical dysplasia with disorganization of cortical layering and abundant heterotopic neurons in the white matter. The patient made a quick recovery from surgery and had no deficits. An MRI performed after surgery revealed a gross removal of the lesion (Fig. 24B) with possibly some residual extent of dysplasia in the surgical cavity. She had a seizure 35 days after surgery similar to her habitual preoperative pattern and has continued to have seizures at the same frequency as before surgery except for a four month period when she was seizure free.

The persistence of seizures in this patient is either due to a remnant of the MRI visible cortical dysplastic lesion which was not resected or to additional dysplastic cortex located outside the recognized lesion and too subtle to be detected. Often areas of cortical dysplasia do not have sharply demarcated borders and the lesion may be larger than what can be identified with even the

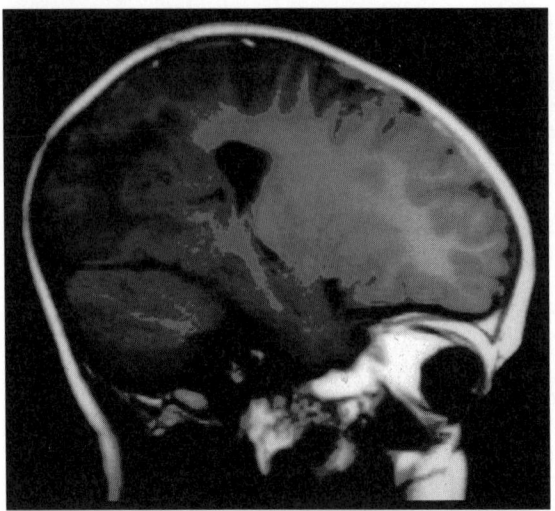

Fig. 25. Case T.C. Preop MRI showing lesion. Extensive area of dysplasia in occipito-parieto-temporal area.

most sophisticated imaging. The striking epileptogenicity of dysplasia is evident by this patient's persistant seizures despite a removal of all of the grossly apparent lesion.

This case illustrates several features in the surgery of cortical dysplasia. First is the need for an intense search for a causative lesion with the appropriate modalities of imaging. Second is the important role of functional imaging and stereotactic image guidance combined to standard preoperative mapping for the safe resection of dysplastic lesions in the central area. Finally this case may indicate that the bulk of the visible lesion was not the actual source of the seizures and that a more subtle distant lesion is the culprit. Reoperation and further removal is not excluded.

Multilobar dysplasia

Patient T.C.
At the time of surgery, T. C. was a five year old girl with intractable epilepsy since two days old. The seizures were manifested by turning of the head to the left, flickering of the eyelids, and stiffening of the left arm and leg. She had many seizures everyday (occasionally up to 40) and her left side would become weaker after a flurry of attacks. The more severe attacks would precipitate a fall. Her neurologic examination showed a left hemianopsia, a paucity of movements and some neglect of the left side of the body. She also walked with a circumduction of the left leg. The MRI showed gross macrogyria of the temporal, parietal and occipital areas on the right (Fig. 25). The white matter in these regions had an abnormally low signal intensity and there was a loss of cortical/medullary differentiation. Scalp EEG demonstrated a severe epileptic abnormality with an abnormal background involving all the right hemisphere. Two seizures were recorded. One arose from the right temporal region and another from the right occipital region.

Since the seizure onset seen on the EEG correlated with the most severe structural abnormality identified on the MRI, a resection of the structurally abnormal region was proposed in an effort to lower the seizure tendency. The patient underwent a temporoparietooccipital craniotomy under general anaesthesia. The boundaries of the lesion identified on MRI were outlined on the surface of the brain using the MRI-guided frameless stereotaxy (Fig. 26A, B). Preresection ECoG demonstrated active diffuse interictal discharges over the right temporoparietooccipital region. Two electrographic seizures were recorded with predominant discharges over the temporal and occipital lobes below the level of the Sylvian fissure. The central area was mapped by cortical stimulation (Fig. 26A, B). (Responses at 4.0 volts: points A, C, and D flexion of all left fingers and point E flexion of 4th and 5th fingers on the left.) A large resection was subsequently performed which encompassed the right temporal, occipital, and lower parietal lobes in addition to a corticectomy of the lower postcentral gyrus. The resection included most of the visible lesion on MRI in addition to the cortex exhibiting the maximal epileptic activity on ECoG (Fig. 26C). Pathology examination demonstrated abnormal large and binucleate neurons throughout the cortical layer and a paucity of myelin in the white matter. After surgery she was seizure free for three months. Some seizures recurred but she has maintained a 90 per cent improvement in seizure frequency for over three years and she no longer has severe attacks with falls.

Chapter 23 Surgical treatment of cortical dysplasias and migration disorders

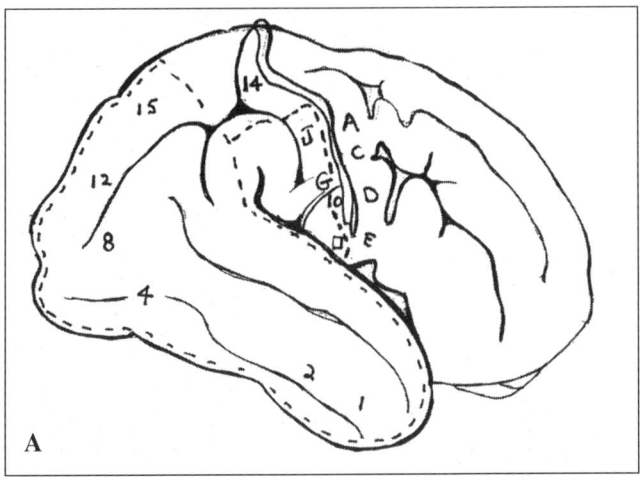

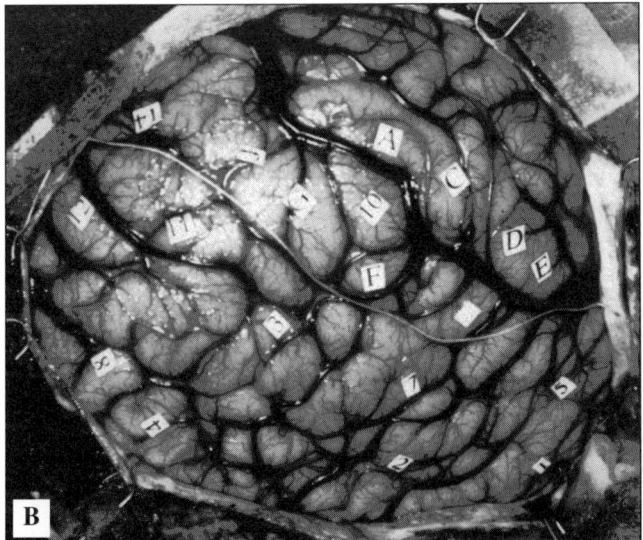

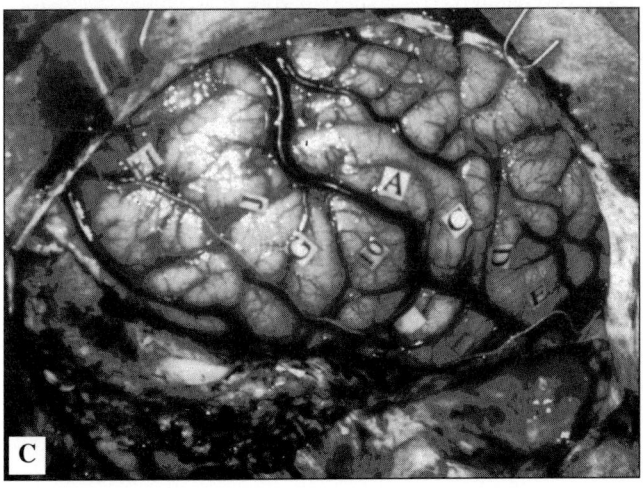

Fig. 26. (A) Case T.C. OR diagram showing physiological responses and extent of resection (dotted line). (B) Case T.C. OR photograph showing physiological responses and extent of removal (white thread) (see fig. 26A for orientation). (C) Case T.C. Operative photograph showing the actual large resection of the occipito-parieto-temporal area (compare with Fig. 26 B).

This case illustrates several of the difficulties in dealing with widespread cortical dysplasia. Incomplete removal does not stop the seizure tendency. However, a subtotal removal of a large area of cortical dysplasia can be beneficial in cases where the area of maximal interictal epileptogenic focus has been identified and resected. Finally, this patient demonstrates that dysplasia may possibly involve an entire hemisphere even though gross imaging changes may be quite localized.

Outcome of surgery

Results of surgery on the seizure tendency are reported according to an outcome classification that we have now used in a personal (A.O.) series of over 1500 patients. (Table 1)

Outcome in temporal lobe resections

Table 2 shows the postoperative seizure outcome in 65 patients with dysplastic lesions including gangliogliomas of the temporal lobe. Among the 36 patients with dysplasias, 69 per cent were seizure free, 20 per cent had a reduction > 90 per cent, and 11 per cent had a reduction of 60–90 per cent of their seizures. Of the 29 patients with gangliogliomas, 80 per cent became seizure free, 17 per cent had a reduction > 90 per cent, and three per cent had a reduction of 60–90 per cent in their seizure tendency.

Outcome in frontal lobe resections

There were 21 patients with frontal dysplasias. Of these, 61 per cent became seizure-free, 17 per cent had a reduction > 90 per cent, and nine per cent had a reduction of 60–90. Thus 87 per cent were improved and 13 per cent had a reduction of less than 60 per cent in their seizure tendency. Among the three patients with frontal gangliogliomas two became seizure-free and one had a reduction of 60–90 per cent. (Table 3)

Outcome in extratemporal and extra-frontal resections

Table 4 shows that of the 12 patients in the parietal group, 42 per cent became seizure free and 50 per cent had a reduction > 90 per cent and eight per cent had a reduction of 60–90 per cent. Of the seven patients with occipital lesions, 28 per cent had > 90 per cent reduction and 72 per cent became seizure-free. Nine patients were operated in the central area (some on several occasions). Four became seizure free and four patients had a reduction > 90 per cent and one had a reduction of 60–90 per cent. All were improved. (Table 4.)

Outcome of callosotomy

Twelve patients were operated for diffuse dysplastic conditions giving rise to drop attacks such as bilateral perisylvian dysplasia and double cortex. None became seizure free but eight patients had a reduction > 90 per cent and four had a reduction of 60–90 per cent.

Complications of surgery for treatment of cortical dysplasias

Complications have been few. In the 129 patients reported here, complications are reported as follows: mortality 0, permanent hemiparesis 0, infection 0, transient dysphasia one and dysarthria one. The transient dysphasia was encountered in a patient who underwent removal of the left first frontal gyrus including part of the supplementary motor area. One patient with intractable status epilepticus had a series of three operations culminating in an 'en-bloc' central resection with the purpose of saving her life. This procedure, as expected, was followed by severe hemiparesis but probably saved her life by complete control of her seizures. One patient who underwent an additional lower central resection had over 90 per cent control of his intractable seizures but developed increased difficulty with the pronounciation of long words and especially those starting with the letter S.

Table 1. A. O. Classification of seizure outcome

Class I:	100% Reduction
Class II:	> 90 % Reduction
Class III:	60–90% Reduction
Class IV:	< 60% Reduction
Class V:	No improvement
Class VI:	Worse

Table 2. Postoperative seizures outcome in 65 patients with temporal dysplastic lesions

Lesion type	Cases	I (%)	II (%)	III (%)	IV (%)	Improved
Dysplasias	36	69	20	11	0	100
Gangliogliomas	29	80	17	3	0	100
Total	65	74.5	18.5	7	0	100

Table 3. Postperative seizure outcome in 24 patients with frontal dysplastic lesions

Lesion type	Cases	I (%)	II (%)	III (%)	Improved	IV (%)
Dysplasias	21	61	17	9	87	13
Gangliogliomas	3	67	0	33	100	0
Total	24	64	8.5	21	93.5	6.5

Table 4. Postperative seizure outcome in patients with extratemporal and extra-frontal dysplastic lesions

Regions	Cases	I (%)	II (%)	III (%)	Improved	IV (%)
Central	9	45	44	11	100	0
Parietal	12	42	50	8	100	0
Occipital	7	72	28	0	100	0
Total	28	53	41	6	100	0
Callosotomy	12	0	75	25	100	0

Discussion

Traditional neuropathology and modern MR imaging have revealed a widespread variety of cortical dysplasias and migration disorders. These anomalies may involve all cortical areas of the brain i.e. central, frontal, temporal, insular and parietal. Migration lesions may involve not only the cortex, but the subcortical white matter and the paraventricular area. They may be focal, bilateral, nodular, laminar or diffuse.

Specific problems characterize the surgery of dysplasias, namely the size of the visible lesion, the location and relationship with the electrical focus and their potential association with brain tumours.

Size of lesions

Areas of cortical dysplasia may be very small or cryptic. Others may be large or widespread. When small, these morphological anomalies may be very hard to detect on MRI and may be missed. When small areas of dysplasias are difficult to detect on MRI, they may be totally impossible to find at operation. The boundaries of the larger zones of dysplasia may be very hard to delineate even on MRI. They can also be impossible to recognize when the cortex is exposed at surgery since there is no clear line of demarcation between normal and abnormal cortex. Furthermore their extent may be quite variable and this may cause considerable difficulty in centering a bone flap for craniotomy.

Location of lesions

Since cortical dysplasia frequently involves crucial areas of the brain such as the posterior frontal lobe and the central, insular and parietal cortex, the technical challenge of dealing with the primary motor and sensory cortex or with speech related centers is often considerable. This situation may be compounded by the fact that the anatomy and actual function of the involved cortex may be altered by the presence of dysplasia even though considerable function may be retained in dysplastic tissue.

Relationship of dysplastic lesions to tumour

In some instances areas of cortical dysplasia have been clearly associated with a definite tumoural process. This has often been seen in tuberous sclerosis in which the classical tubers are convolutional foci of sclerosis where the gliosis is associated with gross disturbance of cell architecture and with abnormal (so-called balloon cells) cell forms. Tumours associated with tuberous sclerosis are usually circumscribed and represent a distinct form of benign giant cell astrocytoma.

The distinction between hamartoma and neoplasm is sometimes unclear. Gangliogliomas which contain dysplastic neurons also appear as a tumoral variety of cortical dysplasias. Recent data have confirmed a relationship between additional tumour types and cortical dysplasia (Prayson et al., 1993). The presence of dysplastic cortical areas within or around a tumour such as a ganglioglioma or a dysembryoplastic neuroepithelial tumour suggests a congenital developmental origin for these hamartomatous lesions. Dysplastic cortex and heterotopias were found in association with gangliogliomas in a high percentage in a recent series (Prayson et al., 1993). A congenital origin is also suggested for gangliogliomas by the relatively high incidence of other congenital abnormalities (Haddad et al., 1992; Russell & Rubinstein, 1989) and by a close anatomical relationship with temporo-mesial structures, where prolonged postmature neurocytogenesis has been documented (Gueneau et al., 1982).

Well defined masses of ectopic grey matter may be encountered in the centrum semi-ovale. Aside from their possible clinical significance as epileptogenic foci they are of considerable interest because they could provide an explanation for those hamartomatous lesions detected in locations where neurones are not normally present.

A variety of surgical modalities have been used in the treatment of dysplasias ranging from lesionectomy to cortical resections, to hemispherectomy and to cortical transection. Often the condition has necessitated staged interventions. When a lesion is located in a silent area, it should be removed by lesionectomy and corticectomy. Whenever feasible, all abnormal looking or thickened cortex must be resected.

As shown in previous report (Olivier et al., 1996) and with the present series of patients, the advent of image guided surgery with 2-D and 3-D MRI reconstruction has brought considerable improvement to the surgical management of cortical dysplasia. Since these lesions are better seen on MRI scans than at surgery, the frameless stereotaxic technique using a pointer during craniotomy is now routinely used to locate and delineate the malformation (Olivier *et al.*, 1996; Olivier *et al.*, 1994). Several recent studies have now shown the high intrinsic epileptogenicity of dysplasia (Avoli *et al.*, 1996; Mattia *et al.*, 1995; Munari *et al.*, 1996; Palmini *et al.*, 1996). By combining functional and electrical data to image guided surgery it is now easier to resect the lesion and primary focus.

Conclusion

With the advent of MRI cortical dysplasias are more frequently recognized as a cause of surgically treatable epilepsies. However even with excellent MRI pictures it may be extremely difficult to confirm a suspicion of dysplasia either because of the small size of the lesions which are often buried at the base of sulci or because a dysplastic gyrus may look so much like a normal one. MRI may show the gross boundaries of the lesion but not necessarily demonstrate its full extent. Thus the main surgical difficulty is in evaluating with accuracy the location and extent of the lesion, preoperatively and during surgery and identifying the electrical focus during surgery. Newer technical strategies with three dimensional MRI reconstruction are most promising. Lesions which have been radically removed such as gangliogliomas had excellent results. Incomplete removals because of location, extent or bilaterality of the lesions lead to less satisfactory outcome. By applying the standard principles of epilepsy surgery, morbidity can be kept low.

References

Andermann, F., Olivier A., Melanson D. & Robitaille Y. (1987): Epilepsy due to focal cortical dysplasia with macrogyria and forme fruste: a study of 15 cases. In: *Advances in Epileptology,* eds. P. Wolf & M. Dam, **16**, pp. 35–38. New York: Raven Press.

Avoli, M., Hwa, G.G.C., Mattia, D., Villemure, J.-G. & Olivier, A. (1996): Microphysiology of human neocortex in vitro. In: *Dysplasias of cerebral cortex and epilepsy,* eds. R. Guerrini *et al.*, pp. 35–42. Phildelphia: Lippincott-Raven.

Bruton, J.J. (1988): *The neuropathology of temporal lobe epilepsy*. Institute of Psychiatry, Mandsky Monographs, vol. 31. Oxford: Oxford University Press.

Daumas-Duport, C. (1993): Dysembryoplastic neuroepithelial tumours. *Brain Pathol.* **3**, 283–295.

Gueneau, G., Privat, A., Drouet, J. *et al.* (1982): Subgranular zone of the dentate gyrus of young rabbits as a secondary matrix. A high-resolution autoradiographic study. *Dev. Neurosci.* **5**, 345–358.

Haddad, S.F., Moore, Sa., Menezes, A.H., *et al.* (1992): Ganglioglioma: 13 years of experience. *Neurosurgery* **31**, 171–178.

Hardiman, O., Burke, T., Philips, J. *et al.* (1988): Microdysgenesis in resected temporal cortex: Incidence and clinical significance in focal epilepsy. *Neurology* **38**, 1041–1047.

Janota, I. & Polkey, C.E. (1985): Focal dysplasia of the cerebral cortex, in surgery for epilepsy. *Neuropathol. Appl. Neurobiol.* **11**, 325–326.

Janota, I. & Polkey, C.E. (1992): Cortical dysplasia in epilepsy : a study of material from surgical resections for intractable epilepsy. In: *Recent Advances in Epilepsy,* ed. T.A. Pedley & B.S. Meldrum, pp. 37–49. Edinburgh: Churchill Livingstone.

Khajavi, K., Comair, Y.G. & Hahn, J.F. (1994): Completeness of tumour resection determines seizure outcome in children with medically intractable epilepsy and gangliogliomas. *J. Neurosurg.* **80**, 396A (abstract).

Kuzniecki. R., Andermann, F., Fusco, L. *et al.* (1990): Corpus callosotomy in the management of the congenital bilateral perisylvian syndrome. *Epilepsia* **31**, 639.

Mathieson, G. (1975): Pathologic aspects of epilepsy with special reference to the surgical pathology of focal cerebral seizures. In: *Advances in Neurology,* eds. D.P. Purpura, J.K. Penry & R.D. Walter, vol. 8, pp. 107–138. New York: Raven Press.

Mattia, D., Olivier, A. & Avoli, M. (1995): Seizure-like discharges recorded in the human dysplastic neocortex maintained *in vitro*. *Neurology* **45 (7)**, 1391–1395.

Munari, C., Francione, S., Kahane, P., Tassi, L., Hoffman, D., Garrel, S. & Pasquier, B. (1996): Usefulness of stereo EEG investigations in partial epilepsy associated with cortical dysplastic lesions and gray matter heterotopia. In: *Dysplasias of cerebral cortex and epilepsy,* eds. R. Guerrini *et al.*, pp. 383–394. Phildelphia: Lippincott-Raven.

Norman, R.M. (1967): Malformations of the nervous system. Birth injury and diseases of early life. In: *Greenfield's Neuropathology,* eds. W. Blackwood, W. McMenemey, A. Meyer, R.M. Norman & D. Russell, pp. 324–440. London: Edward Arnold Ltd.

Olivier, A., Andermann, F., Palmini, A. & Robitaille, Y. (1996): Surgical treatment of cortical dysplasias. In: *Dysplasias of cerebral cortex and epilepsy,* eds. R. Guerrini *et al.,* pp. 351–361. Philadelphia: Lippincott-Raven.

Olivier, A., Germano, I.M., Cukiert, A. & Peters, T. (1994): Frameless stereotaxy for surgery of the epilepsies: preliminary experience. Technical note. *J. Neurosurg.* **84,** 629–635.

Palmini, A., Gambardella, A., Andermann, F., Olivier, A. *et al.* (1996): Outcome of surgical treatment in patients with localized cortical dysplasia & intractable epilepsy. In: *Dysplasias of cerebral cortex and epilepsy,* eds. R. Guerrini *et al.,* pp. 367-374. Phildelphia: Lippincott-Raven.

Palmini, A., Andermann, F. & Olivier, A. (1991): Focal neuronal migration disorders and intractable partial epilepsy. Results of surgical treatment. *Ann. Neurol.* **30(6),** 750–757.

Palmini, A., Gambardella, A., Andermann, F., Olivier, A. *et al.,* (1995): Outcome of surgical treatment in patients with localized cortical dysplasia and intractable epilepsy. *Ann. Neurol.* **37(4),** 476–487.

Perot, P., Weir, B. & Rasmussen, T. (1966): Tuberous sclerosis: surgical therapy for seizures. *Ann. Neurol.* **15,** 498–506.

Prayson, R.A., Estes, M.L. & Morris, H.H. (1933): Coexistence of neoplasia and cortical dysplasia in patients presenting with seizures. *Epilepsia* **34 (4),** 609–615.

Robain, A. (1996): Introduction to the pathology of cerebral cortical dysplasia. In: *Dysplasias of cerebral cortex and epilepsy,* eds. R. Guerrini *et al.,* pp. 1–9. Phildelphia: Lippincott-Raven.

Russell, D.S. & Rubinstein, L.J. (1989): In: *Pathology of tumours of the nervous system,* 5th ed. Baltimore, MD: Williams & Wilkins.

Staunton, T., Andermann, F., Melanson, D. *et al.* (1983): Focal macrogyria: a recognizable developmental disorder presenting with intractable focal seizures. *Ann. Neurol.* **14,** 152.

Talairach, J., Bancaud, J., Szikla, G. *et al.* (1974): Approche nouvelle de la chirurgie de l'épilepsie. *Neurochirurgie,* Tome **20, (Suppl. 1)** Paris: Masson.

Taylor, D.C., Falconer, M.A., Bruton, C.J. *et al.* (1971): Focal dysplasia of the cerebral cortex in epilepsy. *J. Neurol. Neurosurg. Psych.* **34,** 369–387.

Chapter 24

Surgical management of severe partial epilepsy symptomatic of neuronal migration disorders: physiopathological considerations and perspectives of research

Claudio Munari[1,2], Lorella Minotti[3], Laura Tassi[1],
Stefano Francione[1], Philippe Kahane[3], Carlo Alberto Galli[1],
Nadia Colombo[1], Emilia Berta[1], Basile Pasquier[3],
Giorgio Lo Russo[1], Dominique Hoffmann[3],
Alim Louis Benabid[3], Roberto Spreafico[4]

[1]*Dipartimento di Scienze Neurologiche, Centro Regionale per la Chirurgia dell'Epilessia, Ospedale Niguarda Ca' Granda, Piazza Ospedale Maggiore 3, 20162 Milan, Italy;*
[2]*Istituto di Clinica Neurochirurgica, Università di Genova, Italy;*
[3]*Service d'Anatomie Pathologique, Centre Hospitalier Régional et Universitaire CHU, B.P. 217X, 38043, Grenoble Cedex 9, France;*
[4]*Divisione di Neurofisiologia Sperimentale ed Epilettologia, Istituto Nazionale Neurologico 'C. Besta', Via Celoria 11, 20133, Milan, Italy*

Introduction

Since the original definition of Penfield & Erickson (1941), severe partial epilepsies have been divided in two groups: 'symptomatic' (when the aetiological lesion is evident) and cryptogenetic (when a lesion should exist, but it is not clearly evident). These two subgroups have been included, among other criteria, also in the last International Classification of Epilepsies and related syndromes (ILAE Commission Classification 1989). Some large series have been published including analytical data on the aetiological lesions found during surgical interventions aiming to suppress drug-resistant partial seizures (Talairach *et al.*, 1974; Rasmussen, 1983; Wolf & Wiestler, 1993; Pasquier *et al.*, 1996). The most important differences existing between these reports can be explained by several factors:

- the duration of the period during which patients are included can vary from several decades (Talairach et al., 1974; Rasmussen, 1983) to a few years (Wolf & Wiestler, 1993; Pasquier *et al.*, 1996);
- the criteria for selecting patients as candidates for surgical treatment (Lindsay et al., 1984);
- the age of the investigated population;

- the type of presurgical neurophysiological and neuroradiological investigations;
- more or less recent recognition of some neuropathological entities (e.g. dysembryoplastic neuroepithelial tumour (DNT): Daumas-Duport *et al.*, 1988).

Current MRI utilization is progressively showing that neuronal migration disorders (NMDs) represent one of the most frequent aetiological factors in patients with severe, drug-resistant, partial epilepsy. Literature data suggest that the extent of the surgical removal of this type of epileptogenic lesion is often decided on the basis of either the macroscopically identified alteration or the electro-cortico-graphic (acute or chronic) findings (Palmini *et al.*, 1996), or both.

Among the different possible surgical options, the simple 'lesionectomy' is preferred by many surgical teams since this procedure is apparently simple to perform, without the need for complex and time- and money-consuming presurgical investigations. However, the results obtained with this simplified approach, particularly regarding seizure suppression, are relatively dishomogeneous. Several factors can theoretically play an important role in the surgical result: the existence of familiar antecedents of epilepsy, age at the onset of seizures, the duration of epilepsy, the neurological status at intervention and so on. Last but not least, the type of the lesion, its extent and its topographic location play a part.

In this short paper we will discuss, on the basis of our surgical experience, the possible relationships between the MRI evidence of a NMD and the extent of the epileptogenic zone (EZ) defined according to the previously described criteria (Munari & Bancaud, 1985; Lüders et al., 1993).

Patients and methods

During the period from March 1990 to June 1997, 360 consecutive patients were operated on (at the Grenoble and Milano Epilepsy Surgery Centers) according to the previously described methodology (Munari, 1987; Munari *et al.*, 1994, 1996a). For this study only 30 patients were selected (8.3 per cent) in whom the histological examination of surgical specimen obtained at the intervention proved the existence of a NMD.

Seizure frequency was daily, or more, in half of them. Seizures started at a mean age of 6.5 years (< 1 in 7, < 5 in 19, < 10 in 24). Mean epilepsy duration was 16.3 years. Only two very young children were operated on after less than two years from seizure onset.

Non-invasive presurgical investigations

Spontaneous seizures were recorded during video-EEG intensive monitoring in almost all patients. Interictal SPECT and PET were only occasionally performed outside the double blind research protocols (Lucignani *et al.*, 1996). Functional MRI was performed only in a few patients presenting with some peculiar aspects (see below, the case with bilateral opercular dysplasia: BOD).

Preoperative MRI

- was 'normal' in 10,
- only showed a cryptic vascular malformation in two (contralateral in one), and
- suggested a NMD in the other 18 (bilateral in two).

Invasive presurgical procedures

Stereotactic neuroradiological procedures in stereoscopic conditions (Munari *et al.*, 1987) were performed in all patients. A stereo-EEG investigation, with 9–15 multilead stereotactically introduced intracerebral electrodes (DIXI, Besançon), was performed in 24/30 patients (80 per cent), since the relationship between the MRI evident lesion and the electroclinical findings of the scalp-

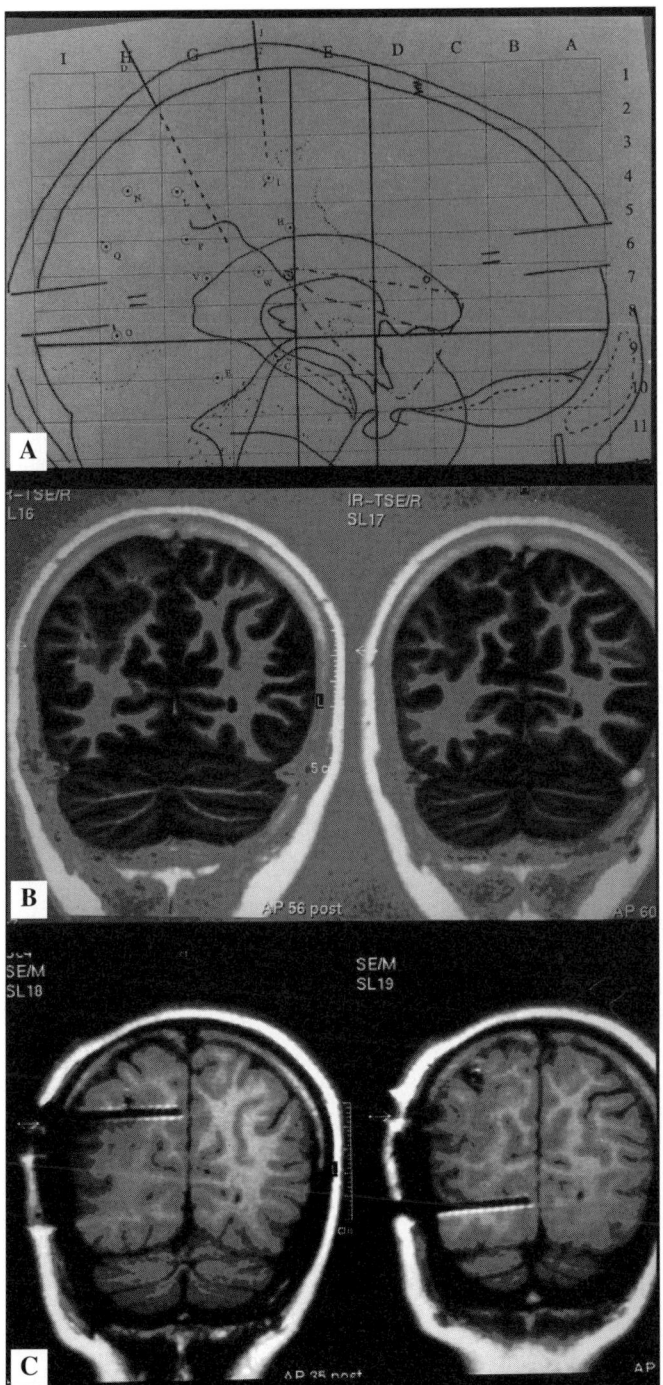

Fig. 1. (A) Stereo-EEG study, by means of 13 stereotactically implanted electrodes (lateral view of the skull), exploring the right parieto-occipito-temporal region, in a patient with neuroradiologically diagnosed NMD; (B) Inversion recovery (coronal view) brain MRI of the same patient as (A) showing altered gyri and thickness of the grey matter; (C) T1 (coronal view) in the same plane as (B) showing electrode position.

EEG recorded seizures was not sufficiently clear to define the extent of the surgical removal. The aim of this procedure was to investigate not only the evident NMD, but also the cortical areas (not necessarily immediately adjacent) possibly involved by the ictal discharges (Fig. 1)

Surgical intervention

The mean age at the time of operation was 22.9 years (2–44). The boundaries of the surgical intervention were defined on the basis of the anatomo-electro-clinical findings. In stereo-EEG investigated patients, the EZ was either totally or partially removed, considering the functional value of the epileptogenic cortex.

In the two patients with bilateral NMD, the unilateral intervention was performed after the demonstration that ictal discharges originated in one side only. In the patient with BOD, scalp-EEG recorded seizures strongly suggested a right-sided centro-parietal origin of the seizures. The SEEG, individually adapted to her characteristics, also assessed by functional MRI, confirmed the existence of a unique, opercular parietal EZ in the right hemisphere, which was removed. In the other one, a child of 10 years with a bioccipital cortical dysplasia, several spontaneous seizures recorded during video-EEG monitoring invariably started in the right occipital lobe, which was therefore removed without invasive recordings.

All the removed cerebral cortex (lesional and epileptogenic) was histologically examined. Immunohistochemical studies were also performed on part of the ablated specimens using different antibodies addressed to recognize cytoskeletal components and neuronal markers (for detailed procedure see Spreafico et al., 1998).

Postoperative follow-up

Clinical, cognitive, EEG and MRI postoperative controls were performed at one, six, 12, 24 months, and then every 12 months. Postoperative follow-up was > 12 months (17–70 months; mean: 40) in 19 patients (Grenoble).

Two-step surgery and reoperations

Three patients underwent two operations. In one, only the temporal neocortical NMD was initially removed (see case Z.R. in Chapter 20 in this volume). Since she was clinically unchanged, the SEEG defined EZ was then removed ('two-step' surgery). In one case (R.M.) the surgical removal of both the frontal mesial NMD and the EZ was initially incomplete. The second operation was radical.

In the remaining one (B.M.), the first operation was performed at the age of two: only the suprasylvian opercular part of a multilobar cortical dysplasia was removed, according to the predominant ictal clinical symptomatology. The reoperation was performed after stereo-EEG recordings.

Results

Topography and extent of the epileptogenic zone

The EZ was considered as 'multilobar' in 13 cases (four with 'normal' MRI), temporal in 11, frontal in four ('normal' MRI in one), right parietal in one with bilateral opercular dysplasia, and right occipital in one with bilateral occipital dysplasia.

Seizure frequency

Nineteen patients had a postoperative follow-up > 12 months. Eleven (57.8 per cent) were completely seizure-free (Class IA of Engel, 1987); more specifically: 3/10 patients with multilobar, 3/3 with frontal, 4/4 with temporal and 1/1 with occipital EZ.

The patient with the BOD was seizure-free for 17 months, then she presented two seizures, but now she has been seizure-free for three months. The child with bilateral occipital dysplasia, operated on the right side, is still seizure-free 51 months after the intervention. The first two patients who underwent 'two-step' surgery did not present any seizures afterwards. In the third one (B.M.), seizure frequency dropped from 80 to 10/day after the first operation, and 25 to 30/month, only occurring during sleep, after the second, stereo-EEG-guided operation.

Neuropathological alterations

Different degrees of histopathological abnormalities were found not only in the specimens obtained from the MRI evident lesion but also outside the MRI apparent limits of the dysplasia, in the stereo-EEG identified EZ. Dysplastic tissue was also found in the EZ of some patients with apparently normal MRI and thus considered, before the intervention, as presenting with a 'cryptogenetic' epilepsy.

Using immunocytochemical procedures, different types of morphological abnormalities were found according to the different groups of dysplasia shown by MRI. However, in the so-called focal dysplasia, the observed immunocytochemical abnormalities suggested different etiological factors (Spreafico et al., 1998; see also Chapter 20 in this volume).

In addition, using antibodies against neuronal markers, such as GABA and calcium binding proteins, some possible basic mechanisms leading to epilepsy, at least in patients with severe pharmaco-resistant partial epilepsy, were suggested.

Chapter 24 Surgery of epilepsy symptomatic of NMDs

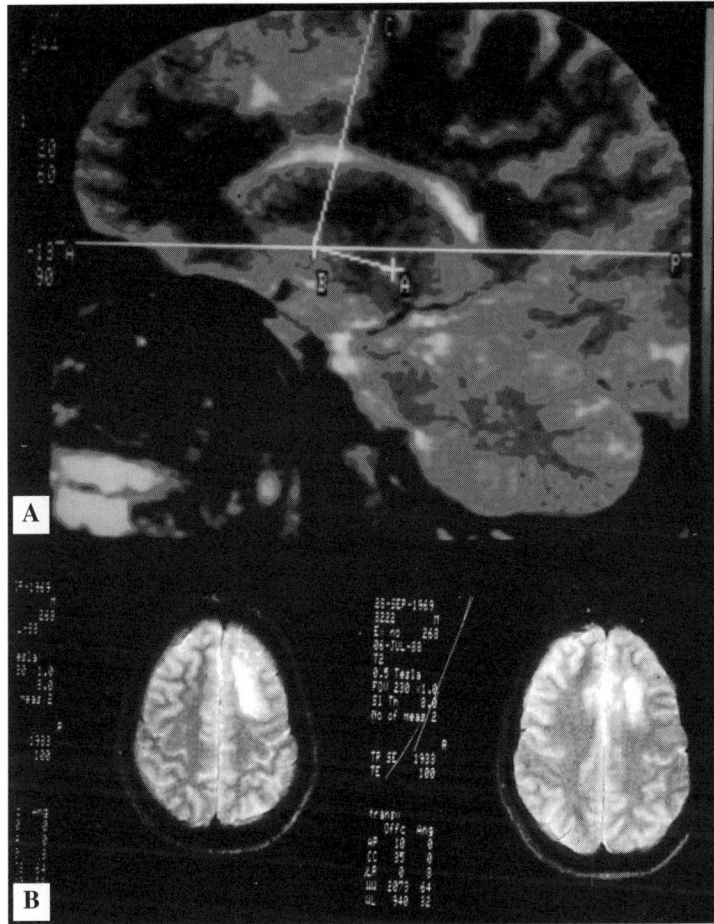

Fig. 2. R.M. Cerebral MRI showing a left frontal mesial hyperintense lesion in T2 weighted images: (A) sagittal view; (B) axial view.

Illustrative cases

R.M.

This patient was 21 years old when admitted for the first time to the CHU INSERM U318 in Grenoble in 1990. He had started having seizures at the age of four with speech and motor arrest, staring, right arm elevation (hypertonic, with dystonic hand) and right turning of the head. Falls were caused by hypertonus of the right leg. At seven years he began to experience a subjective sensation, preceding the described motor signs: fear, a warm sensation rising from the abdomen to the face, tachicardia, sometimes associated with paresthesias located in the genital region or in the right hand. Cerebral MRI showed a left frontal mesial hyperintense lesion in T2 weighted images (Fig. 2). He had about 8–10 seizures/day, during sleep or when awake.

During the hospitalization he first underwent video-EEG and, after implantation of intracerebral depth electrodes, stereo-video-EEG recordings (Fig. 3). Anatomo-electro-clinical data were consistent with left mesial frontal seizures, involving the supplementary motor area. A first left mesial frontal cortectomy was performed in January 1991. Histopathological diagnosis was cortical dysplasia (Fig. 4, post-operative MRI). After three months, seizures recurred with the same subjective and objective symptomatology, less intense and almost only during sleep or on awakening, without falls. One year after this operation his total I.Q. increased from 87 to 99. A second stereo-EEG study was performed in January 1994, investigating the rectus gyrus, F3 anterior, F2, area 24 (ante-

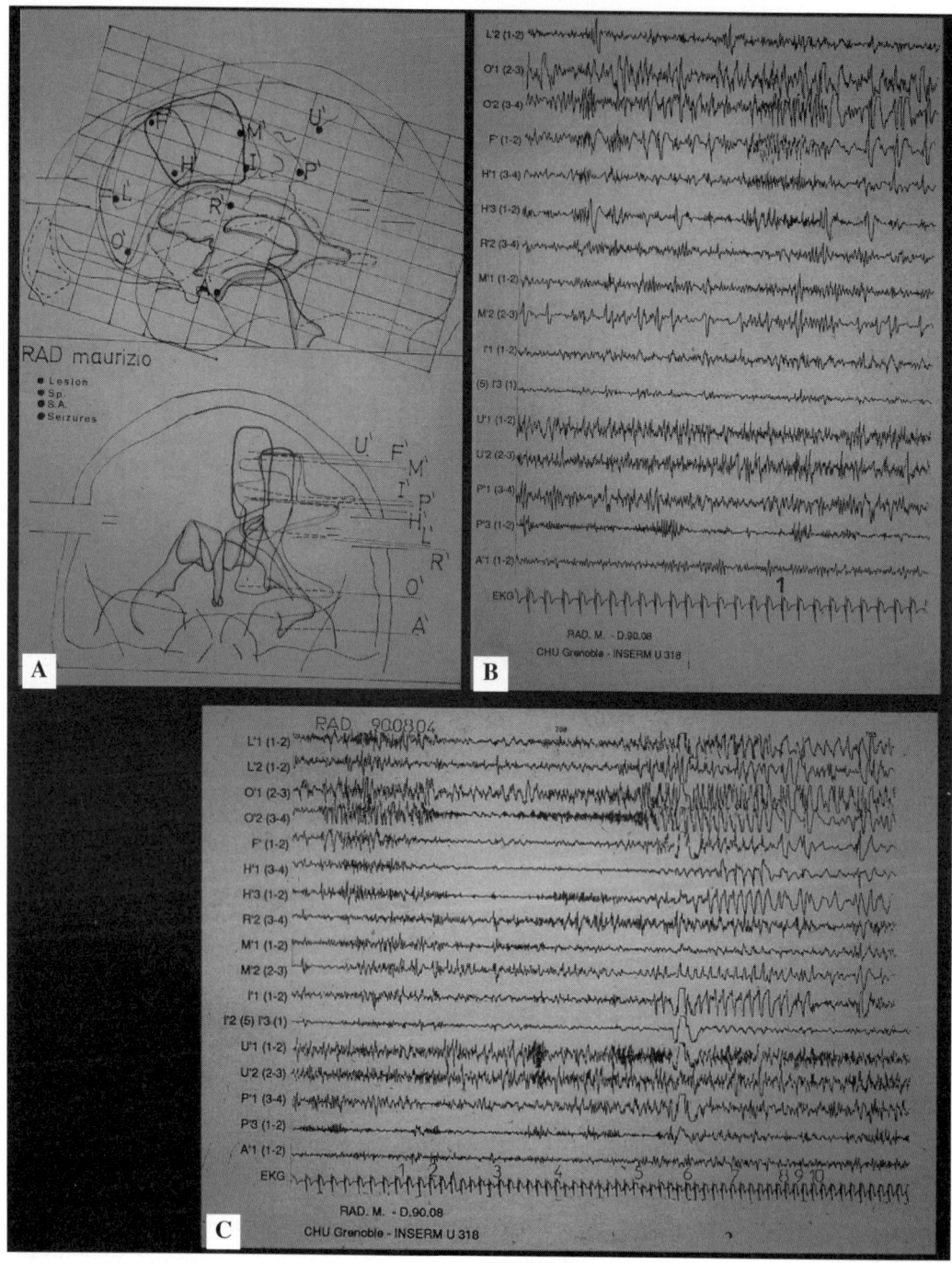

Fig. 3. R.M. (A) First stereo-EEG study, by means of 10 stereotactically implanted electrodes (lateral and frontal view of the skull). Although we attributed the sensation of fear to discharges involving the prefrontal mesial cortex, we also explored the corpus amygdaloideum to exclude, as the recordings found, a secondary involvement of this structure; (B) seizures objectively characterized by only speech arrest and bilateral down stretching of the lips; (C) as (B) plus right arm elevation.

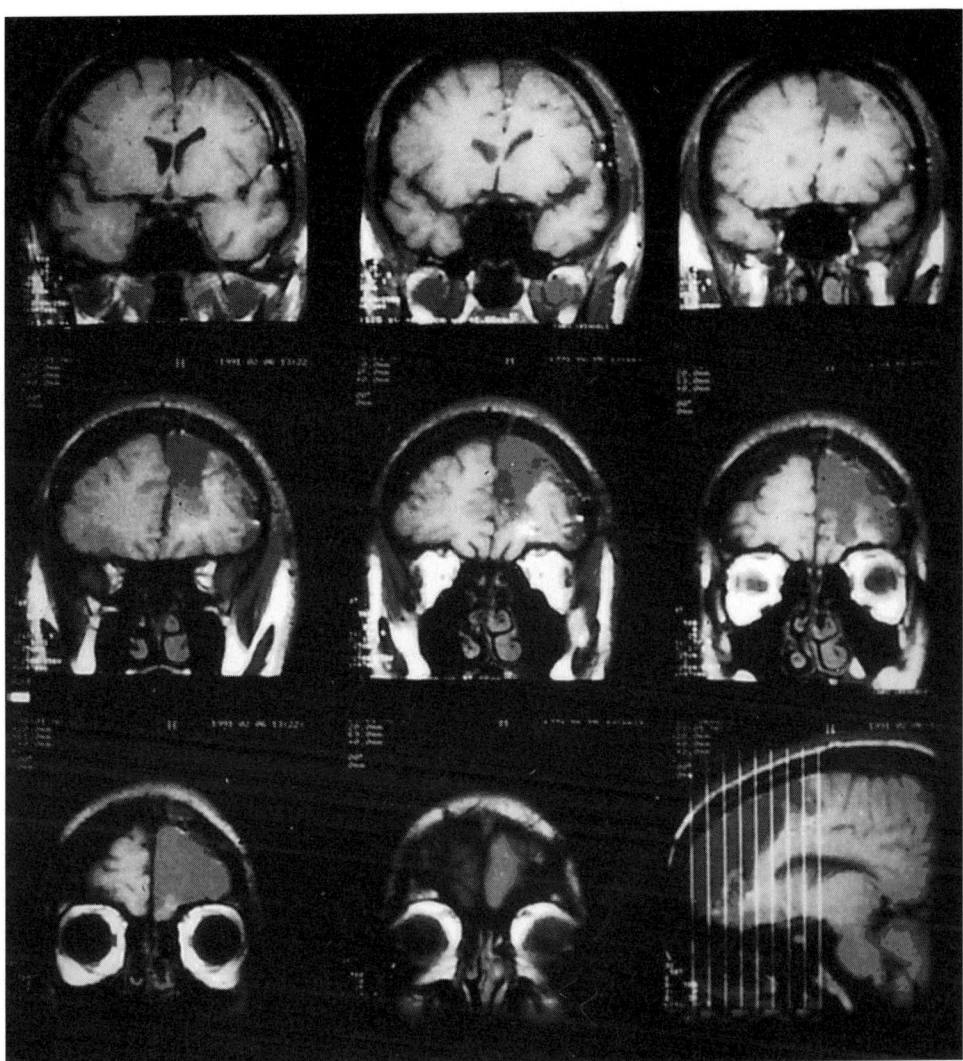

Fig. 4. R.M. Cerebral MRI, coronal and sagittal (T1 weighted) views, showing extension of the first cortectomy.

rior cingular gyrus), the posterior border of the first cortectomy (mesial aspect), the pre-central cortex (mesial and lateral aspects), the post-central cortex and the paracentral lobule, the post-central lateral cortex and the parietal cingular gyrus. Seizures were found to originate anteriorly, posteriorly and laterally in the boundaries of the first operation, but also to involve, secondarily, cortical motor and language areas (Wada test: left hemisphere dominant for language).

A second cortectomy with removal of the anterior part of rectus gyrus, frontal pole, area 24, and F1 and F2 as far as the pre-central sulcus was performed in March 1994 (Fig. 5, MRI performed after the second operation). Immediately after the operation he had aphemia and a mild motor inertia of the right arm (related to the SSMA removal) which completely cleared after ten days. After the second operation the patient has been seizure-free. After being seizure-free for two years he began tapering antiepileptic drugs: Carbamazepine, initially 1400 mg/day, was withdrawn, but he is still taking Phenobarbital, 150 mg/day.

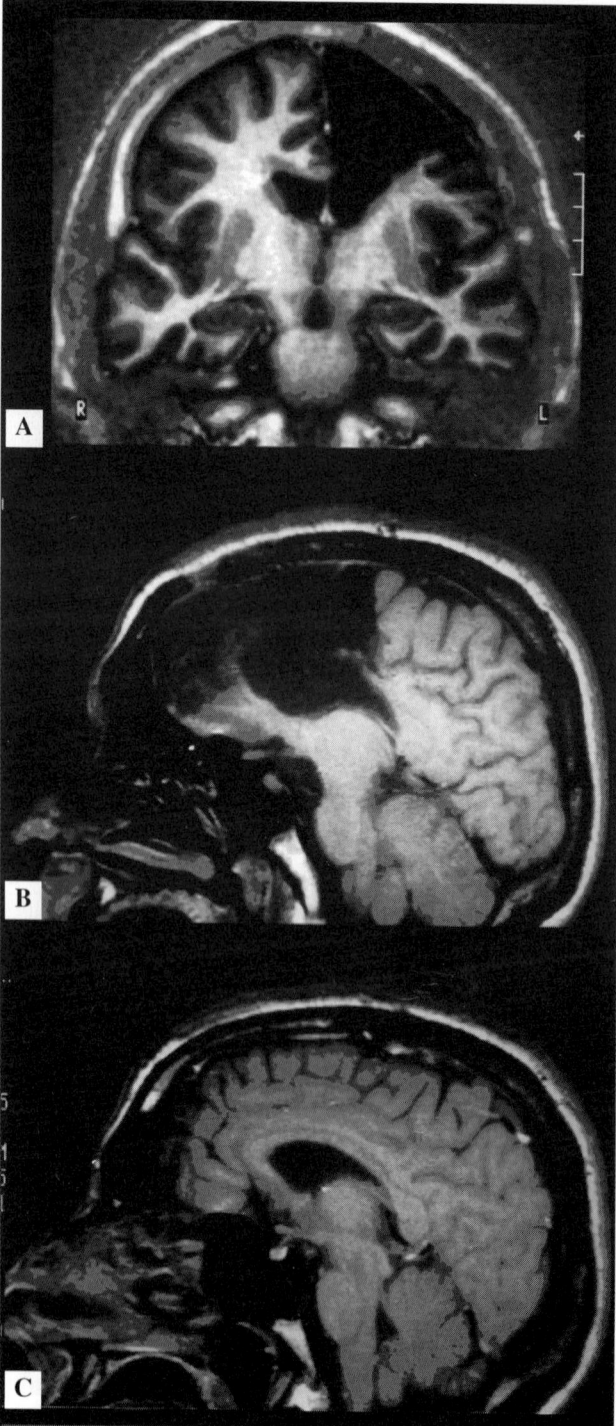

B.M.

This patient was two years old when admitted to CHU in Grenoble in March 1993. He had two second cousins with epilepsy during infancy. Seizures started when he was 10 days old with left deviation of the lip corner, eyelids and left-limb clonic jerks that were occasionally followed by a tonic phase. He had 15–85 seizures/day, during sleep but also in the awake state. His daily therapy included Phenytoin 160 mg, Phenobarbital 45 mg, Valproic Acid 220 mg, Clobazam 10 mg and Vigabatrin 800 mg. The neurological examination showed a calm baby that had not yet started talking, but could not stay seated without help, and presented a left hemiparesis, more severe at the upper limb. Cerebral MRI showed a slight right 'hemiatrophy', with decreased representation of the white matter in the centro-parietal regions (Fig. 6). According to the anatomo-electro-clinical data, (video-EEG recording showed a right central ictal discharge) in April 1993 he had a partial lesionectomy plus cortectomy including the pre- and post- central right opercular regions and the arm region of the right central motor cortex. Histopathological diagnosis was cortical dysplasia. Figure 7A–C shows, by post-operation MRI, the extension of the resection and the persistence of an altered signal in the right centro-parietal region.

After one year the child could walk autonomously, spoke some words and had a fairly good comprehension. He still had about 2–10 seizures/day mostly during sleep or on awakening. His parents sought a second surgical opinion in January 1996. At this time he had:

(a) 'milder' seizures: a subjective sensation during which he looked for support, then slowly fell to the ground, laughing; these seizures lasted a few seconds;

Fig. 5 R.M. Cerebral MRI: (A) coronal (inversion recovery) view showing extension of the second cortectomy; (B) sagittal (T1 weighted) views showing removal also of the 24 (cingulate gyrus) area; (C) the sparing of the corpus callosum.

Chapter 24 Surgery of epilepsy symptomatic of NMDs

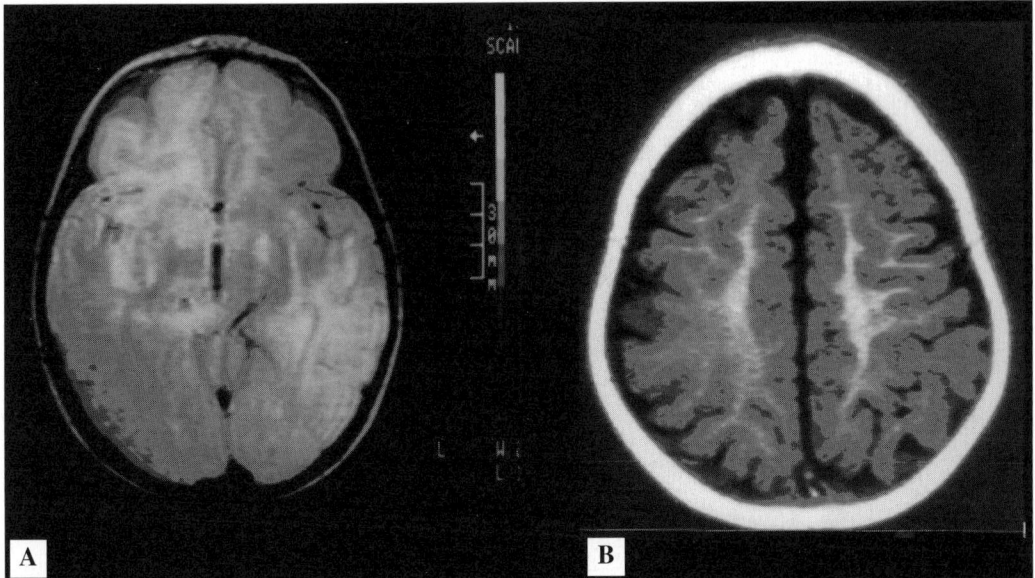

Fig. 6. B.M. Cerebral MRI before the first operation showing a decreased representation of the white matter in the right centro-parietal region: (A) PD weighted; (B) T1 weighted images (axial view).

(b) 'stronger' seizures, almost always during sleep: awakening, staring, red face, screaming, hypertonia of the left limbs, his right hand beat the head, pedalling with the right leg, then he became pale and had chewing and swallowing movements.

Video-EEG recordings showed an extended right fronto-central ictal discharge.

In October 1996 he underwent a stereo-video EEG study (Fig. 7 D). The spontaneous ictal discharges, could start everywhere from the electrodes exploring the dysplastic region, but also in the central part of the cingular gyrus (deep leads of electrode Z). Electrical intracerebral stimulation of the frontal cingular gyrus (mesial leads of the electrode G) also elicited seizures.

In December 1996 he underwent a lesionectomy plus corticotomy including right central and parietal regions and the posterior portion of the first temporal gyrus. Fig. 8 shows the post-operation MRI. Histopathological diagnosis was severe cortical dysplasia with balloon cells and giant neurones. No worsening of the left motor deficit was noted after the operation. The only surgery complication was a subgaleal CS fluid collection that spontaneously resolved in two months.

At follow-up after 18 months the child had improved his cognitive acquisitions, speech and motor performances. He still had about 25–30 seizures/month, only occurring during sleep. He is taking Barbiturate 75 mg/day and Carbamazepine 750 mg/day.

Z.R.

This patient was a right handed 19-year-old girl when hospitalized in Grenoble to study her partial epilepsy in 1993. Seizures started at the age of nine; she heard music (always the same music) with a voice singing, but she could not understand the words. She could rarely talk during the subjective

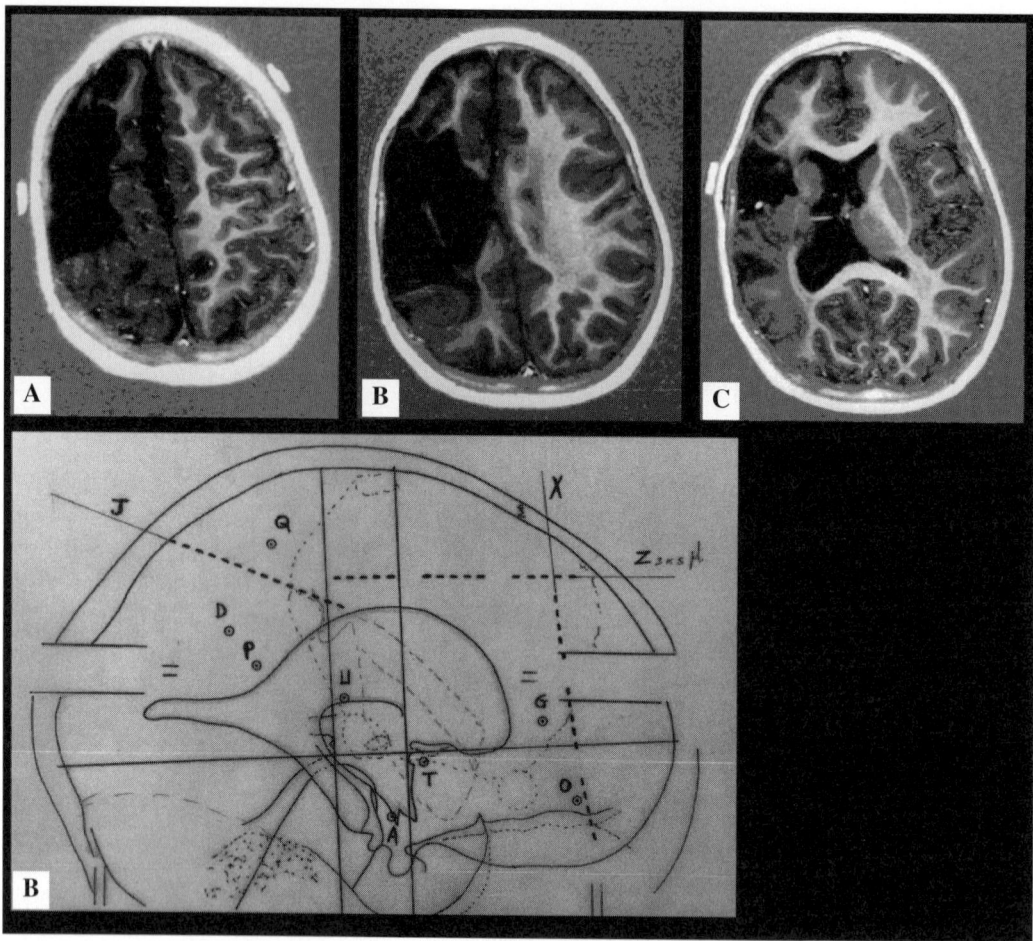

Fig. 7. B.M. (A, B, C) Cerebral MRI (inversion recovery, axial views) showing extension of the first operation and persistence of a 'thick' cortex with decreased white matter representation in the right centro-parietal region. (D) Stereo-EEG study, by means of 11 stereotactically implanted electrodes (lateral view of the skull), exploring the fronto-temporo-parietal region, with particular attention to the boundaries of the residual 'dysplastic' (posterior) region.

sensation. If the seizure went on she could have clonic jerks of the lips and eyelids. Impairment of contact appeared only after adolescence and characterized 50 per cent of her seizures; she never had language problems at recovery of contact. Seizure frequency was about 10/day.

Interictal EEG showed slow and paroxysmal abnormalities on the right temporal derivations. Brain MRI showed an inhomogeneous signal (hypointense in T1 and hyperintense in T2) in the first temporal convolution (Fig. 9). She underwent stereotactic seriated biopsies of the right temporal lesion. Histopathological diagnosis was: hamartoma? DNT? After this procedure, seizure frequency decreased.

A 'two step' surgery was proposed. The 'first step', a simple lesionectomy, was performed in January 1995. Histopathological diagnosis was cortical dysplasia. Figure 10 A, B shows the post-operation MRI. Seizures with identical features reappeared soon after surgery.

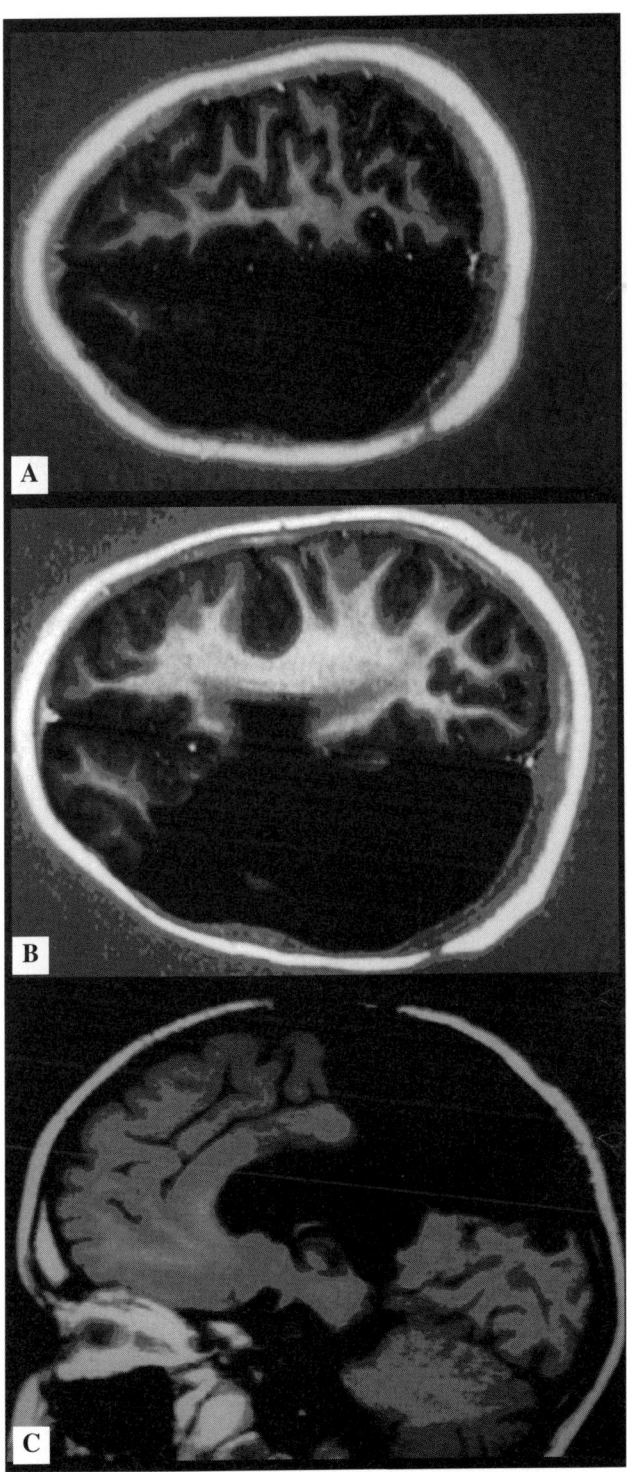

Fig. 8. B.M. (A, B) Cerebral MRI, axial (inversion recovery) and (C) sagittal (T1 weighted) views, showing the extension of the second resection.

After video-EEG recording (ictal discharges involved the anterior and middle temporal region, but also the suprasylvian region) she underwent a SEEG study investigating the right temporo-opercular-parietal region (Fig. 10 C). In October 1996 she underwent the 'second step' with removal of the EZ as defined by the stereo-EEG study. Figure 11 shows the extension of the second operation including the temporal pole, T1, T2, T3, T4, the uncus, the amygdaloid nucleus, and the anterior part of both the hippocampus and the gyrus parahippocampi. Since then (22 months), she has been seizure-free. After eighteen months of being seizure-free she began tapering antiepileptic drugs: Clonazepam 6 mg/day was withdrawn, but she is still taking Phenobarbital 150 mg/day.

Discussion

The current utilization of high resolution MRI techniques does allow the continuously increasing recognition of anatomical alterations in patients with severe drug-resistant partial epilepsies. When these patients are candidates for surgical treatment of their epilepsy, the identification of an anatomical lesion represents only the first step of an often sophisticated diagnostic procedure. In fact, whereas some authors claim that 'the lesion is guilty until proved innocent' (Cascino et al., 1992), results of the so-called 'pure' ('simple' would be better, in our opinion) lesionectomy are relatively disappointing in several types of epileptogenic lesions (Simard et al., 1986; Palmini et al., 1991; Haddad et al., 1992). In order to improve the indications of a simple lesionectomy, we believe that, whatever the type of the aetiological lesion, a surgical decision should be taken, in each individual patient, after answering the following questions:

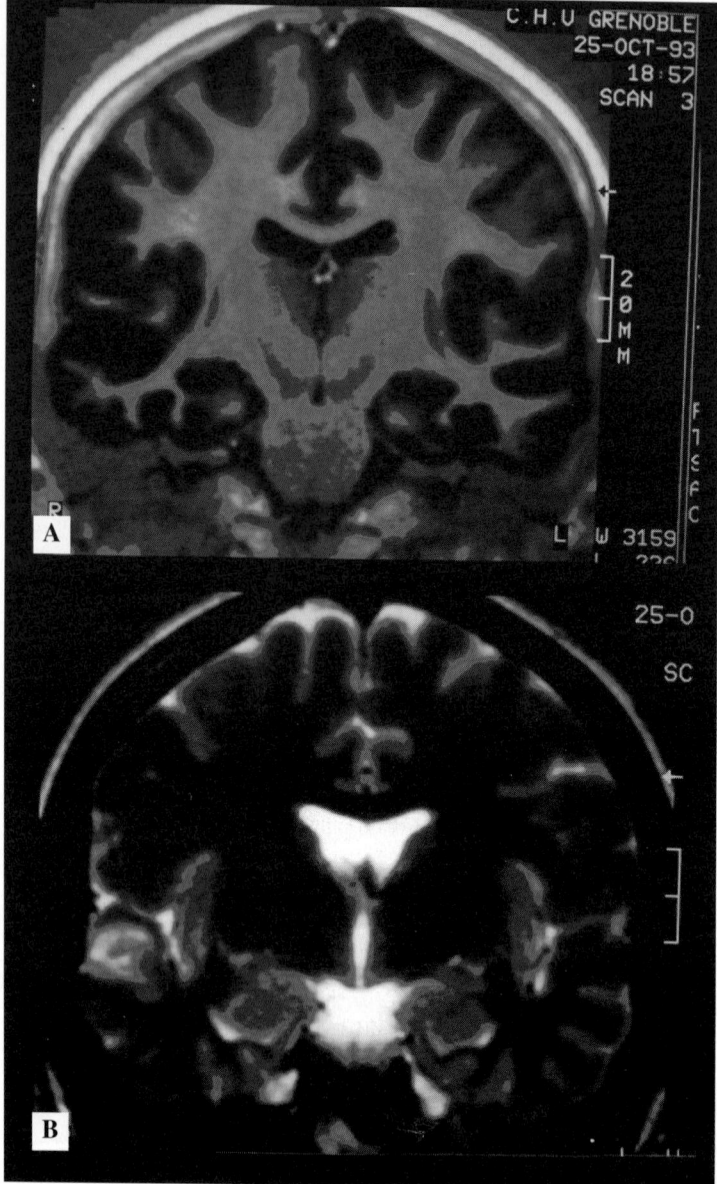

Fig. 9. Z.R. Cerebral MRI before lesionectomy: (A) inversion recovery and (B) T2 weighted images (coronal views) showing an altered signal in the first right temporal gyrus.

- are initial ictal discharges only intra-lesional or can they also start outside of the lesion? (Francione et al., 1994)
- is the clinical ictal symptomatology only linked to ictal discharges strictly confined to the lesion?

These questions are obviously valid also in patients with NMDs, even though it is still undemonstrated that all the NMDs are systematically epileptogenic *in toto*.

Video-EEG-recorded seizures can be very helpful to decide the surgical treatment (also in patients with bilateral lesions): when the topography of the ictal discharges is strictly coincident with the site of the NMD and when the clinical ictal semeiology does not conflict with this localization, a simple lesionectomy can be proposed.

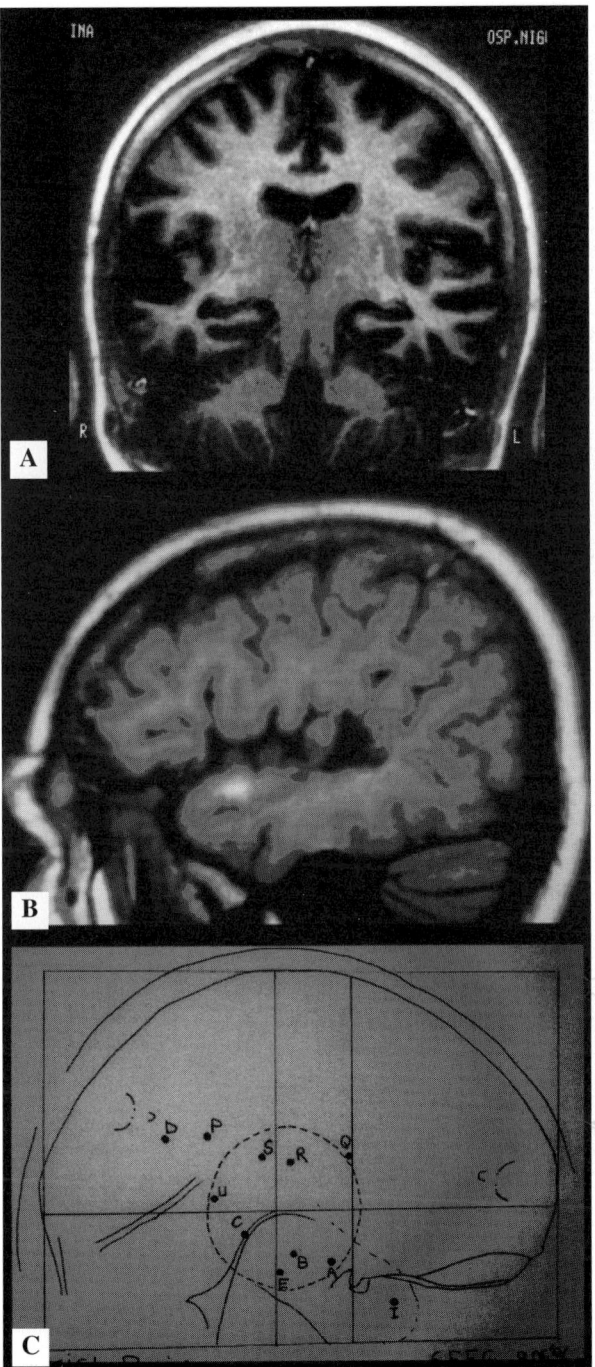

Fig. 10. Z.R. Cerebral MRI after lesionectomy: (A) inversion recovery-coronal view and (B) T1 weighted-sagittal view) showing the extension of the 'lesionectomy'. (C) Stereo-EEG study, by means of 11 stereotactically implanted electrodes (lateral view of the skull), exploring the temporo-parietal region, with particular care for the limits of the first lesionectomy.

However, our data show that there is a frequent apparent discrepancy between the MRI evidence of the NMD and the three-dimensional organization of the EZ as defined by stereo-EEG (Munari et al., 1996b). Moreover, the surgical decision about the amount of the apparently extra-lesional cortex must be taken considering that the same patient may present seizures with variable extension (of the cortical regions involved), length and 'intensity' of the ictal discharges, to which may correspond a variation in the ictal clinical symptomatology (see Fig. 3, patient R. M.).

When we have been able to remove all the EZ, also outside MRI apparent limits of the dysplasia, seizures disappeared. Supporters of the simple lesionectomy could object that, at least in some cases, we cannot demonstrate that the simple removal of the MRI-evident NMD would not have produced the same result. Some fully informed patients accept a 'two-step' surgery programme:

- at the first operation, we just remove the MRI evident lesion, as could be done in other Epilepsy Surgery Centers;

- if seizures persist, then the stereo-EEG-defined EZ is removed (see case Z.R. in Chapter 21 in this volume).

This kind of strategy presents a two-fold advantage:

- it avoids unnecessary removal of cortical tissue;

- it validates, in patients not cured after the first surgical step, stereo-EEG data on the extent of the EZ.

Microscopical alterations, as revealed by the systematic examination of all the specimens, are often much more extensive than the MRI alterations, thus explaining, at least partially, the apparent discrepancy between the MRI data and the stereo-EEG neurophysiopathological findings. Conversely, the results obtained in the two patients with bilateral NMD strongly suggest that:

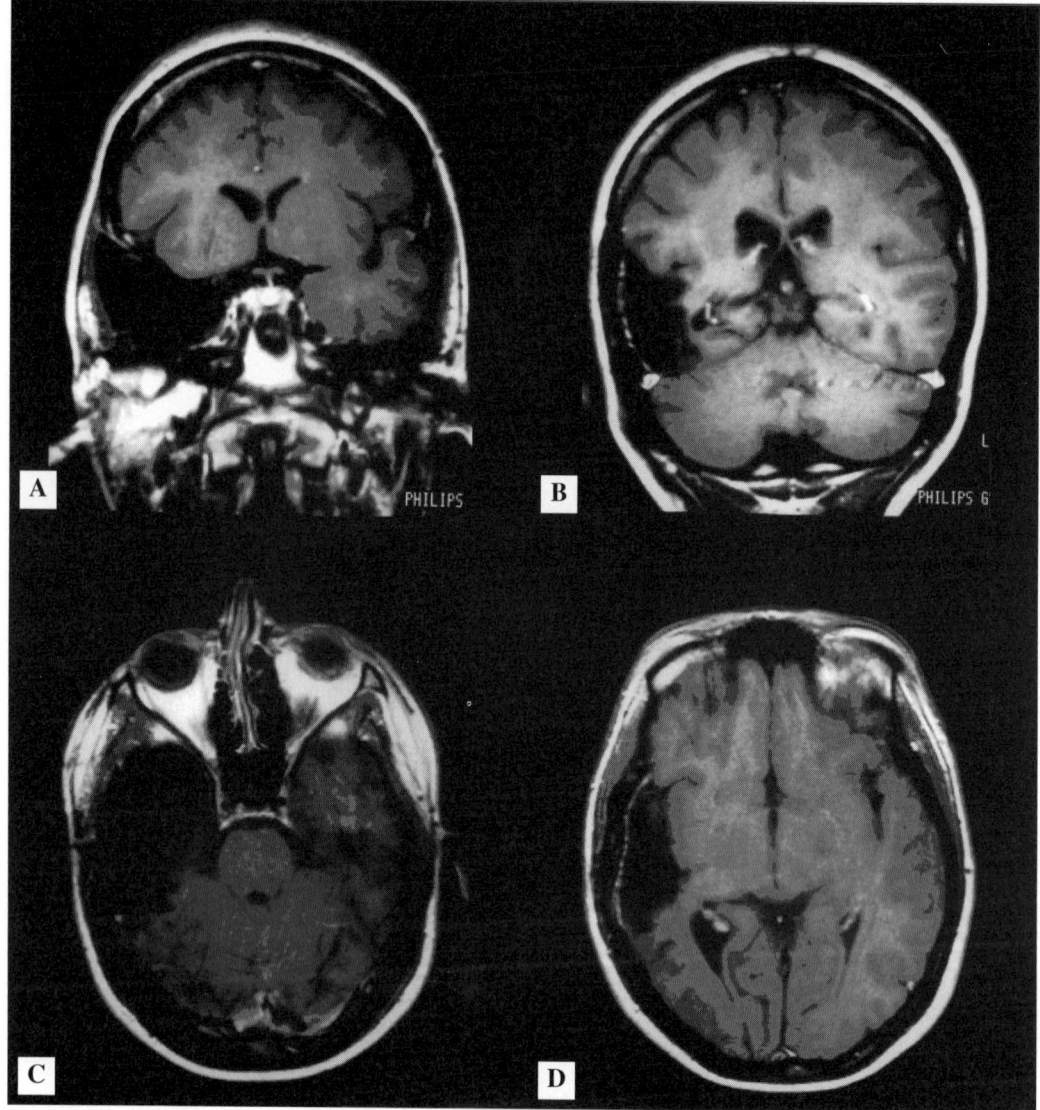

Fig. 11. Z.R. Cerebral MRI after right temporal cortectomy: T1 weighted coronal (A, B) and axial (C, D) views.

- Patients with bilateral NMD can just suffer from a unilateral epilepsy;
- EZ can be, in some cases, more limited than the MRI anatomical alterations.

In other words, the topographical and functional relationships between MRI-revealed NMD and EZ are far from being clear and unequivocal: neither all the NMDs nor all the components of a NMD are necessarily epileptogenic.

Stereo-EEG-recorded seizures seem to be very helpful for an individually adapted definition of the extent of the surgical removal in patients with NMDs.

The possible epileptogenic role of balloon cells and giant neurons, outside the MRI boundaries of some NMDs, needs to be further investigated, since immunocytochemical studies could suggest different possible basic mechanisms leading to epilepsy, at least in patients with severe pharmaco-resistant partial epilepsy.

References

Cascino, D.G., Kelly, P.J., Sharbrough, F.W., Hulihan, J.F., Hirschorn, K.A. & Trenerry, M.R. (1992): Long-term follow-up of stereotactic lesionectomy in partial epilepsy: predictive factors and electroencephalographic results. *Epilepsia* **33**, 639–644.

Commission on Classification and Terminology of the International League against Epilepsy (1989): Proposal for revised classification of epilepsies and epileptic syndromes. *Epilepsia* **30**, 389–399.

Daumas-Duport, C., Monsaingeon, V., Vedrenne, C., Munari, C., Bancaud, J. & Chodkiewicz, J.P. (1988): Complex neuro-epithelial tumours in epilepsy surgery. A series of 20 cases. In : *The rational basis of the surgical treatment of epilepsies.*, ed. G. Broggi, pp. 149–167. London: John Libbey.

Engel Jr., J. (1987): Outcome with respect to epileptic seizures. In: *Surgical treatment of the epilepsies*, ed. J. Engel, Jr., pp. 553–571. New York: Raven Press.

Francione, S., Kahane, P., Tassi, L., Hoffmann, D., Durisotti, C., Pasquier, B. & Munari, C. (1994): Stereo-EEG recorded interictal and ictal electrical activity of a histologically proved heterotopic gray matter associated with partial epilepsy. *Electroenceph. Clin. Neurophysiol.* **90**, 284–290.

Haddad, S.F., Moore, S.A., Menezes, A.H., Van Gilder, J.C. & Sutton, L.N. (1992): Ganglioglioma: 13 years of experience. *Neurosurgery* **31**, 171–178.

Lindsay, J., Ounsted, C. & Richards, P. (1984): Long term outcome in children with temporal lobe seizures. V: indications and contra-indications for neurosurgery. *Dev. Med Child Neuro.* **26**, 25–32.

Lucignani, G., Tassi, L., Fazio, F., Galli, L., Grana, C., Del Sole, A., Hoffmann, D., Francione, S., Minicucci, F., Kahane, P., Messa, C. & Munari, C. (1996): Double-blind stereo-EEG and FDG PET study in severe partial epilepsies: are the electric and metabolic findings related? *Eur. J. Nucl. Med.* **23**, 1498–1507.

Lüders, H.O., Engel Jr., J. & Munari, C. (1993): General principles. In: *Surgical treatment of the epilepsies*, ed. J. Engel, Jr., pp.137–153. New York: Raven Press.

Munari, C. (1987): Depth electrodes implantation at Hopital Sainte Anne, Paris. In: *Surgical treatment of the epilepsies*, ed. J. Engel, Jr., pp. 583–588. New York: Raven Press.

Munari, C. & Bancaud, J. (1985): The role of the stereo-EEG in evaluation of partial epileptic seizures. In: *The epilepsies*, eds. P.L. Morselli & R.J. Porter, pp. 267–306. London: Butterworths.

Munari, C., Giallonardo, A.T., Musolino, A., Brunet, P., Chodkiewicz, J.P., Bancaud, J. & Talairach, J. (1987): Epileptic neuroradiological examinations necessary for stereotactic procedures. In: *Methods of presurgical evaluation of epileptic patients*, eds. H.G. Wieser & C.E. Elger, pp. 141–145. Berlin: Springer-Verlag.

Munari, C., Hoffmann, D., Francione, S., Kahane, P., Tassi, L., Lo Russo, G. & Benabid, A.L. (1994): Stereo-electroencephalography methodology: advantages and limits. *Acta Neurol. Scand.* **152 (Suppl.)**, 56–67.

Munari, C., Cardinale, F., Tassi, L., Mai, R., Colombo, N., Bottini, G., Lo Russo, G. & Francione, S. (1996a): Le epilessie temporali curabili chirurgicamente. *Chirurgia Italiana* **48**, 1–64.

Munari, C., Francione, S., Kahane, P., Tassi, L. & Hoffmann D. (1996b): Usefulness of stereo-EEG investigations in partial epilepsy associated with cortical dysplastic lesions and gray matter heteropia. In: *Dysplasias of cerebral cortex and epilepsy*, eds. R. Guerrini, F. Andermann, R. Canapicchi, J. Roger, B.G. Zifkin & P. Pfanner, pp. 383–394. Philadelphia: Lippincott-Raven.

Palmini, A., Andermann, F., Olivier, A., Tampieri, D. & Robitaille Y. (1991): Focal neuronal migration disorders and intractable partial epilepsy: results of surgical treatment. *Ann. Neurol.* **30**, 750–757.

Palmini, A., Gambardella, A., Andermann, F., Olivier, A., Costa Da Costa, J., Tampieri, D., Robitaille, Y., Paglioli, E., Paglioli-Neto, E. & Coutinho, L. (1996): Outcome of surgical treatment in patients with localized cortical dysplasia and intractable epilepsy. In: *Dysplasias of cerebral cortex and epilepsy*, eds. R. Guerrini, F. Andermann, R. Canapicchi, J. Roger, B.G. Zifkin & P. Pfanner, pp. 367–374. Philadelphia: Lippincott-Raven.

Pasquier, B., Bost, F., Peoc'h, M., Barnoud, R. & Pasquier D. (1996): Données neuropathologiques dans l'épilepsie partielle pharmaco-résistante: rapport d'une série de 195 cas. *Ann. Pathol.* **16,** 174–181.

Penfield, W. & Erickson T.C. (1941): *Epilepsy and cerebral localization.* Springfield, IL: Charles C. Thomas Publishers.

Rasmussen, T.B. (1983): Surgical treatment of complex partial seizures: results, lesson, and problems. *Epilepsia* **24 (Suppl.),** S65–S76.

Simard, J.M., Garcia-Bengochea, F., Ballinger, W.E., Mickle, J.P. & Quisling, R.G. (1986): Cavernous angioma: a review of 126 collected and 12 new clinical cases. *Neurosurgery* **18,** 162–172.

Spreafico, R., Pasquier, B., Minotti, L., Garbelli, R., Kahane, P., Grand, S., Benabid, A.L., Tassi, L., Avanzini, G., Battaglia, G. & Munari C. (1998): Immunocytochemical investigation on dysplastic human tissue from epileptic patients. *Epilepsy Res.* 32, 34–48

Talairach, J., Bancaud, J., Szikla, G., Bonis, A., Geier, S. & Vedrenne C. (1974): Approche nouvelle de la neurochirurgie de l'épilepsie. Méthodologie stéréotaxique et résultats thérapeutiques. *Neurochirurgie* **20 (Suppl. 1),** 1–240.

Wolf, H.K. & Wiestler O.D. (1993): Surgical pathology of chronic epileptic seizure disorders. *Brain Pathology* **3,** 371–380.

Index

A

acquired factors	187-8
acquired neonatal encephalopathies	35-51
acquired white matter damage with sparing of gray matter	41-7
subpial haemorrhage with EGLM damage	36-41
acute lesions	37, 43
age-related factors	69-72
agyria	41, 49, 203, 266
Aicardi syndrome	191-2, 263
axonal differentiation in callosal connections development	57-8

B

band heterotopia	13, 16, 17, 161-2, 171, 204, 209, 220-1, 223-4
see also heterotopia, subcortical band	
Baraitser-Winter syndrome	266-7
bilateral perisylvian syndrome	177
brain damage, seizure-induced	71-2

C

callosal connections	56-9
callosotomy	298
cell proliferation, migration and death	81-7
cell-intrinsic versus extrinsic determinants of callosal connections	58-9
central area	283-9
central nervous system development	77-80
foetal	83-7
morphogenetic disturbances	80-1
cerebral cortex	23-31
chronic (repaired) lesions	41, 46-7
congenital bilateral perisylvian syndrome	165, 209
congenital nephrosis syndrome	212
cortex	148-54
cortical connections	55-60
axonal differentiation	57-8
callosal connections	56-9
cell-intrinsic versus extrinsic determinants	58-9
cortical dysplasia	3-17, 49, 51, 178, 220, 228-35
acquired white matter damage with sparing of gray matter	46, 47
band heterotopia	162
patients, materials and methods	228
polymicrogyria	165
results	228-33
schizencephaly	174
cortical malformations and epilepsy	145-6
cortical microgyria and epileptogenesis	133-41
neocortical slices	134-45
reorganization of excitatory connectivity within paramicrogyral zone	135-9
site of origin of epileptogenic discharge	135
cortical neurones connectivity in tish rat brain	147-8

319

cortical physiological properties,
  maturation of   63-73
  age-related factors   69-70, 71-2
    postnatal developmental
      changes in neocortex   64-9
  cortical rhythms   68-9
  firing characteristics   66-8
  morphology   64
  passive properties   64
  receptor-mediated activities   68
  voltage dependent channels   64-6
cortical rhythms   68-9
corticogenesis   77-87
  cell proliferation, migration
    and death   81-7
  central nervous system
    development   77-80
  central nervous system, morphogenetic
    disturbances of   80-1
diffuse heterotopia
  see band heterotopia
dormant basket cell hypothesis   72
double cortex syndrome
  see band heterotopia
Duchenne Muscular Dystrophy   91, 92
dysembryoplastic neuroepithelial
  tumours   236-7
dysplasia   203, 268
  bilateral   276
  bilateral occipital   306
  bilateral opercular   306
  of central area   283-9
  cortical   171, 184, 187, 249, 257, 268
  ectodermal
  focal   177, 306
  focal cortical
            168, 177-9, 198, 203, 209, 245, 248
  of frontal area   277-82
  multilobar   296-8
  of occipital area   290-1
  of parietal area   292-5
  parieto-occipital cortical   210
  septo-optic   173, 256

  of temporal area   276-7
  see also cortical dysplasia
  dysplastic lesions and tumours   300-1

E

EGLM damage   36-41
Ehlers-Danlos syndrome   205, 212
electrophysiological evidence   124-7
encephalopathies see acquired neonatal
epidermal nevus syndrome   163
epilepsy
  and cortical malformations   145-6
  and polymicrogyria   191-9
  and schizencephaly   187
  and tish rat   154
epileptogenesis see
  cortical microgyria and epileptogenesis
epileptogenic dysplastic tissue:
  immunocytochemical studies   241-9
  methods   242-3
  results   243-7
ethanol-exposed rats   92-5, 98-101
evoked potentials see neuronal migration
  disorders and evoked potentials
excessively bursting behaviour   129-30
excitatory connectivity reorganization
  within paramicrogyral zone   135-9
excitatory synaptic reorganization   72
extra-frontal resections   298
extratemporal resections   298

F

firing characteristics   66-8, 121, 124-127, 129
Foetal Alcohol Syndrome   91-92
foetal central nervous system   83-7
frontal area   277-82
frontal lobe resections   298
frontonasal dysplasia syndrome   212

G

genetic factors   187-8, 211-14

see also neuronal migration disorders: genetic basis

H

hamartoma	275, 300
hypothalamic	16, 17
hemimegalencephaly	5, 162-5, 177, 178, 179, 203, 209, 236
hemipareses	196-7
heterotopia	128, 220, 222-3, 235, 275, 300
X-linked bilateral periventricular nodular	204
X-linked subcortical band	204
bilateral	210, 211
bilateral diffuse periventricular nodular	206
bilateral periventricular nodular	222, 265
bilateral subcortical	122, 145
cerebral	203
classical bilateral periventricular nodular	268-9
cortical	118, 171, 175
see also neuronal development and cortical heterotopia	
diffuse	211
focal	204, 219
focal periventricular nodular	207
focal subcortical	171, 174
generalized	204
gray matter	204, 208
hippocampal	110, 118, 123, 129
laminar	204
leptomeningeal	35, 41
marginal	41
neuronal	117, 122
nodular	204
nodular bilateral periventricular	184
partial band	163
periventricular	117-18, 123, 129, 171, 174-6, 204
subcortical	11, 16, 121, 123
subcortical band	146, 154, 178, 266, 267-8
subcortical neuronal	110
subcortical nodular	204, 209
subependymal	171
symmetric	211
unilateral	211
unilateral nodular	225
unilateral periventricular	223
unilateral periventricular nodular	118
unilateral subependymal nodular	175
see also band heterotopia; periventricular nodular heterotopia	
heterotopic neurogenesis in tish cortex	152-4
holoprosencephaly	179
homeobox genes and neuronal migration disorders	253-7
human development brain dysgeneses *see* methylazoxymethanol (MAM) treated rats	
hyperplasia	236
hypoplasia	196
cerebellar	212, 261, 264, 265, 268
neocortical	117
neopallial	264
optic nerve	173, 256
unilateral cerebral	210
unilateral cortical	210
hypsarrhythmia	71, 179

I

immunocytochemical studies	241-9
immunohistochemical experiments on mdx mice	93-4
infancy	70-1, 177-9

L

Lennox-Gastaut syndrome	71, 178, 194, 195-6
lesions, location of	300
lesions, size of	300
lissencephaly	13, 178, 179, 219, 220, 221, 223, 225, 261
X-linked	267-8
with cerebellar hypoplasia	265
classical	162, 265, 266-7
partial	234

321

M

macrogyria	296
mdx mice	93-4, 95-7, 100-1
megalencephaly	203
methylazoxymethanol (MAM) treated rats and human development brain dysgeneses	109-18
administration	110
morphological analysis	110-15
tract tracing experiments	112, 115-17
methylazoxymethanol (MAM) treated rats and neuronal migration disorders	121-30
double MAM treatment	124-8
electrophysiological evidence	124-7
morphological features	127-8
excessively bursting behaviour	129-30
increased neuronal excitability	122-3
pyramidal neurone phenotypes and connectivity	128-9
transplacental MAM treatment	123
MH syndrome	268-9
microcephaly	87, 123, 257, 261-4
microgyria	38-39, 41, 133, 135, 137-139, 141
see also cortical microgyria	
microlissencephaly	87, 261-4, 265
micropolygyria	14, 17
Miller-Dieker syndrome	212, 266-7
morphogenetic disturbances	80-1
mossy fibre sprouting	72
motor and somatosensory cortices, preferential impairment of	91-102
mdx mice	95-7, 100-1
ethanol-exposed rats	94-5, 98-100
immunohistochemical experiments on mdx mice	93-4
quantitative evaluations	94
tract tracing experiments on ethanol-exposed rats	93

N

neocortex, postnatal developmental changes in	64-9
neocortical slices	134-5
neoplasia	203
neuronal development and cortical heterotopia	145-54
cortical malformations and epilepsy	145-6
cortical neurones connectivity in tish rat brain	147-8
heterotopic neurogenesis in tish cortex	152-4
tish brain and cortex	148
tish cortex development	148-52
tish rat as animal model	146-7
tish rat and epilepsy	154
neuronal excitability, increased	122-3
neuronal migration in developing cerebral cortex	23-31
methodological tools	24-5
morphogenetic events and cell identity	25-8
neuronal migration disorders: genetic basis	261-9
X-linked lissencephaly and subcortical band heterotopia (XLIS) and LIS1	267-8
classical bilateral periventricular nodular heterotopia/MH syndrome	268-9
classical lissencephaly and subcortical band heterotopia	266-7
lissencephaly with cerebellar hypoplasia	265
microcephaly with simplified gyral patterns and microlissencephaly	261-4
new classification and recent progress	261
neuronal migration disorders and epilepsy in infancy	177-9
and evoked potentials	219-2
heterotopia	222-3
pachygyria	223-4
patients	220
polymicrogyria	222
recording	221
sensory evoked potentials	221
visual evoked potentials	221
and homeobox genes	253-7
and increased neuronal excitability	122-3

see also methylazoxymethanol
(MAM) treated rats
neuroradiology 161-8, 171-6, 187
Norman-Roberts syndrome 264

O

occipital area 290-1

P

pachygyria 49, 220, 221, 223-4, 225, 266
  acquired white matter damage
    with sparing of gray matter 41
  band heterotopia 161
  cortical 179
  generalized 14
  periventricular nodular heterotopia 203
  polymicrogyria 167, 191
  paramicrogyral zone 135-9
  parietal area 292-5
  passive properties 64
  periventricular nodular
    heterotopia 11, 16, 203-14, 220, 221
    bilateral focal 214
    genetics and biology 211-14
    malformations description 204-8
    prevalence, clinical findings and
      epileptogenicity 208-11
    unilateral 214
polymicrogyria
  165-8, 171, 191-9, 220, 222, 225, 235
  Aicardi syndrome 192
  bilateral anterior parietal 165
  bilateral medial parietal occipital 165
  bilateral occipital 165
  bilateral parasagittal parieto-occipital 194-5
  bilateral perisylvian 167, 192-4, 195-6
  bilateral posterior parietal 165, 166
  bilateral symmetrical 166
  bilateral symmetrical frontal 165
  cortical dysplasias 15
  cortical microgyria 133-4, 139-40
  corticogenesis 80

four-layered 191, 193, 198
infancy 177, 179
multilobar 197
parasagittal 222
parietal 222
parietal bilateral 225
parieto-occipital 195-6
peri-rolandic 167
periventricular nodular
  heterotopia 203, 213-14
schizencephaly 172, 174
unilateral 196-9
unlayered 191
porencephaly 171, 173
postnatal developmental changes
  in neocortex 64-9
Proteus syndrome 163
pyramidal neurone phenotypes
  and connectivity 128-9

R

receptor-mediated activities 68

S

schizencephaly 171-2, 181-8, 191, 256-7, 265
  bilateral 182, 185-6, 187
  closed lip
    171, 172-3, 181, 182, 184, 185, 187, 257
  and epilepsy 187
  genetic versus acquired factors 187-8
  neuroradiological findings and
    clinical outcome 187
  open lip 171, 173-4, 181, 182, 184, 187, 257
  unilateral 182, 184-5, 187
seizure-induced brain damage 71-2
short gut syndrome 212
subacute (healing) lesions 37, 41, 43-6
subpial haemorrhage with EGLM damage 36-41
surgical management of severe
  partial epilepsy symptomatic
  of neuronal migration disorders 303-17
  illustrative cases 307-13

323

invasive presurgical procedures 304-5
neuropathological alterations 306
non-invasive presurgical investigations 304
postoperative follow-up 306
preoperative magnetic resonance imaging 304
seizure frequency 306
surgical intervention 305-6
topography and extent of
   epileptogenic zone 306
two-step surgery and reoperations 306
surgical treatment 275-301
   callosotomy 298
   complications 298-9
   distribution according to regions
      and pathology 276
   dysplasia of central area 283-9
   dysplasia of frontal area 277-82
   dysplasia of occipital area 290-1
   dysplasia of parietal area 292-5
   dysplasia of temporal area 276-7
   dysplastic lesions and tumours 300-1
   extratemporal and
      extra-frontal resections 298
   frontal lobe resections 298
   lesions, location of 300
   lesions, size of 300
   multilobar dysplasia 296-8
   temporal lobe resections 298

T

temporal area 276-7
temporal lobe resections 298
tish rats 145, 146-8
   brain and cortex 148
   cortex 152-4
   cortex development 148-52
   and epilepsy 154
tract tracing experiments 93, 112, 115-17
tuberous sclerosis 228-33, 235-7
   patients, materials and methods 228
   results 228-33
tumours
   7, 49, 171, 175, 227-29, 233, 236, 275, 299-301

V

voltage dependent channels 64-6

W

West Syndrome 71

X

X-linked lissencephaly and subcortical
   band heterotopia (XLIS) 265-8